Handbook of Cancer Chemotherapy

SIXTH EDITION

Handbook of Cancer Chemotherapy

SIXTH EDITION

Edited by

ROLAND T. SKEEL, M.D.
Professor of Medicine
Medical College of Ohio
and
Chief of Hematology and Oncology
Department of Medicine
Medical College Hospital
Toledo, Ohio

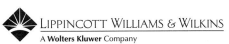

LIPPINCOTT WILLIAMS & WILKINS
A **Wolters Kluwer** Company
Philadelphia • Baltimore • New York • London
Buenos Aires • Hong Kong • Sydney • Tokyo

Acquisitions Editor: Jonathan Pine
Developmental Editor: Tanya Lazar
Production Editor: Emmeline A. Parker
Manufacturing Manager: Colin Warnock
Cover Illustration by: Patricia Gast
Compositor: Circle Graphics
Printer: RR Donnelley/Crawfordsville

© 2003 by LIPPINCOTT WILLIAMS & WILKINS
530 Walnut Street
Philadelphia, PA 19106 USA
LWW.com

First Edition, 1982   Fourth Edition, 1995
Second Edition, 1987 Fifth Edition, 1999
Third Edition, 1991

Printed in the USA

Library of Congress Cataloging-in-Publication Data

Handbook of cancer chemotherapy / edited by Roland T. Skeel. — 6th ed.
    p. ; cm.
  Includes bibliographical references and index.
  ISBN 0-7817-3629-3
    1. Cancer—Chemotherapy—Handbooks, manuals, etc. I. Skeel, Roland T.
  [DNLM: 1. Neoplasms—drug therapy—Handbooks. 2. Antineoplastic Agents—administration & dosage—Handbooks. QZ 39 H2355 2003]
  RC271.C5 H36 2003
  616.94′4061—cd21

                                                            2002043060

Care has been taken to confirm the accuracy of the information presented and to describe generally accepted practices. However, the authors, editor, and publisher are not responsible for errors or omissions or for any consequences from application of the information in this book and make no warranty, expressed or implied, with respect to the currency, completeness, or accuracy of the contents of the publication. Application of this information in a particular situation remains the professional responsibility of the practitioner.

The authors, editor, and publisher have exerted every effort to ensure that drug selection and dosage set forth in this text are in accordance with current recommendations and practice at the time of publication. However, in view of ongoing research, changes in government regulations, and the constant flow of information relating to drug therapy and drug reactions, the reader is urged to check the package insert for each drug for any change in indications and dosage and for added warnings and precautions. This is particularly important when the recommended agent is a new or infrequently employed drug.

Some drugs and medical devices presented in this publication have Food and Drug Administration (FDA) clearance for limited use in restricted research settings. It is the responsibility of the health care provider to ascertain the FDA status of each drug or device planned for use in their clinical practice.

10 9 8 7 6 5 4 3

Contents

Section I.
Basic Principles and Considerations
of Rational Chemotherapy

Section II.
Chemotherapeutic and Biotherapeutic Agents
and Their Use

Section III.
Chemotherapy of Human Cancer

Section IV.
Selected Aspects of Supportive Care of Patients with Cancer

Appendices

Contributing Authors

Haitham S. Abu-Lebdeh, M.D. *Consultant, Department of Internal Medicine, Mayo Clinic; Assistant Professor of Medicine, Mayo Medical School, Rochester, Minnesota*

Tracy T. Batchelor, M.D., M.P.A. *Assistant Professor, Department of Neurology, Harvard Medical School; Executive Director of the Brain Tumor Center, Department of Neurology, Massachusetts General Hospital, Boston, Massachusetts*

Robert S. Benjamin, M.D. *Department of Sarcoma / Medical Oncology, University of Texas Cancer Center, Houston, Texas*

Al B. Benson III, M.D. *Professor of Medicine, Northwestern University, Chicago, Illinois*

Charles S. Cleeland, M.D. *McCullough Professor of Cancer Research and Chairman, Department of Symptom Research, University of Texas, M.D. Anderson Cancer Center, Houston, Texas*

Daniel Y. Danso, M.D. *Formerly Assistant Professor of Medicine, Medical College of Ohio, Ruppert Health Center, Toledo, Ohio, Currently Private Practice, East Central Oncology Associates, Midland, Michigan*

Ronald C. DeConti, M.D. *Professor, Department of Inter-disciplinary Oncology, University of South Florida; Medical Director, Department of Interdisciplinary Oncology, H. Lee Moffitt Cancer Center and Research Institute, Tampa, Florida*

Andrew M. Evens, D.O. *Fellow, Division of Hematology / Oncology, Northwestern University Feinberg School of Medicine, Chicago, Illinois*

Michael J. Fisch, M.D., M.P.H. *Assistant Professor of Medicine, Palliative Care and Rehabilitation, University of Texas M.D. Anderson Cancer Center, Houston, Texas*

Kathleen S. N. Franco-Bronson, M.D. *Adjunct Professor, Department of Psychiatry, Medical College of Ohio, Toledo; Director of Consultation-Liason, Department of Psychiatry and Psychology, Cleveland Clinic Foundation, Cleveland, Ohio*

Walter H. Gajewski, M.D. *Associate Professor, Department of Obstetrics and Gynecology, Brown University; Associate Director, Program in Women's Oncology, Providence, Rhode Island*

Mary Gordinier, M.D. *Assistant Professor, Program in Women's Oncology, Department of Ob-Gyn, Women and Infants Hospital, Providence, Rhode Island*

C. O. Granai, M.D.   *Associate Professor and Director, Program in Women's Oncology, Brown University–Women and Infants Hospital, Providence, Rhode Island*

John P. Greer, M.D.   *Associate Professor of Medicine and Pediatrics, Department of Hematology and Oncology; Clinical Director, Department of Hematology and Stem Cell Transplant, Vanderbilt University, Nashville, Tennessee*

Tien Hoang, M.D.   *Clinical Instructor, Department of Medicine/Medical Oncology, University of Wisconsin Medical School, Madison, Wisconsin*

Chatchada Karanes, M.D.   *Medical Director, National Marrow Program, Minneapolis, Minnesota*

Samir N. Khleif, M.D.   *Senior Investigator, National Cancer Institute, Bethesda, Maryland; Director General, King Hussein Cancer Center, Amman, Jordan*

Benjamin E. Lawler, M.D.   *Instructor in Neurology, Harvard Medical School, Boston, Massachusetts*

Robert D. Legare, M.D.   *Assistant Professor, Director, Cancer Risk Assessment and Prevention Program, Department of Ob-Gyn, Women and Infants Hospital, Providence, Rhode Island*

Rodger D. MacArthur, M.D.   *Associate Professor of Medicine, Division of Infectious Diseases, Wayne State University, Detroit, Michigan*

Iman Mohamed, M.D., M.R.C.P. (UK).   *Assistant Professor, Medical College of Ohio; Medical Director of Breast Center, Department of Medical Oncology, Medical College of Ohio Hospital, Toledo, Ohio*

David S. Morgan, M.D.   *Associate Professor of Medicine, Vanderbilt Medical Center, Nashville, Tennessee*

Craig R. Nichols, M.D.   *Professor of Medicine, Departments of Medicine, Hematology, and Oncology, Oregon Health Sciences University, Portland, Oregon*

Martin M. Oken, M.D.   *Clinical Professor, Department of Medicine, University of Minnesota Medical School; Research Director, Virginia Piper Cancer Institute, Minneapolis, Minnesota*

Diely A. Pichardo, M.D.   *Fellow, Division of Hematology and Oncology, Northwestern University Medical School and Northwestern Memorial Hospital, Chicago, Illinois*

Walter D.Y. Quan, Jr., M.D.   *Assistant Professor, Department of Medicine, East Carolina University; Director of Immunotherapy, Leo Jenkins Cancer Institute, Greenville, North Carolina*

Scott B. Saxman, M.D.   *Senior Investigator, Cancer Therapy Evaluation Program, National Cancer Institute, Bethesda, Maryland*

Joan H. Schiller, M.D.   *Professor, Department of Medicine, University of Wisconsin, Madison, Wisconsin*

Roland T. Skeel, M.D.   *Professor, Department of Medicine, Medical College of Ohio; Chief of Hematology and Oncology, Department of Medicine, Medical College Hospital, Toledo, Ohio*

Mary R. Smith, M.D.   *Professor, Department of Medicine and Pathology, Medical College of Ohio, Toledo, Ohio*

Richard S. Stein, M.D.   *Associate Professor of Medicine, Division of Hematology and Oncology, Vanderbilt Medical Center, Nashville, Tennessee*

NurJehan Stutz, M.D.   *Assistant Professor and Director of Blood Bank, Department of Pathology, Medical College of Ohio; Medical Director, Department of Blood Services, American Red Cross, Western Lake Erie Region, Toledo, Ohio*

Martin S. Tallman, M.D.   *Professor of Medicine, Division of Hematology and Oncology, Northwestern University Feinberg School of Medicine; Attending Physician, Department of Medicine, Northwestern Memorial Hospital, Chicago, Illinois*

Janelle M. Tipton, M.S.N., R.N., A.O.C.N.   *Oncology Clinical Nurse Specialist and Adjunct Instructor of Nursing, Medical College of Ohio, Cancer Institute, Toledo, Ohio*

Neeraja L. Varanasi, M.D.   *Staff Physician, Oakwood Hospital Medical Center, Dearborn, Michigan*

Jamie H. Von Roenn, M.D.   *Professor of Medicine, Division of Hematology and Oncology, Northwestern University, The Feinberg School of Medicine, and the Robert H. Lurie Comprehensive Cancer Center; Medical Director, Palliative Care and Home Hospice Program, Northwestern Memorial Hospital, Chicago, Illinois*

Peter White, M.D.   *Emeritus Professor of Medicine, Medical College of Ohio, Richard D. Ruppert Health Center, Toledo, Ohio*

Kristi S. Williams, M.D.   *Associate Professor, Department of Psychiatry, Medical College of Ohio, Toledo, Ohio*

Preface

This edition of the *Handbook of Cancer Chemotherapy* has been updated to keep it the most useful chemotherapy handbook available. The chapter on the biologic and pharmacologic basis of cancer chemotherapy has been expanded to include clinically relevant new understanding of cellular mechanisms that direct cancer cell growth and its potential control with molecular targeted therapy. The chapter on high-dose chemotherapy with progenitor cell and cytokine support has been extensively revised in recognition of the growing understanding of the potential and limitations of peripheral blood stem cell transplant, particularly in solid tumors, and new concepts such as nonmyeloablative allogeneic stem cell transplants. Primary indications, usual dosage and schedule, and expected toxicities have been added for new drugs and biologic agents that oncologists have begun to use in the last 5 years, and new data added to the information for many of the older agents.

Each of the chapters dealing with specific cancer sites has been revised to reflect current best medical practice and to point the way toward future advances. The section on supportive care has been updated to highlight those issues and pharmacologic agents that are most essential to the daily care of patients with cancer. Because cancer screening is so important to reducing the number of cancer deaths, current American Cancer Society screening guidelines have been continued in the appendix, as well as an expanded list of helpful internet addresses for cancer information.

The *Handbook* continues to be a practical pocket or desk reference, with a wealth of information for oncology specialists, nononcology physicians, house officers, oncology nurses, pharmacists, and medical students. It can even be read and understood by many patients and their families who want to be able to find practical information about their cancer and its treatment. Unlike many other books, the *Handbook* combines in one place the most current rationale and the specific details necessary to safely administer chemotherapy for most adult cancers.

The hope for a more specific, radically improved medical treatment for cancer, which has been stimulated by the tremendous recent increase in information on the molecular basis of cancer, and a few new highly effective molecularly targeted agents, is just beginning to become realized. Rituximab and trastuzumab, which 5 years ago were just entering the clinical practice arena, have been joined by other molecular targeted therapies, including both antibodies and small molecules that inhibit specific enzymes, such as receptor tyrosine kinases (RTKs). The highly effective imatinib mesylate (Gleevec) and other signal transduction inhibitors are only the first drugs in an ever growing group of new biologic agents based on the explosion of knowledge about the biologic basis for cancer cell development and growth and metastasis.

Cure of cancer with chemotherapy or other less toxic systemic treatment has been a long-term aspiration for many people: those engaged in cancer research, physicians who daily are faced with anxious patients who have cancer, and others in the health professions. It has also been a fervent hope of patients and their families. Although cure is possible for some common tumors, particularly when there is only micrometastasis, and for some more advanced tumors such as lymphomas, for many patients chemotherapy remains palliative, at best. When curing and minimizing the cancer can no longer be achieved, then expert, compassionate supportive care becomes the essential and appropriate focus of the oncology team.

Progress is always slower than patients, physicians, and basic scientists would like. Current trials, which are exploring new molecular targeted therapy alone and combined with chemotherapy, continue to offer a realistic expectation of accelerated progress in the control of cancer in the decades ahead.

R.T.S.

Basic Principles and Considerations of Rational Chemotherapy

1

Biologic and Pharmacologic Basis of Cancer Chemotherapy

Roland T. Skeel and Samir N. Khleif

I. General mechanisms by which chemotherapeutic agents control cancer. The purpose of treating cancer with chemotherapeutic agents is to prevent cancer cells from multiplying, invading, metastasizing, and ultimately killing the host (patient). Most agents currently in use appear to exert their effect primarily on cell proliferation. Because cell multiplication is a characteristic of many normal cells as well as cancer cells, most cancer chemotherapeutic agents also have toxic effects on normal cells, particularly those with a rapid rate of turnover, such as bone marrow and mucous membrane cells. The goal in selecting an effective drug, therefore, is to find an agent that has a marked growth-inhibitory or controlling effect on the cancer cell and a minimal toxic effect on the host. In the most effective chemotherapeutic regimens, the drugs are capable not only of inhibiting but also of completely eradicating all neoplastic cells while sufficiently preserving normal marrow and other target organs to permit the patient to return to normal, or at least satisfactory, function and quality of life.

Ideally, the cell biologist, pharmacologist, and medicinal chemist would like to look at the cancer cell, discover how it differs from the normal host cell, and then design a chemotherapeutic agent to capitalize on that difference. In practice, often less rational means have been used for most of the chemotherapeutic agents that are now in use. The effectiveness of agents has been discovered by treating either animal or human neoplasms, after which the pharmacologist attempts to discover why the agent works as well as it does. With few exceptions, the reasons why chemotherapeutic and biologic agents are more effective against cancer cells than against normal cells have been poorly understood. With the rapid expansion of information about cell biology and the factors within the neoplastic cell that control cell growth, the strictly empiric method of discovering effective new agents is changing. For example, antibodies against the protein product of the overexpressed *HER2/neu* oncogene have been demonstrated to have definite (though limited) effectiveness in controlling metastatic breast cancer. Discovery of the constitutively activated Bcr-Abl tyrosine kinase created as a consequence of the chromosomal translocation in chronic myelogenous leukemia (CML) has led to an exciting new era of orally administered small molecular inhibitors of critical molecular changes in cancer cells. This increased understanding of cancer cell biology promises to provide more specific and selective ways of controlling cancer cell growth in the next 10 years.

Inhibition of cell multiplication and tumor growth can take place at several levels within the cell and its environment:

1. Macromolecular synthesis and function
2. Cytoplasmic organization and signal transduction

3. Cell membrane and associated cell surface receptor synthesis, expression, and function
4. Environment of cancer cell growth

A. Classic chemotherapy agents. Most agents currently in use, with the exception of immunotherapeutic agents and other biologic response modifiers, appear to have their primary effect on either macromolecular synthesis or function. This effect means that they interfere with the synthesis of deoxyribonucleic acid (DNA), ribonucleic acid (RNA), or proteins or with the appropriate functioning of the preformed molecule. When interference in macromolecular synthesis or function in the neoplastic cell population is sufficiently great, a proportion of the cells die. Some cells die because of the direct effect of the chemotherapeutic agent. In other instances, the chemotherapy may trigger differentiation, senescence, or apoptosis, the cell's own mechanism of programmed death.

Cell death may or may not take place at the time of exposure to the drug. Often, a cell must undergo several divisions before the lethal event that took place earlier finally results in the death of the cell. Because only a proportion of the cells die as a result of a given treatment, repeated doses of chemotherapy must be used to continue to reduce the cell number (Fig. 1-1). In an ideal system, each time the dose is repeated, the same proportion of cells—not the same absolute number—is killed. In the example shown in Fig. 1-1, 99.9% (3 logs) of the cancer cells are killed with each treatment, and there is a 10-fold (1-log) growth between treatments, for a net reduction of 2 logs with each treatment. Starting at 10^{10} cells (about 10 g or 10 cm^3 leukemia cells), it would take five treatments to reach fewer than 10^0, or 1, cell. Such a model makes certain assumptions that rarely are strictly true in clinical practice:

1. All cells in a tumor population are equally sensitive to a drug.
2. Drug accessibility and cell sensitivity are independent of the location of the cells within the host and of local host factors such as blood supply and surrounding fibrosis.
3. Cell sensitivity does not change during the course of therapy.

The lack of curability of most initially sensitive tumors is probably a reflection of the degree to which these assumptions do not hold true.

B. Biologic response modifiers and molecular targeted therapy. Within individual cells and cell populations are intricate interrelated mechanisms that promote or suppress cell proliferation, facilitate invasion or metastasis when the cell is malignant, lead to cell differentiation, promote (relative) cell immortality, or set the cell on the path to inevitable death (apoptosis). These activities are controlled in large part by normal genes and, in the case of cancer, by mutated cancer promoter genes, tumor suppressor genes, and their products. Included in these products are a host of cell growth factors that control the machinery of the cell. Some of these factors that affect normal cell growth have been biosynthesized and are now used to enhance the production of normal cells (e.g., epoetin and filgrastim) and to treat cancer (e.g., interferon [IFN]).

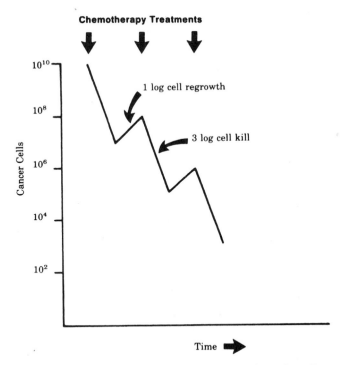

Fig. 1-1.   The effect of chemotherapy on cancer cell numbers. In an ideal system, chemotherapy kills a constant proportion of the remaining cancer cells with each dose. Between doses, cell regrowth occurs. When therapy is successful, cell killing is greater than cell growth.

The recent expansion of our understanding of the biologic control of normal cells and tumor growth at the molecular level has only begun to offer improved therapy for cancer, though it has helped to explain differences in response among populations of patients. New discoveries in cancer cell biology have provided insights into apoptosis, cell cycling control, angiogenesis, metastasis, cell signal transduction, cell surface receptors, differentiation, and growth factor modulation. New drugs in clinical trials have been designed to block growth factor receptors, prevent oncogene activity, block the cell cycle, restore apoptosis, inhibit angiogenesis, restore lost function of tumor suppressor genes, and selectively kill tumors containing abnormal genes. Further understanding of each of these holds a great potential for providing powerful and more selective means to control neoplastic cell growth and may lead to effective cancer treatments in the next decade.

   II.   Tumor cell kinetics and chemotherapy. Cancer cells, unlike other body cells, are characterized by a growth process whereby their sensitivity to normal controlling factors has been partially or completely lost. As a result of this uncontrolled growth, it was once thought that cancer cells grew or multiplied faster than normal cells and that this growth rate was responsible for the sensitivity of cancer cells to chemotherapy. Now it is known that most cancer cells grow less rapidly than the more active normal cells such as bone marrow. Thus, although the growth rate of many cancers is faster than that of normal surrounding tissues, growth rate alone cannot explain the greater sensitivity of cancer cells to chemotherapy.

A. **Tumor growth.** The growth of a tumor depends on several interrelated factors.

1. **Cell cycle time,** or the average time for a cell that has just completed mitosis to grow, redivide, and again pass through mitosis, determines the maximum growth rate of a tumor but probably does not determine drug sensitivity. The relative proportion of cell cycle time taken up by the DNA synthesis phase may relate to the drug sensitivity of some types (S phase specific) of chemotherapeutic agents.

2. **Growth fraction,** or the fraction of cells undergoing cell division, contains the portion of cells that are sensitive to drugs whose major effect is exerted on cells that are dividing actively. If the growth fraction approaches 1 and the cell death rate is low, the tumor-doubling time approximates the cell cycle time.

3. **Total number of cells in the population** (determined at some arbitrary time at which the growth measurement is started) is clinically important because it is an index of how advanced the cancer is; it frequently correlates with normal organ dysfunction. As the total number of cells increases, so does the number of resistant cells, which in turn leads to decreased curability. Large tumors may also have greater compromise of blood supply and oxygenation, which can impair drug delivery to the tumor cells as well as impair sensitivity to both chemotherapy and radiotherapy.

4. **Intrinsic cell death rate** of tumors is difficult to measure in patients but probably makes a major and positive contribution by slowing the growth rate of many solid tumors.

B. **Cell cycle.** The cell cycle of cancer cells is qualitatively the same as that of normal cells (Fig. 1-2). Each cell begins its growth during a *postmitotic period,* a phase called G_1, during which enzymes necessary for DNA production, other proteins, and RNA are produced. G_1 is followed by a period of DNA *synthesis* (S), in which essentially all DNA synthesis for a given cycle takes place. When DNA synthesis is complete, the cell enters a *premitotic period* (G_2), during which further protein and RNA synthesis occurs. This gap is followed immediately by *mitosis* (M), at the end of which actual physical division takes place, two daughter cells are formed, and each cell again enters G_1. G_1 phase is in equilibrium with a *resting state* called G_0. Cells in G_0 are relatively inactive with respect to macromolecular synthesis and are consequently insensitive to many chemotherapeutic agents, particularly those that affect macromolecular synthesis.

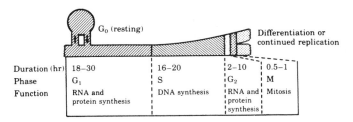

Duration (hr)	18–30	16–20	2–10	0.5–1
Phase	G_1	S	G_2	M
Function	RNA and protein synthesis	DNA synthesis	RNA and protein synthesis	Mitosis

Fig. 1-2.   Cell cycle time for human tissues has a wide range (16 to 260 h), with marked differences among normal and tumor tissues. Normal marrow and gastrointestinal lining cells have cell cycle times of 24 to 48 h. Representative durations and the kinetic or synthetic activity are indicated for each phase.

C.   Phase and cell cycle specificity. Most classic chemotherapeutic agents can be grouped according to whether they depend on cells being in cycle (i.e., not in G_0) and, if they depend on the cell being in cycle, whether their activity is greater when the cell is in a specific phase of the cycle. Most agents cannot be assigned to one category exclusively. Nonetheless, these classifications can be helpful for understanding drug activity.

    1.   Phase-specific drugs. Agents that are most active against cells in a specific phase of the cell cycle are called *cell cycle phase–specific drugs*. A partial list of these drugs is shown in Table 1.1.

        a.   Implications of phase-specific drugs. Phase specificity has important implications for cancer chemotherapy.

            (1)   Limitation to single-exposure cell kill. With a phase-specific agent, there is a limit to the number of cells that can be killed with a single instantaneous (or very short) drug exposure because only those cells in the sensitive phase are killed. A higher dose kills no more cells.

            (2)   Increasing cell kill by prolonged exposure. To kill more cells requires either prolonged exposure to, or repeated doses of, the drug to allow more cells to enter the sensitive phase of the cycle. Theoretically, all cells could be killed if the blood level or, more importantly, the intracellular concentration of the drug remained sufficiently high while all cells in the target population passed through one complete cell cycle. This theory assumes that the drug does not prevent the passage of cells from one (insensitive) phase to another (sensitive) phase.

            (3)   Recruitment. A higher number of cells could be killed by a phase-specific drug if the proportion of cells in the sensitive phase could be increased (recruited).

        b.   Cytarabine. One of the best examples of a phase-specific agent is cytarabine (ara-C), which is an inhibitor of DNA synthesis and thus is active only in the S phase (at standard doses). When used in doses of 100 to 200 mg/m^2 daily (i.e., not "high-dose ara-C"), ara-C is rapidly deaminated *in vivo* to an inactive compound, ara-U, and rapid

Table 1.1. Cell cycle phase–specific chemotherapeutic agents

Phase of greatest activity	Class	Type	Characteristic agents
Gap 1 (G_1)	Natural product	Enzyme	Asparaginase
	Hormone	Corticosteroid	Prednisone
G_1/S junction	Anti-metabolite	Purine analog	Cladribine
DNA synthesis (S)	Anti-metabolite	Pyrimidine analog	Cytarabine, fluorouracil, gemcitabine
	Anti-metabolite	Folic acid analog	Methotrexate
	Anti-metabolite	Purine analog	Thioguanine, fludarabine
	Natural product	Topoisomerase I inhibitor	Topotecan
	Miscellaneous	Substituted urea	Hydroxyurea
Gap 2 (G_2)	Natural product	Antibiotic	Bleomycin
	Natural product	Topoisomerase II inhibitor	Etoposide
	Natural product	Microtubule polymerization and stabilization	Paclitaxel (Taxol)
Mitosis (M)	Natural product	Mitotic inhibitor	Vinblastine, vincristine, vindesine, vinorelbine

injections result in very short effective levels of ara-C. As a result, single doses of ara-C are nontoxic to the normal hematopoietic system and are generally ineffective for treating leukemia. If the drug is given as a daily rapid injection, some patients with leukemia respond well but not nearly as well as when ara-C is given every 12 h. The apparent reason for the greater effectiveness of the 12-h schedule is that the S phase (DNA synthesis) of human acute non-lymphocytic leukemia cells lasts about 18 to 20 h. If the drug is given every 24 h, some cells that have not entered the S phase when the drug is first administered will not be sensitive to its effect. Therefore, these cells can pass all the way through the S phase before the next dose is administered and will completely escape any cytotoxic effect. However, when the drug is given every 12 h, no cell that is "in cycle" will be able to escape exposure to ara-C because none will be able to get through one complete S phase without the drug being present.

If all cells were in active cycle, that is, if none were resting in a prolonged G_1 or G_0 phase, it would be theoretically possible to kill any cells in a population by a continuous or scheduled exposure equivalent to one complete cell cycle. Experiments with patients who have acute leukemia have shown that if tritiated thymidine is used to label cells as they enter DNA synthesis, it may be 7 to 10 days before the maximum number of leukemia cells have passed through the S phase. This means that, barring permutations caused by itself or other drugs, for ara-C to have a maximum effect on the leukemia, the repeated exposure must be continued for a 7- to 10-day period. Clinically, continuous infusion or administration of ara-C every 12 h for 5 days or longer appears to be most effective for treating patients with newly diagnosed acute nonlymphocytic leukemia. However, even with such prolonged exposure, it appears that a few of the cells do not pass through the S phase.

2.   Cell cycle–specific drugs. Agents that are effective while cells are actively in cycle but that are not dependent on the cell being in a particular phase are called *cell cycle–specific* (or *phase-nonspecific*) *drugs*. This group includes most of the alkylating agents, the antitumor antibiotics, and some miscellaneous agents, examples of which are shown in Table 1.2. Some agents in this group are not totally phase-nonspecific; they may have greater activity in one phase than in another, but not to the degree of the phase-specific agents. Many agents also appear to have some activity in cells that are not in cycle, although not as much as when the cells are rapidly dividing.

3.   Cell cycle–nonspecific drugs. A third group of drugs appears to be effective whether cancer cells are in cycle or are resting. In this respect, these agents are similar to photon irradiation; that is, both types of therapy are effective irrespective of whether or not the cancer cell is in cycle. Drugs in this category are called *cell cycle–nonspecific drugs* and include mechlorethamine (nitrogen mustard) and the nitrosoureas (see Table 1.2).

Table 1.2.   Cell cycle–specific and cell cycle–nonspecific chemotherapeutic agents

Class	Type	Characteristic agents
Cell cycle–specific		
Alkylating agent	Nitrogen mustard	Chlorambucil, cyclophosphamide melphalan
	Alkyl sulfonate	Busulfan
	Triazene	Dacarbazine
	Metal salt	Cisplatin, carboplatin
	Antibiotic	Dactinomycin, daunorubicin, doxorubicin, idarubicin
Cell cycle–nonspecific		
Alkylating agent	Nitrogen mustard	Mechlorethamine
	Nitrosourea	Carmustine, lomustine

D.   Changes in tumor cell kinetics and therapy implications. As cancer cells grow from a few cells to a lethal tumor burden, certain changes occur in the growth rate of the population and affect the strategies of chemotherapy. These changes have been determined by observing the characteristics of experimental tumors in animals and neoplastic cells growing in tissue culture. Such model systems readily permit accurate cell number determinations to be made and growth rates to be determined. (Because tumor cells cannot be injected or implanted into humans and permitted to grow, studies of growth rates of intact tumors in humans must be limited largely to observing the growth rate of macroscopic tumors.)

   1.   Stages of tumor growth. Immediately after inoculation of a tissue culture or an experimental animal with tumor cells, there is a *lag phase,* during which there is little tumor growth; presumably, the cells in this phase are becoming accustomed to the new environment and are preparing to enter into cycle. The lag phase is followed by a period of rapid growth called the *log phase,* during which there are repeated doublings of the cell number. In populations in which the growth fraction approaches 100% and the cell death rate is low, the population doubles within a period approximating the cell cycle time. As the cell number or tumor size becomes macroscopic, the doubling time of the tumor cell population becomes prolonged and levels off (*plateau phase*). Most clinically measurable human cancers are probably in the plateau phase, which may account, in part, for the slow doubling time observed in many human cancers (30 to 300 days). Because the rate of change in the slope of the growth curve during the premeasurable period is unknown for most human cancers, extrapolation from two points when the mass is measurable to estimate the onset of the growth of the malignancy is subject to considerable error. The prolongation in tumor-doubling time in the plateau phase may be due to a smaller growth fraction, a change in the cell cycle time, an increased intrinsic death rate (predominantly apoptosis, which is a programmed and highly orchestrated cell death that occurs both naturally and under the influence of many types of chemotherapy), or a combination of these factors. Factors responsible for these changes include decreased nutrients or growth promotion factors, increased inhibitory metabolites or inhibitory growth factors, and inhibition of growth by other cell–cell interactions.

   2.   Growth rate and effectiveness of chemotherapy. Chemotherapeutic agents are most effective during the period of logarithmic growth. As might be expected, this result is particularly true for the antimetabolites, which are largely S phase specific. As a result, when human tumors become macroscopic, the effectiveness of many chemotherapeutic agents is reduced because only part of the cell population is dividing actively. Theoretically, if the cell population could be reduced sufficiently by other means such as surgery or radiotherapy, chemotherapy would be more effective because a higher fraction of the remaining cells would be in logarithmic growth. The validity of this theoretical premise is supported by the varying degrees of success of surgery plus chemotherapy or radiotherapy plus chemotherapy in the treatment of breast cancer, colon cancer, Wilms' tumor, ovarian cancer, small cell anaplastic cell carcinoma of the lung, non–small cell carcinoma of the lung, head and neck cancers, and osteosarcomas.

III.   Combination chemotherapy. Combinations of drugs are frequently more effective in producing responses and prolonging life than are the same drugs used sequentially. Combinations are likely to be more effective than single agents for several reasons.

A.   Reasons for effectiveness of combinations

1.   Prevention of resistant clones. If 1 in 10^5 cells is resistant to drug A and 1 in 10^5 cells is resistant to drug B, it is likely that treating a macroscopic tumor (which generally would have more than 10^9 cells) with either agent alone would result in several clones of cells that are resistant to that drug. If, after treatment with drug A, a resistant clone has grown to macroscopic size (if the same mutant frequency persists for drug B), resistance to that agent will also emerge. If both drugs are used at the outset of therapy or in close sequence, however, the likelihood of a cell being resistant to both drugs (excluding, for a moment, the situation of pleiotropic drug resistance) is only 1 in 10^{10}. Thus, the combination confers considerable advantage against the emergence of resistant clones. Compounding the problem of pre-existing resistant clones is the resistance that develops through spontaneous mutation in the absence of drug exposure. The use of multiple drugs with independent mechanisms of action or alternating non–cross-resistant combinations (as well as the use of surgery or radiotherapy to eliminate macroscopic tumor) theoretically minimizes the chances for outgrowth of resistant clones and increases the likelihood of remission or cure.

2.   Cytotoxicity to resting and dividing cells. The combination of a drug that is cell cycle specific (phase nonspecific) or cell cycle nonspecific with a drug that is cell cycle phase specific can kill cells that are dividing slowly as well as those that are dividing actively. The use of cell cycle–nonspecific drugs can also help recruit cells into a more actively dividing state, which results in their being more sensitive to the cell cycle phase–specific agents.

3.   Biochemical enhancement of effect

a.   Combinations of individually effective drugs that affect different biochemical pathways or steps in a single pathway can enhance each other. This may apply to some newer agents whereby blocking more than one molecular target in the interacting signal transduction pathways may magnify the interference of cell proliferation compared with that seen with either agent alone.

b.   Combinations of an active agent with an inactive agent can potentially result in beneficial effects by several mechanisms.

(1)   An intracellular increase in the drug or its active metabolites, by either increasing influx or decreasing efflux (e.g., calcium channel inhibitors with multiple agents affected by multidrug resistance [MDR] due to P-glycoprotein overexpression).

(2)   Reduced metabolic inactivation of the drug (e.g., inhibition of cytidine deaminase inactivation of ara-C with tetrahydrouridine).

(3)   Cooperative inhibition of a single enzyme or reaction (e.g., leucovorin enhancement of fluorouracil inhibition of thymidylate synthetase).

(4)   Enhancement of drug action by inhibition of competing metabolites (e.g., *N*-phosphonacetyl-L-aspartic acid inhibition of *de novo* pyrimidine synthesis with resultant increased incorporation of 5-fluorouridine triphosphate into RNA).

4.   Sanctuary access. Combinations can be used to provide access to sanctuary sites for reasons such as drug solubility or affinity of specific tissues for a particular drug type.

5.   Rescue. Combinations can be used in which one agent rescues the host from the toxic effects of another drug (e.g., leucovorin administration after high-dose methotrexate).

B.   Principles of agent selection. When selecting appropriate agents for use in a combination, the following principles should be observed:

1.   Choose individually active drugs. Do not use a combination in which one agent is inactive when used alone unless there is a clear, specific biochemical or pharmacologic reason to do so, for example, high-dose methotrexate followed by leucovorin rescue or leucovorin followed by fluorouracil. *This principle is not applicable to the combined use of chemotherapeutic agents with biologic response modifiers or molecular targeted agents* because the cooperativity of chemotherapy and these drugs may not depend on the independent cytotoxic effect of these nonclassic agents.

2.   When possible, choose drugs in which the dose-limiting toxicities differ qualitatively or in time of occurrence. Often, however, two or more agents that have marrow toxicity must be used, and the selection of a safe dose of each is critical. As a starting point, two cytotoxic drugs in combination can usually be given at two-thirds of the dose used when the drugs are given alone. Whenever a new drug combination is tried, a careful evaluation of both expected and unanticipated toxicities must be carried out. Unexpected results such as the increased cardiotoxicity of the combination of trastuzumab with doxorubicin may occur, and this latter case has precluded the use of these agents together.

3.   Select agents for a combination for which there is a biochemical or pharmacologic rationale. Preferably, this rationale has been tested in an animal tumor system and in the appropriate model system, and the combination has been found to be better than either agent alone.

4.   Be cautious when attempting to improve on a successful two-drug combination by adding a third, fourth, or fifth drug simultaneously. Although this approach may be beneficial, two undesirable results may be seen:

a.   An intolerable level of toxicity that leads to excessive morbidity and mortality.

b.   Unchanged or reduced antitumor effect because of the necessity to reduce the dose of the most effective drugs to a level below which antitumor responses are not seen, despite the theoretical advantages of the combination. Therefore, the addition of each new agent to a combination must be considered carefully, the principles of combination therapy closely followed, and controlled clinical trials carried out to compare the efficacy of any new regimen with a more established (standard) treatment program.

C.   Clinical effectiveness of combinations. Combinations of drugs have been clearly demonstrated to be better than single agents for treating many, but not all, human cancers. The survival benefit of combinations of drugs compared with that of the same drugs used sequentially has been marked in diseases such as acute lymphocytic and acute nonlymphocytic leukemia, Hodgkin's lymphoma, non-Hodgkin's lymphomas with more aggressive behavior (intermediate and high grade), breast carcinoma, anaplastic small cell carcinoma of the lung, colorectal carcinomas, ovarian carcinoma, and testicular carcinoma. The benefit is less evident in cancers such as non–small cell carcinoma of the lung, non-Hodgkin's lymphomas with favorable prognoses, head and neck carcinomas, carcinoma of the pancreas, and melanoma, although reports exist for each of these tumors in which combinations are better in one respect or another than single agents.

IV.   Resistance to antineoplastic agents. Resistance to antineoplastic chemotherapy is a combined characteristic of a specific drug, a specific tumor, and a specific host whereby the drug is ineffective in controlling the tumor without excessive toxicity. Resistance of a tumor to a drug is the reciprocal of selectivity of that drug for that tumor. The problem for the medical oncologist or pharmacologist is not simply to find an agent that is cytotoxic but to find one that selectively kills neoplastic cells while preserving the essential host cells and their function. Were it not for the problem of resistance of human cancer to antineoplastic agents or, conversely, the lack of selectivity of those agents, cancer chemotherapy would be similar to antibacterial chemotherapy in which complete eradication of infection is regularly observed. Such a utopian state of cancer chemotherapy has not yet been achieved for most human cancers. The problem of resistance and ways to overcome or even exploit it remain an area of major interest for the chemotherapist.

Resistance to antineoplastic chemotherapeutic agents may be either natural or acquired. *Natural resistance* refers to the initial unresponsiveness of a tumor to a given drug, and *acquired resistance* refers to the unresponsiveness that emerges after initially successful treatment. There are three basic categories of resistance to chemotherapy: kinetic, biochemical, and pharmacologic.

A.   Cell kinetics and resistance. Resistance based on cell population kinetics relates to cycle and phase specificity, growth fractions and the implications of these factors for responsiveness to specific agents, and schedules of drug administration. A particular problem with many human tumors is that they are in a plateau growth phase with a small growth fraction. This factor renders many of the cells insensitive to the antimetabolites and relatively unresponsive to many of the other chemotherapeutic agents. Strategies to overcome resistance due to cell kinetics include the following:

1. Reducing tumor bulk with surgery or radiotherapy
2. Using combinations to include drugs that affect resting populations (with many G_0 cells)
3. Scheduling of drugs to prevent phase escape or to synchronize cell populations and increase cell kill

B.   Biochemical causes of resistance. Resistance can occur for biochemical reasons including the inability of a tumor to convert a drug to its active form, the ability of a tumor to inactivate a drug, or the location of a tumor at a site where substrates are present that bypass an otherwise lethal blockade. How cells become resistant is only partially understood. There can be decreased drug uptake, increased efflux, changes in the levels or structure of the intracellular target, reduced intracellular activation or increased inactivation of the drug, or increased rate of repair of damaged DNA. In one pre–B-cell leukemia cell line, *bcl-2* overexpression or decreased expression of the homolog *bax* renders cells resistant to several chemotherapeutic agents. Because bcl-2 blocks apoptosis, it has been proposed that its overexpression blocks chemotherapy-induced apoptosis. The interrelationship between mutations of *p53, HER2,* and a host of other oncogenes and tumor suppressor genes and resistance to the cytotoxic effects of radiotherapy, chemotherapeutic, hormonal, and biologic agents, when better understood, may further our understanding of resistance and provide new therapeutic strategies.

MDR, also called *pleiotropic drug resistance,* is a phenomenon whereby treatment with one agent confers resistance not only to that drug and others of its class but also to several other unrelated agents. MDR is commonly mediated by an enhanced energy-dependent drug efflux mechanism that results in lower intracellular drug concentrations. With this type of MDR, overexpression of a membrane transport protein called *P-glycoprotein* (P meaning pleiotropic or permeability) is observed commonly. Other MDR proteins are the multidrug resistance protein found in human lung cancer lines and the lung resistance protein. These proteins appear to have differing expression in different sets of neoplasms. Drugs that are effective in reversing resistance to P-glycoprotein do not reverse multidrug resistance protein. Combination chemotherapy can overcome biochemical resistance by increasing the amount of active drug intracellularly as a result of biochemical interactions or effects on drug transport across the cell membrane. Calcium channel blockers, antiarrhythmics, cyclosporin A analogs (e.g., PSC-833, a nonimmunosuppressive derivative of cyclosporin D), and other agents have been found to modulate the MDR effect *in vitro,* and some beneficial effects have been observed clinically.

The use of a second agent to rescue normal cells may also permit the use of high doses of the first agent, which can overcome the resistance caused by a low rate of conversion to the active metabolite or a high rate of inactivation. Another way to overcome resistance is to follow marrow-lethal doses of chemotherapy by posttherapy infusion of stem cells obtained from the peripheral blood or bone marrow. This experimental technique shows some promise for the treatment of lymphomas, chronic granulocytic leukemia, multiple myeloma, and a few other cancers. A more widely applicable technique may be to combine high-dose chemotherapy with blood cell growth factors, for example, granulocyte colony-stimulating factor (G-CSF) and granulocyte–macrophage colony-stimulating factor (GM-CSF) or oprelvekin (interleukin [IL]-11) to stimulate platelets. These and other marrow-protective and marrow-stimulating agents are being used increasingly and may enhance the effectiveness of chemotherapy in the treatment of several types of cancer. High-dose therapy is discussed more extensively in Chapter 5.

C.   Pharmacologic causes of resistance. Apparent resistance to cancer chemotherapy can result from poor or erratic absorption, increased excretion or catabolism, and drug interactions, all leading to inadequate blood levels of the drug. Strictly speaking, this result is not true resistance; but to the degree that the insufficient blood levels are not appreciated by the clinician, resistance appears to be present. The variation from patient to patient at the highest tolerated dose has led to dose modification schemes that permit dose escalation when the toxicities of the chemotherapy regimen are minimal or nonexistent as well as dose reduction when toxicities are great. This regulation is particularly important for some chemotherapeutic agents for which the dose–response curve is steep. Selection of the appropriate dose on the basis of predicted pharmacologic behavior is essential for some agents not only to avoid serious toxicity but also to optimize effectiveness. This has been applied successfully to dose selection of carboplatin by predicting the time × concentration product (area under the curve) based on the individual patient's creatinine clearance.

True pharmacologic resistance is caused by the poor transport of agents into certain body tissues and tumor cells. For example, the central nervous system (CNS) is a site that many drugs do not reach well. Several drug characteristics favor transport into the CNS, including high lipid solubility and low molecular weight. For tumors that originate in the CNS or metastasize there, the drugs of choice should be those that achieve effective antitumor concentration in the brain tissue and that are also effective against the tumor cell type being treated.

D.   Nonselectivity and resistance. Nonselectivity is not a mechanism for resistance but rather an acknowledgment that for most cancers and most drugs, the reasons for resistance and selectivity are only partially understood. Given a limited understanding of the biochemical differences between normal and malignant cells prior to the last 10 years, it is gratifying that chemotherapy has been as successful as frequently as it has. With the burgeoning of knowledge about the cancer cell, there is reason to hope that in 20 years, we will view current chemotherapy regimens as a fledgling—if not crude—beginning and will have found many more tumor molecular target–directed agents that have a high potential for curing the human cancers that now resist effective treatment.

V.   Molecular targeted therapy
A.   Introduction. Molecular targeted therapy is a new approach to cancer treatment. This approach is the result of the advances that have occurred in the last 20 years in the understanding of the molecular causes of malignant transformation. Agents in this type of therapy are vastly different from the traditional chemotherapeutic agents that you will be reading about throughout the chapters of this book, in that they are designed with the intention to specifically target cancer cells and spare the normal ones. This is because agents that qualify as molecular target therapeutics take advantage of the special molecular characteristics of cancer cells to exert their mechanism of action.
B.   An ideal molecule for targeted therapy should have the following characteristics:

1. Uniquely expressed in cancer cells; hence the agent will specifically target the cancer and not the normal cells.
2. Important for the maintenance of the malignant phenotype; therefore, once the target has been effectively hit, the cancer cell will not be able to develop resistance against the medication by suppressing the function of or expelling the molecule from the cell.

C.   Strategies. There are two main strategies to approach molecular targeted therapy development:
   1.   Functional therapy. This is a strategy that is intended to restore the normal function or abrogate the abnormal function of the defective molecule in the tumor cell. This could be accomplished by reinstituting the normal molecule, inhibiting the production of the defective molecule, or aborting, altering, or reversing the new acquired function. Examples of this approach include gene therapy, antisense, and small-molecule therapy.
   2.   Phenotype-directed therapy. This is a therapeutic strategy that is intended to target the unique phenotype of the cancer cell. Such agents include monoclonal antibodies (MoAbs), immunotoxins, and vaccine therapy.
      There are many molecular targeted therapies and compounds that are under development in clinical trials. Because of the unique and emerging role of molecular targeted therapy, examples of various types are shown below. In the section that follows, agents under each category that are either already in the clinic or close to being introduced into the clinic are presented.
D.   Functional therapy
   1.   Imatinib mesylate (Gleevec). Imatinib mesylate is a small molecule that functions as a protein kinase inhibitor. Its molecular formula is $C_{29}H_{31}N_7O \cdot CH_4SO_3$ with a relative molecular weight of 589.7. Imatinib mesylate is designed to inhibit Bcr-Abl tyrosine kinase, which is the resultant product of the Bcr-Abl translocation in CML. Through the inhibition of the Bcr-Abl tyrosine kinase, imatinib mesylate induces apoptosis in Bcr-Abl–positive cells. Imatinib mesylate is indicated for the treatment of patients with CML blast crisis, accelerated phase of CML, or chronic phase CML. Clinical

studies have demonstrated that imatinib mesylate can lead to 95% hematologic response and 76% cytogenetic response when given to patients with newly diagnosed chronic-phase CML.

In vitro studies have demonstrated that this agent is not exclusively selective for the Bcr-Abl tyrosine kinase; it is has also been found to inhibit the receptor kinases for platelet-derived growth factors, stem cell factor, and c-Kit. Therefore, indications in other diseases, including the rare gastro-intestinal stromal tumor, are currently under testing.

2.   ZD1839 (Iressa). ZD1839 is another example of a small molecule with selective molecular effect. This molecule is designed to effectively inhibit the tyrosine kinase domain of the epidermal growth factor receptor. This compound is being studied in clinical trials, and it will probably enter the clinic in the near future. In Phase I studies, toxicity was manageable. Most common side effects seen were acne-like skin rash (seen more in responders than nonresponders), nausea, vomiting, and diarrhea. In those and subsequent studies, clinical responses have been observed in patients with various malignant tumors including colon cancer, non–small cell carcinoma of the lung, breast cancer, ovarian cancer, colorectal cancer, and head and neck cancer.

ZD1839 has also been found to exert some synergy in combination with chemotherapeutic agents. It has been demonstrated that the combination of ZD1839 with taxanes, folate antagonists, or platinum compounds can markedly enhance their antitumor activity. ZD1839 is currently in Phase III clinical development for the treatment of advanced non–small cell carcinoma of the lung. In addition, further trials are ongoing or planned in a number of other tumor types.

E.   Phenotype-directed therapy

1.   Monoclonal antibodies. MoAbs are biologic agents that are designed with the intention to specifically target membrane proteins that carry an extracellular domain. The MoAbs can exert their antitumor effect through multiple potential mechanisms including blocking the targeted receptor and preventing its function in transmitting proliferative signals to the nucleus, activating antibody-dependent cellular cytotoxicity, or helping in internalizing the receptor and hence delivering toxic agents into the cells. The MoAb technology has been very much improved, in the last decade, by humanizing these biologic agents to form chimeric antibodies. Substitution with the human Fc portion of the molecule for the murine equivalent leads to significant decrease in the ability to generate human anti-mouse antibody (HAMA), though human anti-chimera antibodies (HACAs) may still occur. This has made these biologic agents more usable in the treatment of cancer, particularly when repetitive dosing is needed. MoAbs may be used alone or as a delivery system for cellular toxins, radionuclides, or chemotherapy.

a.   Trastuzumab (Herceptin). Trastuzumab is a humanized (chimeric) MoAb that binds the HER2/neu receptor. It was approved by the U.S. Food and Drug Administration (FDA) in 1998 for the use in patients with metastatic breast cancer with tumors that overexpress the HER2/neu protein. *HER2/neu* (*c-erbB2*) is an oncogene that encodes a 185-kDa epidermal growth factor receptor protein with tyrosine kinase activity. It is found to be overexpressed in many epithelial cancers including colon, pancreas, genitourinary, and breast.

In a large, multicenter Phase III study in patients with metastatic breast cancer that overexpressed HER2, it was demonstrated that trastuzumab, when used as first-line therapy in combination with chemotherapy (with either the combination of anthracyclines and cyclophosphamide or paclitaxel as a single agent), can significantly increase both the duration of response and the overall survival. Trastuzumab is used in breast cancer patients in two settings: as a single agent for second-line therapy or in combination with paclitaxel as first-line therapy. Whereas the mechanism of action of trastuzumab is not entirely clear, it is believed to act through one or more of the following mechanisms: binding to the receptor, thereby inhibiting the tyrosine kinase signaling pathway; activating antibody-dependent cellular cytotoxicity; and enhancing chemotherapy-induced cytotoxicity.

Trastuzumab has certain expected side effects. Cardiotoxicity is one of its most serious side effects. Heart failure associated with this therapy has been reported in 7% to 10% of patients and may be severe; therefore, it is important to observe patients for any indications of cardiac dysfunction. Precaution also should be exercised in patients with pre-existing cardiac conditions. Other side effects include hypersensitivity reaction and severe pulmonary events in a small percentage of patients.

b.   Rituximab (Rituxan). This is an IgG1 kappa murine–human chimeric MoAb that is generated against the CD20 antigen. CD20 is expressed on the cell surface of the B cells and hence on the surface of B-cell lymphoma. Rituximab is indicated for the treatment of relapsed or refractory B-cell non-Hodgkin's lymphoma and chronic lymphocytic leukemia that expresses CD20 marker. Rituximab is also being increasingly used in combination with chemotherapy (e.g., cyclophosphamide, vincristine, doxorubicin, and prednisone), particularly in the more aggressive non-Hodgkin's lymphomas.

Severe hypersensitivity reactions may occur with the infusion of rituximab, typically within 30 to 120 min of starting the infusion. Therefore, caution should be taken if any symptoms or signs of hypersensitivity reaction arise; anaphylactic treatment medication should be kept on the bedside. Tumor lysis syndrome is another condition that the treating physician has to be aware of when using rituximab.

c.   Alemtuzumab (Campath). This is a humanized IgG1 kappa murine–human chimeric MoAb that is directed against CD52 cell surface glycoprotein. CD52 is expressed on the surface of normal and malignant B and T cells, natural killer cells, monocytes, and macrophages. Alemtuzumab is indicated for the treatment of B-cell chronic lymphocytic leukemia in patients who have failed fludarabine. The dose of alemtuzumab is 3 mg daily administered IV over 2 h. Side effects expected with alemtuzumab include flu-like symptoms and gastrointestinal disturbances in addition to neutropenia and thrombocytopenia, which occur in most of the patients treated with this agent. Therefore, complete blood count should be monitored on a weekly basis while alemtuzumab is administered to the patient. Patients who have recently been treated with this MoAb should not receive any live viral vaccines because of the immune suppression effect of the medication.

d.   Gemtuzumab ozogamicin (Mylotarg). Gemtuzumab is a humanized IgG4 kappa antibody against the CD33 antigen conjugated with calicheamicin. Calicheamicin is a cytotoxic agent that is isolated from fermentation of the bacterium *Micromonospora echinospora* ssp *calichensis.* The CD33 antigen is a sialic acid–dependent adhesion protein that is expressed on the surface of immature cells of the myelomonocytic lineage and the surface of leukemic blast cells but not on the normal pluripotent hematopoietic stem cells. When this fusion antibody binds to the CD33 receptors, it gets internalized into the cell, after which the calicheamicin is cleaved and released. The calicheamicin in turn binds to the minor grooves of the DNA, leading to DNA breaks and apoptosis.

Gemtuzumab is indicated for the treatment of the first relapse of myeloid leukemia that expresses CD33 in older patients (over 60 years old) who are not candidates for chemotherapy. Clinical trials have shown that, when given as single agent, gemtuzumab may lead to 16% complete response and 30% overall response with a median time to remission of 60 days. Common side effects for this medication include neutropenia and thrombocytopenia in almost all patients (the time for neutrophil recovery is around 40 days), fever and chills in more than 70% of patients, in addition to nausea, vomiting, and diarrhea.

e.   Cetuximab (IMC-C225, C225). Cetuximab is a chimeric MoAb that binds to the external ligand-binding domain of epidermal growth factor. Cetuximab binds to the epidermal growth factor receptor with much higher affinity than does epidermal growth factor or transforming growth factor-α. This MoAb is currently in Phase II and III trials and may enter the clinic in the near future, alone or in combination with chemotherapy or radiation therapy.

Preclinical data have shown that combining cetuximab with chemotherapy or radiation therapy enhances the antitumor effects of many of these agents. Accordingly, several Phase I and II clinical trials have been conducted evaluating cetuximab in combination with chemotherapy or radiation in patients with solid tumors. In this setting, treatment with C225 resulted in acceptable safety profile, and it has shown some degree of antitumor activity when combined with radiation therapy or cisplatin in head and neck tumors and non–small cell lung carcinoma. Similarly, cetuximab has also been combined with either irinotecan (CPT-11) or gemcitabine in advanced colorectal cancer and pancreatic cancer, respectively. In both of these cases, investigators have reported tolerable side effects with some antitumor activity. A Phase III clinical trial is also underway to evaluate cetuximab in combination with cisplatin in patients with head and neck carcinoma.

2.   Immunotoxins

a.   Denileukin diftitox (Ontak).

Denileukin diftitox is a recombinant construct that includes a fragment of the interleukin (IL)-2 protein (Ala_1- Thr_{133}) linked to a fragment of the diphtheria toxin fragment A and B (Met_1-Thr_{387}). This construct is designed to bind to the CD25 component of the IL-2 receptor (IL-2R) on the surface of the targeted cells that express the receptor; in turn, the complex becomes internalized into the cytoplasm and releases the toxin to exhibit its damaging effect. The high-affinity IL-2R is normally present on the activated T and B lymphocytes and activated macrophages. However, cutaneous T-cell lymphoma (CTCL) also expresses high-affinity IL-2R, which forms an appropriate target.

In two different clinical studies, investigators have shown that 30% of patients with CTCL demonstrate clinical response, including around 10% complete response. Therefore, the indications for this agent include persistent or recurrent CTCL that expresses the IL-2R CD25. Side effects expected from denileukin diftitox include hypersensitivity reaction in more than two-thirds of patients, regardless of the cycle. When this occurs, decreasing the rate, interruption, or termination of the infusion should be done, according to the severity of the symptoms. Also, antianaphylactic medications should be prepared at the bedside. Vascular leak syndrome was also reported in around 27% of the patients, a small percentage of whom required hospitalization. Therefore, special caution needs to be taken for patients with pre-existing conditions such as cardiovascular diseases.

3.   Radioimmunoconjugates

a.   Ibritumomab tiuxetan (Zevalin, IDEC-Y2B8).

Ibritumomab is a murine monoclonal anti-CD20 antibody conjugated to tiuxetan that chelates to the pure beta-emitting yttrium-90 (^{90}Y). The mechanism of action includes antibody-mediated cytotoxicity and cellularly targeted radiotherapy (radioimmunotherapy [RIT]). It is indicated for use in non-Hodgkin's lymphoma, follicular B cell, CD20 positive, which is rituximab refractory. Experimentally it is used in non-Hodgkin's lymphoma that has relapsed or is refractory to other agents, but not refractory to rituximab. It should be used with caution in patients with 25% or greater marrow involvement with lymphoma, prior external beam radiotherapy to 25% or greater of the bone marrow, or a history of HAMAs or HACAs. Because the drug does not emit gamma radiation, hospitalization is not required. Neutropenia and thrombocytopenia are common and are related to the radionuclide dose. At the higher end of the dosing, 25% of patients will develop nadir neutrophil counts of less than 500/μL. Low-grade nausea and vomiting are common.

Infusion-related fever, chills, dizziness, asthenia, headache, back pain, arthralgia, and hypotension are occasional.

b. ^{131}**I-Tositumomab (Bexxar).** ^{131}I-Tositumomab is a murine IgG2a monoclonal anti-CD20 antibody radiolabeled with ^{131}I, an emitter of both beta and gamma radiation. The mechanism of action includes antibody-mediated cytotoxicity and cellularly targeted radiotherapy (RIT). It is indicated in non-Hodgkin's lymphoma, chemotherapy refractory, CD20 positive, low grade, or transformed low grade. Before dosimetric and therapeutic doses, patients are premedicated with acetaminophen 650 mg and diphenhydramine 50 mg. A saturated solution of potassium iodide, 2 to 3 drops orally three times daily, is given beginning 24 h before the dosimetric dose and continuing for 14 days after the therapeutic dose to prevent uptake of ^{131}I by the thyroid. It must be used with caution in patients with 25% marrow involvement with lymphoma, prior external beam radiotherapy to 25% of the bone marrow, or a history of HAMAs or HACAs.

Myelosuppression is universal, with about 20% of patients having grade 4 thrombocytopenia or neutropenia. The nadir counts occur at a median of 5 to 6 weeks, with recovery to baseline by 10 weeks. Nausea is common; vomiting, abdominal pain, and anorexia are occasional. HAMAs or HACAs may develop (5% to 10%). Infusion-related fever, chills, dizziness, asthenia, wheezing or coughing, nasal congestion, headache, back pain, arthralgia, and hypotension are occasional to common, more with dosimetric than therapeutic dosing. Most commonly these are self-limited and mild to moderate in severity. Fatigue or asthenia is common. Cough and edema are occasional; dyspnea is uncommon. Thyroid suppression is uncommon when prophylaxis with potassium iodide is used. Myelodysplasia is occasionally seen 20 to 40 months after treatment.

VI. Biologic therapies
A. Bone marrow–supportive agents
1. Erythrocyte growth factors
a. **Epoetin** is a recombinant growth factor, identical to endogenous human erythropoietin, that promotes the proliferation and differentiation of committed erythroid precursors. It is indicated to be used in patients with nonhematologic malignancies who have chemotherapy-induced anemia to minimize transfusion requirements during therapy. It is not indicated in these patients when they have anemia due to other causes such as iron deficiency, bleeding, or hemolysis. Erythropoietin takes time to work, and a decision on the effectiveness should not be made prior to 4 to 8 weeks. If transfusion requirement does not change after 8 weeks, the dose may be increased. The dose should be withheld if the hematocrit increases to more than 40% and resumed with 25% reduction when the hematocrit is reduced to 36%. If the patient fails to show improvement after increasing the dose to 60,000 U (900 U/kg)/week, it is unlikely that the patient will respond and other causes of the anemia should be looked for carefully. Rarely it may

induce pure red cell aplasia with associated neutralizing anti-erythropoietin antibodies.

b.   Darbepoetin is an erythropoiesis-stimulating protein closely related to erythropoietin that has a threefold longer terminal half-life than epoetin. Its indications are similar to epoetin.

2.   Myeloid–monocytic growth factors

a.   Granulocyte colony-stimulating factor (filgrastim). G-CSF is a 175–amino acid growth factor with proliferative activity for bone marrow progenitors committed to the neutrophil line. As discussed elsewhere in this volume, G-CSF is widely used in the setting of cytotoxic chemotherapy for solid tumors and leukemia to accelerate recovery of neutrophils and lessen the risk of bacterial infection. Guidelines for its use include the following:

- The reduction of a likelihood of first-cycle neutropenia when this likelihood is otherwise 40% or higher (primary prophylaxis)
- In further cycles of chemotherapy after occurrence of febrile neutropenia, when maintenance of dose intensity rather than dose reduction is appropriate (secondary prophylaxis)
- After high-dose chemotherapy followed by peripheral blood stem cell or autologous bone marrow support
- Rarely, in the treatment of established febrile neutropenia, generally only when the infection is life threatening or is expected to require prolonged antibiotic or antifungal therapy

b.   Granulocyte–macrophage colony-stimulating factor (sargramostim). GM-CSF is a 127—amino acid growth factor that exhibits its predominant proliferative effects on multipotent stem cells, inhibits neutrophil migration, potentiates the functions of neutrophils and macrophages, and results in production of a spectrum of cytokines from these activated cells. GM-CSF is used mainly for the following indications: to shorten neutrophil recovery time after induction therapy in acute myelogenous leukemia and accelerate myeloid recovery after bone marrow transplantation.

3.   Megakaryocyte growth factor; interleukin-11 (oprelvekin). IL-11 is a 177–amino acid growth factor that is a member of the same family of growth factors as G-CSF. IL-11 is a thrombopoietic growth factor that stimulates the proliferation of megakaryocyte progenitor cells and induces megakaryocyte maturation, leading to increase in platelets. Therefore, it is indicated to accelerate the recovery of platelets after cytotoxic chemotherapy and has been approved for clinical use for that indication.

B.   Biologic therapy for cancer

1.   Interleukin-2 (Proleukin). IL-2 is a cytokine that is secreted by the activated T cells. IL-2 binds to a specific cell surface receptor on activated T lymphocytes and leads to T-cell proliferation. In addition, IL-2 can also activate natural killer cells. Through these mechanisms and perhaps others, IL-2 has been found to exhibit antitumor properties. In clinical trials, it has been found that IL-2 has antitumor activity when used alone in high doses in patients with renal cell carcinoma and malignant melanoma. High-dose IV therapy with IL-2 given as a single agent has received FDA approval for the treatment of patients with metastatic renal cell carcinoma and metastatic melanoma. Careful selection of patients for such an intensive therapy is mandatory, especially for the cardiopulmonary status. This therapy is associated with significant toxicity and should be administered only by physicians experienced in its use. Intermediate SC doses have been investigated and found to be effective in the same diseases; however, this way of administration has not been approved yet for such an indication.

2.   Interferon-α (IFN-alfa-2a, IFN-alfa-2b). The IFNs are a family of small molecular weight proteins and glycoproteins that are secreted by activated T cells and other cells secondary to viral infection. There are three major types of IFNs: α, β, and γ. IFN-α is produced by T cells, B cells, and macrophages when exposed to the appropriate antigens, IFN-β is produced by fibroblasts when exposed to viral infection, and IFN-γ is produced by T cells after stimulation with IL-2 or specific or nonspecific antigens. Here, we will be discussing IFN-α, which is the only one of the IFNs that is approved by the FDA for human cancer therapy. Approved indications include hairy cell leukemia, melanoma with high risk of recurrence after resection, follicular lymphoma as initial treatment for the aggressive types, in combination with anthracyclines, and acquired immune deficiency syndrome–related Kaposi's sarcoma. Side effects of IFN-α are dependent on the dose and the route given. Flu-like symptoms are the universal side effect for this reagent; the severity is dependent on the dose. Other side effects include liver function disturbances and bone marrow toxicity.

SELECTED READINGS

Baguley BC, Holdaway KM, Fray LM. Design of DNA intercalators to overcome topoisomerase II-mediated multi-drug resistance. *JNCI* 1990;82:398–402.

Barinaga M. From bench top to bedside. *Science* 1997;278:1036–1039.

Baselga J, Pfister D, Cooper MR, et al. Phase I studies of anti-epidermal growth factor receptor chimeric antibody C225 alone and in combination with cisplatin. *J Clin Oncol* 2000;18:904–914.

Baserga R. The cell cycle. *N Engl J Med* 1981;304:453–459.

Ciardiello F, Caputo R, Bianco R, et al. Antitumor effect and potentiation of cytotoxic drugs activity in human cancer cells by ZD-1839 (Iressa), an epidermal growth factor receptor-selective tyrosine kinase inhibitor. *Clin Cancer Res* 2000;6:2053–2063.

Clarkson B, Fried J, Strife A, et al. Studies of cellular proliferation in human leukemia. 3. Behavior of leukemic cells in three adults with acute leukemia given continuous infusions of 3H-thymidine for 8 or 10 days. *Cancer* 1970;25:1237–1260.

Dalton WS, Grogan TM, Meltzer PS, et al. Drug-resistance in multiple myeloma and non-Hodgkin's lymphoma: detection of P-glycoprotein and potential circumvention by addition of verapamil to chemotherapy. *J Clin Oncol* 1989;7:415–424.

Endicott JA, Ling U. The biochemistry of P-glycoprotein-mediated multidrug resistance. *Annu Rev Biochem* 1989;58:137–171.

Fan Z, Baselga J, Masui H, et al. Antitumor effect of anti-epidermal growth factor receptor monoclonal antibodies plus cis-diamine-dichloroplatinum on well established A431 cell zenografts. *Cancer Res* 1993;53:4637–4642.

Friedland ML. Combination chemotherapy. In: Perry MC, ed. *The chemotherapy source book.* Baltimore: Williams & Wilkins, 1996: 63–78.

Goldie JH. Drug resistance. In: Perry MC, ed. *The chemotherapy source book.* Baltimore: Williams & Wilkins, 1992:54–66.

Goldie JH, Coldman AJ. A mathematical model for relating drug sensitivity of tumors to their spontaneous mutation rate. *Cancer Treat Rep* 1979;63:1727–1733.

Kinzler KW, Vogelstein B. Cancer therapy meets p53. *N Engl J Med* 1994;331:49–50.

Ranson M, Hammond LA, Ferry D, et al. ZD1839, a selective oral epidermal growth factor receptor–tyrosine kinase inhibitor, is well tolerated and active in patients with solid, malignant tumors: results of a phase I trial. *J Clin Oncol* 2002;20:2240–2250.

Robert F, Ezekiel MP, Spencer SA, et al. Phase I study of anti-epidermal growth factor receptor antibody cetuximab in combination with radiation therapy in patients with advanced head and neck cancer. *J Clin Oncol* 2001;19:3234–3243.

Schabel FM Jr. The use of tumor growth kinetics in planning "curative" chemotherapy of advanced solid tumors. *Cancer Res* 1969;29: 2384–2398.

Schlessinger J. Cell signaling by receptor tyrosine kinases. *Cell* 2000; 103:211–225.

Sikic BI. Modulation of multidrug resistance: at the threshold. *J Clin Oncol* 1993;11:1629–1635.

Simon MA. Receptor tyrosine kinases: specific outcomes from general signals. *Cell* 2000;103:13–15.

Slingerland JM, Tannock IF. Cell proliferation and cell death. In: Tannock IF, Hill RP, eds. *The basic science of oncology.* New York: McGraw-Hill, 1998:134–165.

Van Noorden CFJ, Meade-Tollin LC, Bosman FT. Metastasis. *Am Scientist* 1998;86:130–141.

Walker RA. The erbB/HER type 1 tyrosine kinase receptor family. *J Pathol* 1998;185:234–235.

Yarbro JW. The scientific basis of cancer chemotherapy. In: Perry MC, ed. *The chemotherapy source book.* Baltimore: Williams & Wilkins, 1996:3–18.

Yarden Y, Shwkowski MX. Untangling the ErbB signalling network. *Nat Rev Mol Cell Biol* 2001;2:127–137.

Systematic Assessment of the Patient with Cancer and Long-Term Medical Complications of Treatment

Roland T. Skeel

I. Establishing the diagnosis

A. Pathologic diagnosis is critical. Although it might seem obvious that the diagnosis of cancer must be firmly established before chemotherapy or any other treatment is administered, the critical nature of an accurate diagnosis warrants a reminder. As a rule, there must be cytologic or histologic evidence of neoplastic cells together with a clinical picture consistent with the diagnosis of the cancer under consideration. Commonly, patients present to their physician with a complaint such as a cough, bleeding, pain, or a lump; through a logical sequence of evaluation, the presence of cancer is revealed on a cytologic or histologic specimen. Less frequently, lesions are discovered fortuitously during routine examination, evaluation of an unrelated disorder, or systematic screening for cancer. With some types of cancer, pathologists can establish the diagnosis based on small amounts of material obtained from needle biopsies, aspirations, or tissue scrapings. Other cancers require larger pieces of tissue for special staining, immunohistologic evaluation, flow cytometry, examination by electron microscopy, or more sophisticated studies such as evaluation for gene rearrangement or genetic profiles.

It is often helpful to confer with the pathologist before obtaining a specimen to determine what kind and size of specimen is adequate to establish the complete diagnosis. When a tissue diagnosis of cancer is made by the pathologist, it is incumbent on the clinician to review the material with the pathologist. This practice is good medicine (and good learning); it also allows the clinician to tell the patient that he or she has actually seen the cancer. In addition, it prevents the physician from administering chemotherapy without a firm pathologic diagnosis. The pathologist often gives a better consultation—not just a tissue diagnosis— when the clinician shows a personal interest.

B. Pathologic and clinical diagnosis must be consistent. Once the tissue diagnosis is established, the clinician must be certain that the pathologic diagnosis is consistent with the clinical findings. If the two are not consistent, a search must be made for additional information, clinical or pathologic, that allows the clinician to make a unified diagnosis. A pathologic diagnosis, like a clinical diagnosis, is also an opinion with varying levels of certainty. The first part of the pathologic diagnosis—and usually the easier part—is an opinion about whether the tissue examined is neoplastic. Because most pathologists rarely render a diagnosis of cancer unless the degree of certainty is high, a positive diagnosis of cancer is generally reliable. The clinician must be more cautious if the diagnosis rendered states that the tissue is "highly suggestive of" or "consistent with the diagnosis of." Absence of definitively diagnosed cancer in a specimen does not mean that cancer is not present, however; it means only that it could not be diagnosed on the tissue obtained, and clinical circumstances must establish if additional tissue sampling is necessary. A second part of the pathologist's diagnosis is an opinion about the type of cancer and the tissue of origin. This determination is not necessary in all circumstances but is usually helpful in selecting the most appropriate therapy and making a determination of prognosis.

C.   Treatment without a pathologic diagnosis. There are rare circumstances in which treatment is undertaken before a pathologic diagnosis is established. Such circumstances are clearly exceptions, however, and involve less than 1% of all patients with cancer. Therapy is begun without a pathologic diagnosis only when the following conditions are met:

1.   Withholding prompt treatment or carrying out the procedures required to establish the diagnosis would greatly increase a patient's morbidity or risk of mortality.
2.   The likelihood of a benign diagnosis is remote.

Two examples of such circumstances are a primary tumor of the midbrain and superior vena cava syndrome with no accessible supraclavicular nodes and no endobronchial disease found on bronchoscopy in a patient in whom the risk of bleeding from mediastinoscopy is deemed greater than the risk of administering radiotherapy for a disease of uncertain nature.

II.   Staging. Once the diagnosis of cancer is firmly established, it is important to determine the anatomic extent or stage of the disease. The steps taken for staging vary considerably among cancers because of the differing natural histories of the tumors.

A.   Staging system criteria. For most cancers, a system of staging has been established based on the following factors:

1.   Natural history and mode of spread of the cancer
2.   Prognostic import for the staging parameters used
3.   Value of the criteria used for decisions about therapy

B.   Staging and therapy decisions. In the past, surgery and radiotherapy were used to treat patients with cancer in early stages, and chemotherapy was used when surgery and radiotherapy were no longer effective or when the disease was in an advanced stage at presentation. In such circumstances, chemotherapy was only palliative (except for gestational choriocarcinoma), and in the absence of exquisitely sensitive tumors or strikingly potent drugs, the likelihood of increasing the survival was low. As knowledge has increased about the genetic determinants of cancer growth, tumor cell kinetics, and the development of resistance, the value of early intervention with chemotherapy has been transposed from animal models to human cancers. To plan this intervention and evaluate its effectiveness, careful staging has become increasingly important. Only when the exact extent of disease has been established can the most rational plan of treatment for the individual patient be devised, whether it is surgery, radiotherapy, chemotherapy, or biologic therapy alone or in combination.

Although no single staging system is universally used for all cancers, the system developed jointly by the American Joint Committee on Cancer (AJCC) and the TNM Committee of the International Union Against Cancer (IUCC) is most widely used for staging solid tumors. It is based on the status of the primary tumor (T), regional lymph nodes (N), and distant metastasis (M). For most cancers, tumor grade (G) is also taken into account. The stage of the tumor is based on a condensation of the total possible TNM and G categories to create stage groupings, usually stages 0, I, II, III, and IV, which are relatively homogeneous with respect to prognosis. When relevant to the specific cancers whose chemotherapy is discussed in Section III of this handbook, the staging system or systems most commonly used for that cancer are discussed.

III.   Performance status. The performance status refers to the level of activity of which a patient is capable. It is an independent measure (independent of the anatomic extent or histologic characteristics of the cancer) of how much the cancer or co-morbid conditions have affected the patient and a prognostic indicator of how well the patient is likely to respond to treatment.

A.   Types of performance status scales. Two performance status scales are in wide use:

1.   The Karnofsky Performance Status Scale (Table 2.1) has 10 levels of activity. It has the advantage of allowing discrimination over a wide scale but the disadvantages of being difficult to remember easily and perhaps of making discriminations that are not clinically useful.

2.   The Eastern Cooperative Oncology Group (ECOG) Performance Status Scale (Table 2.2) has the advantages of being easy to remember and making discriminations that are clinically useful.

3.   According to the criteria of each scale, patients who are fully active or have mild symptoms respond more frequently to treatment and survive longer than patients who are less active or have severe symptoms. A clear designation of the performance status distribution of patients in therapeutic clinical trials is thus critical in determining the comparability and generalizability of trials and the effectiveness of the treatments used.

B.   Use of performance status for choosing treatment. In the individualization of therapy, the performance status is often a useful parameter to help the clinician decide whether the patient will benefit from treatment or will be made worse. For example, unless there is some reason to expect a dramatic response of a cancer to chemotherapy, treatment is often withheld from patients with an ECOG Performance Status Scale score of 4 because responses to therapy are infrequent and toxic effects of the treatment are likely to be great.

C.   Quality of life. A related but partially independent measure of performance status can be determined based on patients' own perceptions of their quality of life (QOL). QOL evaluations have been shown to be independent predictors of tumor response and survival in some cancers, and they are important compo-

Table 2.1. Karnofsky performance status scale

Functional capability	Level of activity
Able to carry on normal activity; no special care needed	100%—Normal; no complaints, no evidence of disease 90%—Able to carry on normal activity; minor signs or symptoms of disease 80%—Normal activity with effort; some signs or symptoms of disease
Unable to work; able to live at home; cares for most personal needs; needs varying amount of assistance	70%—Cares for self; unable to carry on normal activity or to do active work 60%—Requires occasional assistance but is able to care for most of own needs 50%—Requires considerable assistance and frequent medical care
Unable to care for self; requires equivalent of institutional or hospital care	40%—Disabled; requires special medical care and assistance 30%—Severely disabled; hospitalization indicated, although death not imminent 20%—Very sick; hospitalization necessary; active supportive treatment necessary 10%—Moribund; fatal processes progressing rapidly 0%—Dead

Table 2.2. Eastern Cooperative Oncology Group performance status scale

Grade	Level of activity
0	Fully active; able to carry on all predisease performance without restriction (Karnofsky 90%–100%)
1	Restricted in physically strenuous activity but ambulatory and able to carry out work of a light or sedentary nature, e.g., light housework, officework (Karnofsky 70%–80%)
2	Ambulatory and capable of all self-care but unable to carry out any work activities; up and about >50% of waking hours (Karnofsky 50%–60%)
3	Capable of only limited self-care; confined to bed or chair >50% of waking hours (Karnofsky 30%–40%)
4	Completely disabled; cannot carry on any self-care; totally confined to bed or chair (Karnofsky 10%–20%)

nents in a comprehensive assessment of response to therapy. For some cancers, improvement in QOL measures early in the course of treatment is the most reliable indicator of survival.

IV.   Response to therapy. Response to therapy may be measured by survival, objective change in tumor size or in tumor product (e.g., immunoglobulin in myeloma), and subjective change.

A.   Survival. One goal of cancer therapy is to allow patients to live as long and with the same QOL as they would have if they did not have the cancer. If this goal is achieved, it can be said that the patient is cured of the cancer (though biologically the cancer may still be present). From a practical standpoint, we do not wait to see if patients live a normal life span before saying that a given treatment is capable of achieving a cure, but we follow a cohort of patients to see if their survival within a given time span is different from that in a comparable cohort without the cancer. For the evaluation of response to *adjuvant therapy* (additional treatment after surgery or radiotherapy that is given to treat potential nonmeasurable, micrometastatic disease) or *neoadjuvant therapy* (chemotherapy or biologic therapy given as initial treatment before surgery or radiotherapy), survival analysis (rather than tumor response) must be used as the definitive objective measure of anti-neoplastic effect. With neoadjuvant therapy, tumor response and resectability are also partial determinants of effectiveness.

It is, of course, possible that a patient may be cured of the cancer, that is, the cancer that was treated, but die early owing to complications associated with the treatment, including second cancers. Even with complications (unless they are acute ones such as bleeding or infection), survival of patients who have been cured of the cancer is likely to be longer than if the treatment had not been given, though shorter than if the patient had never had the cancer.

If cure is not possible, the reduced goal is to allow the patient to live longer than if the therapy under consideration were not given. It is important for physicians to know if, and with what likelihood, any given treatment will result in a longer life. Such information helps physicians to choose whether to recommend treatment and the patient to decide whether to undertake the recommended treatment program.

It is usually helpful to learn from the patient what his or her goals of therapy are and to have a frank discussion about whether those goals are realistic. This can avoid unnecessary surprises and anger at some later time, which can occur when the patient has set a goal that is not realistic and the physician has not discussed what may or may not reasonably be expected as a consequence of therapy.

B.   Objective response. Although survival is important to the individual patient, it is determined not only by the treatment undertaken but also by biologic determinants of the patient's individual cancer and subsequent treatment; thus, survival does not give an early measurement of treatment effectiveness. Tumor regression, on the other hand, frequently occurs early in the course of effective treatment and is therefore a readily used measurement of treatment benefit. Tumor regression can be determined by a decrease in size of a tumor or the reduction of tumor products.

   1. Tumor size. When tumor size is measured, responses are usually classified by the new Response Evaluation Criteria in Solid Tumors (RECIST) methodology published in the *Journal of the National Cancer Institute* in 2000 (Therasse et al., 2000).

   a. Baseline lesions are characterized as "measurable" (20 mm or more in longest diameter with conventional techniques, 10 mm or more in longest diameter with spiral computed tomography scan) or "nonmeasurable" (smaller lesions and truly nonmeasurable lesions). To assess response, all measurable lesions up to a maximum of 5 per organ and 10 in total are designated as "target" lesions and measured at baseline. Only the longest diameter of each lesion is measured. The sum of the longest diameters of all target lesions is designated the "baseline sum longest diameter." There are a variety of lesions in cancer that cannot be measured. These include many metastatic lesions to the bone, effusions, lymphangitic disease of the lung or skin, and lesions that have necrotic or cystic centers.

   b. Response categories are based on measurement of target lesions:

   (1) Complete response is the disappearance of all target lesions.

   (2) Partial response is a decrease of at least 30% in sum of the longest diameters of target lesions, using as reference the baseline sum longest diameter.

   (3) Progressive disease is an increase of 20% or more in sum of the longest diameters of target lesions, taking as reference the smallest sum longest diameter recorded since the treatment started, or the appearance of one or more new lesions.

   (4) Stable disease is when there is neither sufficient shrinkage to qualify for partial response nor sufficient increase to qualify for progressive disease.

   c. Time to progression is an additional indicator that is often used. It takes into account the fact that from the patient's perspective, complete response, partial response, and stable disease may be meaningless distinctions so long as the tumor is not causing symptoms or impairment of function. It also takes into account that some agents result in disease stability for a substantial period, despite failure to produce measurable disease shrinkage. Time to progression can also be used as an indicator of disease status when there was no measurable disease at the outset of therapy or when the therapeutic modalities were not comparable. For example, if one wanted to compare the results of surgery alone with those of chemotherapy alone, time to progression from the onset of treatment would allow a valid comparison of the effectiveness of the treatments, whereas the traditional tumor response criteria would not. Time to progression thus places each of the agents or modalities on an even basis.

   d. If survival curves of patient populations having different categories of response are compared, those patients with a complete response frequently survive longer than those with a lesser response. If a sizable number of complete responses occur with a treatment regimen, the survival rate of patients treated with that regimen is likely to be significantly greater than that of patients who are untreated. When the number of complete responders in a population rises to about 50%, the possibility of cure for a small number of patients begins to appear. With increasing percentages of complete responders, the frequency of cures is likely to increase correspondingly.

Although patients who have partial response to a treatment usually survive longer than those who have stable disease or progression, it is often not easy to demonstrate that the overall survival of the treated population is better than that of a comparable untreated group. In part, this difficulty may be due to a phenomenon of small numbers. If only 15% to 20% of a population respond to therapy, the median survival rate may not change at all, and the numbers may not be high enough to demonstrate a significant difference in survival duration of the longest surviving 5% to 10% of patients (the "tail" of the curves) for treated and untreated populations. It is also possible that the patients who achieve a partial response to therapy are those who have less aggressive disease at the outset of treatment and thus will survive longer than the nonresponders regardless of therapy. These caveats notwithstanding, most clinicians and patients welcome even a partial response as a sign that offers hope for longer survival and improved QOL.

2.   Tumor products. For many cancers, objective tumor size changes are difficult or impossible to document. For some of these neoplasms, tumor products (hormones, antigens, antibodies) may be measurable and may provide a good, objective way to evaluate tumor response. Two examples of such markers that closely reflect tumor cell mass are the abnormal immunoglobulins (M proteins) produced in multiple myeloma and the human chorionic gonadotropin (β-hCG) produced in choriocarcinoma and testicular cancer. Other markers such as prostate-specific antigen may be less reliable and less helpful measures of response of tumor to therapy.

3.   Evaluable disease. Other objective changes may occur but are not easily quantifiable. When these changes are not easily measurable, they may be termed *evaluable*. For example, neurologic changes secondary to primary brain tumors cannot be measured with a caliper, but they can be evaluated using neurologic testing. An arbitrary system of grading the degree of severity of the neurologic deficit can be devised to permit surrogate evaluation of tumor response. Evaluable disease is not a category of the RECIST criteria.

4.   Performance status changes may also be used as a measure of objective change, although in many respects, the performance status is more representative of the subjective than the objective status of the disease.

C.   Subjective change and quality-of-life considerations. A subjective change is one that is perceived by the patient but not necessarily by the physician or others around the patient. Subjective improvement and an acceptable QOL are often of far greater importance to the patient than objective improvement: If the cancer shrinks, but the patient feels worse than before treatment, he or she is not likely to believe that the treatment was worthwhile. It is not valid to look at subjective change in isolation, however, because temporary worsening in the perceived state of well-being may be necessary to achieve subsequent long-term improvement.

This point is particularly well illustrated by the combined-modality treatment in which chemotherapy is used to treat micrometastases after surgical removal of the macroscopic tumor. In such a circumstance, the patient is likely to feel entirely well after the primary surgical procedure, but the side effects of chemotherapy increase the symptoms and make the patient feel subjectively worse for the period of treatment. The winner's stakes are valuable, however, because if the chemotherapy treatment of the micrometastases is successful, the patient will be cured of the cancer and can be expected to have a normal or near-normal life expectancy rather than dying from recurrent disease. Most patients agree that the temporary subjective worsening is not only tolerable but well worth the price if cure of the cancer is a distinct possibility. This judgment depends on the severity and duration of symptoms, functional impairment, and perceptions of illness during the acute phase of the treatment; the expected benefit (increased likelihood of survival) anticipated as a result of the treatment; and the potential long-term adverse consequences of the treatment.

When chemotherapy is given with a palliative intent, patients (and less often physicians) may be unwilling to tolerate significant side effects or subjective worsening. Fortunately, subjective improvement often accompanies objective improvement, so those patients in whom there is measurable improvement of the cancer also feel better. The degree of subjective worsening that each patient is willing to tolerate varies, and the patient and physician together must discuss and evaluate whether the chemotherapy treatment program is worth continuing. Such discussions should include a clear presentation of the scientific facts that include objective survival and tumor response data together with whatever QOL information has been documented for the treatment proposed. Moreover, the expressed desires and the social, economic, psychological, and spiritual situations of the patient and his or her family must be sensitively considered.

A word of caution about discussions of response and survival is important. Patients can more easily understand the notion of response rates than survival probabilities. For example, a 50:50 chance of the cancer shrinking helps them to understand the goals and expectations of therapy and does not lead to undue anxiety over time. On the other hand, providing median or expected survival estimates is more problematic intellectually and, more particularly, emotionally. It is therefore usually best to give the patient a range of expected survival rather than a number. For example, the physician can say, "Some patients may have progression of their disease and possibly die within 6 months, but others may go on feeling fairly well and functioning well for 2 or more years." This helps the patient and family not to focus on a single number ("They said I only had 13 months to live") and to avoid some of the feeling of impending doom.

V.   Toxicity

A.   Factors affecting toxicity. One of the characteristics that distinguishes cancer chemotherapeutic agents from most other drugs is the frequency and severity of anticipated side effects at usual therapeutic doses. Because of the severity of the side effects, it is critical to monitor the patient carefully for adverse reactions so that therapy can be modified before the toxicity becomes life-threatening. Most toxicity varies according to the following factors:

1. Specific agent
2. Dose
3. Schedule of administration
4. Route of administration
5. Predisposing factors in the patient, which may be known and predictive for toxicity or unknown and resulting in unexpected toxic effects

B.   Clinical testing of new drugs for toxicity. Before the introduction of any agent into wide clinical use, the agent must undergo testing in carefully controlled clinical trials. The first set of clinical trials are called Phase I trials. They are carried out with the express purpose of determining toxicity in humans and establishing the maximum tolerated dose, although with anti-neoplastic agents, they are done only in patients who might benefit from the drug. Such trials are undertaken only after extensive tests in animals have been completed. Much human toxicity is predicted by animal studies, but because of significant species differences, initial doses used in human studies are several times lower than doses at which toxicity is first seen in animals. Phase I trials are carried out using several schedules, and the dose is escalated in successive groups of patients once the toxicity of the prior dose has been established.

At the completion of Phase I trials, there is usually a great deal of information about the spectrum and anticipated severity of acute drug effects (toxicity). However, because patients in Phase I trials often do not live long enough to undergo many months of treatment, chronic or cumulative effects may not be discovered. Discovery of these toxicities may occur only after widespread use of the drug in Phase II trials (to establish the spectrum of effectiveness of the drug), in Phase III trials (to compare the new drug or combination with standard therapy), or from postmarketing reports (when even larger numbers and less rigorously selected patients are treated).

C.   Common acute toxicities. Some toxicities are relatively common among cancer chemotherapeutic agents. Common acute toxicities include the following:

1. Myelosuppression with leukopenia, thrombocytopenia, and anemia
2. Nausea, vomiting, and other gastrointestinal effects
3. Mucous membrane ulceration
4. Alopecia

Aside from nausea and vomiting and acute cholinergic gastrointestinal effects, most of these toxicities occur because of the cytotoxic effects of chemotherapy on rapidly dividing normal cells of the bone marrow and epithelium (e.g., mucous membranes, skin, and hair follicles).

D. Selective toxicities. Other toxicities are less common and are specific to individual drugs or classes of drugs. Examples of drugs and their related toxicities include the following:

1. Anthracyclines and anthracenediones: cardiomyopathy
2. Asparaginase: anaphylaxis (allergic reaction)
3. Bleomycin: pulmonary fibrosis
4. Cisplatin: renal toxicity, neurotoxicity
5. Fludarabine, cladribine, pentostatin: prolonged suppression of cellular immunity with heightened risk for opportunistic infection
6. Ifosfamide and cyclophosphamide: hemorrhagic cystitis
7. Ifosfamide: central nervous system toxicity
8. Mitomycin: hemolytic–uremic syndrome
9. Monoclonal antibodies (e.g., rituximab, trastuzumab): hypersensitivity reactions
10. Paclitaxel: neurotoxicity, acute hypersensitivity reactions
11. Procarbazine: food and drug interactions
12. Vinca alkaloids: neurotoxicity

E. Recognition and evaluation of toxicity. Anyone who administers chemotherapeutic agents *must* be familiar with the expected and the unusual toxicities of the agent the patient is receiving, be prepared to avert severe toxicity when possible, and be able to manage toxic complications when they cannot be avoided. The specific toxicities of commonly used individual chemotherapeutic agents are detailed in Chapter 4.

For the purpose of reporting toxicity in a uniform manner, *criteria* are often established to grade the severity of the toxicity. For many years, a simplified set of criteria was used by several National Cancer Institute–supported clinical trial groups for the most common toxic manifestations. Although this document was helpful, it was, in many respects, incomplete. To address this issue, a new set of more comprehensive toxicity criteria was developed and is now available on the Internet. A sample showing one section (for blood and bone marrow) from the new Common Toxicity Criteria (CTC) is shown in Table 2.3. The complete CTC, generic reporting forms, and a host of other helpful information can be obtained on the Internet (*http://ctep.cancer.gov/*). The complete set of criteria and generic reporting forms can be downloaded as needed. All new clinical trials approved by the NCI Cancer Therapy Evaluation Program (CTEP) will use these new toxicity criteria. Such standardization is important in the evaluation of the toxicity of cancer treatment. Small flipbooks with the CTC can be obtained from the NCI CTEP by sending an e-mail request to *ncictephelp@ctep.nci.nih.gov.* Other general information about the program can be obtained from *info@ctep.nci. nih.gov.*

F. Acute toxicity management. Prevention and treatment of bone marrow suppression can be partially achieved using filgrastim, sargramostim, epoetin, and oprelvekin. Treatment of its infectious, bleeding, and anemia consequences is discussed in Chapters 27 and 28. Management of nausea and vomiting, mu-

(text continues on page 42)

Table 2.3. Representative section from cancer therapy evaluation program (CTEP) common toxicity criteria, version 2.0, March 1998

Category	Blood/bone marrow toxity grade				
	0	1	2	3	4
Bone marrow cellularity	Normal for age	Mildly hypocellular or 25% reduction from normal cellularity for age	Moderately hypocellular or >25% to ≤50% reduction from normal cellularity for age or >2 but <4 wk to recovery of normal bone marrow cellularity	Severely hypocellular or >50% to ≤75% reduction in cellularity for age or 4–6 wk to recovery of normal bone marrow cellularity	Aplasia or >6 wk to recovery of normal bone marrow cellularity

Normal ranges:
Children (≤18 yr) 90% cellularity average
Younger adults (19–59 yr) 60%–70% cellularity average
Older adults (≥60 yr) 50% cellularity average

Note: Grade bone marrow cellularity only for changes related to treatment not disease.

CD4 count	WNL	<LLN to 500/mm³	200 to <500/mm³	50 to <200/mm³	<50/mm³
Haptoglobin	Normal	Decreased	—	Absent	—
Hemoglobin	WNL	<LLN – 10.0 g/dL	8.0 – <10.0 g/dL	6.5 – <8.0 g/dL	<6.5 g/dL
		<LLN – 100 g/L	80 – <100 g/L	65 – 80 g/L	<65 g/L
		<LLN – 6.2 mmol/L	4.9 – <6.2 mmol/L	4.0 – <4.9 mmol/L	<4.0 mmol/L

Note: The following criteria may be used for leukemia studies or bone marrow infiltrative/myelophthisic process if the protocol so specifies.

For leukemia studies or, bone marrow, infiltrative/ myelophthisic processes	WNL	10% to <25% decrease from pretreatment	25% to <50% decrease from pretreatment	50% to <75% decrease from pretreatment	≥75% decrease from pretreatment
Hemolysis (e.g., immune hemolytic anemia, drug-related hemolysis, other)	None	Only laboratory evidence of hemolysis [e.g., direct antiglobulin test (DAT, Coombs') schistocytes]	Evidence of red cell destruction and ≥2-g decrease in hemoglobin, no transfusion	Requiring transfusion and/or medical intervention (e.g., steroids)	Catastrophic consequences of hemolysis (e.g., renal failure, hypotension, bronchospasm, emergency splenectomy)

Also consider Haptoglobin, Hemoglobin.

continued

Table 2.3. Continued

Category	Blood/bone marrow toxicity grade				
	0	1	2	3	4
Leukocytes (total WBC)	WNL	<LLN to 3.0×10^9/L <LLN to 3,000/mm³	≥2.0 to <3.0×10^9/L 2,000 to <3,000/mm³	≥1.0 to <2.0×10^9/L 1,000 to <2,000/mm³	<1.0×10^9/L <1,000/mm³
For BMT studies, if specified in the protocol:	WNL	≥2.0 to <3.0×10^9/L 2,000 to <3,000/mm³	≥1.0 to <2.0×10^9/L, ≥1,000 to <2,000/mm³	≥0.5 to <1.0×10^9/L ≥500 to <1,000/mm³	<0.5×10^9/L <500/mm³
For pediatric BMT studies (using age, race, and sex normal values), if specified in the protocol		*≥75% to <100% LLN*	*≥50 to <75% LLN*	*≥25% to 50% LLN*	*<25% LLN*
Lymphopenia	WNL	<LLN to 1.0×10^9/L <LLN to 1,000/mm³	≥0.5 to <1.0×10^9/L ≥500 to <1,000/mm³	<0.5×10^9/L <500/mm³	—
For pediatric BMT studies (using age, race and sex normal values), if specified in the protocol		*≥75% to <100% LLN*	*≥50% to <75% LLN*	*≥25% to <50% LLN*	*<25% LLN*
Neutrophils/granulocytes (ANC/AGC)	WNL	≥1.5 to <2.0×10^9/L ≥1,500 to <2,000/mm³	≥1.0 to <1.5×10^9/L ≥1,000 to <1,500/mm³	≥0.5 to <1.0×10^9/L ≥500 to <1,000/mm³	<0.5×10^9/L <500/mm³

For BMT studies, if specified in the protocol	WNL	≥1.0 to <1.5 × 10⁹/L ≥1,000 to <1,500/mm³	≥0.5 to <1.0 × 10⁹/L ≥500 to <1,000/mm³	≥0.1 to <0.5 × 10⁹/L ≥100 to <500/mm³	<0.1 × 10⁹/L <100/mm³
For leukemia studies or bone marrow infiltrative/myelophthisic process, if specified in the protocol	WNL	10% to <25% decrease from baseline	25% to <50% decrease from baseline	50% to <75% decrease from baseline	≥75% decrease from baseline
Platelets	WNL	<LLN to <75.0 × 10⁹/L <LLN to 75,000/mm³	≥50.0 to <75.0 × 10⁹/L ≥50,000 to <75,000/mm³	≥10.0 to <50.0 × 10⁹/L ≥10,000 to <50,000/mm³	<10.0 × 10⁹/L <10,000/mm³
For BMT studies, if specified in the protocol	WNL	≥50.0 to <75.0 × 10⁹/L ≥50,000 to <75,000/mm³	≥20.0 to <50.0 × 10⁹/L ≥20,000 to <50,000/mm³	≥10.0 to <20.0 × 10⁹/L ≥10,000 to <20,000/mm³	<10.0 × 10⁹/L <10,000/mm³
For leukemia studies or bone marrow infiltrative/myelophthisic process, if specified in the protocol	WNL	10% to <25% decrease from baseline	25% to <50% decrease from baseline	50% to <75% decrease from baseline	≥75% decrease from baseline
Transfusion: platelets	None	—	—	Yes	Platelet transfusions and other measures required to improve platelet increment; platelet

continued

Table 2.3. *Continued*

	Blood/bone marrow toxicity grade				
Category	0	1	2	3	4
					transfusion refractoriness associated with life-threatening bleeding. (e.g., HLA or cross-matched platelet transfusions)
For BMT studies, if specified in the protocol	None	1 platelet transfusion in 24 h	2 platelet transfusions in 24 h	≥3 platelet transfusions in 24 h	Platelet transfusions and other measures required to improve platelet increment; platelet transfusion refractoriness associated with life-threatening bleeding (e.g., HLA or cross-matched platelet transfusions)

Also consider Platelets.

	None	Mild	Moderate	Severe	Life-threatening or disabling
Transfusion: pRBCs				Yes	
For BMT studies, if specified in the protocol	None	≤2 U pRBCs ($\leq 15\ cm^3/kg$) in 24 h elective or planned	3 U pRBCs ($>15\ to\ \leq 30\ cm^3/kg$) in 24 h elective or planned	≥4 U pRBCs ($>30\ cm^3/kg$) in 24 h	Hemorrhage or hemolysis associated with life-threatening anemia; medical intervention required to improve hemoglobin
For pediatric BMT studies if specified in the protocol	None	≤15 mL/kg in 24 h elective or planned	>15 to ≤30 mL/kg in 24 h elective or planned	>30 mL/kg in 24 h	Hemorrhage or hemolysis associated with life-threatening anemia; medical intervention required to improve hemoglobin

Also consider Hemoglobin.

	None	Mild	Moderate	Severe	Life-threatening or disabling
Blood/Bone Marrow-Other (Specify, _____)	None	Mild	Moderate	Severe	Life-threatening or disabling

WNL, within normal limits; LLN, lower limit of normal; DAT, direct antiglobulin test; WBC, white blood cell count; BMT, bone marrow transplantation, ANC/AGC, HLA, human leukocyte antigen; pRBCs, packed red blood cells;

From Cancer Therapy Evaluation Program. *Common Toxicity Criteria document* (http://ctep.cancer.gov/reporting/ctc.html), revised March 23, 1998 (publish date April 30, 1999), which provides an alphabetical listing of adverse events with associated descriptions of grade severity.

cositis, and alopecia as well as diarrhea, nutrition problems, and drug extravasation are discussed in Chapter 26. Other acute toxicities are discussed with the individual drugs in Chapter 4. Long-term medical problems are a special issue and are highlighted in the section that follows.

VI. Late physical effects of cancer treatment

A. Late organ toxicities. Late organ toxicities may be minimized by limiting doses when thresholds are known. In most instances, however, individual patient effects cannot be predicted. Treatment is primarily symptomatic.

1. Cardiac toxicity (e.g., congestive cardiomyopathy) is most commonly associated with high total doses of the anthracyclines (doxorubicin, daunorubicin, epirubicin). In addition, high-dose cyclophosphamide as used in transplantation regimens may contribute to congestive cardiomyopathy. When mediastinal irradiation is combined with these chemotherapeutic agents, cardiac toxicity may occur at lower doses. Although evaluation of ventricular ejection fraction with echocardiography or nuclear radiography studies has been useful for acutely monitoring the effects of these agents on the cardiac ejection fraction, studies have reported late onset of congestive heart failure during pregnancy or after the initiation of vigorous exercise programs in adults who were previously treated for cancer as children or young adults. The cardiac reserve in these previously treated cancer patients may be marginal. It is probable that there are some changes that take place even at low doses, and it is only because of the great reserve in cardiac function that effects are not measurable until higher doses have been used. Mediastinal irradiation also may accelerate atherogenesis and lead to premature symptomatic coronary artery disease.

Because of the large number of women with breast cancer who are treated with doxorubicin as part of an adjuvant chemotherapy regimen, this group is of special concern and warrants ongoing clinical follow-up.

2. Pulmonary toxicity has been classically associated with high doses of bleomycin (more than 400 U). However, a number of other agents have been associated with pulmonary fibrosis (e.g., alkylating agents, methotrexate, nitrosoureas). Premature respiratory insufficiency, especially with exertion, may become evident with aging.

3. Nephrotoxicity is a potential toxicity of several agents (e.g., cisplatin, methotrexate, nitrosoureas). These agents can be associated with both acute and chronic toxicities. Other nephrotoxic agents such as amphotericin or aminoglycosides may exacerbate the problem. Even usually benign agents such as the bisphosphonates may be a problem. Rarely, some patients may require hemodialysis as a result of chronic toxicity.

4. Neurotoxicity has been particularly associated with the vinca alkaloids, cisplatin, oxaliplatin, epipodophyllotoxins, and taxanes. Peripheral neuropathy can cause considerable sensory and motor disability. Autonomic dysfunction may produce debilitating postural hypotension. Whole-brain irradiation, with or without chemotherapy, can be a cause of progressive dementia and dysfunction in some long-term survivors. This is particularly a problem for patients with primary brain tumors and for some patients with small cell lung cancer who have received prophylactic therapy. Survivors of childhood leukemia have developed a variety of neuropsychological abnormalities related to central nervous system prophylaxis that included whole-brain irradiation.

It has become evident over the last several years that some patients (up to one in five) who have received adjuvant chemotherapy for carcinoma of the breast also have measurable cognitive deficits such as difficulties with memory or concentration. This appears to be greater for women who have received high-dose chemotherapy than for those women who have received standard-dose chemotherapy, and in both groups, the incidence is higher than in control women. It is not uncommon for patients to refer to the effects of chemotherapy with complaints about memory being worse than it was, not being able to calculate numbers in their head, or just having "chemo-brain."

5. Hematologic and immunologic impairment is usually acute and temporally related to the cancer treatment (e.g., chemotherapy or radiation therapy). In some instances, however, there can be persistent cytopenias, as with alkylating agents. Immunologic impairment is a long-term problem for patients with Hodgkin's disease, which may be due to the underlying disease as well as to the treatments that are used. Fludarabine, cladribine, and pentostatin cause profound suppression of CD4 and CD8 lymphocytes and render patients treated susceptible to opportunistic infections. Patients who have undergone splenectomy are also at risk of overwhelming bacterial infections. Complete immunologic reconstitution may take 2 years after marrow-ablative therapy requiring stem cell reconstitution.

B. Second malignancies

1. Acute myelogenous leukemia may occur secondary to combined modality treatment (e.g., radiation therapy and chemotherapy in Hodgkin's disease) or prolonged therapy with alkylating agents or nitrosoureas (e.g., for multiple myeloma). In general, this form of treatment-related acute leukemia arises in the setting of myelodysplasia and is refractory even to intensive treatment. Treatment with the epipodophyllotoxins also has been associated with the development of acute nonlymphocytic leukemia. This may be the result of a specific gene rearrangement between chromosome 9 and chromosome 11 that creates a new cancer-causing oncogene: ALL-1/AF-9. The peak time of occurrence of secondary acute leukemia in patients with Hodgkin's disease is 5 to 7 years after treatment, with an actuarial risk of 6% to 12% by 15 years. Thus, a slowly developing anemia in a survivor of Hodgkin's disease should alert the clinician to the possibility of a secondary myelodysplasia or leukemia.

Fortunately, the risk of secondary leukemias in women treated with standard adjuvant therapy for breast cancer (e.g., cyclophosphamide, methotrexate, and fluorouracil) is not much higher than that in the general population. Treatments using higher-than-standard doses of cyclophosphamide (with doxorubicin) or nonstandard drugs (such as mitoxantrone) as adjuvant therapy in breast cancer and high-dose chemotherapy as used as preparative therapy for autologous peripheral blood progenitor cell transplant have been associated with increased risk of acute nonlymphocytic leukemia and myelodysplasia.

2.   Solid tumors and other malignancies are seen with increased frequency in survivors who have been treated with chemotherapy or radiation therapy. Non-Hodgkin's lymphomas have been reported as a late complication in patients treated for Hodgkin's disease or multiple myeloma. Patients treated with long-term cyclophosphamide are at risk of bladder cancer. Patients who have received mantle irradiation for Hodgkin's disease have an increased risk of breast cancer, thyroid cancer, osteosarcoma, bronchogenic carcinoma, colon cancer, and mesothelioma. In these cases, the second neoplasm is usually in the irradiated field. In general, the risk of solid tumors begins to increase during the second decade of survival after Hodgkin's disease. As a result, young women who have received mantle irradiation for Hodgkin's disease should be screened more carefully for breast cancer, starting at an age earlier than what is advised in standard screening recommendations.

C. Other sequelae

  1.   Endocrine problems may result from cancer treatment. Patients receiving radiation therapy to the head and neck region may develop subclinical or clinical hypothyroidism. This is a particular risk in patients receiving mantle irradiation for Hodgkin's disease. Biennial assessment of thyroid-stimulating hormone should be undertaken in these patients. Thyroid replacement therapy should be given if the thyroid-stimulating hormone level rises, to decrease the risk of thyroid cancer. Short stature may be a result of pituitary irradiation and growth hormone deficiency.

  2.   Premature menopause may occur in women who have received certain chemotherapeutic agents (e.g., alkylating agents, procarbazine) or abdominal and pelvic irradiation. The risk is age related, with women older than 30 years at the time of treatment having the greatest risk of treatment-induced amenorrhea and menopause. Early hormone replacement therapy should be considered in such women, if not otherwise contraindicated, to reduce the risk of accelerated osteoporosis and premature heart disease from estrogen deficiency.

  3.   Gonadal failure or dysfunction can lead to infertility in both male and female cancer survivors during their peak reproductive years. Azoospermia is common, but the condition may improve over time after the completion of therapy. Retroperitoneal lymph node dissection in testicular cancer may produce infertility due to retrograde ejaculation. Psychological counseling should be provided to these patients to help them adjust to these long-term sequelae of therapy. Cryopreservation of sperm before treatment should be considered in men. For women, there are limited means available to preserve ova or protect against ovarian failure associated with treatment. Abdominal irradiation in young girls can lead to pregnancy loss due to decreased uterine capacity.

4. The musculoskeletal system can be affected by radiation therapy, especially in children and young adults. Radiation may injure the growth plates of long bones and lead to muscle atrophy. Short stature may be a result of direct injury to bone.

Acknowledgment: The author is indebted to Dr. Patricia A. Ganz who contributed to previous editions of this chapter. Most of the section on the late consequences of cancer treatment represents Dr. Ganz's work and has been included verbatim in this revision of the handbook.

SELECTED READINGS

American Joint Committee on Cancer. *AJCC Cancer Staging Manual.* 6th ed. New York: Springer, 2002.

Cancer Therapy Evaluation Program. *Common Toxicity Criteria document. http://ctep.cancer.gov/reporting/ctc.html.* 1999.

Curtis RE, Boice J-D Jr, Stovall M, et al. Risk of leukemia after chemotherapy and radiation treatment for breast cancer. *N Engl J Med* 1992;326:1745–1751.

Goldhirsch A, Gelber PD, Simes RJ, et al. Costs and benefits of adjuvant therapy in breast cancer: a quality-adjusted survival analysis. *J Clin Oncol* 1989;7:36–44.

Kennealey GT, Mitchell MS. Factors that influence the therapeutic response. In: Becker FF, ed. *Cancer: a comprehensive treatise. Vol. 5.* New York: Plenum, 1977.

Loescher LJ, Welch-McCaffrey D, Leigh SA, et al. Surviving adult cancers. Part 1: physiologic effects. *Ann Intern Med* 1989;111:411–432.

Pedersen-Bjergaard J, Sigsgaard TC, Nielsen D, et al. Acute monocytic or myelomonocytic leukemia with balanced chromosome translocations to band 11q23 after therapy with 4-epidoxorubicin and cisplatin or cyclophosphamide for breast cancer. *J Clin Oncol* 1992;10:1444–1451.

Perry MC. Toxicity: ten years later. *Semin Oncol* 1992;19:453–457.

Pui CH, Ribeiro RC, Hancock ML, et al. Acute myeloid leukemia in children treated with epipodophyllotoxins for acute lymphoblastic leukemia. *N Engl J Med* 1991;325:1682–1687.

Schagen SB, van Dam FS, Muller MJ, et al. Cognitive deficits after postoperative adjuvant chemotherapy for breast carcinoma. *Cancer* 1999;85:640–650.

Tallman MS, Gray R, Bennett JM, et al. Leukemogenic potential of adjuvant chemotherapy for early-stage breast cancer: the Eastern Cooperative Oncology Group experience. *J Clin Oncol* 1995;13:1557–1563.

Therasse P, Arbuck SG, Eisenhauer EA, et al. New guidelines to evaluate the response to treatment in solid tumors. *JNCI* 2000;92:205–216.

van Leeuwen FE, Klokman JW, Hagenbeek A, et al. Second cancer risk following Hodgkin's disease: a 20-year follow-up study. *J Clin Oncol* 1994;12:312–325.

3

Selection of Treatment for the Patient with Cancer

Roland T. Skeel

I. Setting treatment goals

A.   Patient perspective. Although most often patients come to the physician looking for the medical perspective on what can be done about their cancer, it is critical that physicians and other health care professionals remember that unless we know what the patient's goals are, our ideas and our plans of therapy may not address the patient's needs. As a consequence, it is critical for the physician to ask the patient to share in setting treatment goals because it is the patient who must undergo the rigors of treatment and be willing to abide by its consequences. Whereas the physician's medical recommendations most commonly are accepted, some patients reject them as inappropriate for them for a variety of reasons. Some ask the physician for another recommendation, and others seek the opinion of a second physician. The physician must clearly present the reasons for the treatment recommendations and why they seem to be the best ways to achieve the treatment objective. The physician has the obligation to make a treatment recommendation, but the patient always has the right to reject that advice without fear that the physician will be upset, dislike the patient, or refuse to continue to give the patient care.

B.   Medical perspective. Before a physician decides on a course of treatment to recommend for a patient with cancer, an achievable medical goal of treatment must be clearly defined. If the goal is to cure the patient of cancer, the strategy of therapy is likely to be different from the strategy chosen if the purpose is to prolong life or to relieve symptoms. To propose the goal of therapy, the physician must be

- familiar with the natural history and behavior of the cancer to be treated
- knowledgeable about the principles and practice of therapy for each of the treatment modalities that may be effective in that cancer
- well grounded in the ethical principles of the treatment of patients with cancer
- familiar with the theory and use of antineoplastic agents
- informed about the particular therapy for the cancer in question
- aware of the patient's individual circumstances, including stage of disease, performance status, social situation, and concurrent illnesses

Armed with this information and with the treatment goals in mind, the physician can develop a course of treatment and make a recommendation to the patient.

Components of the treatment plan include the following:

1. Should the cancer be treated at all, and, if so, is the treatment to be designed for cure, prolongation of life, or palliation of symptoms?
2. How aggressive should the therapy be to achieve the defined objective?
3. Which modalities of therapy will be used and in what sequence?
4. How will the treatment efficacy be determined?
5. What are the criteria for deciding the duration of therapy?

II.   Choice of cancer treatment modality

A.   Surgery. The oldest, most established, and still most effective way to cure most cancers is surgery. Surgery is selected as the treatment if the cancer is limited to one area and if it is anticipated that all cancer cells can be removed without unduly compromising vital structures. If it is believed that the patient can survive the operation and return to a worthwhile life, surgery is recommended. Surgery is not recommended if the risk of surgery is greater than the risk of the cancer, if metastasis always occurs despite complete removal of the primary tumor, or if the patient will be left so debilitated, disfigured, or otherwise impaired that although cured of cancer he or she feels that life is not worthwhile. If metastasis regularly (or always) occurs despite complete removal of the primary tumor, the benefits of removal of the gross tumor should be clearly defined before surgery is undertaken.

Most commonly, surgery is reserved for treatment of the primary neoplasm, although at times it may be used effectively to remove isolated metastases (e.g., in lung, brain, liver) with curative intent. Surgery is also used palliatively, such as for decompression of the brain in patients with glioma or biliary bypass in patients with carcinoma of the pancreas. In nearly all nonhematologic cancers, a surgeon should be consulted to determine the role of surgery in the optimal treatment of the patient.

B.   Radiotherapy. Radiotherapy is used for the treatment of local or regional disease when surgery cannot completely remove the cancer or when it would unduly disrupt normal structures or functions. In the treatment of some cancers, radiotherapy is as effective as surgery for eradicating the tumor. In this circumstance, factors such as the anticipated side effects of the treatment, the expertise and experience of local oncologists, and the preference of the patient may influence the choice of treatment.

One determinant of the appropriateness of radiotherapy is the inherent sensitivity of the cancer to ionizing radiation. Some kinds of cancer (e.g., the lymphomas and seminomas) are highly sensitive to radiotherapy. Other kinds (e.g., melanomas and sarcomas) tend to be less sensitive. Such considerations do not preclude the use of radiotherapy, however, and it is helpful to obtain the evaluation of the radiotherapist before initiating treatment so that treatment planning can take into consideration the possible contribution of this modality.

Although radiotherapy is frequently used as the primary or curative mode of therapy, it is also well suited to palliative management of problems such as bone metastases, superior vena cava syndrome, and local nodal metastases. The use of radiotherapy in the management of spinal cord compression and superior vena cava syndrome is discussed in Chapter 29.

C.   Chemotherapy. Chemotherapy has as its primary role the treatment of disease that is no longer confined to one site or region and has spread systemically. In the earliest days of chemotherapy, this interpretation directed its use to diseases that regularly presented in a disseminated form (e.g., leukemia) or after disease recurred following primary management with surgery or radiotherapy. It is now understood that widespread systemic micrometastases commonly occur early in cancer. These metastases are associated with certain predictive factors such as the axillary node metastases of carcinoma of the breast and the large tumor size and poorly differentiated histologic features of sarcomas or the cancer's genetic profile. Therefore, chemotherapy is now applied earlier to treat systemic disease. When this treatment is used for micrometastases, the response of an individual patient cannot be measured, unless the chemotherapy is used as a "neoadjuvant," that is, before surgery or radiotherapy. Then tumor response may predict more important endpoints such as time to treatment failure and survival. More commonly, when the chemotherapy is used as an adjuvant after removal of visible disease, the effectiveness of therapy must be determined by comparing the survival of high-risk patients who receive therapy with that of similar (control) patients who do not receive therapy for the micrometastases. Chemotherapy also has a role in the treatment of localized or regional disease. These specialized uses are discussed in Chapter 30.

D.   Biologic response modifiers. It has long intrigued cancer biologists that cancer does not occur randomly but preferentially selects specific populations: the young, the elderly, the immunosuppressed (certain types of cancer only), and those with a strong family history of cancer. These observations have led cancer biologists to postulate that some kind of biologic control over or proclivity toward the emergence of cancer exists, which some people have and others do not, at least at the time the cancer becomes established. One prime candidate for the mechanism of biologic control of cancer has been immunity. That immunity plays some role in controlling the development of cancer has been clearly demonstrated in animal models and a few, though not most, human neoplasms. Other biologic factors, including those controlled by oncogenes and tumor suppressor genes and their protein products that affect the cancer cell directly or its environment, are becoming better defined and are, in all likelihood, even more important than classic immunity in the development of cancer.

In an attempt to exploit and enhance the biologic control that is presumed to exist to some degree in everyone, a variety of agents called *biologic response modifiers* have been used in the treatment of cancer. Two classes of biologic response modifiers, the interferons and lymphokines (of which interleukin-2 is an example), have been studied intensively, and there is evidence of their substantial activity in some types of cancer. Related, but separate, are molecular targeted agents that inhibit the activity of abnormally expressed protein products such as the constitutively activated Bcr-Abl tyrosine kinase in chronic myelogenous leukemia or other unique components of the cancer cell. This area of intensive research promises to provide an important contribution to effective cancer therapy.

E. Combined-modality therapy. Neither surgery, radiotherapy, biotherapy, nor chemotherapy alone is appropriate for the treatment of all cancers. Frequently, patients present with cancer in which there is a bulky primary lesion, macroscopically evident regional disease, and presumed microscopic or submicroscopic systemic disease. For this reason, oncologists have turned to a multidisciplinary approach to the treatment of cancer, selecting two or more modalities of therapy for sequential or simultaneous use. This approach requires close cooperation among the surgical oncologist, radiation oncologist, and medical oncologist to provide the patient with the best overall treatment plan. Although combined-modality therapy is neither effective nor desirable for all kinds or stages of cancers, the regular practice of a multidisciplinary approach provides the best opportunity to exploit the advantages of each mode of treatment. "Tumor Boards" often serve as the format for ensuring that patients will regularly have the benefit of various treatment perspectives.

III. Palliative care. The medical oncologist, who is also an internist, is often seen as the coordinator of cancer treatment. In this role, although the cancer is focused on, the broader perspective of the oncologist as a coordinator of the patient's care—in partnership with the patient—should not become obscured. Decisions about what therapy to use and how aggressively to treat the cancer are critically important to medically sound patient care. Decisions about when to stop active cancer treatment are also vitally important and may be among the most difficult responsibilities for the oncologist. Quality of life is often enhanced in patients responding to chemotherapy and other cancer treatments; it just as surely deteriorates more rapidly when the tumor does not respond to therapy and the patient experiences the toxicity of treatment along with the pain, fatigue, cachexia, and other symptoms of the cancer. For the 50% of patients with cancer who are not cured, the decision to stop antineoplastic therapy is just as important as the selection of chemotherapy regimens earlier in the disease. There comes a time when the best advice a physician can give is for the patient to forgo additional chemotherapy or any other active cancer treatment.

The introduction and rapid acceptance of hospice programs throughout the United States during the last 30 years reflect the need for this kind of care. Hospice programs have effectively addressed the special physical, psychological, social, and spiritual needs of patients approaching the end of life and have provided the unique skills required to maintain the best possible quality of life as long as possible. More recently, acute care hospitals have recognized that they, too, have patients who are at the end of life and need a special focus on the palliative aspects of their care. Yet too often physicians are reluctant to "give up" and are unable to recognize or to accept when the patient will be helped more by an acknowledgment that active cancer therapy will not improve survival or enhance quality of life.

Oncologists and others caring for patients with cancer who have been trained as acute care physicians can learn specific techniques to enhance the quality of life from those who are expert in palliative care. For example, one might compare the quality of death in hospitalized patients given "maintenance" IV hydration with that of hospice home care patients offered oral fluids and mouth care to assuage thirst. The former method may result in an overhydrated, edematous patient who dies with an uncomfortable-sounding "death rattle" that is disconcerting to family and staff; the latter usually results in a visibly more comfortable patient who is more likely to die with less edema and without as much apparent respiratory distress.

Legitimate questions also can be raised about medical costs toward the end of life that are incurred when physicians give "futile" and "marginal" care. Development of guidelines by physicians and hospitals that define futile care, along with thoughtful consideration of when the therapy offered patients has marginal value, may enable physicians to improve the quality of life for patients and at the same time hold down one component of the rising spiral of health care costs.

SELECTED READINGS

Brody H, Campbell ML, Faber-Langendoen K, et al. Withdrawing intensive life-sustaining treatment—recommendations for compassionate clinical management. *N Engl J Med* 1997;336:6.

Emanuel EJ, et al. Ethics of randomized clinical trials. *J Clin Oncol* 1998;16:365–366.

Lundberg GO. American health care system management objectives: the aura of inevitability becomes incarnate. *JAMA* 1993; 269:2254–2255.

Skeel RT. Measurement of Quality of Life Outcomes. Berger, Portnoy, and Weissman. *Principles and practice of palliative care and supportive oncology 2nd ed.* Philadelphia: Lippincott, Williams & Wilkins, 2002:1107–1122.

Taylor LM, Feldstein ML, Skeel RT, et al. Fundamental dilemmas of the randomized clinical trial process: results of a survey of the 1737 Eastern Cooperative Oncology Group investigators. *J Clin Oncol* 1994;12:1776–1805.

Chemotherapeutic and Biotherapeutic Agents and Their Use

Antineoplastic Drugs and Biologic Response Modifiers: Classification, Use, and Toxicity of Clinically Useful Agents

Roland T. Skeel

I. Classes of drugs. Chemotherapeutic agents are customarily divided into several classes. For two of the classes, the *alkylating agents* and the *antimetabolites,* the names indicate the mechanism of cytotoxic action of the drugs in their class. For the *hormonal agents,* the name designates the physiologic behavior of the drug, and for the *natural products,* the name reflects the source of the agents. The *biologic response modifiers* include agents that mimic, stimulate, enhance, inhibit, or otherwise alter the host responses to the cancer. Several new agents have emerged that affect defined and putative abnormalities in the cancer cell and its environment and can best be classed as *molecularly targeted agents.* Drugs that do not fit easily into other categories are grouped together as *miscellaneous agents.* Data for individual agents are given in Section II of this chapter.

Within each class are several types of agents (Table 4.1). As with the criteria for separating into class, the types are also grouped according to the mechanism of action, biochemical structure or derivation, and physiologic action. In some instances, these groupings into classes and types are arbitrary, and some drugs seem to fit into either more than one category or none. However, the classification of chemotherapeutic agents in this fashion is helpful in several respects. For example, because the antimetabolites interfere with purine and pyrimidine metabolism and the formation of deoxyribonucleic acid (DNA) and ribonucleic acid (RNA), they are all at least cell cycle–specific and in some instances primarily cell cycle phase–specific. The nitrosourea group of alkylating agents, on the other hand, contains drugs that are predominantly or entirely cell cycle–nonspecific. Such knowledge can be helpful in planning therapy for tumors when sufficient kinetic information permits a rational selection of agents and when drugs are selected for use in combination.

The classification scheme also may help to predict cross-resistance between drugs. Tumors that are resistant to one of the nitrogen mustard types of alkylating agents thus would be likely to be resistant to another of that same type, but not necessarily to one of the other types of alkylating agents such as the nitrosoureas or the metal salts (e.g., cisplatin). The classification system does not help in predicting multidrug resistance, which may have several phenotypes.

Table 4.1.   **Useful chemotherapeutic agents**

Class and type	Agents
Alkylating agents	
Alkyl sulfonate	Busulfan
Ethylenimine derivative	Thiotepa (triethylenethiophosphoramide)
Metal salt	Carboplatin, cisplatin, oxaliplatin
Nitrogen mustard	Chlorambucil, cyclophosphamide, estramustine, ifosfamide, mechlorethamine, melphalan
Nitrosourea	Carmustine, lomustine, streptozocin
Triazene	Dacarbazine, temozolamide
Antimetabolites	
Antifolates	Methotrexate, pemetrexed,[a] raltitrexed,[a] trimetrexate
Purine analogs	Mercaptopurine, thioguanine, pentostatin, cladribine, fludarabine
Pyrimidine analogs	Azacitidine,[a] capecitabine, cytarabine, floxuridine, fluorouracil, gemcitabine
Natural products	
Antibiotics	Bleomycin, dactinomycin, daunorubicin, doxorubicin, epirubicin, idarubicin, mitomycin, mitoxantrone, valrubicin
Enzyme	Asparaginase
Microtubule polymer stabilizer	Docetaxel, paclitaxel
Mitotic inhibitor	Vinblastine, vincristine, vindesine,[a] vinorelbine
Topoisomerase I inhibitors	Irinotecan, topotecan
Topoisomerase II inhibitors	Etoposide, teniposide
Hormones and hormone antagonists	
Androgen	Fluoxymesterone and others
Androgen antagonist	Bicalutamide, flutamide, nilutamide
Aromatase inhibitor	Aminoglutethimide, anastrozole, letrozole, exemestane
Corticosteroid	Dexamethasone, prednisone
Estrogen	Diethylstilbestrol
Estrogen antagonist (selective estrogen receptor modulator)	Fulvestrant, raloxifene, tamoxifen, toremifene
Luteinizing hormone–releasing hormone agonist	Goserelin, leuprolide, triptorelin
Progestin	Megestrol acetate, medroxyprogesterone acetate
Thyroid hormones	Levothyroxine, liothyronine

Table 4.1. *Continued*

Class and type	Agents
Molecularly targeted agents	
Gene expression modulators	Retinoids, rexinoids
Monoclonal antibody	Alemtuzumab, cetuximab[a], gemtuzumab, ibritumomab tiuxetan, trastuzumab (Herceptin), rituximab, ^{131}I-tositumomab
Tyrosine kinase inhibitor (includes receptor tyrosine kinase inhibitors)	Imatinib mesylate, semaxanib (SU5416),[a] ZD1839 (gefitinib, Iressa)[a]
Biologic response modifiers	
Interferons	Interferon-α_{2a}, interferon-α_{2b}
Interleukins	Aldesleukin (interleukin-2), oprelvekin, denileukin diftitox
Myeloid- and erythroid-stimulating factors	Epoetin, filgrastim, sargramostim
Nonspecific immuno-modulation	Thalidomide
Miscellaneous agents	
Adrenocortical suppressant	Mitotane
Bisphosphonates	Pamidronate, zoledronic acid
Cytoprotector (reactive species antagonists)	Amifostine, dexrazoxane, mesna
Growth factor–binding inhibitor	Suramin[a]
Methylhydrazine derivative	Procarbazine
Photosensitizing agents	Porfimer
Platelet-reducing agent	Anagrelide
Salt	Arsenic trioxide
Somatostatin analog	Octreotide
Substituted melamine	Altretamine (hexamethylmelamine)
Substituted urea	Hydroxyurea

A. Alkylating agents

1. General description. The alkylating agents are a diverse group of chemical compounds capable of forming molecular bonds with nucleic acids, proteins, and many molecules of low molecular weight. The compounds either are electrophiles or generate electrophiles *in vivo* to produce polarized molecules with positively charged regions. These polarized molecules then can interact with electron-rich regions of most cellular molecules. The cytotoxic effect of the alkylating agents appears to relate primarily to the interaction between the electrophiles and DNA. This interaction may result in substitution reactions, cross-linking reactions, or strand-breaking reactions. The net effect of the alkylating agent's interaction with DNA is to alter the information coded in the DNA molecule. This alteration results in inhibition or inaccurate replication of DNA, with resultant mutation or cell death. One implication of the mutagenic capability of alkylating agents is the possibility that they are teratogenic and carcinogenic. Because they interact with preformed DNA, RNA, and protein, the alkylating agents are not phase-specific, and at least some are cell cycle–nonspecific.

   2.   Types of alkylating agents
      a.   Nitrogen mustards. These compounds produce highly reactive carbonium ions that react with the electron-rich areas of susceptible molecules. They vary in reactivity from mechlorethamine, which is highly unstable in aqueous form, to cyclophosphamide, which must be biochemically activated in the liver.
      b.   Ethylenimine derivatives. Triethylenethiophosphoramide (thiotepa) is the only compound in this group that has much clinical use. Ethylenimine derivatives are capable of the same kinds of reactions as the nitrogen mustards.
      c.   Alkyl sulfonates. Busulfan is the only clinically active compound in this group. It appears to interact more with cellular thiol groups than with nucleic acids.
      d.   Triazines. Dacarbazine, the only agent of this type, was originally thought to be an antimetabolite because of its resemblance to 5-aminoimidazole-4-carboxamide. Dacarbazine is now known to act as an alkylator after 5-aminoimidazole-4-carboxamide is cleaved from active diazomethane.
      e.   Nitrosoureas. The nitrosoureas undergo rapid, spontaneous activation in aqueous solution to form products capable of alkylation and carbamoylation. They are unique among the alkylating agents with respect to not being cross-resistant with other alkylating agents, being highly lipid soluble, and having delayed myelosuppressive effects (6 to 8 weeks).
      f.   Metal salts. Cisplatin, carboplatin, and oxaliplatin inhibit DNA synthesis probably through the formation of intrastrand cross-links in DNA and formation of DNA adducts. They also react with DNA through chelation or binding to the cell membrane.

B.   Antimetabolites
   1.   General description. The antimetabolites are a group of low-molecular-weight compounds that exert their effect by virtue of their structural or functional similarity to naturally occurring metabolites involved in nucleic acid synthesis. Because they are mistaken by the cell for normal metabolites, they either inhibit critical enzymes involved in nucleic acid synthesis or become incorporated into the nucleic acid and produce incorrect codes. Both mechanisms result in inhibition of DNA synthesis and ultimate cell death. Because of their primary effect on DNA synthesis, the antimetabolites are most active in cells that are actively growing and are largely cell cycle phase–specific.

2.   Types of antimetabolites

a.   Folic acid analogs. Methotrexate, the dominant member of this group and the only one in wide clinical use, inhibits the enzyme dihydrofolate reductase. This inhibition blocks the production of the reduced N-methylenetetrahydrofolate, the co-enzyme in the synthesis of thymidylic acid. Other metabolic processes in which there is one–carbon unit transfer are also affected but are probably of less importance in the cytotoxic action of methotrexate. Ralitrexed (Tomudex) is a quinazoline antifolate that is an inhibitor of thymidylate synthase. Pemetrexed is a multitargeted pyrrolopyrimidine-based antifolate that, when polyglutamated, inhibits dihydrofolate reductase, thymidylate synthase, and glycinamide ribonucleotide formyltransferase.

b.   Pyrimidine analogs. These compounds inhibit critical enzymes necessary for nucleic acid synthesis and may become incorporated into DNA and RNA.

c.   Purine analogs. The specific site of action for the purine analogs is less well defined than for most pyrimidine analogs, although it is well demonstrated that they interfere with normal purine interconversions and thus with DNA and RNA synthesis. Some of the analogs also are incorporated into the nucleic acids. The adenosine deaminase inhibitor pentostatin increases the intracellular concentration of deoxyadenosine triphosphates in lymphoid cells and inhibits DNA synthesis, probably by blocking ribonucleotide reductase. Among the metabolic alterations is nicotinamide adenine dinucleotide depletion, which may result in cell death. Cladribine accumulates in cells as the triphosphate, is incorporated into DNA, and inhibits DNA repair enzymes and RNA synthesis. As with pentostatin, nicotinamide adenine dinucleotide levels are also depleted.

C.   Natural products

1.   General description. The natural products are grouped together not on the basis of activity but because they are derived from natural sources. The clinically useful drugs are plant products, fermentation products of various species of the soil fungus *Streptomyces,* and bacterial products.

2.   Types of natural products

a.   Mitotic inhibitors. Vincristine, vinblastine, and their semisynthetic derivatives vindesine and vinorelbine are derived from the periwinkle plant (*Catharanthus roseus*), a species of myrtle. They appear to act primarily through their effect on microtubular protein with a resultant metaphase arrest and inhibition of mitosis.

b.   *Podophyllum* derivatives. Etoposide and teniposide, semisynthetic podophyllotoxins derived from the root of the May apple plant (*Podophyllum peltatum*), form a complex with topoisomerase II, an enzyme that is necessary for the completion of DNA replication. This interaction results in DNA strand breakage and arrest of cells in late S and early G_2 phases of the cell cycle.

c.   Camptothecins. These agents are analogs of camptothecin (CPT), a derivative of the Chinese tree *Camptotheca accuminata.* The primary target of the two clinically active agents, irinotecan (CPT-11) and topotecan, is DNA topoisomerase I.

d. Antibiotics. The antitumor antibiotics are a group of related antimicrobial compounds produced by *Streptomyces* species in culture. Their cytotoxicity, which limits their antimicrobial usefulness, has proved to be of great value in treating a wide range of cancers. All of the clinically useful antibiotics affect the function and synthesis of nucleic acids.

   (1) Dactinomycin, the anthracyclines (doxorubicin, daunorubicin, epirubicin, and idarubicin), and the anthracenedione mitoxantrone cause topoisomerase II–dependent DNA cleavage and intercalate with the DNA double helix.

   (2) Bleomycins cause DNA strand scission. The resulting fragmentation is believed to underlie the drug's cytotoxic activity.

   (3) Mitomycin causes cross-links between complementary strands of DNA that impair replication.

e. Enzymes. Asparaginase, the one example of this type of agent, catalyzes the hydrolysis of asparagine to aspartic acid and ammonia and deprives selected malignant cells of an amino acid essential to their survival.

D. Hormones and hormone antagonists

   1. General description. The hormones and hormone antagonists that are clinically active against cancer include steroid estrogens, progestins, androgens, corticoids and their synthetic derivatives, nonsteroidal synthetic compounds with steroid or steroid-antagonist activity, hypothalamic–pituitary analogs, and thyroid hormones. Each agent has diverse effects. Some effects are mediated directly at the cellular level by the drug binding to specific cytoplasmic receptors or by inhibition or stimulation of the production or action of the hormones. These agents may also act by stimulating or inhibiting natural autocrine and paracrine growth factors (e.g., epidermal growth factor, transforming growth factors-α and -β). The relative roles of the various actions of hormones and hormone antagonists are only partially understood and probably vary among tumor types. For estrogen receptor antagonists such as tamoxifen, which, when bound to the estrogen receptor, ultimately controls the promoter region of genes that affect cell growth, there are a host of modulating factors including some 20 receptor-interacting proteins and 50 transcription-activating factors as well as many response elements. Other effects are mediated through indirect effects on the hypothalamus and its anterior pituitary–regulating hormones. The final common pathway in most circumstances appears to lead to the malignant cell, which has retained some sensitivity to direct or indirect hormonal control of its growth. An exception to this mechanism is the effect of corticosteroids on leukemias and lymphomas, in which the steroids appear to have direct lytic effects on abnormal lymphoid cells that have high numbers of glucocorticoid receptors.

   2. Types of hormones and hormone antagonists

   a. Androgens may exert their antineoplastic effect by altering pituitary function or directly affecting the neoplastic cell.

b.   Antiandrogens inhibit nuclear androgen binding.

c.   Corticosteroids cause lysis of lymphoid tumors that are rich in specific cytoplasmic receptors and may have other indirect effects as well.

d.   Estrogens suppress testosterone production (through the hypothalamus) in males and alter breast cancer cell response to prolactin.

e.   Progestins appear to act directly at the level of the malignant cell receptor to promote differentiation.

f.   Estrogen antagonists compete with estrogen for binding on the cytosol estrogen receptor protein in cancer cells. The receptor/hormone complex ultimately controls the promoter region of genes that affect cell growth.

g.   Aromatase inhibitors are nonsteroidal inhibitors of the aromatization of androgens to estrogens. Aminoglutethimide is relatively nonselective, having many biochemical sites of inhibition of steroidogenesis. Its use requires corticosteroid replacement. In contrast, the selective aromatase inhibitors such as anastrozole or letrozole primarily block the conversion of adrenally generated androstenedione to estrone by aromatase in peripheral tissues without inhibition of progesterone or corticosteroid synthesis.

h.   Hypothalamic hormone analogs, such as the luteinizing hormone–releasing hormone agonists leuprolide or goserelin, can inhibit luteinizing hormone and follicle-stimulating hormone (after initial stimulation) and the production of testosterone or estrogen by the gonads.

i.   Thyroid hormones inhibit the release of thyroid-stimulating hormone, thus inhibiting growth of well-differentiated thyroid tumors.

E.   Molecularly targeted agents

1.   General. This classification is a new one in oncology that has become possible because of maturation of knowledge about the molecular events that are responsible for the development of cancer. Understanding of the genetic changes in the cancer cell, the downstream molecular events that follow as a consequence, and the mechanisms by which these events regulate cell growth and death has led to a host of possibilities for the control of cancer growth.

2.   Tyrosine kinase inhibitors. The first clinical example of this is the signal transduction inhibitor imatinib mesylate, which inactivates the constitutively active fusion product tyrosine kinase arising from the Philadelphia chromosome found in chronic myelogenous leukemia, Bcr-Abl, as well as c-kit kinase, which is overexpressed in gastrointestinal stromal tumors. A second promising target is the EGFR–associated tyrosine kinase, because of its overexpression in a large variety of cancers. A number of small-molecule inhibitors of its enzymatic activity are in development. One of these, ZD1839 (Iressa), is an orally active, selective quinazoline derivative that has demonstrated considerable promise in Phase II and III trials. Other receptors such as vascular endothelial growth factor receptor are stimulated by an increase in vascular endothelial growth factor, which in turn is stimulated by hypoxia and tumor cell products. The result is to increase angiogenesis and facilitate further tumor growth. Inhibitors of vascular endothelial growth factor receptor tyrosine kinases are in clinical trials.

3.   Monoclonal antibodies. Monoclonal antibodies have emerged over the last 5 to 10 years as useful adjuncts to the medical oncologist's armamentarium. These agents, which are derived from murine antibodies, may have varying levels of humanization (chimerism) and may be unconjugated (alemtuzumab, cituximab, rituximab, trastuzumab) or conjugated with radionuclides (ibritumomab tiuxetan, tositumomab) or another toxic moiety (gemtuzumab).

4.   Other agents. Other agents affect nuclear activity, such as the binding of all-*trans*-retinoic acid with cytoplasmic proteins, which in turn interact with nuclear retinoic acid receptors that affect expression of genes that control cell growth and differentiation.

F.   Miscellaneous agents. Miscellaneous agents are listed in Table 4.1. Descriptions of specific agents are found in Section III, below.

II.   Clinically useful chemotherapeutic and biologic agents. Section III of this chapter contains an alphabetically arranged description of the chemotherapeutic and biologic agents that are recognized to be clinically useful. Each drug is listed by its generic name, with other common names or tradenames included. A brief description is given of the probable mechanism of action, clinical uses, recommended doses and schedules, precautions, and side effects.

A.   Recommended doses: CAUTION. Although every effort has been made to ensure that the drug dosages and schedules given here are accurate and in accord with published standards, readers are advised to check the product information sheet included in the package of each U.S. Food and Drug Administration (FDA)–approved drug. For drugs not yet approved for general use, FDA–National Cancer Institute (NCI) guidelines and any current medical literature should be used to verify recommended dosages, contraindications, and precautions and to review potential toxicity.

B.   Dose selection and designation. The doses are listed using body surface area (square meters) as the base for nearly all the agents included. Adult doses from the literature, which are expressed using a weight base, have been converted by multiplying the milligram-per-kilogram dose by 37 to give the milligram-per-square-meter dose. Doses using a weight base, which have been taken from the pediatric literature, have been converted using a factor of 25. Because many of the drugs are given in combination with other agents, doses most commonly used in popular combinations may also be indicated. These data should not be used as the sole source of information for any of the drugs but rather should be used as a guide to confirm and compare dose ranges and schedules and to identify potential problems. For some agents, the area-under-the-curve (AUC) method of dose calculation seems to be most reliable for achieving the most accurate dosing and balance between efficacy and toxicity; when that is the standard, the AUC dose is used.

C.   Drug toxicity: frequency designation. The designation of the frequency of toxic side effects is indicated as follows (probability of occurrence equals percentage of patients):

1.   Universal (90% to 100%)
2.   Common (15% to 90%)
3.   Occasional (5% to 15%)
4.   Uncommon (1% to 5%)
5.   Rare (<1%)

These designations are meant only to be guides, and the likelihood of a side effect in each patient depends on that patient's physical status, including co-morbidities, treatment history, dose, schedule, and route of drug administration, and other concurrent treatment.

D.   Dose modification

   1.   Philosophy. The optimal dose and schedule of a drug are those that give maximum benefit with tolerable toxicity. Most chemotherapeutic agents have a steep dose–response curve; therefore, if no toxicity is seen, as a rule, a higher dose should be given to get the best possible therapeutic benefit. If toxicity is great, however, the patient's life may be threatened or the patient may decide that the treatment is worse than the disease and refuse further therapy. How much toxicity the patient and the physician are willing to tolerate depends on the likelihood that more intensive treatment will make a major therapeutic difference (e.g., cure versus no cure) and on the patient's physical and psychological tolerance for adverse effects.

   The general grading scheme for all toxicity is as follows:

0—None
1—Mild
2—Moderate
3—Severe
4—Life threatening

   2.   Guidelines

      a.   Nonhematologic toxicity

         (1)   Acute effects. Acute drug toxicity that is limited to 1 to 2 days and is not cumulative is not usually a cause of dose modification unless it is of grade 3 or 4, that is, severe or life threatening (see *Common Toxicity Criteria Document,* NCI Cancer Therapy Evaluation Program, on the Internet at **http://ctep.cancer.gov/reporting/ctc.html** for individual toxicities and Table 2.3 for an example of hematologic toxicity criteria). Occasionally, repeating a dose that caused intractable nausea and vomiting or a temperature higher than 40°C (104°F) is warranted, but for most other grade 3 or 4 toxicity, the subsequent doses should be reduced by 25% to 50%. If the acute drug effects (e.g., severe paresthesias or abnormalities of renal or liver function) last longer than 48 h, the subsequent doses should be reduced by 35% to 50%.

         A recurrence of the grade 3 or 4 side effects at the reduced doses would be an indication either to reduce by another 25% to 50% or to discontinue the drug altogether. Non–dose-related toxicity such as anaphylaxis is an indication to discontinue the offending drug. Lesser degrees of hypersensitivity can often be dealt with effectively by increasing the dose of protective agents (like dexamethasone or diphenhydramine) or slowing the rate of infusion. For some biologic agents, such as Herceptin (HER2-directed monoclonal antibody), physiologic effects that look like hypersensitivity reactions occur primarily on first or second doses of treatment and diminish with continued treatment.

(2)   Chronic effects. Chronic or cumulative toxicity such as pulmonary function changes with bleomycin or decreased cardiac function with doxorubicin is nearly always an indication to discontinue the responsible agent. Chronic or cumulative neurotoxicity due to vincristine, cisplatin, paclitaxel, or other agents may require no dose change, reduction, or discontinuation, depending on the severity of the resultant neurologic dysfunction and the patient's ability to tolerate it.

b.   Hematologic toxicity. The degree of myelosuppression and attendant risk of infection and bleeding that are acceptable depend on the cancer, the duration of the myelosuppression, the goals of therapy, and the general health of the patient. In addition, one must consider the relative benefit of less aggressive or more aggressive therapy. For example, with acute nonlymphocytic leukemia, remission is unlikely unless sufficient therapy is given to cause profound pancytopenia for at least 1 week. Because there is little benefit with lesser treatment, grade 4 leukopenia and thrombocytopenia are acceptable toxicities in this circumstance. Grade 4 myelosuppression is also acceptable when the goal is cure of a cancer that does not involve the marrow, such as testicular carcinoma. With breast cancer, on the other hand, responses are seen with less aggressive treatment, and prolonged pancytopenia may not be acceptable, particularly if chemotherapy is being used palliatively or in an adjuvant setting in which the proportion of patients expected to benefit from chemotherapy is relatively small and excessive toxicity would pose an unacceptable risk. (Whether higher doses might increase cure is currently under investigation.)

With these caveats in mind, the dose modification schemes shown in Tables 4.2 and 4.3 can serve as a guide to reasonable dose changes for drugs whose major toxicity is myelosuppression. Separate schemes are given for the nitrosoureas and for drugs that have more prolonged myelosuppression.

III.   Data for clinically useful chemotherapeutic and biologic agents. *Note:* Although every effort has been made to ensure that the drug dosage and schedules herein are accurate and in accord with published standards, users are advised to check the product information sheet included in the package of each FDA-approved drug and FDA-NCI guidelines for drugs that are not yet approved for general use (see Table 4.1) to verify recommended dosages, contraindications, and precautions.

Agents that have not yet been approved by the FDA are included because they either have some demonstrated usefulness or are widely used in investigational studies. As their efficacy and toxicity are more firmly established, it is expected that some will be approved by the FDA for general use, whereas others will remain investigational or be dropped from further study.

Table 4.2.   Dose modifications for myelosuppressive drugs with a nadir[a] at less than 3 weeks

Degree of suppression	ANC (WBC)/μL on day of scheduled treatment[b]		Platelets/μL on day of scheduled treatment	Dose as percentage of immediately preceding cycle
Minimal	≥1,500 (≥3,500)	*and*	≥100,000	100
Mild	1,200–1,500 (3,000–3,500)	*or*	75,000–100,000	75
Moderate	1,000–1,200 (2,500–3,000)	*or*	50,000–75,000	50
Severe	<1,000 (<2,500)	*or*	<50,000	0 (delay 1 wk)

ANC, absolute neutrophil count; WBC, white blood cell count.

[a] If the nadir of ANC is <1,000/μL and is associated with fever of >38.3°C (101°F) or the nadir of platelets is <40,000/μL, decrease dose by 25% in subsequent cycles. If the dose is already to be reduced on the basis of the ANC or platelet count on the day of treatment as per this table, do not reduce further because of the nadir count.

[b] ANC is the preferred parameter, if available. If counts are rising at the end of a treatment cycle, it is often appropriate to delay 1 wk and then treat according to the dose modification scheme shown here.

Table 4.3.   Dose modifications for myelosuppressive drugs[a] with a nadir at 3 weeks or later

Point in time	ANC (WBC)/μL		Platelets/μL	Dose as percentage of immediately preceding cycle
I. On day of scheduled treatment[b]	≥1,800 (≥3,500)	and	≥100,000	Dose modified for nadir only
	<1,800 (<3,500)	or	<100,000	0[c]
II. At last nadir	>750	and	>75,000	100
	500–750	or	40,000–75,000	75
	<500	or	<40,000	50
III. After 2-wk delay	≥1,800 (≥3,500)	and	≥100,000	Dose modified for nadir only
	1,200–1,800 (2,500–3,500)	or	75,000–100,000	75
	<1,200	or	<75,000	Continue to hold

ANC, absolute neutrophil count; WBC, white blood cell count.
[a] Nitrosoureas or other agents with prolonged nadir.
[b] ANC is the preferred parameter to use.
[c] Withhold treatment and repeat count in 2 wk. At 2 wk, treat on basis of lowest dose indicated by nadir (II) or delay (III) section of table.

ALDESLEUKIN

Other names. Interleukin-2 (IL-2), Proleukin.

Mechanism of action. Enhances mitogenesis of T cells, natural killer cells, and lymphokine-activated killer cells; augments cytotoxicity of natural killer and lymphokine-activated killer cells; induces interferon-γ.

Primary indications.
1. Renal cell carcinoma.
2. Melanoma.

Usual dosage and schedule. A wide range of doses and routes (IV or SC) have been used. In any of the schedules, therapy may be stopped prematurely for severe constitutional symptoms or for cardiovascular, renal, hepatic, neurologic, pulmonary, or hematologic toxicity.

1. 600,000 IU/kg (22×10^6 IU/m^2) as a 15-min IV infusion every 8 h for up to 14 doses on days 1 to 5. Repeat on days 15 to 19. Repeat cycle in 6 to 12 weeks if stable or responding disease.
2. 18×10^6 IU/m^2/24 h as a continuous IV infusion daily for up to 5 days. Repeat in 2 weeks. Repeat cycle in 6 to 12 weeks if stable or responding disease.
3. 22×10^6 IU/m^2 SC or as a 15-min IV infusion for 5 consecutive days for 2 successive weeks. Repeat every 3 to 6 weeks as tolerated. In some regimens, it is preceded by 3 days with a single dose of low-dose cyclophosphamide 350 mg/m^2 IV push.
4. 9×10^6 IU/m^2 daily by continuous IV infusion on days 1 to 4 (96 h), together with chemotherapy (cisplatin, vinblastine, dacarbazine) and interferon in melanoma.

Schedules 1, 2, and 4 require hospitalization. Schedule 3 can be given in an outpatient setting but may require several hours of observation after treatment.

Special precautions. Patients must be carefully monitored after treatment using any of the dosing regimens. Outpatient regimens require that patients have cardiovascular status observed for up to 5 h, particularly after the first several doses. With higher doses, capillary leak syndrome resulting in hypotension, pulmonary edema, myocardial infarction, arrhythmias, azotemia, and alterations in mental status may occur. Intensive care, controlled volume replacement, and intubation may be required. The lower doses can be given in an outpatient setting.

Toxicity. All are dose dependent.

1. *Myelosuppression and other hematologic effects.* Uncommon at lower doses and common but rarely serious at higher doses. Anemia requiring transfusion is common at higher doses. Thrombocytopenia is common at higher doses.
2. *Nausea, vomiting, and other gastrointestinal effects.*
   a. Anorexia, nausea, vomiting, and diarrhea are common.
   b. Transient liver function abnormalities including hyperbilirubinemia, hypoalbuminemia, and elevation of the prothrombin time and partial thromboplastin time are common.
   c. Colonic perforations are rare.
3. *Mucocutaneous effects.* Mucositis is occasional to common. Alopecia is uncommon. Pruritic erythematous rash is common.

4. *Cardiovascular effects.*
    a. Arrhythmias are common and dose related.
    b. Hypotension is dose related but is occasionally seen at the lower-dose schedules.
    c. Myocardial injury is seen primarily at the higher-dose schedules.
    d. Pulmonary edema from capillary leak syndrome is common with intensive-dose regimens.
    e. Weight gain is common from edema, particularly in more intensive-dose regimens.
5. *Neuropsychiatric effects.*
    a. Mental status changes are common, with dose-related severity.
    b. Dizziness or light-headedness is common.
    c. Blurry vision and other visual disturbances are occasional.
    d. Seizures are uncommon to rare at lower-dose regimens.
6. *Renal function impairment.* Common but reversible. More frequent laboratory abnormalities include creatinine elevation, hypomagnesemia, acidosis, hypocalcemia, hypophosphatemia, hypokalemia, hypouricemia, and hypoalbuminemia.
7. *Fever.* With or without chills; universal and may be severe.
8. *Bacterial infection.* Occasional. Probably related to chemotactic defect induced in granulocytes.
9. *Myalgias and arthralgias.* Occasional to common.
10. *Malaise and fatigue.* Common and dose related.

Prophylaxis of acute toxicity.
1. Acetaminophen 650 to 1,000 mg PO 1 h before therapy and every 3 h for two doses.
2. Cimetidine 800 mg PO or other histamine H_2-receptor antagonist before therapy and daily for duration of treatment.
3. Antiemetics such as granisetron, ondansetron or other $5HT_3$ antagonist, metoclopramide, and prochlorperazine may be used. Do not use dexamethasone.
4. Meperidine 25 to 50 mg IV, when chills start after first dose. For subsequent doses, meperidine 150 mg PO 1.5 h before chills are predicated to start, based on the first treatment.
5. Diphenhydramine 50 mg PO every 3 h for three doses may be substituted for meperidine in patients who tolerate the latter drug poorly.
6. Diphenoxylate with atropine (Lomotil) 1 tablet up to eight times daily for diarrhea.
7. Hydroxyzine 25 to 50 mg PO every 4 to 6 h for itching.

ALEMTUZUMAB

Other names. Campath, Campath-1H.

Mechanism of action. Alemtuzumab is a chimeric (murine and human) monoclonal antibody directed against the CD52 antigen found on the surface of 95% of B and T lymphocytes. It is also expressed in other normal cells found in the peripheral blood and marrow and some other somatic cells. Cellular cytotoxicity is mediated through complement-mediated lysis, antibody-dependent cellular cytotoxicity, and induction of apoptosis.

Primary indications.
1. B-Cell chronic lymphocytic leukemia that has previously been treated with alkylating agents and has failed fludarabine therapy.
2. T-Cell prolymphocytic leukemia.

Usual dosage and schedule.
1. *Initiation.* 3 mg as a 2-h IV infusion daily.
2. *Escalation.* When infusion-related toxicities are less than grade 2, the dose is escalated to 10 mg as a 2-h IV infusion daily. When the 10-mg dose is tolerated, maintenance therapy is initiated.
3. *Maintenance.* 30 mg as a 2-h IV infusion three times a week, on alternate days, for 12 weeks.

Infusion-related events (see below) are ameliorated by pretreatment with antihistamines, acetaminophen, and antiemetics as well as incremental dose escalation.

Special precautions.
1. Must not be administered as IV push or bolus dose.
2. Single doses of greater than 30 mg and cumulative doses of more than 90 mg/week should not be given.
3. If therapy is interrupted for 7 or more days, the dose initiation and escalation scheme is required to avert toxicity.
4. Alemtuzumab is contraindicated in patients who have active systemic infections, underlying immunodeficiency, or known type I hypersensitivity or anaphylactic reactions to the drug or any of its components.

Toxicity.
1. *Myelosuppression and other hematologic effects.* Lymphopenia is universal. Neutropenia, anemia, and thrombocytopenia are common and often severe (grade 3 or greater). Opportunistic and other infections, including pneumonia and sepsis, are seen in 10% to 15% of patients. Autoimmune hemolytic anemia and thrombocytopenia are uncommon (1% to 2%). Pancytopenia and marrow hypoplasia are uncommon but may require permanent discontinuation of therapy. Because of the high incidence of opportunistic infections, anti-herpes and anti–*Pneumocystis carinii* pneumonia prophylaxis is recommended. For *P. carinii* pneumonia prophylaxis: trimethoprim-sulfamethoxazole DS 1 PO b.i.d. Monday, Wednesday, and Friday. If allergic, use Dapsone 100 mg Monday, Wednesday, and Friday. For herpes zoster prophylaxis: famciclovir 500 mg PO b.i.d. or valacyclovir 500 mg t.i.d.
2. *Nausea, vomiting, and other gastrointestinal effects.* Nausea and vomiting are common; diarrhea, abdominal pain, and dyspepsia are occasional.
3. *Mucocutaneous effects.* Rash, urticaria, pruritus, and increased sweating are common. Stomatitis is occasional.
4. *Infusion-related events.* Rigors, fever, nausea and vomiting, and rash—including urticaria—are common. Shortness of breath, hypotension, bronchospasm, headache, pruritus, and diarrhea are occasional. Angioedema is uncommon.
5. *Miscellaneous effects.*
   a. Dyspnea, cough, and bronchitis are common. Pneumonia, pharyngitis, bronchospasm, and rhinitis are occasional.

   b. Hypotension is common, hypertension occasional. Tachycardia and supraventricular tachycardia are occasional but usually not severe. Syncope is uncommon.
   c. Hypersensitivity reactions to alemtuzumab may occur (2%) and result in hypersensitivity to other monoclonal antibodies.
   d. Insomnia, depression, and somnolence are occasional. Headache, dysesthesias, dizziness, and tremor are occasional.

ALITRETINOIN

Other names. 9-*cis*-Retinoic acid, Panretin Gel.
Mechanism of action. Binds to cytoplasmic retinoic acid–binding proteins and then is transported to the nucleus where it interacts with nuclear retinoic acid receptors. These then affect expression of the genes that control cell growth and differentiation.
Primary indication. Acquired immune deficiency syndrome (AIDS)–related cutaneous Kaposi's sarcoma.
Usual dosage and schedule. Apply sufficient gel (0.1%) to cover lesion with a generous coating two to four times daily, according to individual lesion tolerance. Allow to dry for 3 to 5 min before covering with clothing.
Special precautions.
   1. Women are advised to avoid becoming pregnant because of potential fetal risk.
   2. Minimize exposure to ultraviolet rays from sun or sun lamps.
Toxicity.
   1. *Myelosuppression and other hematologic effects.* None.
   2. *Nausea, vomiting, and other gastrointestinal effects.* None.
   3. *Mucocutaneous effects.* Skin reactions with erythema, scaling, irritation, redness, rash, or other dermatitis are common. Pruritus, exfoliative dermatitis, and other erosive or draining skin lesions are occasional.
   4. *Miscellaneous effects.*
      a. Neurologic complaints of burning or pain are common.
      b. Edema is occasional.

ALTRETAMINE

Other names. Hexamethylmelamine, Hexalen, HXM.
Mechanism of action. Unknown. Although it structurally resembles the known alkylating agent triethylenemelamine, it has some antimetabolite characteristics.
Primary indications. Carcinoma of the ovary, persistent or recurrent after first-line therapy.
Usual dosage and schedule.
   1. 260 mg/m^2 PO daily in three or four divided doses after meals and at bedtime for 14 or 21 days every 4 weeks when used as a single agent.
   2. 150 to 200 mg/m^2 PO daily in three or four divided doses for 2 of 3 or 4 weeks when used in combination.
Special precautions.
   1. Concurrent altretamine and antidepressants of the monoamine oxidase inhibitor class may cause severe orthostatic hypotension.
   2. Cimetidine may increase toxicity.

Toxicity.
1. *Myelosuppression and other hematologic effects.* Dose-limiting leukopenia and thrombocytopenia are uncommon, though lesser degrees are common. Anemia is common.
2. *Nausea, vomiting, and other gastrointestinal effects.* Mild to moderate nausea, vomiting, and other gastrointestinal occur in about 30% of patients and are rarely severe. Tolerance may develop.
3. *Mucocutaneous effects.* Alopecia, skin rash, and pruritus are rare.
4. *Miscellaneous effects.*
   a. Peripheral sensory neuropathies are common and may be ameliorated by pyridoxine, but tumor response may be compromised.
   b. Central nervous system (CNS) effects including agitation, confusion, hallucinations, depression, and Parkinsonian-like symptoms are uncommon with recommended intermittent schedule.
   c. Decreased renal function is occasional.
   d. Increased alkaline phosphatase level is occasional.
   e. Diarrhea is occasional.

AMIFOSTINE

Other name. Ethyol.
Mechanism of action. The prodrug, amifostine, is dephosphorylated to an active free thiol metabolite that can reduce the toxic effects of cisplatin. The differential activity between normal and cancer tissue is thought to be related to higher capillary alkaline phosphatase activity and better vascularity of normal tissue. Pretreatment reduces cumulative renal toxicity from cisplatin.
Primary indications.
1. For reduction of cumulative renal toxicity associated with repeated administration of cisplatin in patients with advanced cancer.
2. For reduction of moderate to severe xerostomia from radiation of the head and neck where the radiation port includes a substantial portion of the parotid glands.
Usual dosage and schedule.
1. *Reduction of cumulative renal toxicity with chemotherapy.* 910 mg/m^2 IV over 15 min once daily, starting 30 min before cisplatin chemotherapy.
2. *Reduction of xerostomia from radiation of the head and neck.* 200 mg/m^2 administered once daily as a 3-min IV infusion, starting 15 to 30 min prior to standard fraction radiation therapy (1.8 to 2.0 Gy).
Special precautions. To minimize hypotension during the infusion, patients should be adequately hydrated prior to the amifostine infusion and kept in a supine position during the infusion. Blood pressure should be monitored every 5 min during the infusion and thereafter as clinically indicated. Interrupt the infusion if the decrease in systolic pressure is more than 20% to 25% of the baseline systolic pressure.
Toxicity.
1. *Myelosuppression and other hematologic effects.* Not increased by amifostine.

2. *Nausea, vomiting, and other gastrointestinal effects.* Nausea and vomiting are common and may be severe.
3. *Mucocutaneous effects.* Skin rash is rare.
4. *Miscellaneous effects.*
   a. Transient hypotension during the infusion is common. Loss of consciousness may occur but is usually easily reversed.
   b. Flushing and feeling of warmth are occasional.
   c. Chilling and feeling of coldness are occasional.
   d. Dizziness, somnolence, hiccups, and sneezing are occasional.
   e. Allergic reactions are rare but have included anaphylactic reactions.
   f. Hypocalcemia is rare.
   g. Seizures are rare.

AMINOGLUTETHIMIDE

Other name. Cytadren.

Mechanism of action. Inhibits aromatization and cytochrome P-450 hydroxylating enzymes, thereby blocking the conversion of androgens to estrogens and the biosynthesis of all steroid hormones. This drug causes, in effect, a reversible chemical adrenalectomy.

Primary indications. Adrenocortical carcinoma, ectopic Cushing's syndrome. Previously used in breast cancer, but uncommonly now because of more specific aromatase inhibitors.

Usual dosage and schedule. 1,000 mg daily in four divided doses.

Special precautions. Hydrocortisone must be given concomitantly to prevent adrenal insufficiency, particularly if used in breast cancer. Suggested dose is 100 mg daily in divided doses for 2 weeks, then 40 mg daily in divided doses.

Toxicity.
1. *Myelosuppression and other hematologic effects.* Leukopenia and thrombocytopenia are rare, and if they occur, they resolve rapidly when the drug is stopped.
2. *Nausea, vomiting, and other gastrointestinal effects.* Occasional and usually mild.
3. *Mucocutaneous effects.* A morbilliform rash is commonly seen during the first week of treatment, but it usually disappears within 1 week.
4. *Hormonal effects.*
   a. Adrenal insufficiency is common without replacement hydrocortisone in patients with normal adrenal glands.
   b. Hypothyroidism is uncommon.
   c. Masculinization is possible.
5. *Neurologic effects.*
   a. Lethargy is common. Although usually mild and transient, it is occasionally severe.
   b. Vertigo, nystagmus, and ataxia are occasional.
6. *Miscellaneous effects.*
   a. Facial flushing is uncommon.
   b. Periorbital edema is uncommon.
   c. Cholestatic jaundice is rare.
   d. Fever is uncommon.

ANAGRELIDE

Other names. Imidazo(2,1-b)quinazolin-2-one, Agrelin.
Mechanism of action. Mechanism for thrombocytopenia unknown but may be due to impaired megakaryocyte function. Inhibitor of platelet aggregation but not at usual therapeutic doses.
Primary indications. Uncontrolled thrombocytosis in chronic myeloproliferative disorders such as essential thrombocythemia, chronic granulocytic leukemia, and polycythemia rubra vera.
Usual dosage and schedule. Supplied as 0.5- and 1-mg capsules.
1. 0.5 mg PO q.i.d. or 1 mg PO b.i.d. Increase by 0.5 mg/day every 5 to 7 days if no response. Maximum daily dose is 10 mg/day. Maximum single dose is 2.5 mg. Higher doses cause postural hypotension.
2. Alternative dosing schedules:
    a. *Elderly.* 0.5 mg PO daily; increase by 0.5 mg each week.
    b. *Abnormal renal or hepatic function.* 0.5 mg PO b.i.d.
Special precautions.
1. Contraindicated in pregnancy.
2. Use with caution in patients with heart disease. Tachycardia and forceful heartbeat may be exacerbated by caffeine; consumption of caffeine should be avoided for 1 h before and after anagrelide is taken.
3. Use other drugs that inhibit platelet aggregation (such as nonsteroidal anti-inflammatory drugs) with caution. Monitor platelet count every few days during first week, then weekly until the maintenance dose is reached.
Toxicity.
1. *Myelosuppression and other hematologic effects.* White cell count is none. Anemia is common (36%) but mild. Thrombocytopenic hemorrhage is uncommon (2%).
2. *Nausea, vomiting, and other gastrointestinal effects.* Nausea is occasional (15%); vomiting is uncommon. Diarrhea (26%), gas, and abdominal pain are common; pancreatitis is rare. Lactase supplementation eliminates diarrhea (anagrelide formulated with lactose).
3. *Mucocutaneous effects.* Rash, including urticaria, is occasional (8%). Hyperpigmentation is rare. Sun sensitivity is possible.
4. *Miscellaneous effects.*
    a. Palpitations (26%), forceful heartbeat, and tachycardia are common. Congestive heart failure is uncommon, but fluid retention or edema is common (21%). Tachyarrhythmias (including atrial fibrillation and premature atrial beats) are occasional. Angina, cardiomyopathy, and other severe cardiovascular effects are rare, although there are somewhat more frequent (8%) episodes of chest pain. Drinking alcoholic beverages may cause flushing. Higher than recommended single doses cause postural hypotension. Cardiovascular effects appear to result from vasodilation, positive inotropy, and decreased renal blood flow.
    b. Headaches are common (44%) and occasionally are severe; they usually diminish in about 2 weeks. Weakness (asthenia) is common (22%). Dizziness is occasional.

    c. Pulmonary infiltrates are rare but are a reason to stop anagrelide and treat with steroids.

    d. Hepatic enzyme elevation is rare, but caution is recommended when there is evidence of hepatic dysfunction.

ANASTROZOLE

Other name. Arimidex.

Mechanism of action. Decreases estrogen biosynthesis by selective inhibition of aromatase (estrogen synthetase).

Primary indications.
1. Carcinoma of the breast (advanced) as first-line treatment in women with hormone receptor–positive or unknown cancers.
2. Carcinoma of the breast after progression in patients previously responsive to tamoxifen therapy.

Usual dosage and schedule. 1 mg PO daily.

Special precaution. Potential hazard to fetus if given during pregnancy.

Toxicity.
1. *Myelosuppression and other hematologic effects.* No dose-related myelosuppression. Thromboembolic events are uncommon (3% to 4%).
2. *Nausea, vomiting, and other gastrointestinal effects.* Nausea is occasional; vomiting is uncommon. Diarrhea and constipation are occasional.
3. *Mucocutaneous effects.* Rash is uncommon. Hot flushes are common (25% to 30%). Vaginal dryness and leukorrhea are uncommon.
4. *Miscellaneous effects.*
    a. Asthenia is common.
    b. Musculoskeletal pain is occasional.
    c. Headache and dizziness are occasional.
    d. Arthralgia is occasional.
    e. Peripheral edema and weight gain are occasional (lower than with megestrol).
    f. Dyspnea and cough are occasional.
    g. Hypercalcemia is rare.
    h. Uterine bleeding appears less commonly than with tamoxifen.
    i. Osteoporosis and fractures are more common than with tanioxifen.

ANDROGENS

Other names. Fluoxymesterone (Halotestin), testolactone (Teslac), others.

Mechanism of action. Mechanism of antitumor effects is not clear.

Primary indications.
1. Anemia of myelodysplastic syndromes.
2. Breast carcinoma (in combination with other agents).

Usual dosage and schedule.
1. *Fluoxymesterone.* 20 to 40 mg PO daily in four divided doses.
2. *Testolactone.* 1,000 mg PO daily in four divided doses.

Special precaution. Hypercalcemia may occur with initial therapy.

Toxicity.
1. *Myelosuppression and other hematologic effects.* None. Erythropoiesis is stimulated.
2. *Nausea, vomiting, and other gastrointestinal effects.* Mild and dose related.
3. *Mucocutaneous effects.* Acne.
4. *Miscellaneous effects.*
    a. Masculinization—including an increase in facial and body hair, deepening of voice, acne, baldness, and clitoral hypertrophy—is common in females but may be minimized by dose attenuation.
    b. Intrahepatic biliary stasis with hyperbilirubinemia is uncommon but may occur at high androgen doses (17-methyl derivatives only).
    c. Fluid retention is occasional, although it is less severe with androgens than with estrogens.

ARSENIC TRIOXIDE

Other name. Trisenox.
Mechanism of action. Although the mechanism is incompletely understood, effects of arsenic trioxide include morphologic changes and DNA fragmentation characteristic of apoptosis and alteration of the fusion protein PML-RAR-α.
Primary indication. Acute promyelocytic leukemia that is refractory to retinoid and anthracycline therapy and has t(15;17) translocation or *PML/RAR*-α gene expression.
Usual dosage and schedule.
1. *Induction.* 0.15 mg/kg IV daily until marrow remission. Maximum of 60 doses.
2. *Consolidation.* 0.15 mg/kg IV daily for 25 doses over a period of up to 5 weeks. Consolidation is started 3 to 6 weeks after completion of induction therapy.
Special precautions.
1. Tachycardia and prolonged QT interval are common. This may lead to complete atrioventricular block with fatal ventricular arrhythmia. Electrolyte (including magnesium) abnormalities should be corrected prior to initiation of therapy, and patients with prolonged QT intervals should have measures taken to reduce this prolongation prior to treatment with arsenic trioxide. A QT value greater than 500 msec during therapy is an indication to suspend arsenic trioxide treatment and to initiate measures to correct other risk factors that may be contributing to the prolongation of the QT.
2. Acute promyelocytic leukemic differentiation syndrome, similar to that observed with retinoic acid, may be seen and is potentially fatal. This syndrome consists of fever, dyspnea, weight gain, pulmonary infiltrates, and pleural or pericardial effusions with or without leukocytosis. High-dose corticosteroids (e.g., dexamethasone 10 mg b.i.d.) should be started at the first signs of this syndrome and continued until it has subsided.
Toxicity.
1. *Myelosuppression and other hematologic effects.* Anemia, thrombocytopenia, and neutropenia are occasional. Leuko-

cytosis is common. Disseminated intravascular coagulation is occasional and may be severe. Infections and neutropenic fever are occasional.

2. *Nausea, vomiting, and other gastrointestinal effects.* Nausea, vomiting, diarrhea, and abdominal pain are common (over 50%). Gastrointestinal bleeding with or without diarrhea is occasional (8%). Constipation, anorexia, and other abdominal distress are occasional.

3. *Mucocutaneous effects.* Sore throat is common (40%). Dermatitis, pruritus, and ecchymosis are also common. More severe mucocutaneous reactions including local exfoliation, urticaria, and oral blistering are occasional to uncommon. Epistaxis is common (25%). Eye irritation and injection are occasional.

4. *Miscellaneous effects.*

   a. Tachycardia and prolonged QT interval are common. This may lead to complete atrioventricular block with fatal ventricular arrhythmia.

   b. Acute promyelocytic leukemic differentiation syndrome, similar to that seen with retinoic acid, may be seen. This consists of fever, dyspnea, weight gain, pulmonary infiltrates, and pleural or pericardial effusions with or without leukocytosis. This syndrome may be fatal.

   c. Headache and insomnia are common. Edema and pleural effusion are common (though not commonly serious), and general weight gain is occasional. Drug hypersensitivity is uncommon. Injection site edema, erythema, and pain are occasional.

   d. Hypokalemia, hypomagnesemia, and hyperglycemia are common (45% to 50%). Hyperkalemia is occasional to common (18%), as are elevated transaminases, hypocalcemia, and hypoglycemia.

   e. Cough and dyspnea are common (over 50%). Pleural effusion, hypoxia, wheezing, and asymptomatic auscultatory findings are occasional to common (8% to 20%).

   f. Renal failure is occasional.

ASPARAGINASE

Other names. L-Asparaginase, Elspar, Kidrolase, pegaspargase, Oncaspar.

Mechanism of action. Hydrolysis of serum asparagine occurs, which deprives leukemia cells of the required amino acid and inhibits protein synthesis. Normal cells are spared because they generally have the ability to synthesize their own asparagine. Pegaspargase is a chemically modified formulation of asparaginase in which the L-asparaginase is covalently conjugated with monomethoxypolyethylene glycol. This modification increases its half-life in the plasma by a factor of 4 to about 5.7 days and reduces its recognition by the immune system, which allows the drug to be used in patients previously hypersensitive to native L-asparaginase.

Primary indication. Acute lymphocytic leukemia, primarily for induction therapy.

Usual dosage and schedule. Both schedules are usually used in combination with other drugs. The schedules listed are only two of many acceptable dosing schedules.

1. *L-Asparaginase.* 6,000 to 18,500 IU/m^2 IV daily for up to 14 days.
2. *Pegaspargase.* 2,500 IU/m^2 IM (or IV) once every 14 days in patients who have developed hypersensitivity to native forms of asparaginase.

Special precautions. Asparaginase is contraindicated in patients with pancreatitis or a history of pancreatitis. Asparaginase is contraindicated in patients who have had significant hemorrhagic events associated with prior L-asparaginase therapy. Pegaspargase is also contraindicated in patients who have had previous serious allergic reactions such as generalized urticaria, bronchospasm, laryngeal edema, hypotension, or other unacceptable adverse reactions to prior pegaspargase.

1. Be prepared to treat anaphylaxis at each administration of the drug. Epinephrine, antihistamines, corticosteroids, and life-support equipment should be readily available.
2. Giving concurrently with or immediately before vincristine may increase vincristine toxicity.
3. The IM route is preferred for pegaspargase because of a lower incidence of hepatotoxicity, coagulopathy, and gastrointestinal and renal disorders compared with the IV route of administration.

Toxicity.

1. *Myelosuppression and other hematologic effects.* Occasional.
2. *Nausea, vomiting, and other gastrointestinal effects.* Occasional and usually mild.
3. *Mucocutaneous effects.* No toxicity occurs except as a sign of hypersensitivity.
4. *Anaphylaxis.* Mild to severe hypersensitivity reactions, including anaphylaxis, occur in 20% to 30% of patients. Such reaction is less likely to occur during the first few days of treatment. It is particularly common with intermittent schedules or repeat cycles. If the patient develops hypersensitivity to the *Escherichia coli*–derived enzyme (Elspar), *Erwinia*-derived asparaginase may be safely substituted because the two enzyme preparations are not cross-reactive. Note that hypersensitivity may also develop to *Erwinia*-derived asparaginase, and continued preparedness to treat anaphylaxis must be maintained.

    If administered IM, asparaginase should be given in an extremity so that a tourniquet can be applied to slow the systemic release of asparaginase should anaphylaxis occur.

    Approximately 30% of patients previously sensitive to L-asparaginase will have a hypersensitivity reaction to pegaspargase, whereas only 10% of those who were not hypersensitive to the native form will have a hypersensitivity reaction to the polyethylene glycol–modified drug.
5. *Miscellaneous effects.*
    a. Mild fever and malaise are common and occasionally progress to severe chills and malignant hyperthermia.
    b. Hepatotoxicity is common and occasionally severe. Abnormalities observed include elevations of serum glutamic–oxaloacetic transaminase (SGOT), alkaline phosphatase, and bilirubin, depressed levels of hepatic-

derived clotting factors and albumin, and hepatocellular fatty metamorphosis.
c. Renal failure is rare.
d. Pancreatic endocrine and exocrine dysfunction, often with manifestations of pancreatitis, occasionally occurs. Nonketotic hyperglycemia is uncommon.
e. CNS effects (depression, somnolence, fatigue, confusion, agitation, hallucinations, or coma) are seen occasionally. They are usually reversible following discontinuation of the drug.

BEXAROTENE (CAPSULES)

Other name. Targretin.
Mechanism of action. A member of the subclass of retinoids (rexinoid) that selectively activates retinoid X receptors. These receptors are distinct from retinoic acid receptors but also act as transcription factors that regulate the expression of genes that control cellular differentiation and proliferation. The exact mechanism in cutaneous T-cell lymphoma is unknown.
Primary indications. Cutaneous manifestations of cutaneous T-cell lymphoma in patients refractory to at least one prior systemic therapy.
Usual dosage and schedule. 300 mg/m^2/day to start as a single oral daily dose taken with a meal. Dosage is adjusted downward by 100-mg/m^2/day decrements for toxicity or upward to 400 mg/m^2/day if there have been no response and good tolerability after 8 weeks of treatment. Treatment may be continued for up to 2 years.
Special precaution. Avoid use in pregnant women because of marked teratogenic potential.
Toxicity.
1. *Myelosuppression and other hematologic effects.* Mild to moderate leukopenia is occasional to common with a time of onset of 4 to 8 weeks. Severe or worse leukopenia is occasional.
2. *Nausea, vomiting, and other gastrointestinal effects.* Mild nausea, abdominal pain, and diarrhea are occasional. Vomiting and anorexia are uncommon.
3. *Mucocutaneous effects.* Skin reactions are occasional to common. They include redness, dryness, and pruritus of the skin and mucous membranes, possible vesicle formation, exfoliative dermatitis, cheilitis, and conjunctivitis. There also may be increased skin photosensitivity (e.g., to sun), and the nails may become brittle. Alopecia is uncommon.
4. *Miscellaneous effects.*
   a. Cataracts and corneal ulcerations or opacities are uncommon.
   b. Arthralgias, bone pain, and muscle aches are occasional. Fever, chills, and headache (flu syndrome) are occasional.
   c. Hypertriglyceridemia (80%) and hypercholesterolemia (35% to 40%) are common. Hypertriglyceridemia is usually more severe. These are reversible with discontinuation of therapy and may be reduced by antilipemic therapy.

d.   Headache is common. Lethargy, fatigue, confusion, and mental depression are uncommon; pseudotumor cerebri is rare.
e.   Inflammatory bowel disease and pancreatitis (associated with hypertriglyceridemia) are rare.
f.   Hepatotoxicity with increased lactate dehydrogenase, SGOT, serum glutamic–pyruvic transaminase (SGPT), γ-glutamyl transpeptidase, and alkaline phosphatase is occasional.
g.   Hypothyroidism is common, with decreased T_4 and thyroid-stimulating hormone.
h.   Peripheral edema is occasional.
i.   Hypernatremia is rare.

BEXAROTENE (GEL)

Other name. Targretin gel (1%).

Mechanism of action. A member of the subclass of retinoids (rexinoid) that selectively activates retinoid X receptors. These receptors are distinct from retinoic acid receptors but also act as transcription factors that regulate the expression of genes that control cellular differentiation and proliferation. The exact mechanism in cutaneous T-cell lymphoma is unknown.

Primary indications. Cutaneous manifestations of cutaneous T-cell lymphoma (stage IA and IB) in patients who have refractory or persistent disease after other therapies or who have not tolerated other therapies.

Usual dosage and schedule. The gel is applied once every other day for the first week. The frequency is then increased at weekly intervals as tolerated to once daily, twice daily, and up to four times daily, according to individual lesion tolerance. Treatment frequency should be reduced or treatment suspended for severe local irritation.

Special precaution. Avoid use in pregnant women because of marked teratogenic potential.

Toxicity.

1.   *Myelosuppression and other hematologic effects.* Uncommon.
2.   *Nausea, vomiting, and other gastrointestinal effects.* Not expected.
3.   *Mucocutaneous effects.* Skin reactions are occasional to common. They include pain, redness, dryness, and pruritus of the skin, possible vesicle formation, and exfoliative dermatitis. There also may be increased skin photosensitivity (e.g., to sun).
4.   *Miscellaneous effects.*
     a.   Hypertriglyceridemia is occasional.
     b.   Headache and paresthesias are occasional.
     c.   Peripheral edema is occasional.

BICALUTAMIDE

Other name. Casodex.

Mechanism of action. A nonsteroidal antiandrogen that is a competitive inhibitor of androgens at the cellular androgen receptor in target tissues such as the prostate.

Primary indications. Carcinoma of the prostate, often in combination with luteinizing hormone–releasing hormone agonist.

Usual dosage and schedule. 50 mg daily, in morning or evening.
Special precautions. Rare cases of severe liver injury have been
reported. Bicalutamide should be used with caution in patients
with moderate to severe hepatic impairment.
Toxicity.
1. *Myelosuppression and other hematologic effects.* No myelosuppression. May interact with warfarin and increase international normalized ratio.
2. *Nausea, vomiting, and other gastrointestinal effects.* Nausea,
   diarrhea, flatulence, and constipation are occasional; vomiting is uncommon.
3. *Mucocutaneous effects.* Mild skin rash is occasional.
4. *Miscellaneous effects.*
   a. Secondary pharmacologic effects including breast ten-
      derness, breast swelling, hot flashes (49%), impotence,
      and loss of libido are common but reversible after ces-
      sation of therapy.
   b. Elevated liver function tests are uncommon.
   c. Adverse cardiovascular events are similar to those seen
      with orchiectomy.
   d. Dizziness or vertigo is occasional.

BLEOMYCIN

Other name. Blenoxane.
Mechanism of action. Bleomycin binds to DNA, causes single-
and double-strand scission, and inhibits further DNA, RNA, and
protein synthesis.
Primary indications.
1. Testis, head and neck, penis, cervix, vulva, anus, and skin
   carcinomas.
2. Hodgkin's and non-Hodgkin's lymphomas.
3. Pleural effusions—used as sclerosing agent.
Usual dosage and schedule.
1. 10 to 20 U/m² IV or IM once or twice a week *or*
2. 30 U IV push weekly for 9 to 12 weeks in combination with
   other drugs for testis cancer.
3. 60 U in 50 mL of normal saline instilled intrapleurally.
Special precautions.
1. In patients with lymphoma, a test dose of 1 or 2 U should be
   given IM prior to the first dose of bleomycin because of the possibility of anaphylactoid, acute pulmonary, or severe hyper-
   pyretic responses. If no acute reaction occurs within 4 h,
   regular dosing may begin.
2. Reduce dose for renal failure:

Serum creatinine	% of full dose
2.5–4.0	25
4.0–6.0	20
6.0–10.0	10

3. The cumulative lifetime dose should not exceed 400 U because of the dose-related incidence of severe pulmonary fibrosis. Smaller limits may be appropriate for older patients
   or those with pre-existing pulmonary disease. Frequent
   evaluation of pulmonary status including symptoms of
   cough or dyspnea, rales, infiltrates on chest x-ray film, and

pulmonary function studies is recommended to avert serious pulmonary sequelae.
4. Glass containers are recommended for continuous infusion to minimize drug instability.
5. High F_iO_2 (fraction of inspired oxygen; such as might be used during surgery) should be avoided as it exacerbates lung injury, sometimes acutely.

Toxicity.
1. *Myelosuppression and other hematologic effects.* Significant depression of counts is uncommon. This factor permits bleomycin to be used in full doses with myelosuppressive drugs.
2. *Nausea, vomiting, and other gastrointestinal effects.* Occasional and self-limiting.
3. *Mucocutaneous effects.* Alopecia, stomatitis, erythema, edema, thickening of nail bed, and hyperpigmentation and desquamation of skin are common.
4. *Pulmonary effects.*
   a. Acute anaphylactoid or pulmonary edema–like response is occasional in patients with lymphoma (see Special Precautions, above).
   b. Dose-related pneumonitis with cough, dyspnea, rales, and infiltrates, progressing to pulmonary fibrosis.
5. *Fever.* Common. Occasionally severe hyperpyrexia, diaphoresis, dehydration, and hypotension have occurred and resulted in renal failure and death. Antipyretics help control fever.
6. *Miscellaneous effects.*
   a. Lethargy, headache, and joint swelling are rare.
   b. IM or SC injection may cause pain at injection site.

BUSULFAN

Other names. Myleran, Busulfex.
Mechanism of action. Bifunctional alkylating agent. Its effect may be greater on cellular thiol groups than on nucleic acids.
Primary indications.
1. *Standard doses.* Chronic granulocytic (myelogenous) leukemia.
2. *High doses with stem cell rescue.* Acute leukemia, lymphoma, chronic granulocytic leukemia.
Usual dosage and schedule.
1. 3 to 4 mg/m² PO daily for remission induction in adults until the leukocyte count is 50% of the original level, then 1 to 2 mg/m² PO daily. Busulfan may be given continuously or intermittently for maintenance.
2. For high doses with stem cell rescue, consult specific protocols. Not recommended outside research setting. Typical dose is 1 mg/kg PO q6 h for 4 consecutive days. Alternative dosing of IV form (Busulfex) is 0.8 mg/kg of ideal body weight (or actual if lower) as a 2-h infusion through a central catheter every 6 h for 4 days (16 doses). High-dose therapy requires pretreatment with phenytoin.
Special precautions. Obtain complete blood count weekly while patient is on therapy. If leukocyte count falls rapidly to less than 15,000/μL, discontinue therapy until nadir is reached and rising counts indicate a need for further treatment.

Toxicity.
1. *Myelosuppression and other hematologic effects.* Dose limiting. A fall in the leukocyte count may not begin for 2 weeks after starting therapy, and it is likely to continue for 2 weeks after therapy has been stopped. Recovery of marrow function may be delayed for 3 to 6 weeks after the drug has been discontinued. High-dose therapy requires stem cell rescue (e.g., bone marrow transplantation).
2. *Nausea, vomiting, and other gastrointestinal effects.* Rare.
3. *Mucocutaneous effects.* Hyperpigmentation occurs occasionally, particularly in skin creases.
4. *Pulmonary effects.* Interstitial pulmonary fibrosis is rare and is an indication to discontinue drug. Corticosteroids may improve symptoms and minimize permanent lung damage.
5. *Metabolic effects.* Adrenal insufficiency syndrome is rare. Hyperuricemia may occur when the leukemia cell count is rapidly reduced. Ovarian suppression and amenorrhea are common.
6. *Miscellaneous effects.*
   a. Secondary neoplasia is possible.
   b. Fatal hepato-veno-occlusive disease with high-dose therapy is occasional.
   c. Seizures after high-dose therapy are occasional.

CAPECITABINE

Other name. Xeloda.
Mechanism of action. An orally administered prodrug that is converted to fluorouracil intracellularly. When this is converted to the active nucleotide, 5-fluoro-2-deoxyuridine monophosphate, it inhibits the enzyme thymidylate synthetase and blocks DNA synthesis. The triphosphate may also be mistakenly incorporated into RNA, which interferes with RNA processing and protein synthesis.
Primary indications.
1. Metastatic breast cancer that is resistant to anthracycline- and paclitaxel-containing chemotherapy regimens. May also be used in patients in whom anthracyclines are contraindicated.
2. Colorectal carcinoma, particularly in situations where continuous infusion of fluorouracil might have been used.
3. Pancreatic carcinoma.
Usual dosage and schedule. Generally taken with water, twice daily (about 12 h between doses) within 30 min after a meal.
1. $1,250 \text{ mg/m}^2$ PO twice daily for 2 weeks, followed by a 1-week rest, given as 3-week cycles.
2. $1,000–1,250 \text{ mg/m}^2$ PO twice daily for 2 weeks, in combination with docetaxel 75 mg/m^2 IV over 1 h once every 3 weeks. Two weeks of treatment are followed by a 1-week rest to complete the 3-week cycle.
3. 800 to 825 mg/m^2 PO twice daily for 5 or 7 days a week as a radiosensitizer for the duration of the radiotherapy unless toxicity prohibits continuation.
Special precautions. Patients with moderate renal impairment ($C_{Cr} = 30$ to 50 mL/min) require a 25% dosage reduction. Diarrhea

may be severe and require fluid and electrolyte replacement. Incidence and severity may be worse in patients 80 years of age or older. Therapy may need to be interrupted and subsequent doses decreased for severe or repeated toxicity. Increase in prothrombin time (PT) and international normalized ratio (INR) may be seen in patients previously stable on oral anticoagulants. Monitor PT/INR more frequently when patient is on capecitabine.

Toxicity.

1. *Myelosuppression and other hematologic effects.* Common, but when used as a single agent, these usually are mild to moderate, with anemia predominating. Neutropenia is common when used in combination and may be associated with neutropenic fever.

2. *Nausea, vomiting, and other gastrointestinal effects.* Both nausea (45%) and vomiting (35%) are common but usually not severe. Diarrhea is common (55%); in up to 15% of patients, it is severe to life threatening. Gastrointestinal motility disorders including ileus may be seen, and necrotizing enterocolitis has been reported. Abdominal pain is occasional to common. Anorexia is occasional to common (26%). Hyperbilirubinemia is common (48%) but only occasionally severe or life threatening.

3. *Mucocutaneous effects.* Hand-and-foot syndrome is common (54%) and may be severe. Dermatitis is also common (27%), as is stomatitis, but it is uncommon that these are severe. Eye irritation and increased lacrimation are occasional.

4. *Miscellaneous effects.*
   a. Fatigue is common.
   b. Paresthesias are occasional.
   c. Fever is occasional.
   d. Headache or dizziness is occasional.
   e. Cardiotoxicity is possible, as with any fluorinated pyrimidine.

5. Hand-and-foot syndrome and diarrhea may be ameliorated by celecoxib 200 mg PO b.i.d.

CARBOPLATIN

Other names. Paraplatin, CBDCA.

Mechanism of action. Covalent binding to DNA.

Primary indications. Ovarian, endometrial, and lung cancers and other cancers in which cisplatin is active.

Usual dosage and schedule. Area-under-the-curve (AUC) dosing (Calvert formula) is generally preferred.

1. Target AUC is commonly 4 to 6, depending on previous treatment and other drugs to be used. Administration dose (mg) = (target AUC) × ([creatinine clearance] + 25). Administration dose is given by IV infusion over 15 to 60 min and repeated every 3 to 4 weeks.

2. 300 to 400 mg/m^2 IV by infusion over 15 to 60 min or longer, repeated every 3 to 4 weeks.

3. Higher doses up to 1,600 mg/m^2 divided over several days have been used followed by stem cell rescue (e.g., bone marrow transplantation).

Special precautions.
1. Much less renal toxicity than cisplatin, so there is no need for a vigorous hydration schedule or forced diuresis. If AUC dosing is not used, reduce dose to 250 mg/m^2 for creatinine clearance of 41 to 59 mL/min; reduce to 200 mg/m^2 for clearance of 16 to 40 mL/min.
2. Anaphylactic-like reactions to carboplatin have been reported and may occur within minutes of carboplatin administration. Epinephrine, corticosteroids, and antihistamines have been employed to alleviate symptoms.

Toxicity.
1. *Myelosuppression and other hematologic effects.* Anemia, granulocytopenia, and thrombocytopenia are common and dose limiting. Red blood cell transfusions or epoetin may be required. Thrombocytopenia may be delayed (days 18 to 28).
2. *Nausea, vomiting, and other gastrointestinal effects.* Nausea and vomiting are common, but vomiting (65%) is not as frequent or as severe as with cisplatin and can be controlled with combination antiemetic regimens. Liver function abnormalities are common. Gastrointestinal pain is occasional.
3. *Mucocutaneous effects.* Alopecia is uncommon. Mucositis is rare.
4. *Renal tubular abnormalities.* Elevation in serum creatinine or blood urea nitrogen occurs occasionally. More common is electrolyte loss with decreases in serum sodium, potassium, calcium, and magnesium.
5. *Miscellaneous effects.*
   a. Peripheral neuropathies and central neurotoxicity are uncommon.
   b. Allergic reactions are uncommonly seen with rash, urticaria, pruritus, and rarely bronchospasm and hypotension.
   c. Cardiovascular effects (cardiac failure, embolism, cerebrovascular accidents) are uncommon.
   d. Hemolytic uremic syndrome is rare.

CARMUSTINE

Other names. BCNU, BiCNU, Gliadel wafer (surgically implantable, biodegradable polymer wafer that releases impregnated carmustine from the hydrophobic matrix after implantation).

Mechanism of action. Alkylation and carbamoylation by carmustine metabolites interfere with the synthesis and function of DNA, RNA, and proteins. Carmustine is lipid soluble and easily enters the brain.

Primary indications.
A. *Systemic therapy.*
   1. Hodgkin's and non-Hodgkin's lymphomas.
   2. Brain tumors.
   3. Multiple myeloma.
   4. Melanoma.
B. *Implantable carmustine-impregnated wafer.*
   1. Glioblastoma multiforme.

Usual dosage and schedule.
A. *Systemic therapy.*
   1. 200 to 240 mg/m² IV as a 30- to 45-min infusion every 6 to 8 weeks. Dose often is divided and given over 2 to 3 days. Some recommend limiting the cumulative dose to 1,000 mg/m² to limit pulmonary and renal toxicity.
   2. Higher doses of up to 600 mg/m² have been used with stem cell rescue (e.g., bone marrow or peripheral blood stem cell transplantation).
B. *Implantable carmustine-impregnated wafer.*
   1. Up to 8 wafers, each containing 7.7 mg of carmustine, are applied to the resection cavity surface after removal of the tumor.

Special precautions. For systemic therapy, because of delayed myelosuppression and other hematologic effects (3 to 6 weeks), do not administer drug more often than every 6 weeks. Await a return of normal platelet and granulocyte counts before repeating therapy. Amphotericin B may enhance the potential for renal toxicity, bronchospasm, and hypotension.

Toxicity.
A. *Systemic therapy.*
   1. *Myelosuppression and other hematologic effects.* Delayed and often biphasic, with the nadir at 3 to 6 weeks; it may be cumulative with successive doses. Recovery may be protracted for several months. High-dose therapy requires stem cell rescue.
   2. *Nausea, vomiting, and other gastrointestinal effects.* Effects beginning 2 h after therapy and lasting 4 to 6 h are common.
   3. *Mucocutaneous effects.*
      a. Facial flushing and a burning sensation at the IV site may be due to alcohol used to reconstitute the drug; this is common with rapid injection.
      b. Hyperpigmentation of skin after accidental contact is common.
   4. *Miscellaneous effects.*
      a. Hepatotoxicity is uncommon but can be severe.
      b. Pulmonary fibrosis is uncommon at low doses, but its frequency increases at doses higher than 1,000 mg/m².
      c. Secondary neoplasia is possible.
      d. Renal toxicity is uncommon at doses of less than 1,000 mg/m².
      e. With high-dose therapy, encephalopathy, hepatotoxicity, and pulmonary toxicity are common and dose limiting. Hepato-veno-occlusive disease also occurs (occasional).
B. *Implantable carmustine impregnated wafer.* Limited toxicity beyond that expected from craniotomy is seen. Serious intracranial infection was seen in 4% of patients compared with 1% of placebo-treated patients. Brain edema not responsive to steroids may also be seen in a similar percentage of patients. Abnormal wound healing may occur. Remnants of the wafer may be seen for many months after implantation.

CETUXIMAB (INVESTIGATIONAL)

Other names. Epidermal growth factor receptor (EGFr) antibody, C225, Erbitux.

Mechanism of action. Epidermal growth factor receptor antibody that blocks the ligand-binding site and inhibits proliferation of cells. It is thought potentially most useful in those tumors that overexpress epidermal growth factor receptor.

Primary indications.
1. Carcinoma of head and neck.
2. Lung cancer.

Usual dosage and schedule. 400 mg/m^2 IV loading dose administered over 2 h on day 1. Then 250 mg/m^2 IV maintenance doses administered over 1 h weekly thereafter. May be administered in combination with other agents.

Special precautions. Severe anaphylactoid reactions may occur.

Toxicity.
1. *Myelosuppression and other hematologic effects.* Leukopenia and anemia are occasional.
2. *Nausea, vomiting, and other gastrointestinal effects.* Nausea is occasional to common. Diarrhea is occasional.
3. *Mucocutaneous effects.* Acne-like rash is common. Stomatitis is occasional.
4. *Miscellaneous effects.*
   a. Asthenia is common.
   b. Allergic or hypersensitivity reactions are occasional but may be severe.
   c. Chills are occasional.
   d. Human antichimeric antibodies (HACAs) are uncommon.

CHLORAMBUCIL

Other name. Leukeran.

Mechanism of action. Classic alkylating agent, with primary effect on preformed DNA.

Primary indications.
1. Chronic lymphocytic leukemia.
2. Low-grade non-Hodgkin's lymphoma.

Usual dosage and schedule.
1. 3 to 4 mg/m^2 PO daily until a response is seen or cytopenias occur; then, if necessary, maintain with 1 to 2 mg/m^2 PO daily.
2. 30 mg/m^2 PO once every 2 weeks (with or without prednisone 80 mg/m^2 PO on days 1 to 5).

Special precaution. Increased toxicity may occur with prior barbiturate use.

Toxicity.
1. *Myelosuppression and other hematologic effects.* Dose limiting and may be prolonged.
2. *Nausea, vomiting, and other gastrointestinal effects.* May be seen with higher doses but are uncommon.
3. *Mucocutaneous effects.* Rash is uncommon.
4. *Miscellaneous effects.*
   a. Liver function abnormalities are rare.
   b. Secondary neoplasia is possible.

   c. Amenorrhea and azoospermia are common.
   d. Drug fever is uncommon.
   e. Pulmonary fibrosis is rare.
   f. CNS effects including seizure and coma may be seen at very high doses (higher than 100 mg/m^2).

CISPLATIN

Other names. *cis*-Diamminedichloroplatinum (II), DDP, CDDP, Platinol.

Mechanism of action. Similar to alkylating agents with respect to binding and cross-linking strands of DNA.

Primary indications. Usually used in combination with other cytotoxic drugs.
1. Testis, ovary, endometrial, cervical, bladder, head and neck, gastrointestinal, and lung carcinomas.
2. Soft tissue and bone sarcomas.
3. Non-Hodgkin's lymphoma.

Usual dosage and schedule.
1. 40 to 120 mg/m^2 IV on day 1 as infusion every 3 weeks.
2. 15 to 20 mg/m^2 IV on days 1 to 5 as infusion every 3 to 4 weeks.

Special precautions. Do not administer if serum creatinine level is more than 1.5 mg/dL. Irreversible renal tubular damage may occur if vigorous diuresis is not maintained, particularly with higher doses (higher than 40 mg/m^2), and with additional concurrent nephrotoxic drugs such as the aminoglycosides. At higher doses, diuresis with mannitol with or without furosemide plus vigorous hydration are mandatory.
1. An acceptable method for hydration in patients without cardiovascular impairment for cisplatin doses up to 80 mg/m^2 is as follows:
   a. Have patient void, and begin infusion of 5% dextrose in half-normal saline with KCl 20 mEq/L and MgSO$_4$ 1 g/L (8 mEq/L); run at 500 mL/h for 1.5 to 2.0 L.
   b. After 1 h of infusion, give 12.5 g of mannitol by IV push.
   c. Immediately thereafter, start the cisplatin (mixed in normal saline at 1 mg/mL) and infuse over 1 h through the sidearm of the IV line while continuing the hydration.
   d. Give additional mannitol (12.5 to 50.0 g by IV push) if necessary to maintain urinary output of 250 mL/h over the duration of the hydration. If patient gets more than 1 L behind on urinary output or signs or symptoms of congestive heart failure develop, 40 mg of furosemide may be given.
2. For doses of more than 80 mg/m^2, a more vigorous hydration is recommended.
   a. Have patient void, and begin infusion of 5% dextrose in half-normal saline with KCl 20 mEq/L and MgSO$_4$ 1 g/L (8 mEq/L); run at 500 mL/h for 2.5 to 3.0 L.
   b. After 1 h of infusion, give 25 g of mannitol by IV push.
   c. Continue hydration.
   d. After 2 h of hydration, if urinary output is at least 250 mL/h, start the cisplatin (mixed in normal saline at 1 mg/mL) and infuse over 1 to 2 h (1 mg/m^2/min) through the sidearm of the IV line while continuing the hydration.

e.   Give additional mannitol (12.5 to 50 g by IV push) if
necessary to maintain urinary output of 250 mL/h over
the duration of the hydration. If patient gets more than
1 L behind on urinary output or signs or symptoms of
congestive heart failure develop, 40 mg of furosemide
may be given.
3.   For patients with known or suspected cardiovascular impairment (ejection fraction under 45%), a less vigorous rate
of hydration may be used, provided the dose of cisplatin is
limited (e.g., less than 60 mg/m²). An alternative is to give
carboplatin.
Toxicity.
1.   *Myelosuppression and other hematologic effects.* Mild to moderate, depending on the dose. Relative lack of myelosuppression and other hematologic effects allows cisplatin to be used
in full doses with more myelosuppressive drugs. Anemia is
common and may have a hemolytic component. Anemia often
is amenable to epoetin therapy.
2.   *Nausea, vomiting, and other gastrointestinal effects.* Severe
and often intractable vomiting regularly begins within 1 h
of starting cisplatin and lasts 8 to 12 h. Prolonged nausea,
vomiting, and other gastrointestinal effects occur occasionally. These effects may be minimized by the use of a combination antiemetic regimen, for example, dexamethasone,
ondansetron or granisetron, and lorazepam (see Chapter 26).
3.   *Mucocutaneous effects.* None.
4.   *Renal tubular damage.* Acute reversible and occasionally
irreversible nephrotoxicity may occur, particularly if adequate
attention is not given to achieving sufficient hydration and
diuresis. Nephrotoxic antibiotics increase risk of acute
renal failure.
5.   *Ototoxicity.* High-tone hearing loss is common, but significant hearing loss at vocal frequencies occurs only occasionally. Tinnitus is uncommon.
6.   *Severe electrolyte abnormalities.* These abnormalities, for
example, marked hyponatremia, hypomagnesemia, hypocalcemia, and hypokalemia, may be seen up to several days
after treatment.
7.   *Anaphylaxis.* May occur after several doses. Responds to
epinephrine, antihistamines, and corticosteroids.
8.   *Miscellaneous effects.*
a.   Peripheral neuropathies are clinically significant signs
and symptoms common at cumulative doses over
300 mg/m².
b.   Hyperuricemia is uncommon and parallels renal failure.
c.   Autonomic dysfunction with symptomatic postural hypotension is occasional.

CLADRIBINE

Other names. 2-Chlorodeoxyadenosine, Leustatin.
Mechanism of action. Deoxyadenosine analog with high cellular
specificity for lymphoid cells. Resistant to effect of adenosine deaminase. Accumulates in cells as triphosphate, is incorporated into
DNA, and inhibits DNA repair enzymes and RNA synthesis. Also
results in NAD depletion. Effect is independent of cell division.

Primary indications.
1. Hairy-cell leukemia.
2. Chronic lymphocytic leukemia.
3. Waldenström's macroglobulinemia.
4. Possibly other lymphoid neoplasms.

Usual dosage and schedule.
1. 0.09 mg/kg (3.33 mg/m^2) IV daily as a continuous 7-day infusion.
2. 0.14 mg/kg (5.2 mg/m^2) IV as a 2-h infusion daily for 5 days.
3. 0.14 mg/kg (5.2 mg/m^2) SC daily for 5 days.

Special precautions.
1. Give allopurinol 300 mg daily as prophylaxis against hyperuricemia.
2. Opportunistic infections occur occasionally and should be watched for closely.

Toxicity.
1. *Myelosuppression and other hematologic effects.* Moderate granulocyte suppression is common. Marrow suppression with leukopenia and thrombocytopenia may be prolonged for over a year. Serious infection is common. Profound suppression of CD4 and CD8 counts is common and often prolonged for over 1 year. Opportunistic infections including herpes, fungus, and *Pneumocystis* infection may occur and should be watched for. Some routinely use prophylaxis against one or more of these infections, including acyclovir 400 mg b.i.d. and trimethoprim-sulfamethoxazole 1 double-strength tablet twice daily on 2 or 3 days a week.
2. *Nausea, vomiting, and other gastrointestinal effects.* Mild nausea with decrease in appetite is common, but no vomiting is expected.
3. *Mucocutaneous effects.* Rash is common.
4. *Miscellaneous effects.*
   a. Fever, possibly due to release of pyrogens from tumor cells, is common.
   b. Headache, dizziness, insomnia, fatigue, myalgia, and arthralgia are occasional.
   c. Edema and tachycardia are occasional.
   d. Cough, shortness of breath, and abnormal breath sounds are occasional.

CORTICOSTEROIDS

Other names. Prednisone, dexamethasone (Decadron), and others.
Mechanism of action. Unknown but apparently related to the presence of glucocorticoid receptors in tumor cells. Mediated in part by *bcl-2* gene and promotion of apoptotic cell death.
Primary indications.
1. Acute and chronic lymphocytic leukemia.
2. Hodgkin's and non-Hodgkin's lymphomas.
3. Multiple myeloma.
4. Carcinoma of the breast.
5. Cerebral edema or spinal cord injury (compression).
6. Nausea and vomiting from chemotherapy.

Usual dosage and schedule.
1. *Prednisone.* Dose varies with neoplasm and combination. Typical regimen, *except* for acute lymphocytic leukemia, is as follows:
    a. 40 mg/m^2 PO days 1 to 14 every 4 weeks *or*
    b. 100 mg/m^2 PO days 1 to 5 every 4 weeks.
2. *Prednisone.* For acute lymphocytic leukemia, 40 to 50 mg/m^2 PO daily for 28 days.
3. *Dexamethasone.* For cerebral edema or spinal cord injury, 10 mg IV push; then 16 to 32 mg PO daily. As signs and symptoms are controlled, gradually reduce to lowest effective dose.

Special precaution. Monitor for hyperglycemia.

Toxicity.
1. *Myelosuppression and other hematologic effects.* None.
2. *Nausea, vomiting, and other gastrointestinal effects.* No acute nausea or vomiting. Epigastric pain, extreme hunger, and occasional peptic ulceration with bleeding may occur even with short courses. Antacids or inhibitors of acid secretion are recommended as prophylaxis.
3. *Mucocutaneous effects.* Acne; increased risk for oral, rectal, and vaginal thrush. Thinning of skin and striae develop with continuous use.
4. *Suppression of adrenal–pituitary axis.* May lead to adrenal insufficiency when corticosteroids are withdrawn. This problem is not common with intermittent schedules.
5. *Metabolic effects.* Potassium depletion, sodium and fluid retention, diabetes, increased appetite, loss of muscle mass, myopathy, weight gain, osteoporosis, and development of cushingoid features. Their frequency depends on dose and duration of therapy.
6. *Miscellaneous effects.*
    a. CNS effects, including euphoria, depression, and sleeplessness, are common and may progress to dementia or frank psychosis.
    b. Increased susceptibility to infection is common.
    c. Subcapsular cataracts in patients are uncommon but have been seen even when used for prophylaxis and treatment of drug-induced emesis.

CYCLOPHOSPHAMIDE

Other names. CTX, Cytoxan, Neosar.

Mechanism of action. Metabolism of cyclophosphamide by hepatic microsomal enzymes produces active alkylating metabolites. Cyclophosphamide's primary effect is probably on DNA.

Primary indications.
1. Breast, lung, ovary, testis, and bladder carcinomas.
2. Bone and soft tissue sarcomas.
3. Hodgkin's and non-Hodgkin's lymphomas.
4. Acute and chronic lymphocytic leukemias.
5. Waldenström's macroglobulinemia.
6. Neuroblastoma and Wilms' tumor of childhood.
7. Gestational trophoblastic neoplasms.
8. Multiple myeloma.

Usual dosage and schedule.
1. 1,000 to 1,500 mg/m^2 IV every 3 to 4 weeks *or*
2. 400 mg/m^2 PO days 1 to 5 every 3 to 4 weeks *or*
3. 60 to 120 mg/m^2 PO daily.
4. High-dose regimens (4 to 7 g/m^2 divided over 4 days) are investigational and should be used only with some kind of stem cell rescue (e.g., bone marrow transplantation) and mesna bladder protection.

Special precautions. Give dose in the morning, maintain ample fluid intake, and have patient empty bladder several times daily to diminish the likelihood of cystitis.

Toxicity.
1. *Myelosuppression and other hematologic effects.* Dose limiting. Platelets are relatively spared. Nadir is reached about 10 to 14 days after IV dose with recovery by day 21.
2. *Nausea, vomiting, and other gastrointestinal effects.* Frequent with large IV doses; less common after oral doses. Symptoms begin several hours after treatment and are usually over by the next day.
3. *Mucocutaneous effects.* Reversible alopecia is common, usually starting after 2 to 3 weeks. Skin and nails may become darker. Mucositis is uncommon.
4. *Bladder damage.* Hemorrhagic or nonhemorrhagic cystitis may occur in 5% to 10% of patients treated. It is usually reversible with discontinuation of the drug, but it may persist and lead to fibrosis or death. Frequency is diminished by ample fluid intake and morning administration of the drug. Mesna will protect from this effect.
5. *Miscellaneous effects.*
   a. Immunosuppression is common.
   b. Amenorrhea and azoospermia are common.
   c. Inhibition of antidiuretic hormone is of significance only with very large doses.
   d. Interstitial pulmonary fibrosis is rare.
   e. Secondary neoplasia is possible.
   f. Acute and potentially fatal cardiotoxicity occurs with high-dose therapy. Abnormalities include pericardial effusion, congestive heart failure, decreased electrocardiographic voltage, and fibrin microthrombi in cardiac capillaries with endothelial injury and hemorrhagic necrosis.

CYTARABINE

Other names. Cytosine arabinoside, ara-C, Cytosar-U, DepoCyt (cytarabine, liposomal for intrathecal use only).

Mechanism of action. A pyrimidine analog antimetabolite that, when phosphorylated to arabinosyl-cytosine triphosphate (ara-CTP), is a competitive inhibitor of DNA polymerase.

Primary indications.
1. Acute nonlymphocytic leukemia.
2. Non-Hodgkin's lymphoma (leukemia).
3. Meningeal lymphoma or leukemia.

Usual dosage and schedule.
1. *Induction.* 100 mg/m^2 IV daily as a continuous infusion for 5 to 7 days (in combination with other drugs).

2. *Maintenance.* 100 mg/m^2 SC every 12 h for 4 or 5 days every 4 weeks (with other drugs).
3. *Intrathecally.*
   a. 40 to 50 mg/m^2 of cytarabine, unencapsulated, every 4 days in preservative-free buffered isotonic diluent.
   b. 50 mg of cytarabine liposomal, repeated in 14 to 28 days.
4. *High dose* (tolerated poorly by patient over 70 years old).
   a. *Induction.* 2 to 3 g/m^2 IV over 1 to 2 h every 12 h for up to 12 doses.
   b. *Consolidation.* 3 g/m^2 IV over 3 h every 12 h on days 1, 3, and 5.

Special precautions.
1. None for standard doses. High dose, give in *1- to 3-h infusion.* Longer infusion enhances toxicity.
2. CNS toxicity is increased in patients with a decreased creatinine clearance.
3. Cytarabine liposomal (DepoCyt) should be used only intrathecally.

Toxicity (standard dose only).
1. *Myelosuppression and other hematologic effects.* Dose-limiting leukopenia and thrombocytopenia occur, with nadir at 7 to 10 days after treatment has ended and with recovery during the following 2 weeks, depending on the degree of suppression. Megaloblastosis is common.
2. *Nausea, vomiting, and other gastrointestinal effects.* Common, particularly if the drug is given as a push or rapid infusion.
3. *Mucocutaneous effects.* Stomatitis is seen occasionally.
4. *Miscellaneous effects.*
   a. Flu-like syndrome with fever, arthralgia, and sometimes rash is occasional.
   b. Transient mild hepatic dysfunction is occasional.

Toxicity (high dose).
1. *Myelosuppression and other hematologic effects.* Universal.
2. *Nausea, vomiting, and other gastrointestinal effects.* Nausea, vomiting, and diarrhea are common.
3. *Mucocutaneous effects.* Occasional to common mucositis.
4. *Neurotoxicity.* Cerebellar toxicity is common, particularly in the elderly, but is usually mild and reversible. However, on occasion it has been severe and permanent or fatal.
5. *Conjunctivitis.* Hydrocortisone 2 drops OU q.i.d. for 10 days may ameliorate or prevent keratitis.
6. *Hepatic toxicity with cholestatic jaundice.* Uncommon.

DACARBAZINE

Other names. Imidazole carboxamide, DIC, DTIC-Dome.
Mechanism of action. Uncertain but probably interacts with preformed macromolecules by alkylation. Inhibits DNA, RNA, and protein synthesis.
Primary indications.
1. Melanoma.
2. All soft tissue sarcomas.
3. Hodgkin's lymphoma.
Usual dosage and schedule.
1. 150 to 250 mg/m^2 IV push or rapid infusion on days 1 to 5 every 3 to 4 weeks *or*

2.   400 to 500 mg/m^2 IV push or rapid infusion on days 1 and 2 every 3 to 4 weeks *or*
3.   200 mg/m^2 IV daily as a continuous 96-h infusion.

Special precautions.
1.   Administer cautiously to avoid extravasation, as tissue damage may occur.
2.   Venous pain along the injection site may be reduced by diluting dacarbazine in 100 to 200 mL of 5% dextrose in water and infusing over 30 min rather than injecting rapidly. Ice application may also reduce pain.

Toxicity.
1.   *Myelosuppression and other hematologic effects.* Mild to moderate. This factor allows dacarbazine to be used in full doses with other myelosuppressive drugs.
2.   *Nausea, vomiting, and other gastrointestinal effects.* Common and severe but decrease in intensity with each subsequent daily dose. Onset is within 1 to 3 h, with duration up to 12 h.
3.   *Mucocutaneous effects.*
     a.   Moderately severe tissue damage if extravasation occurs.
     b.   Alopecia is uncommon.
     c.   Erythematous or urticarial rash is uncommon.
4.   *Miscellaneous effects.*
     a.   Flu-like syndrome with fever, myalgia, and malaise lasting several days is uncommon.
     b.   Hepatic toxicity is uncommon.

DACTINOMYCIN

Other names. Actinomycin D, act-D, Cosmegen.
Mechanism of action. Binds to DNA and inhibits DNA-dependent RNA synthesis. Inhibition of topoisomerase II.
Primary indications.
1.   Gestational trophoblastic neoplasms.
2.   Wilms' tumor, childhood rhabdomyosarcoma, and Ewing's sarcoma.

Usual dosage and schedule.
1.   *Children.* 0.40 to 0.45 mg/m^2 (up to a maximum of 0.5 mg) IV daily for 5 days every 3 to 5 weeks.
2.   *Adults.*
     a.   0.40 to 0.45 mg/m^2 IV on days 1 to 5 every 2 to 3 weeks.
     b.   0.5 mg IV daily for 5 days every 3 to 5 weeks.

Special precautions.
1.   Administer by slow IV push through the sidearm of a running IV infusion, being careful to avoid extravasation, which causes severe soft tissue damage.
2.   If given at or about the time of infection with chickenpox or herpes zoster, a severe generalized disease may occur that sometimes results in death.

Toxicity.
1.   *Myelosuppression and other hematologic effects.* May be dose limiting and severe. It begins within the first week of treatment, but the nadir may not be reached for 21 days.
2.   *Nausea, vomiting, and other gastrointestinal effects.* Severe vomiting often occurs during the first few hours after drug administration and lasts up to 24 h.

3. *Mucocutaneous effects.*
   a. Erythema, hyperpigmentation, and desquamation of the skin with potentiation by previous or concurrent radiotherapy are common.
   b. Oropharyngeal mucositis is potentiated by previous or concurrent radiotherapy.
   c. Alopecia is common.
   d. Moderately severe tissue damage occurs with extravasation.
4. *Miscellaneous effects.*
   a. Mental depression is rare.
   b. Hepato-veno-occlusive disease is worse with higher doses and shorter schedules, for example, single dose of 2.5 mg versus 5 days at 0.5 mg/day.

DARBEPOETIN ALFA

Other name. Aranesp.

Mechanism of action. An erythropoiesis-stimulating protein closely related to erythropoietin that is produced in Chinese hamster ovary cells by recombinant DNA technology. It has the same biologic activity, inducing erythropoiesis by stimulating the division and differentiation of committed erythroid progenitor cells. It has a threefold longer terminal half-life than epoetin alfa.

Primary indications.
1. Anemia from chemotherapy in patients with nonmyeloid malignancies.
2. Anemia associated with chronic renal failure.

Usual dosage and schedule. (Chemotherapy patients only.)
1. 2.25 to 4.5 µg/kg (85 to 170 µg/m²) SC weekly or 4.5 to 9 µg/kg (170 to 340 µg/m²) SC every other week. (Available in 40-, 60-, 100-, and 200-µg vials.)
2. Note: 40,000 to 60,000 U of epoetin weekly is equivalent to about 100 µg weekly of darbepoetin.

Special precautions.
1. Contraindicated in patients with uncontrolled hypertension or known hypersensitivity to albumin or mammalian cell–derived products.
2. Iron supplementation may be beneficial if there is any question of body iron stores. If at any time the hematocrit rises above 40%, hold epoetin injections until the hematocrit falls to 36% or less.

Toxicity.
1. *Myelosuppression.* None. Therapeutic effect is increase in hemoglobin.
2. *Nausea, vomiting and other gastrointestinal effects.* Occasional nausea, vomiting, diarrhea, and abdominal pain.
3. *Mucocutaneous effects.* Rare rashes or hives.
4. *Miscellaneous effects.*
   a. Improved energy level, activity level, and self-rated quality-of-life scores occur in patients receiving therapy.
   b. Edema is occasional.
   c. Diarrhea is occasional.
   d. A rise in blood pressure occurs in about 25% of patients. Hypertension may rarely occur in association with a

significant increase in hematocrit; the risk is greatest in patients with pre-existing hypertension. Hypotension may also be seen occasionally.
e. Chest pain and congestive heart failure are uncommon to occasional; edema is occasional. Cardiac arrhythmias are occasional and cardiac arrest has occurred.
f. Seizures, stroke, and myocardial infarction are rare.
g. Flu-like syndrome with fever, myalgias, arthralgia, or back pain is occasional.
h. Thrombotic complications are uncommon.

DAUNORUBICIN

Other names. Daunomycin, rubidomycin, DNR, Cerubidine, liposomal daunorubicin (DaunoXome; see next entry).
Mechanism of action. DNA strand breakage mediated by anthracycline effects on topoisomerase II, DNA intercalation, DNA polymerase inhibition.
Primary indications.
1. Acute nonlymphocytic leukemia and acute lymphocytic leukemia.
2. Kaposi's sarcoma (liposomal daunorubicin).
Usual dosage and schedule.
1. 45 to 60 mg/m^2 IV push on days 1, 2, and 3 every 2 weeks as induction therapy for one or two cycles in combination with other drugs.
2. 45 mg/m^2 IV push on days 1 and 2 every 4 weeks as consolidation therapy for one or two cycles in combination with other drugs.
Special precautions.
1. Administer over several minutes into the sidearm of a running IV infusion, taking precautions to avoid extravasation.
2. Do not give if patient has significantly impaired cardiac function (ejection fraction less than 45%), angina pectoris, cardiac arrhythmia, or recent myocardial infarction.
3. Do not exceed cumulative dosage of 550 mg/m^2 (400 mg/m^2 if given previous radiation therapy that has encompassed the heart).
4. Reduce dose if patient has impaired liver or renal function:

Serum bilirubin (mg/dL)	Serum creatinine (mg/dL)	% of full dose
1.2–3.0	–	75
> 3.0 *or*	> 3.0	50

Toxicity.
1. *Myelosuppression and other hematologic effects.* Dose-limiting pancytopenia with nadir at 1 to 2 weeks.
2. *Nausea, vomiting, and other gastrointestinal effects.* Nausea and vomiting occur on the day of administration in one-half of patients.
3. *Mucocutaneous effects.* Alopecia is common, but stomatitis is rare. Severe local tissue damage may progress to skin ulceration, and necrosis may occur with SC extravasation.
4. *Cardiac effects.* Potentially irreversible congestive heart failure may occur owing to cardiomyopathy. The incidence is highly dependent on the lifetime cumulative dose, which

should not exceed 550 mg/m^2 (400 mg/m^2 if patient was given previous radiotherapy that encompassed the heart). Discontinue drug if there is clinical congestive heart failure or if the ejection fraction falls on the radionuclide angiogram:
   a.   To less than 45% *or*
   b.   To less than 50% if the total decrease is 10% or more (e.g., falls from 59% to 49%).
         If repeat ejection fraction determination shows return of function, drug may be cautiously restarted, but ejection fraction should be measured before each dose. Transient electrocardiographic changes are common and are not usually serious.
   5.   *Miscellaneous effects.*
      a.   Red urine caused by the drug and its metabolites is common.
      b.   Chemical phlebitis and phlebothrombosis of veins used for injection are common.

DAUNORUBICIN, LIPOSOMAL

Other name. DaunoXome.
Mechanism of action. Daunorubicin, liposomal, which is designed to be protected from removal by the reticuloendothelial system, has a prolonged circulation time compared with unprotected drug. The agent penetrates tumor tissue and releases the active ingredient daunorubicin. The active drug causes DNA strand breakage mediated by anthracycline effects on topoisomerase II, DNA intercalation, and DNA polymerase inhibition.
Primary indication. Advanced Kaposi's sarcoma, associated with human immunodeficiency virus (HIV).
Usual dosage and schedule. 40 mg/m^2 IV over 60 min every 2 weeks.
Special precautions.
   1.   Must be diluted to a concentration of 1 mg/mL with 5% dextrose for injection. Liposomal daunorubicin should be considered an irritant, and care should be taken to avoid extravasation.
   2.   Do not give if the patient has significantly impaired cardiac function.
   3.   Do not exceed a lifetime cumulative dose of 550 mg/m^2 (400 mg/m^2 if the patient was given prior chest radiotherapy). Patients with HIV may experience a decrease in left ventricular ejection fraction and congestive heart failure at lower doses than those without.
   4.   Reduce or hold dose in patients with impairment of liver function. A 25% dose reduction is recommended if the serum bilirubin is 1.2 to 3 mg/dL. One-half the normal dose is recommended in patients with serum bilirubin concentration greater than 3 mg/dL.
Toxicity. Effects that are a result of liposomal daunorubicin have been somewhat difficult to determine with certainty because most patients have been on several other agents that may cause marrow or other toxicity.
   1.   *Myelosuppression and other hematologic effects.* Common and dose related. May be severe.

2. *Nausea, vomiting, and other gastrointestinal effects.* Nausea, vomiting, and diarrhea are common.
3. *Mucocutaneous effects.* Alopecia is occasional. Stomatitis is occasional.
4. *Miscellaneous effects.*
    a. Cardiac events including cardiomyopathy or congestive heart failure may occur and are dose dependent (see Special Precautions above).
    b. Acute infusion-associated reactions with back pain, flushing, and tightness in the chest and throat, alone or in combination, have occurred in approximately 14% of patients treated with liposomal daunorubicin. They usually occur with the first infusion and are not likely to occur later if the first infusion is given without a reaction. They generally occur during the first 5 min of the infusion and subside with interruption of the infusion. Some patients tolerate restarting at a lower rate of infusion. Most patients are able to continue therapy.
    c. Fatigue is common.
    d. Fever is common.
    e. Pain at the injection site is likely after extravasation.

DENILEUKIN DIFTITOX

Other name. Ontak.

Mechanism of action. Denileukin diftitox is produced by genetically fusing protein from the diphtheria toxin to interleukin-2 (IL-2). This stable fusion protein targets cells with receptors for IL-2 on their surfaces, including malignant cells and some normal lymphocytes, resulting in cell death. Efficacy in patients without the CD25 receptor is not known.

Primary indications. Persistent or recurrent cutaneous T-cell lymphoma that expresses the CD25 component of IL-2 receptor.

Usual dosage and schedule. 9 or 18 µg/kg/day (350 to 700 mg/m^2/day) IV over at least 15 min for 5 consecutive days every 21 days.

Special precaution. Acute hypersensitivity reactions occur commonly.

Toxicity.

1. *Myelosuppression and other hematologic effects.* Lymphopenia is common.
2. *Nausea, vomiting, and other gastrointestinal effects.* Nausea, vomiting, and diarrhea are common. Dehydration as a consequence is occasional.
3. *Mucocutaneous effects.* Rashes—including generalized macropapular, petechial, vesicular bullous, urticarial, and eczematous—may be seen, with both acute and delayed onset.
4. *Miscellaneous effects.*
    a. Severe infections are common.
    b. Acute hypersensitivity reactions occur commonly, including hypotension, back pain, dyspnea, vasodilation, rash, chest pain or tightness, and tachycardia. Syncope is uncommon; anaphylaxis is rare.
    c. Vascular leak syndrome is common.
    d. Hypoalbuminemia is common.
    e. Arterial and venous thrombosis is uncommon.

    f. Flu-like symptoms with chills, fever, headache, and weakness are common. Myalgias and arthralgias are occasional.

    g. Fluid retention.

DEXRAZOXANE

Other names. Zinecard, ICRF-187.

Mechanism of action. Probably by means of conversion of dexrazoxane intracellularly to a chelating agent that interferes with iron-mediated free radical generation, which is thought to be responsible, in part, for anthracycline-related cardiomyopathy. Appears to protect against myocardial toxicity without impairment of tumor response.

Primary indication. Prophylaxis of cardiomyopathy in patients who have received a cumulative dose of doxorubicin of 300 mg/m^2 or greater and who are believed to benefit from continued therapy with this drug.

Usual dosage and schedule. 10 mg of dexrazoxane for every 1 mg of doxorubicin, for example, 600 mg/m^2 of dexrazoxane for 60 mg/m^2 of doxorubicin. Repeat whenever doxorubicin is to be repeated. Administered as a slow injection or rapid infusion over 15 to 30 min.

Special precautions. None.

Toxicity. Most side effects encountered with dexrazoxane administration are likely to be from the concurrent chemotherapy regimen.

    1. *Myelosuppression and other hematologic effects.* Nadir granulocyte and platelet counts lower than with chemotherapy alone, but duration not prolonged.

    2. *Nausea, vomiting, and other gastrointestinal effects.* No increase observed.

    3. *Mucocutaneous effects.* No increase observed.

    4. *Miscellaneous effects.*

        a. Pain at the injection site is occasional.

        b. Hepatic toxicity is possible.

DOCETAXEL

Other name. Taxotere.

Mechanism of action. Enhanced formation and stabilization of microtubules. Antineoplastic effect may result from nonfunctional tubules or altered tubulin–microtubule equilibrium. Mitotic arrest is seen and is associated with accumulated polymerized microtubules.

Primary indications.

    1. Carcinoma of the breast.

    2. Non–small cell lung cancer.

Usual dosage and schedule.

    1. 60 to 100 mg/m^2 as a 1-h infusion every 3 weeks. Dexamethasone 8 mg PO b.i.d. for 3 days starting 1 day before docetaxel should be given before each course of docetaxel to limit the frequency and severity of hypersensitivity reactions and to reduce the severity of fluid retention.

    2. 35 mg/m^2 as a 1-h infusion weekly. Dexamethasone 8 mg PO b.i.d. 1 day before and 10 mg IV 30 min before should be given

before weeks 1 and 2 of docetaxel to limit the frequency and severity of hypersensitivity reactions. If there are no hypersensitivity reactions in the first 2 weeks, the oral doses given the day prior to docetaxel may be eliminated.

Special precautions.

1. Severe hypersensitivity reactions with flushing and hypotension with or without dyspnea occur in about 1% of patients (even when premedication is used).
2. Should be used with caution in patients with bilirubin above upper limit of normal or other abnormal liver function tests (greater than 1.5 times the upper limit of normal) because of more profound neutropenia.

Toxicity.

1. *Myelosuppression and other hematologic effects.* Severe (grade 4) neutropenia is common and dose related. Many patients have neutropenic fever.
2. *Nausea, vomiting, and other gastrointestinal effects.* Nausea with or without vomiting is common but brief; severe episodes are uncommon. Mild diarrhea is common; severe diarrhea is rare.
3. *Mucocutaneous effects.* Mild mucositis is common; severe mucositis is uncommon. Alopecia is common. Mild to moderate cutaneous reactions such as maculopapular eruptions are common; severe reactions that may be associated with desquamation or bullous eruptions occur only occasionally if systemic prophylaxis is used. Mild to moderate nail changes are common, but severe onycholysis is uncommon.
4. *Hypersensitivity reactions.* Mild to moderate hypersensitivity reactions with flushing, hypotension (or rarely hypertension) with or without dyspnea, and drug fever are occasional with use of the prophylactic regimen recommended. Severe hypersensitivity reactions are uncommon.
5. *Miscellaneous effects.*
   a. Fluid retention syndrome is common and cumulative (more commonly after four courses); can be reduced to occasional frequency (6%) by prophylactic steroids; may limit continuing therapy. May be associated with both pleural and pericardial effusions.
   b. Mild and reversible dysesthesias or paresthesias are common; more severe sensory neuropathies are uncommon.
   c. Reversible increases in transaminase, alkaline phosphatase, and bilirubin.
   d. Local reaction comprises reversible peripheral phlebitis.
   e. Fatigue, weakness (asthenia), and myalgia are common; arthralgia is occasional.
   f. Excessive tearing secondary to anatomic narrowing of nasolacrimal duct is occasional to common.

DOXORUBICIN

Other names. ADR, Adriamycin, Rubex, hydroxyldaunorubicin.

Mechanism of action. DNA strand breakage mediated by anthracycline effects on topoisomerase II, DNA intercalation, and DNA polymerase inhibition.

Primary indications.
1. Breast, bladder, liver, lung, prostate, stomach, and thyroid carcinomas.
2. Bone and soft tissue sarcomas.
3. Hodgkin's and non-Hodgkin's lymphomas.
4. Multiple myeloma.
5. Acute lymphocytic and acute nonlymphocytic leukemias.
6. Wilms' tumor, neuroblastoma, and rhabdomyosarcoma of childhood.

Usual dosage and schedule.
1. 60 to 75 mg/m^2 IV every 3 weeks (or as 96-h continuous infusion).
2. 30 mg/m^2 IV on days 1 and 8 every 4 weeks (in combination with other drugs).
3. 9 mg/m^2 IV daily for 4 days as a continuous infusion (in myeloma).
4. 15 to 20 mg/m^2 IV weekly.
5. 50 to 60 mg instilled into the bladder weekly for 4 weeks, then every 4 weeks for 6 cycles.

Special precautions.
1. Administer over several minutes into the sidearm of a running IV infusion (except when given as a continuous infusion), taking care to avoid extravasation.
2. Do not give if patient has significantly impaired cardiac function (ejection fraction less than 45%), angina pectoris, cardiac arrhythmia, or recent myocardial infarction.
3. Do not exceed a lifetime cumulative dose of 550 mg/m^2 (450 mg/m^2 if patient was given prior chest radiotherapy or concomitant cyclophosphamide) unless there are known risk modifiers such as continuous infusion, weekly dosing, or cardioprotective dexrazoxane and serial measurements of cardiac ejection fraction show minimal change and adequate function.
4. Reduce or hold dose if patient has impaired liver function.
   a. For serum bilirubin of 1.2 to 3.0 mg/dL, give one-half the normal dose.
   b. For serum bilirubin of more than 3.0 mg/dL, give one-fourth the normal dose.

Toxicity.
1. *Myelosuppression and other hematologic effects.* Dose limiting for most patients. Nadir white blood cell and platelet counts occur at 10 to 14 days; recovery by day 21.
2. *Nausea, vomiting, and other gastrointestinal effects.* Mild to moderate in about one-half of patients.
3. *Mucocutaneous effects.*
   a. Stomatitis that is dose dependent.
   b. Alopecia beginning 2 to 5 weeks from start of therapy with recovery following completion of therapy is common.
   c. Recall of skin reaction due to prior radiotherapy is common.
   d. Severe local tissue damage possibly progressing to skin ulceration and necrosis if SC extravasation occurs is common.
   e. Hyperpigmentation of skin overlying veins used for drug injection in which chemical phlebitis has occurred is common.

4. *Cardiac effects.* Potentially irreversible congestive heart failure may occur owing to cardiomyopathy. The incidence is highly dependent on the lifetime cumulative dose, which should not exceed 550 mg/m^2. This limit is lower (450 mg/m^2) if patient has received prior chest radiotherapy or is taking cyclophosphamide concomitantly. Weekly schedule and 96-h infusions are less cardiotoxic, and higher cumulative doses may be tolerable. Congestive heart failure may be predicted by serial measurement of left ventricular function or endomyocardial biopsy. Discontinue drug if there is clinical congestive heart failure or if the ejection fraction falls on the radionuclide angiogram:
   a. To less than 45% *or*
   b. To less than 50% if the total decrease is 10% or more (e.g., falls from 59% to 49%).
   If repeat ejection fraction determination shows return of function, drug may be cautiously restarted, but ejection fraction determination should be done before each dose. Transient electrocardiographic changes are common and are not usually serious.

5. *Miscellaneous effects.*
   a. Red urine caused by drug and its metabolites is common.
   b. Chemical phlebitis and phlebosclerosis of veins used for injection are common, particularly if a vein is used repeatedly.
   c. Fever, chills, and urticaria are uncommon.

DOXORUBICIN, LIPOSOMAL

Other name. Doxil.

Mechanism of action. Doxorubicin, liposomal, which is designed to be protected from removal by the reticuloendothelial system, has a prolonged circulation time compared with unprotected drug. The agent penetrates tumor tissue and releases the active ingredient doxorubicin. The active drug causes DNA strand breakage mediated by anthracycline effects on topoisomerase II, DNA intercalation, and DNA polymerase inhibition.

Primary indications.
1. Advanced Kaposi's sarcoma, associated with HIV.
2. Ovarian carcinoma.
3. Multiple myeloma.

Usual dosage and schedule.
1. 20 mg/m^2 IV infusion at a rate of 1 mg/min for the first dose, then over 30 min for subsequent doses every 2 to 3 weeks for Kaposi's sarcoma.
2. 40–50 mg/m^2 IV infusion at a rate of 1 mg/min for the first dose, then over 1 h every 4 weeks for ovarian carcinoma.
3. 40 mg/m^2 IV infusion at a rate of 1 mg/min for the first dose, then over 1 h every 4 weeks for multiple myeloma, together with vincristine and dexamethasone.

Special precautions.
1. Must be diluted in 250 mL of 5% dextrose for injection. Liposomal doxorubicin is not a vesicant but should be considered an irritant.
2. Initial doses should be given at a rate of 1 mg/min to avoid infusion reactions.

Toxicity. Effects that are a result of liposomal doxorubicin have been somewhat difficult to determine with certainty because most patients have been on several other agents that may cause marrow or other toxicity.

1. *Myelosuppression and other hematologic effects.* Common and dose related. May be severe.
2. *Nausea, vomiting, and other gastrointestinal effects.* Nausea and vomiting are common at the higher doses. Constipation is occasional. Diarrhea is occasional. Anorexia is occasional.
3. *Mucocutaneous effects.* Palmar–plantar erythrodysesthesia is common at the higher doses and is occasionally severe. May be reduced by celecoxib 100 to 200 mg PO b.i.d. Stomatitis is common. Alopecia is occasional. Rash is occasional to common.
4. *Miscellaneous effects.*
    a. Cardiac events, including cardiomyopathy or congestive heart failure, occur in 5% to 10% of patients treated. This is dose dependent and not adequately tested, but appears to be less common than with unincapsulated drug.
    b. Acute infusion-associated reactions with flushing, shortness of breath, facial swelling, headache, chills, back pain, tightness in the chest and throat, or hypotension, alone or in combination, have occurred in approximately 7% of patients treated with liposomal doxorubicin. They usually occur with the first infusion and are not likely to occur later if the first infusion is given without a reaction. Most resolve over the course of several hours to a day.
    c. Asthenia is occasional.
    d. Fever is occasional.
    e. Pain at the injection site is likely after extravasation.

EPIRUBICIN

Other names. Ellence, 4′-Epi-doxorubicin, EPI.
Mechanism of action. DNA strand breakage, mediated by anthracycline effects on topoisomerase II.
Primary indications.
1. Carcinomas of the breast, esophagus, lung, ovary, and stomach.
2. Hodgkin's and non-Hodgkin's lymphoma.
3. Soft tissue sarcomas.

Usual dosage and schedule. 70 to 90 mg/m^2 IV every 3 weeks administered through the sidearm of a freely flowing IV infusion.
Special precautions.
1. Take care to avoid extravasation.
2. Do not exceed a lifetime cumulative dose of 900 mg/m^2 (use a lesser dose for patients with prior chest radiotherapy or prior anthracycline or anthracenedione therapy).
3. Reduce or hold dose if patient has impaired liver function.
    a. For serum bilirubin of 1.2 to 3.0 mg/dL, give one-half the normal dose.
    b. For serum bilirubin of more than 3.0 mg/dL, give one-fourth the normal dose.

Toxicity.
1. *Myelosuppression and other hematologic effects.* Dose-limiting leukopenia with recovery by day 21.

2. *Nausea, vomiting, and other gastrointestinal effects.* Nausea and vomiting are common. Diarrhea and abdominal pain are occasional.
3. *Mucocutaneous effects.*
    a. Stomatitis that is dose dependent.
    b. Alopecia, beginning approximately 10 days after the first treatment, with regrowth when cessation of drug treatment occurs, is common but not universal (25% to 50%).
    c. Flushes, skin and nail hyperpigmentation, photosensitivity, and hypersensitivity to irradiated skin (radiation-recall reaction) have been observed.
    d. Severe local tissue damage possibly progressing to skin ulceration and necrosis if SC extravasation occurs is common.
4. *Cardiac effects.*
    a. Potentially irreversible congestive heart failure may occur owing to cardiomyopathy. The incidence depends on the lifetime dose, which should not exceed 900 mg/m^2. This limit is lower if patient has received prior chest radiotherapy or prior anthracycline or anthracenedione therapy. Congestive heart failure may be predicted by serial measurement of left ventricular function or endomyocardial biopsy.
    b. Transient electrocardiographic changes are similar in type and frequency to those observed after doxorubicin.
5. *Miscellaneous effects.*
    a. Red–orange urine for 24 h after injection owing to drug and its metabolites is common.
    b. Urticaria and anaphylaxis have been reported in patients treated with epirubicin; signs and symptoms of these reactions may vary from skin rash and pruritus to fever, chills, and shock.

EPOETIN

Other names. Recombinant human erythropoietin (rHuEPO), EPO, epoetin-alfa, Epogen, Procrit.
Mechanism of action. Epoetin-alfa is a recombinant glycoprotein that contains 165 amino acids in a sequence identical to that of endogenous human erythropoietin. It has the same biologic activity, inducing erythropoiesis by stimulating the division and differentiation of committed erythroid progenitor cells.
Primary indications.
1. Anemia from chemotherapy in patients with nonmyeloid malignancies.
2. Anemia associated with malignancy, as in multiple myeloma or anemia of chronic disease.
3. Anemia associated with chronic renal failure.
4. Anemia associated with zidovudine therapy in HIV-infected patients.
Usual dosage and schedule.
1. Starting dose is 150 U/kg SC three times a week. The dose may be escalated to 300 U/kg SC three times a week, after a 4- to 8-week trial at the initial dose, in patients who have not responded satisfactorily.

2. Alternative dose is 40,000 U SC once weekly. If there is no
response after 4 to 8 weeks, the dose may be increased to
60,000 U SC once weekly. If no response to this dose, it should
be discontinued.

Special precautions.
1. Contraindicated in patients with uncontrolled hypertension
or known hypersensitivity to albumin or mammalian cell–
derived products.
2. Iron supplementation may be beneficial if there is any question of body iron stores. If at any time the hematocrit rises
above 40%, hold epoetin injections until the hematocrit falls
to 36% or less.

Toxicity.
1. *Myelosuppression and other hematologic effects.* The therapeutic effect is an increase in hemoglobin, and no myelosuppression is to be expected. Rarely it may induce pure red
cell aplasia with associated neutralizing antierythropoietin
antibodies.
2. *Nausea and vomiting.* None.
3. *Mucocutaneous effects.* Rare rashes or hives.
4. *Miscellaneous effects.*
   a. Improved energy level, activity level, and self-rated
   quality-of-life scores occur in patients receiving therapy.
   b. Edema is occasional.
   c. Diarrhea is occasional.
   d. A rise in blood pressure occurs in about 25% of patients.
   Hypertension may rarely occur in association with a
   significant increase in hematocrit; the risk is greatest
   in patients with pre-existing hypertension. Chest pain
   is uncommon; edema is occasional.
   e. Seizures are rare.
   f. Influenza-like syndrome is rare to uncommon. Fever
   alone is occasional.
   g. Thrombotic complications are uncommon.

ESTRAMUSTINE

Other name. Emcyt.
Mechanism of action. A chemical combination of mechlorethamine and estradiol phosphate, estramustine is designed to
selectively enter cells with estrogen receptors and act as an alkylating agent. May promote microtubule disassembly.
Primary indication. Metastatic prostate carcinoma.
Usual dosage and schedule.
1. 400 to 600 mg/m^2 PO daily in two to three divided doses, at
least 1 h before or 2 h after meals.
2. 280 mg PO twice daily days 1 to 5 every 3 weeks in combination with other drugs.

Special precautions. Milk, milk products, and calcium-rich
foods or drugs may impair the absorption.
Toxicity.
1. *Myelosuppression and other hematologic effects.* Occur only
occasionally.
2. *Nausea, vomiting, and other gastrointestinal effects.* Nausea,
usually without vomiting, is commonly seen soon after starting treatment but usually lessens with continued therapy

and antiemetics. If persistent and severe, it may be necessary to discontinue the drug. Diarrhea and other minor gastrointestinal effects are occasional.

3. *Mucocutaneous effects.* Rash with fever is rare.
4. *Miscellaneous effects.*
   a. Congestive heart failure must be watched for in patients with pre-existing cardiac disease, and edema is occasional to common.
   b. Gynecomastia and breast tenderness are common but usually mild.
   c. Vascular effects (thromboembolism, arterial insufficiency) are uncommon.
   d. Elevation of lactate dehydrogenase or SGOT is common.

ESTROGENS

Other names. Diethylstilbestrol (DES), chlorotrianisene (TACE), diethylstilbestrol diphosphate (Stilphostrol), and others.
Mechanism of action. Suppression of testosterone production via negative feedback on hypothalamus.
Primary indication. Prostate carcinoma.
Usual dosage and schedule.
1. DES 1 to 3 mg PO daily.
2. Chlorotrianisene 12 to 25 mg PO daily.
3. Diethylstilbestrol diphosphate 500 to 1,000 mg IV daily for 5 to 7 days, then 250 to 500 mg IV one or two times weekly.
Special precautions.
1. Acute fluid retention and pulmonary edema are possible, particularly with high-dose IV therapy.
2. Hypercalcemia may occur with initial therapy.
Toxicity.
1. *Myelosuppression and other hematologic effects.* None.
2. *Nausea, vomiting, and other gastrointestinal effects.* Nausea with possible vomiting is common at the beginning of therapy but diminishes or stops with continued treatment. Severity may be lessened by beginning treatment with doses lower than those recommended. Diarrhea is uncommon.
3. *Mucocutaneous effects.* Darkening of nipples is common.
4. *Miscellaneous effects.*
   a. Peripheral edema due to sodium retention is common, but congestive heart failure occurs in fewer than 5% of patients.
   b. Any patient taking estrogens may be at higher risk than normal for thromboemboli. An increase in cardiovascular deaths has been seen in male patients given DES at 5 mg daily for prostate carcinoma.
   c. Increased bone pain, tumor pain, and local disease flare are associated with both good tumor response and tumor progression.
   d. Feminization occurs in male patients.

ETOPOSIDE

Other names. Epipodophyllotoxin, VP-16, VP-16-213, VePesid, Etopophos (etoposide phosphate).
Mechanism of action. Interaction with topoisomerase II produces single-strand breaks in DNA. Arrests cells in late S or G_2 phase.

Primary indications.
1. Small cell anaplastic and non–small cell lung carcinomas.
2. Stomach carcinoma.
3. Germ cell cancers.
4. Lymphomas.
5. Acute leukemia.
6. Neuroblastoma.

Usual dosage and schedule.
1. 120 mg/m^2 IV on days 1 to 3 every 3 weeks.
2. 50 to 100 mg/m^2 IV on days 1 to 5 every 2 to 4 weeks.
3. 125 to 140 mg/m^2 IV on days 1, 3, and 5 every 3 to 5 weeks.
4. 50 mg/m^2 PO daily for 21 days. Repeat after 1 to 2 weeks of rest.
5. High-dose therapy (750 to 2,400 mg/m^2) is investigational and should be used only with progenitor cell rescue (e.g., bone marrow or peripheral blood stem cell transplantation).

Special precautions.
1. Administer etoposide as a 30- to 60-min infusion to avoid severe hypotension. Monitor blood pressure during infusion. Etoposide phosphate may be administered as a 5-min bolus infusion.
2. Take care to avoid extravasation.
3. Etoposide must be diluted in 20 to 50 volumes (100 to 250 mL) of isotonic saline before use. Etoposide phosphate vials (100 mg) may be reconstituted in 5 to 10 mL (water, saline, or dextrose) to a concentration of 10 or 20 mg/mL.
4. Decrease dose by 50% for bilirubin levels of 1.5 to 3 mg/dL; decrease by 75% for bilirubin levels of 3 to 5 mg/dL; discontinue drug if bilirubin level is above 5 mg/dL.
5. Decrease dose by 25% for creatinine clearance rate of less than 30 mL/min.

Toxicity.
1. *Myelosuppression and other hematologic effects.* Dose-limiting leukopenia and less severe thrombocytopenia have a nadir at 16 days with recovery by days 20 to 22.
2. *Nausea, vomiting, and other gastrointestinal effects.* Usually mild to moderate nausea and vomiting in about one-third of patients receiving standard doses; common with high-dose therapy. Anorexia is common. Diarrhea is uncommon.
3. *Mucocutaneous effects.*
   a. Alopecia is common.
   b. Stomatitis is uncommon with standard doses and common with high-dose therapy.
   c. Painful rash may occur with high-dose therapy.
   d. Chemical phlebitis is occasional.
4. *Miscellaneous effects.*
   a. Hepatotoxicity is rare.
   b. Peripheral neurotoxicity is rare.
   c. Allergic reaction is rare.
   d. Hemorrhagic cystitis may occur with high-dose therapy.

EXEMESTANE

Other name. Aromasin.

Mechanism of action. Exemestane is an irreversible, steroidal aromatase inactivator that decreases estrogen biosynthesis by selective inhibition of aromatase (estrogen synthetase) in peripheral tissues.

Primary indication. Carcinoma of the breast in postmenopausal women that has progressed following tamoxifen therapy.

Usual dosage and schedule. 25 mg once daily after meal.

Special precaution. Potential hazard to fetus if given during pregnancy.

Toxicity.

1. *Myelosuppression and other hematologic effects.* No dose-related effect. Thromboembolic events are uncommon to rare.
2. *Nausea, vomiting, and other gastrointestinal effects.* Nausea, vomiting, constipation, and diarrhea are uncommon to occasional.
3. *Mucocutaneous effects.* Rash is uncommon.
4. *Miscellaneous effects.*
   a. Fatigue is occasional to common.
   b. Musculoskeletal pain (arthralgia or bone) is occasional to common.
   c. Headache is occasional.
   d. Peripheral edema and weight gain are occasional (lower than with megestrol).
   e. Dyspnea and cough are uncommon to occasional.
   f. Hot flushes are occasional.
   g. Hypercalcemia is rare.

FILGRASTIM

Other names. Granulocyte colony-stimulating factor, G-CSF, Neupogen.

Mechanism of action. Recombinant human G-CSF. Promotes growth and differentiation of myeloid progenitor cells. May improve survival and function of granulocytes.

Primary indications.

1. Prophylaxis of granulocytopenia secondary to intensive chemotherapy.
2. Treatment of granulocytopenia secondary to chemotherapy.
3. Granulocytopenia from primary marrow disorders such as idiopathic neutropenia and aplastic anemia and myelodysplastic syndrome.
4. Granulocytopenia associated with AIDS and its therapy.

Usual dosage and schedule.

1. *Adjunct to chemotherapy.* Commonly 200 to 400 µg/m² (5 to 10 µg/kg) SC daily, starting no sooner than 24 h and no later than 4 days after the last dose of chemotherapy, for 10 to 20 days until the neutrophil count exceeds 10,000/µL after the expected nadir. Because of cost factors, vial size, and comparability of effect with "ballpark" doses, some physicians choose to treat patients weighing less than 75 kg with 300 µg daily and patients weighing more than 75 kg with 480 µg daily.
2. *Other purposes.* 40 to 500 µg/m² SC, IM, or IV daily. Dose and duration are dependent on the purpose of administration.

Special precautions.

1. Use with caution in disorders of myeloid stem cells as it may promote growth of leukemic cells.
2. Contraindicated in patients with known hypersensitivity to *E. coli*–derived proteins.

Toxicity.
1. *Myelosuppression and other hematologic effects.* None (leukocytosis).
2. *Nausea, vomiting, and other gastrointestinal effects.* Rare to uncommon.
3. *Mucocutaneous effects.* Exacerbation of pre-existing dermatologic conditions is occasional; pyoderma gangrenosum is rare.
4. *Miscellaneous effects.* Usually mild and short lived.
   a. Bone pain, musculoskeletal symptoms such as cramps, and back or leg pain are common.
   b. Splenomegaly with prolonged use. Rarely has been associated with splenic rupture.
   c. Exacerbation of pre-existing inflammatory or auto-immune disorders is rare.
   d. Mild elevation of lactate dehydrogenase and alkaline phosphatase.
   e. Allergic-type reactions may occur, including urticaria and anaphylaxis.
   f. Adult respiratory distress syndrome has been reported in neutropenic patients.

FLOXURIDINE

Other name. FUDR.
Mechanism of action. A pyrimidine antimetabolite that, when converted to the active nucleotide, inhibits the enzyme thymidylate synthetase.
Primary indications. Hepatic metastasis of gastrointestinal carcinoma and primary hepatic carcinoma.
Usual dosage and schedule. 4.0 to 6.0 mg/m^2 as a continuous infusion into the hepatic artery daily for 2 weeks, then off for 2 weeks. Administered via continuous-infusion pump.
Special precautions.
1. Reduce dose in patients with compromised liver function.
2. Ulcer-like pain or other significant gastrointestinal symptoms are indications to discontinue intra-arterial therapy, as hemorrhage or perforation may occur.
Toxicity.
1. *Myelosuppression and other hematologic effects.* Uncommon.
2. *Nausea, vomiting, and other gastrointestinal effects.* Nausea and vomiting are uncommon unless the hepatic artery catheter has become displaced and the stomach and duodenum are being infused. Abdominal cramps and pain are common if the catheter is displaced and the stomach and duodenum are being infused. Can progress to frank gastritis or duodenal ulcer. Esophagitis, proctitis, and diarrhea may also occur.
3. *Mucocutaneous effects.*
   a. Stomatitis is an early sign of severe toxicity. It progresses from soreness and erythema to frank ulceration, which may become hemorrhagic in a small number of patients.
   b. Partial alopecia is uncommon.
   c. Hyperpigmentation of skin over face, hands, and the vein used for the infusion is occasional.
   d. Maculopapular rash is uncommon.
   e. Sun exposure tends to increase skin reactions.

4. *Miscellaneous effects.*
   a. Neurotoxicity including headache, minor visual disturbances, and cerebellar ataxia is rare.
   b. Increased lacrimation is uncommon.
   c. Liver function abnormalities and jaundice are common when given by hepatic arterial infusion. Dose should be reduced during subsequent cycle.
   d. Sclerosing cholangitis when given by hepatic artery infusion is uncommon.

FLUDARABINE

Other names. FAMP, Fludara.
Mechanism of action. Inhibition of DNA polymerase and ribonucleotide reductase.
Primary indications.
1. Chronic lymphocytic leukemia.
2. Macroglobulinemia.
3. Indolent lymphomas.
4. Acute leukemia (in combination).
Usual dosage and schedule. 25 mg/m^2 IV as a 30-min infusion daily for 5 days. Other dose schedules, usually less intensive, have been used, often in combinations with other drugs. Repeat every 4 weeks.
Special precautions.
1. If there is the potential for tumor lysis syndrome, administer allopurinol and ensure good hydration and close clinical monitoring.
2. Transfusion-associated graft-versus-host disease may be seen. Therefore, prior irradiation of blood products for transfusion in patients at risk is recommended.
3. Reduce dose by 20% for C_{cr} 30–70 mL/m; do not treat if $C_{cr} < 30$ mL/m.
Toxicity.
1. *Myelosuppression and other hematologic effects.* Granulocytopenia and thrombocytopenia are common, and may be severe, cumulative, and prolonged. Infection, particularly pneumonia, is common during early courses and uncommon after the sixth course.
2. *Nausea, vomiting, and other gastrointestinal effects.* Common (30%) but not usually severe. Diarrhea is occasional.
3. *Mucocutaneous effects.* Occasional mucositis, rash, no alopecia.
4. *Neurotoxicity.* Uncommon at usual dosage. Somnolence or fatigue, paresthesias, and twitching of extremities may be seen. Severe neurologic symptoms including visual disturbances have been common at higher doses than those recommended.
5. *Immune suppression.* Common. Usually seen as a depression in CD4 and CD8 lymphocyte counts. Opportunistic infections may result, and many recommend pneumocystic pneumonia prophylaxis until the CD4 lymphopenia resolves.
6. *Miscellaneous effects.*
   a. Abnormal liver or renal function is rare.
   b. Severe pulmonary toxicity is occasional.
   c. Edema is occasional.
   d. Tumor lysis syndrome is rare.

FLUOROURACIL

Other names. 5-FU, Adrucil, Efudex, Fluoroplex, 5-fluorouracil.

Mechanism of action. A pyrimidine antimetabolite that, when converted to the active nucleotide, inhibits the enzyme thymidylate synthetase and thereby blocks DNA synthesis.

Primary indications.

1. Breast, colorectal, anal, stomach, pancreas, esophagus, liver, head and neck, and bladder carcinomas.
2. Actinic keratosis; basal and squamous cell carcinomas of skin (topically).

Usual dosage and schedule.

1. *Systemic.*
   a. 500 mg/m^2 IV on days 1 to 5 every 4 weeks *or*
   b. 450 to 600 mg/m^2 IV weekly.
   c. 200 to 400 mg/m^2 daily as a continuous IV infusion.
   d. 1,000 mg/m^2 daily for 4 days as a continuous IV infusion every 3 to 4 weeks.
   e. Leucovorin 20 mg/m^2 IV is followed by fluorouracil 425 mg/m^2 IV. The combination is given daily for 5 days. Courses are repeated every 4 weeks.
2. *Intracavitary.* 500 to 1,000 mg for pericardial effusion; 2,000 to 3,000 mg for pleural or peritoneal effusions.
3. *Intra-arterial (liver).* 800 to 1,200 mg/m^2 as a continuous infusion on days 1 to 4, followed by 600 mg/m^2 as a continuous infusion on days 5 to 21.
4. *Topically.* Apply solution or cream twice daily. Use only 5% strength for carcinomas.

Special precautions.

1. Reduce dose in patients with compromised liver function.
2. For intra-arterial infusion, add 5,000 U of heparin to 1 L of 5% dextrose in water together with the daily dose of fluorouracil. The catheter position should be checked with dye injection every few days to ensure that it has not moved and that the hepatic artery has not thrombosed. Ulcer-like pain or other significant gastrointestinal symptoms are indications to discontinue intra-arterial therapy, as hemorrhage or perforation may occur.
3. Precipitation may occur when leucovorin and fluorouracil are mixed in the same bag.

Toxicity.

1. *Myelosuppression and other hematologic effects.* Dose limiting with a nadir at 10 to 14 days after the last dose and recovery by 21 days.
2. *Nausea, vomiting, and other gastrointestinal effects.* Nausea and vomiting may occur but are not usually severe. Diarrhea is common with higher doses, continuous infusion, or when used in combination with leucovorin and irinotecan. Esophagitis and proctitis may also occur.
3. *Mucocutaneous effects.*
   a. Stomatitis is an early sign of severe toxicity. It progresses from soreness and erythema to frank ulceration, which becomes hemorrhagic in a small number of patients.
   b. Partial alopecia is uncommon.
   c. Hyperpigmentation of skin over face, hands, and the veins used for infusion is occasional.

> d. Maculopapular rash is uncommon.
> e. Sun exposure tends to increase skin reactions.
> f. "Hand-and-foot syndrome" with painful erythematous desquamation and fissures of palms and soles is common with continuous infusion and occasional with other schedules or combinations.

4. *Miscellaneous effects.*
   a. Neurotoxicity including headache, minor visual disturbances, and cerebellar ataxia is rare.
   b. Increased lacrimation is uncommon.
   c. Cardiac toxicity including arrhythmias, angina, ischemia, and sudden death is rare. May be more common with continuous infusion and previous history of coronary artery disease.
   d. Hypertriglyceridemia when given in combination with levamisole.

FLUTAMIDE

Other name. Eulexin.

Mechanism of action. Competitive inhibitor of androgens at the cellular androgen receptor in the prostate cancer cells.

Primary indications. Carcinoma of the prostate, most often in combination with luteinizing hormone–releasing hormone agonists.

Usual dosage and schedule. 250 mg PO every 8 h.

Special precautions. Serum transaminase levels should be measured prior to starting treatment with flutamide. Flutamide is not recommended in patients whose serum transaminase values exceed twice the upper limit of normal.

Toxicity.

1. *Myelosuppression and other hematologic effects.* None.
2. *Nausea, vomiting, and other gastrointestinal effects.* Nausea and vomiting are uncommon to occasional. Diarrhea, flatulence, and mild abdominal pain are common.
3. *Mucocutaneous effects.* Mild skin rash is occasional.
4. *Miscellaneous effects.*
   a. Secondary pharmacologic effects including breast tenderness, breast swelling, hot flashes, impotence, and loss of libido are common but reversible after cessation of therapy.
   b. Elevated liver function tests are uncommon; liver failure is rare but may be preceded by flu-like symptoms or right upper quadrant pain and tenderness.
   c. Hypertension is occasional.
   d. Adverse cardiovascular events are similar to those seen with orchiectomy.

FULVESTRANT

Other name. Faslodex.

Mechanism of action. An estrogen receptor antagonist that binds to the estrogen receptor in a competitive manner. It downregulates the estrogen receptor protein in human breast cancer cells. This is associated with a dose-related decrease in the expression of the progesterone receptor and a decrease in the Ki67 labeling index, a marker for cell proliferation. *In vitro* demonstration of reversible inhibition the growth of tamoxifen-resistant as well as estrogen-sensitive human breast cancer cell lines.

Primary indications. Hormone receptor–positive metastatic breast cancer in postmenopausal women with disease progression following antiestrogen therapy. (There are no efficacy data for premenopausal women with advanced breast cancer.)

Usual dosage and schedule. 250 mg IM (into the buttock[s]) as either a single 5-mL injection or two concurrent 2.5-mL injections, repeated once monthly.

Special precautions. Safety has not been evaluated in patients with moderate to severe hepatic impairment.

Toxicity.
1. *Myelosuppression and other hematologic effects.* Anemia is rare.
2. *Nausea, vomiting, and other gastrointestinal effects.* Nausea is common; vomiting, constipation, diarrhea, and anorexia are occasional.
3. *Mucocutaneous effects.* Rash and increased sweating are occasional.
4. *Miscellaneous effects.*
   a. For the body as a whole, headache, back pain, abdominal pain, injection site pain, and pelvic pain are occasional. Occasional patients also experience a flu-like syndrome or fever.
   b. Vasodilation is occasional (18%).
   c. Dizziness, insomnia, paresthesias, depression, and anxiety are uncommon to occasional.
   d. Pharyngitis, dyspnea, and increased cough are occasional.

GEFITINIB

Other names. Iressa, ZD1839.

Mechanism of action. Selectively inhibits tyrosine kinase activity of the epidermal growth factor receptor (EGFR). Epidermal growth factor receptor tyrosine kinase inhibition by gefitinib impairs epidermal growth factor–stimulated autophosphorylation and thus blocks growth signals within the cell.

Primary indication. 1. Carcinoma of the lung, 2. other carcinomas expressing EGFR.

Usual dosage and schedule.
1. 250 to 500 mg daily.
2. 250 to 500 mg daily for 14 consecutive days every 4 weeks.

Special precautions. Diarrhea may be dose limiting and require discontinuation of the drug.

Toxicity.
1. *Myelosuppression and other hematologic effects.* Uncommon, except for anemia, which is occasional and not dose related.
2. *Nausea, vomiting, and other gastrointestinal effects.* Nausea, vomiting, and diarrhea are common. Diarrhea may be dose limiting. Anorexia, constipation, and abdominal pain are also common but usually not severe.
3. *Mucocutaneous effects.* Acne-like or folliculitis-type rash is common, usually appearing by day 14; frequency and sever-

ity are dose related. May be associated with dry skin and itching. Rash usually does not worsen with continued treatment and resolves within a week of discontinuation of the drug. Dry mouth and conjunctivitis are occasional.
4. *Miscellaneous effects.*
   a. Dyspnea is occasional to common.
   b. Asthenia is common.
   c. Headache is occasional.
   d. Somnolence is occasional.
   c. Elevated hepatic transaminases are occasional but may be severe (grade 3 or 4).

GEMCITABINE

Other name. Gemzar.

Mechanism of action. After being metabolized intracellularly to the active diphosphate and triphosphate nucleotides, gemcitabine, a cytidine analog, inhibits ribonucleotide reductase and competes with deoxycytidine triphosphate for incorporation into DNA.

Primary indications.
1. Carcinoma of the pancreas, locally advanced or metastatic.
2. Non–small cell carcinoma of the lung.
3. Carcinomas of the breast, bladder, and ovary.

Usual dosage and schedule.
1. 1,000 mg/m^2 IV over 30 min once weekly for up to 7 weeks when used as a single agent. After 1 week of rest, subsequent cycles are given once weekly for 3 consecutive weeks out of 4.
2. 1,000 to 1,250 mg/m^2 IV over 30 min once weekly for 2 or 3 successive weeks during each 3- to 4-week cycle, when used in combination in lung cancer.

Special precaution. Prolongation of infusion time beyond 60 min increases toxicity.

Toxicity.
1. *Myelosuppression and other hematologic effects.* Myelosuppression is dose related and common.
2. *Nausea, vomiting, and other gastrointestinal effects.* Nausea and vomiting are common but only occasionally severe. Diarrhea and constipation are occasional to common.
3. *Mucocutaneous effects.* Rash, alopecia, and mucositis are occasional.
4. *Miscellaneous effects.*
   a. Transient elevations of serum transaminases and alkaline phosphatase are common.
   b. Mild proteinuria and hematuria are common.
   c. Hemolytic–uremic syndrome is rare (0.25%).
   d. Fever without documented infection is common.
   e. Mild paresthesias are occasional.
   f. Dyspnea is occasional.

GEMTUZUMAB OZOGAMICIN

Other names. Mylotarg, CMA-676.

Mechanism of action. Gemtuzumab is a humanized recombinant monoclonal antibody against the CD33 antigen that is conjugated with the cytotoxic antitumor antibiotic calicheamicin. Once bound to the CD33 antigen, the agent is internalized, calicheamicin is released, and its reactive intermediate binds to DNA and causes DNA double-strand breaks and cell death.

Primary indication. Patients with CD33-positive acute non-lymphocytic leukemia in first relapse who are older than 60 years and are not considered candidates for other cytotoxic chemotherapy.

Usual dosage and schedule. 9 mg/m^2 as a 2-h IV infusion on days 1 and 15.

Special precautions.

1. Infusion-related events may include fever, nausea, chills, hypotension, shortness of breath, and anaphylaxis. Pretreatment with acetaminophen and diphenhydramine may lessen these effects.
2. If dyspnea or significant hypotension occurs, the infusion should be interrupted. Anaphylaxis, pulmonary edema, and acute respiratory distress syndrome usually necessitate discontinuation of therapy.
3. Veno-occlusive disease may occur, even in patients without a history of liver disease or hematopoietic stem cell transplant.
4. Tumor lysis syndrome may occur, particularly when the white blood cell count is higher than 30,000/µL.

Toxicity.

1. *Myelosuppression and other hematologic effects.* Severe to life-threatening granulocytopenia and thrombocytopenia are universal. Severe or worse anemia is common.
2. *Nausea, vomiting, and other gastrointestinal effects.* Nausea, vomiting, and diarrhea are common but only occasionally severe.
3. *Mucocutaneous effects.* Rash, local reaction, petechiae, stomatitis, pharyngitis, and rhinitis are occasional to common. Herpes simplex is common. Alopecia is not seen.
4. *Miscellaneous effects.*
    a. Infusion-related events: chills, fever, nausea, and vomiting are common. Hypotension, hypertension, and headache are occasional. Dyspnea and hypoxia are uncommon (about 5%).
    b. Increased cough, dyspnea, and epistaxis are common. Severe dyspnea or pneumonia is occasional. Pleural effusions, noncardiogenic pulmonary edema, and acute respiratory distress syndrome are rare.
    c. Severe or life-threatening infections are common. These include sepsis, pneumonia, and opportunistic infections.
    d. Hypertension, hypotension, and tachycardia are occasional.
    e. Reversible abnormalities in liver function are common and occasionally severe or life threatening. Fatal liver abnormalities including veno-occlusive disease are rare. Findings that may indicate severe hepatotoxicity include rapid weight gain, right upper quadrant pain, hepatomegaly, ascites, and elevations in liver function tests.

HYDROXYUREA

Other names. Hydrea, Mycocel.

Mechanism of action. Interferes with DNA synthesis, at least in part by inhibiting the enzymatic conversion of ribonucleotides to deoxyribonucleotides.

Primary indications.

1. Head and neck carcinomas.
2. Chronic granulocytic (myelogenous) leukemia, acute lymphocytic and acute nonlymphocytic leukemia with high blast counts.
3. Essential thrombocythemia.
4. Polycythemia rubra vera.
5. Prevention of retinoic acid syndrome in acute promyelocytic leukemia.

Usual dosage and schedule.

1. 800 to 2,000 mg/m^2 PO as a single or divided daily dose *or*
2. 3,200 mg/m^2 PO as a single dose every third day (not for leukemias).

Special precautions. The daily dose must be adjusted for blood count trends. Be careful not to change dose too often because there is a delay in response.

Toxicity.

1. *Myelosuppression and other hematologic effects.* Occurs at doses of more than 1,600 mg/m^2 daily by day 10. Recovery is usually prompt. Increased red cell mean corpuscular volume is common.
2. *Nausea, vomiting, and other gastrointestinal effects.* Nausea is common at high doses. Other gastrointestinal symptoms are uncommon.
3. *Mucocutaneous effects.* Stomatitis is rare. Maculopapular rash may be seen. Inflammation of mucous membranes caused by radiation may be exaggerated.
4. *Miscellaneous effects.*
   a. Temporary renal function impairment or dysuria is uncommon.
   b. CNS disturbances are rare.
   c. May be leukemogenic.

IBRITUMOMAB TIUXETAN

Other names. Zevalin, IDEC-Y2B8.

Mechanism of action. Ibritumomab is a murine monoclonal anti-CD20 antibody conjugated to tiuxetan that chelates to the pure beta-emitting ^{90}Y. The mechanism of action includes antibody-mediated cytotoxicity and cellularly targeted radiotherapy (radioimmunotherapy).

Primary indications.

1. Non-Hodgkin's lymphoma, follicular B-cell, CD-20 positive.
   a. Rituximab refractory.
   b. Relapsed or refractory to other agents but not rituximab refractory (experimental).

Usual dosage and schedule. Rituximab 250 mg/m^2 is given day 1. Within 4 h after completing the infusion, an IV dose of 5 mCi of ^{111}In-ibritumomab tiuxetan is given as an imaging dose over a 10 m period. Imaging is done between 2 and 24 h, between 48 and 72 h, and optionally between 90 and 120 h after the ^{111}In-ibritumomab tiuxetan. If the biodistribution is acceptable, a second dose of rituximab, 250 mg/m^2, is given once, anywhere between days 7 and 9, followed in 4 h by 0.3 to 0.4 mCi/kg IV of ^{90}Y-ibritumomab tiuxetan injected over a 10 m period. The maximum dose is 32 mCi.

Special precautions. Use with caution in patients with 25% or more marrow involvement with lymphoma, prior external beam radiotherapy to 25% or more of the bone marrow, or a history of human antimouse antibodies (HAMAs) or HACAs. Because the drug does not emit gamma radiation, hospitalization is not required.

Toxicity.

1. *Myelosuppression and other hematologic effects.* Neutropenia and thrombocytopenia are common and related to the radionuclide dose. At the higher end of the dosing, 25% will develop nadir neutrophil counts of less than 500/μL.
2. *Nausea, vomiting, and other gastrointestinal effects.* Low-grade nausea and vomiting are common.
3. *Mucocutaneous effects.* Urticaria and pruritus are occasional.
4. *Miscellaneous effects.*
   a. HAMAs or HACAs may develop.
   b. Infusion-related fever, chills, dizziness, asthenia, headache, back pain, arthralgia, and hypotension are occasional.

IDARUBICIN

Other names. 4-Demethoxydaunorubicin, IDA, Idamycin.

Mechanism of action. DNA strand breakage mediated by anthracycline effects on topoisomerase II or free radicals, DNA intercalation, DNA polymerase inhibition.

Primary indications.

1. Acute nonlymphocytic leukemia.
2. Blast crisis of chronic granulocytic (myelogenous) leukemia.
3. Acute lymphocytic leukemia.

Usual dosage and schedule. 12 to 13 mg/m^2 IV daily for 3 days (usually in a combination with cytarabine) during induction; 10 to 12 mg/m^2 IV daily for 2 days during consolidation.

Special precautions. Administer over several minutes into the sidearm of a running IV infusion, taking care to avoid extravasation. Cardiac toxicity may be less than that with daunorubicin. Maximum dose not yet established. Cumulative doses greater than 150 mg/m^2 have been associated with decreased cardiac ejection fraction.

Toxicity.

1. *Myelosuppression and other hematologic effects.* Universal and dose limiting.
2. *Nausea, vomiting, and other gastrointestinal effects.* Nausea, vomiting, and anorexia are common. Diarrhea is occasional to common.
3. *Mucocutaneous effects.* Alopecia is common; mucositis is common but usually not severe.
4. *Hepatic dysfunction.* Common but usually not severe and not clearly due to the idarubicin.

5. *Renal effects.* Common but usually not clinically significant.
6. *Cardiac effects.* Uncommon during induction and consolidation (1% to 5%).
7. *Tissue damage.* Probable if infiltration occurs.
8. *Neurologic effects.* Occasional.

IFOSFAMIDE

Other name. Ifex.

Mechanism of action. Metabolic activation by microsomal liver enzymes produces biologically active intermediates that attack nucleophilic sites, particularly on DNA.

Primary indications.
1. Testicular and lung cancers.
2. Bone and soft tissue sarcomas.
3. Lymphoma.

Special precautions. Must be used with mesna to prevent hemorrhagic cystitis. Mesna dose is at least 20% of the ifosfamide dose (on a weight basis), administered just prior to (or mixed with) the ifosfamide dose and again at 4 and 8 h after the ifosfamide to detoxify the urinary metabolites that cause the hemorrhagic cystitis. Higher doses of ifosfamide may require higher doses and longer durations of mesna. Neither mesna nor its only metabolite, mesna disulfide, affects ifosfamide or its antineoplastic metabolites. Mesna disulfide is reduced in the kidney to a free thiol compound, which then reacts chemically with urotoxic metabolites resulting in their detoxification. Vigorous hydration is also required with a minimum of 2 L of oral or IV hydration daily. Administer as a slow IV infusion over a period of at least 30 min.

Usual dosage and schedule.
1. 1.2 g/m^2 IV over 30 min or more daily for 5 consecutive days every 3 or 4 weeks, usually with other agents. Mesna 120 mg/m^2 is given just before ifosfamide, then mesna 1,200 mg/m^2 as a daily continuous infusion is given until 16 h after the last dose of ifosfamide.
2. 3.6 g/m^2 IV daily as a 4-h infusion for 2 consecutive days, usually with other agents. Mesna is given at a dose of 750 mg/m^2 IV just prior to and at 4 and 8 h after the start of the ifosfamide.
3. Higher dosage schedules have been used experimentally with up to 14 g/m^2 being used per course over a 6-day period, with equal or greater doses of mesna.

Toxicity.
1. *Myelosuppression and other hematologic effects.* Dose limiting. Platelets are relatively spared. Granulocyte nadirs are commonly reached at 10 to 14 days, and recovery is seen by day 21. Thrombocytopenia may be seen with higher doses.
2. *Nausea, vomiting, and other gastrointestinal effects.* Common without standard antiemetics.
3. *Mucocutaneous effects.* Alopecia is common; mucositis is rarely seen at standard doses; dermatitis is rare.
4. *Hemorrhagic cystitis.* Common and dose limiting unless a uroprotective agent such as mesna is used. With mesna, the incidence of hemorrhagic cystitis is 5% to 10%, and gross hematuria is uncommon. Increasing the duration of mesna may alleviate the problem during subsequent cycles.

5. *Miscellaneous effects.*
   a. CNS toxicity (somnolence, confusion, depressive psychosis, hallucinations, disorientation, and uncommonly seizures, cranial nerve dysfunction, or coma) is occasional with doses in the lower range and more common with larger doses.
   b. Infertility is common in men and women, as with other alkylating agents.
   c. Renal impairment is occasional to common. Fanconi syndrome is dependent on dose. May be severe acidosis.
   d. Liver dysfunction is uncommon.
   e. Phlebitis is uncommon.
   f. Fever is rare.
   g. Peripheral neuropathy with high-dose therapy is uncommon.

IMATINIB MESYLATE

Other names. Gleevec, STI-571 (signal transduction inhibitor 571).
Mechanism of action. Inhibitor of the constitutively activated Bcr-Abl tyrosine kinase that is created as a consequence of the (9;22) chromosomal translocation and is required for the transforming function and excess proliferation seen in chronic myelogenous leukemia. It also inhibits platelet-derived growth factor receptor tyrosine kinase and c-Kit tyrosine kinase, the latter of which is activated in gastrointestinal stromal tumors.
Primary indications.
1. Chronic myelogenous leukemia (newly diagnosed) in chronic phase; after failure of interferon-α; or in either the accelerated or the blast phase of the disease.
2. Gastrointestinal stromal tumor.
Usual dosage and schedule.
1. 400 to 600 mg PO daily in the chronic phase of chronic myelogenous leukemia or gastrointestinal stromal tumors.
2. 600 to 800 mg PO daily in the accelerated phase or blast crisis.
Special precautions. None.
Toxicity.
1. *Myelosuppression and other hematologic effects.* Moderate neutropenia and thrombocytopenia are common in all phases, but severe neutropenia or thrombocytopenia is uncommon unless patients are in the accelerated phase or blast crisis of chronic myelogenous leukemia.
2. *Nausea, vomiting, and other gastrointestinal effects.* Nausea, vomiting, abdominal pain, and diarrhea are common, but it is uncommon that they are severe.
3. *Mucocutaneous effects.* Skin rash is common; pruritus and petechiae are occasional.
4. *Miscellaneous effects.*
   a. Fluid retention and edema are common. Pleural effusion and ascites are uncommon.
   b. Musculoskeletal pain or cramps, arthralgia, headache, fever, and fatigue are common, but it is uncommon that they are severe or life threatening.
   c. Dyspnea and cough are occasional.

    d.   Elevated liver function tests or serum creatinine are uncommon to rare. Rare cases of severe hepatotoxicity have been seen.

INTERFERON-α

Other names. Roferon-A (interferon alfa-2a, recombinant alpha-A interferon), Intron A (interferon alfa-2b, recombinant alpha-2 interferon).

Mechanism of action. Believed to involve direct inhibition of tumor cell growth and modulation of the immune response of the host, including activation of natural killer cells, modulation of antibody production, and induction of major histocompatibility antigens.

Primary indications.
1. Chronic myelogenous leukemia.
2. Melanoma (both as adjuvant and metastatic disease therapy).
3. Non-Hodgkin's lymphoma (low grade), mycosis fungoides.
4. Multiple myeloma.
5. Hairy-cell leukemia.
6. Renal cell carcinoma.
7. Other carcinomas in combination with chemotherapy (e.g., fluorouracil in colon carcinoma).
8. Kaposi's sarcoma, associated with HIV.
9. Condyloma acuminatum (intralesional).
10. Chronic hepatitis B and C.

Usual dosage and schedule.
1. 3 to 10×10^6 IU IM or SC in various schedules. Daily dosing is often used for several weeks or months, followed by three-times-a-week dosing.
2. As adjuvant therapy for high-risk melanoma, 20×10^6 IU/m^2 IV 5 consecutive days weekly for 4 weeks, then 10×10^6 IU/m^2 SC three times weekly for 48 weeks.
3. For HIV-related Kaposi's sarcoma, 30×10^6 IU/m^2 SC or IM three times weekly, with dose modifications based upon toxicity.

Investigationally, doses have been higher (up to 50×10^6 IU/m^2 per dose), usually IV at doses higher than 10×10^6 IU/m^2.

Special precautions. May cause or aggravate life-threatening or fatal neuropsychiatric, autoimmune, ischemic, and infectious disorders. Patients with persistently severe or worsening signs or symptoms of these conditions should be withdrawn from therapy.

Toxicity.
1. *Myelosuppression and other hematologic effects.* Common but usually mild to moderate and transient, even with continued therapy. Higher doses may be associated (25% of patients receiving the recommended adjuvant therapy for melanoma) with granulocyte counts of under 750/µL and consequent increased risk for infection.
2. *Nausea, vomiting, and other gastrointestinal effects.* Anorexia and nausea are common, occurring in up to two-thirds of all patients, but vomiting is only occasional. Diarrhea and loose stools are occasional to common.
3. *Mucocutaneous effects.* Rash, dryness, or inflammation of the oropharynx, dry skin or pruritus, and partial alopecia are occasional to common.

4. *Flu-like syndrome.* Syndrome with fatigue, fever, chills, sweating, myalgias, arthralgias, and headache is common to universal with greater severity at higher doses. Tends to diminish with continuing therapy and acetaminophen.

5. *Neurologic effects.*
   a. Occasional paresthesias or numbness in peripheral nervous system.
   b. CNS toxicity is uncommon at lower doses, but with higher doses, there is an increased likelihood of problems including headache, dizziness, somnolence, anxiety, depression (including suicidal behavior), confusion, hallucinations, cerebellar dysfunction, and emotional lability.

6. *General systemic effects.* Fatigue, anorexia, fatigue, and weight loss are common with chronic administration.

7. *Cardiovascular effects.* Mild hypotension is common but rarely symptomatic. Rarely to uncommonly seen are hypertension, chest pain, arrhythmias, and other cardiovascular disorders.

8. *Respiratory effects.* Dyspnea and cough are occasional at higher doses.

9. *Infectious effects.* Exacerbation of herpetic eruptions and nonherpetic cold sores is uncommon.

10. *Miscellaneous effects.* Leg cramps, insomnia, urticaria, hot flashes, and coagulation disorders are uncommon. Visual problems including blurring, diplopia, dry eyes, nystagmus, and photophobia are uncommon. Retinopathy, usually asymptomatic, is rare.

11. *Metabolic effects and laboratory abnormalities.*
    a. Elevated liver enzymes are common.
    b. Mild proteinuria and increase in serum creatinine are occasional.
    c. Hypercalcemia is occasional.
    d. Hypothyroidism and hyperthyroidism with or without antithyroid antibodies.
    e. Hypertriglyceridemia is rare.

12. *Antibody development.* Antibody development (binding and neutralizing) occurs more readily with interferon alfa-2a than with interferon alfa-2b. The significance of this is not clear, though it may be associated with the development of clinical resistance in some patients.

IRINOTECAN

Other names. Camptosar, CPT-11.

Mechanism of action. Irinotecan, a semisynthetic water-soluble derivative of camptothecin, is a prodrug for the lipophilic metabolite SN-38, a potent inhibitor of topoisomerase I, which is an enzyme essential for effective replication and transcription. It binds to the topoisomerase I–DNA cleavable complex, preventing religation after cleavage by topoisomerase I.

Primary indications. Carcinoma of the colon or rectum, either in combination with fluorouracil and leucovorin as primary therapy of metastatic disease or as a single agent after failure of fluorouracil-based therapy.

Usual dosage and schedule.

1. 125 mg/m^2 IV over 90 min weekly for 4 weeks followed by a 2-week rest to complete one cycle when used either as a single agent or in combination with fluorouracil and leucovorin.
2. 180 mg/m^2 IV over 90 min every 2 weeks when used with leucovorin (over 2 h) plus bolus fluorouracil followed by a 22-h infusion of fluorouracil.
3. For severe or worse diarrhea (7 stools or more over pretreatment), doses should be held. When the diarrhea has improved (7 stools or less over pretreatment), treatment may be restarted with doses modified downward by 25 to 30 mg/m^2 during the current and subsequent cycles if there was an increase in stools of 7 to 9 per day and by 50 to 60 mg/m^2 if there was an increase in stools of 10 or more. Doses are also held during treatment and reduced in the same and subsequent cycles for severe neutropenia (absolute neutrophil count under 1,000).

Special precautions.

1. Both early and late diarrhea may occur. That which occurs within 24 h (a cholinergic effect) should be treated with atropine 0.25 to 1 mg IV. Late diarrhea should be treated promptly with loperamide (up to 2 mg every 2 h until the patient is diarrhea-free for 12 h) and prompt fluid and electrolyte replacement as indicated, if the diarrhea becomes severe (increase of seven or more stools per day) or there is dehydration or postural hypotension.
2. Consideration should be given to antibiotic therapy such as with an oral fluoroquinolone, particularly if the patient is neutropenic.
3. A vascular syndrome characterized by sudden unexpected thromboembolic events has also been described.

Toxicity.

1. *Myelosuppression and other hematologic effects.* Neutropenia is common and often severe, particularly in combination therapy; anemia and thrombocytopenia are common but not usually (< 5%) severe.
2. *Nausea, vomiting, and other gastrointestinal effects.* Nausea and vomiting are common and are occasionally severe. Early diarrhea is common but is not usually (< 5%) severe. Late diarrhea is common (85%) and is occasionally severe (15%) to life threatening (5% to 10%). Abdominal cramping is common, occasionally severe. Anorexia is common. Constipation and dyspepsia are occasional. Ileus, colitis, are toxic megacolon are seen rarely.
3. *Mucocutaneous effects.* Alopecia and mucositis are common. Rash and sweating occur occasionally.
4. *Miscellaneous effects.*
   a. Fever is common, rarely severe.
   b. Headache, back pain, chills, and edema are occasional.
   c. Grade 1 to 2 increases in liver function tests are common; it is uncommon for liver function abnormalities to be severe, except in patients with known liver metastasis.

d. Dyspnea, cough, or rhinitis is occasional to common but usually not severe.
e. Insomnia or dizziness is occasional.
f. Flushing is occasional.
g. Anaphylactic reactions are rare.

LETROZOLE

Other name. Femara.
Mechanism of action. Decreases estrogen biosynthesis by selective inhibition of aromatase (estrogen synthetase) in peripheral tissues.
Primary indications. Carcinoma of the breast, advanced or metastatic, that is hormone receptor positive or unknown in postmenopausal women as first-line treatment or in hormone-responsive postmenopausal women with progression following antiestrogen therapy.
Usual dosage and schedule. 2.5 mg PO daily.
Special precaution. Potential hazard to fetus if given during pregnancy.
Toxicity.
1. *Myelosuppression and other hematologic effects.* No dose-related effect. Thromboembolic events are uncommon to rare.
2. *Nausea, vomiting, and other gastrointestinal effects.* Nausea, vomiting, constipation, and diarrhea are uncommon to occasional.
3. *Mucocutaneous effects.* Rash is uncommon.
4. *Miscellaneous effects.*
   a. Fatigue is occasional.
   b. Musculoskeletal pain (arthralgia or bone) is occasional to common.
   c. Headache is occasional.
   d. Peripheral edema and weight gain are occasional (lower than with megestrol).
   e. Dyspnea and cough are uncommon to occasional.
   f. Hot flushes are occasional.
   g. Hypercalcemia is rare.

LOMUSTINE

Other names. CCNU, CeeNU.
Mechanism of action. Alkylation and carbamoylation by lomustine metabolites interfere with the synthesis and function of DNA, RNA, and proteins. Lomustine is lipid soluble and easily enters the brain.
Primary indications.
1. Lung and kidney carcinomas.
2. Hodgkin's and non-Hodgkin's lymphomas.
3. Brain tumors.
Usual dosage and schedule. 100 to 130 mg/m^2 PO once every 6 to 8 weeks (lower dose used for patients with compromised bone marrow function). Some recommend limiting cumulative dose to 1,000 mg/m^2 to limit pulmonary and renal toxicity.
Special precautions. Because of delayed myelosuppression (3 to 6 weeks), do not treat more often than every 6 weeks. Await a return of normal platelet and granulocyte counts before repeating therapy.

Toxicity.
1. *Myelosuppression and other hematologic effects.* Universal and dose limiting. Leukopenia and thrombocytopenia are delayed 3 to 6 weeks after therapy begins and may be cumulative with successive doses.
2. *Nausea, vomiting, and other gastrointestinal effects.* Nausea and vomiting may begin 3 to 6 h after therapy and last up to 24 h.
3. *Mucocutaneous effects.* Stomatitis and alopecia are rare.
4. *Miscellaneous effects.*
   a. Confusion, lethargy, and ataxia are rare.
   b. Mild hepatotoxicity is infrequent.
   c. Secondary neoplasia is possible.
   d. Pulmonary fibrosis is uncommon at doses of less than 1,000 mg/m^2.
   e. Renal toxicity is uncommon at doses of less than 1,000 mg/m^2.

LUTEINIZING HORMONE–RELEASING HORMONE ANALOGS

Other names. Leuprolide (Lupron, Lupron depot, Viadur), goserelin (Zoladex depot), triptorelin pamoate (Trelstar depot).
Mechanism of action. Initial release of follicle-stimulating hormone and luteinizing hormone from the anterior pituitary, followed by diminution of gonadotropin secretion owing to desensitization of the pituitary to gonadotropin-releasing hormone and consequent decrease in the respective gonadal hormones. May also have direct effects on cancer cells, at least in cancer of the breast, in which gonadotropin-releasing hormone–binding sites have been demonstrated.
Primary indications.
1. Metastatic prostate carcinoma.
2. Breast carcinoma in premenopausal and perimenopausal women with metastatic disease (goserelin).
Usual dosage and schedule.
1. Leuprolide depot 7.5 mg IM monthly, 22.5 mg IM every 3 months, or 30 mg IM every 4 months.
2. Goserelin depot, 3.6 mg SC every 4 weeks or 10.8 mg SC every 12 weeks. Use only 3.6-mg implant for breast carcinoma.
3. Triptorelin depot 3.75 mg IM monthly.
Special precaution. Worsening of symptoms may occur during the first few weeks.
Toxicity.
1. *Myelosuppression and other hematologic effects.* Rare if at all.
2. *Nausea, vomiting, and other gastrointestinal effects.* Anorexia, nausea, vomiting, and constipation are uncommon.
3. *Mucocutaneous effects.* Erythema and ecchymosis at the injection site, rash, hair loss, and itching are uncommon.
4. *Cardiovascular effects.* Congestive heart failure, hypertension, and thrombotic episodes are uncommon. Peripheral edema is occasional.
5. *Miscellaneous effects.*
   a. Dizziness, pain, headache, and paresthesias are uncommon.

b. Hot flashes are common; decreased libido is common; gynecomastia with or without tenderness is uncommon; impotence is occasional to common.

c. Bone pain, or "flare," is common on initiation of therapy in patients with bony metastasis. This can be minimized by pretreating with flutamide or another androgen antagonist in men with prostate cancer.

d. Hypersensitivity reactions with rare angioneurotic edema and anaphylaxis have been reported.

MECHLORETHAMINE

Other names. Nitrogen mustard, HN2, Mustargen.

Mechanism of action. Mechlorethamine is a prototype alkylating agent. Its action involves transfer of the alkyl group to amino, carboxyl, hydroxyl, imidazole, phosphate, and sulfhydryl groups within the cell, altering the structure and function of DNA (primarily), RNA, and proteins.

Primary indications.

1. Hodgkin's lymphoma.
2. Malignant pleural and, less commonly, peritoneal or pericardial effusions.
3. Cutaneous T-cell lymphomas (topically).

Usual dosage and schedule.

1. 6 mg/m² IV on days 1 and 8 every 4 weeks (in MOPP regimen for Hodgkin's disease [See Chapter 21]).
2. 8 to 16 mg/m² by intracavitary injection.
3. 10 mg in 60 mL of tap water applied to entire body surface (avoid eyes).

Special precautions.

1. Administer over several minutes into the sidearm of a running IV infusion, taking care to avoid extravasation.
2. Because mechlorethamine is a potent vesicant, extreme care must be exercised while preparing and administering the drug. Gloves and eye glasses are recommended to protect the preparer. If accidental eye contact should occur, institute copious irrigation with normal saline and follow by prompt ophthalmologic consultation. If accidental skin contact occurs, irrigate the affected part immediately with water for at least 15 min and follow by 2.6% sodium thiosulfate solution ($\frac{1}{6}$ M).
3. Mechlorethamine should be used soon after preparation (15 to 30 min) as it decomposes on standing. It *must not* be mixed in the same syringe with any other drug.

Toxicity.

1. *Myelosuppression and other hematologic effects.* Dose limiting, with the nadir at about 1 week and recovery by 3 weeks.
2. *Nausea, vomiting, and other gastrointestinal effects.* Universal. They usually begin within the first 3 h and last 4 to 8 h.
3. *Mucocutaneous effects.* Severe painful inflammation and necrosis are likely if extravasation occurs. May be ameliorated if 2.6% thiosulfate solution ($\frac{1}{6}$ M) is instilled into the area to neutralize active drug and ice packs are applied locally for 6 to 12 h. Maculopapular rash is uncommon.

4. *Miscellaneous effects.*
   a. Phlebitis, thrombosis, or both of the vein used for the injection are common.
   b. Amenorrhea and azoospermia are common.
   c. Hyperuricemia with rapid tumor destruction.
   d. Weakness, sleepiness, and headache are uncommon.
   e. Severe allergic reactions including anaphylaxis are rare.
   f. Secondary neoplasms are possible.

MELPHALAN

Other names. Phenylalanine mustard, L-sarcolysin, L-PAM, Alkeran.

Mechanism of action. Alkylating agent with primary effect on DNA. Amino acid–type structure may result in cellular transport that is different from other alkylating agents.

Primary indications.
1. Multiple myeloma.
2. Breast and ovarian carcinomas.

Usual dosage and schedule.
1. 8 mg/m^2 PO on days 1 to 4 every 4 weeks *or*
2. 10 mg/m^2 PO on days 1 to 4 every 6 weeks *or*
3. 3 to 4 mg/m^2 PO daily for 2 to 3 weeks, then 1 to 2 mg/m^2 PO daily for maintenance.
4. High-dose regimens of 140 to 200 mg/m^2 IV have been used, followed by stem cell rescue (e.g., bone marrow transplantation).
5. 16 mg/m^2 IV every 2 weeks × 4, then every 4 weeks.

Special precautions.
1. Myelosuppression and other hematologic effects may be delayed and prolonged to 4 to 6 weeks.
2. Reduce IV dose by 50% for creatinine levels higher than 1.5 times normal.

Toxicity.
1. *Myelosuppression and other hematologic effects.* Dose limiting; nadir at days 14 to 21.
2. *Nausea, vomiting, and other gastrointestinal effects.* Nausea, vomiting, and diarrhea are uncommon at standard doses but common with high-dose regimens.
3. *Mucocutaneous effects.* Alopecia, dermatitis, and stomatitis are uncommon at standard doses; alopecia and mucositis are common with high-dose regimens.
4. *Miscellaneous effects.*
   a. Acute nonlymphocytic leukemia and myelodysplasia are rare but well documented.
   b. Pulmonary fibrosis is rare.

MERCAPTOPURINE

Other names. 6-Mercaptopurine, 6-MP, Purinethol.

Mechanism of action. A purine antimetabolite that, when converted to the nucleotide, inhibits the formation of nucleotides necessary for DNA and RNA synthesis.

Primary indications. Acute lymphocytic and juvenile chronic granulocytic (myelogenous) leukemias.

Usual dosage and schedule.
1. 100 mg/m^2 PO daily if used alone.
2. 50 to 90 mg/m^2 PO daily if used with methotrexate.

Special precautions.
1. Decrease dose by 75% when used concurrently with allopurinol.
2. Increase interval between doses or reduce dose in patients with renal failure.

Toxicity.
1. *Myelosuppression and other hematologic effects.* Common but mild at recommended doses.
2. *Nausea, vomiting, and other gastrointestinal effects.* Nausea and vomiting are uncommon. Diarrhea is rare.
3. *Mucocutaneous effects.* Stomatitis may be seen with very large doses. Dry, scaling rash is uncommon.
4. *Miscellaneous effects.*
    a. Intrahepatic cholestasis and mild focal centrolobular necrosis with jaundice are uncommon.
    b. Hyperuricemia with rapid leukemia cell lysis is common.
    c. Fever is uncommon.

MESNA

Other name. Mesnex.

Mechanism of action. Mesna disulfide is reduced in the kidney to a free thiol compound, which then reacts chemically with urotoxic metabolites of ifosfamide, resulting in their detoxification.

Primary indication. Prophylaxis for ifosfamide-induced hemorrhagic cystitis.

Usual dosage and schedule. Mesna dose is at least 20% of the ifosfamide dose (on a weight [mg] basis), administered just prior to (or mixed with) the ifosfamide dose and again at 4 and 8 h after the ifosfamide to detoxify the urinary metabolites that cause the hemorrhagic cystitis. Higher doses of ifosfamide may require higher doses and longer durations of mesna.

Special precautions. Contraindicated if patient is sensitive to thiol compounds. Does not prevent or ameliorate any adverse effects of ifosfamide other than hemorrhagic cystitis. Neither mesna nor its only metabolite, mesna disulfide, affects ifosfamide or its antineoplastic metabolites.

Toxicity.
1. *Myelosuppression and other hematologic effects.* None.
2. *Nausea, vomiting, and other gastrointestinal effects.* Nausea, vomiting, and diarrhea are occasional. Nausea and vomiting more commonly from ifosfamide.
3. *Mucocutaneous effects.* Bad taste in the mouth is common.
4. *Miscellaneous effects.*
    a. Headache, fatigue, and limb pain are occasional.
    b. Hypotension and allergic reaction are uncommon to rare.
    c. Gives false-positive test for urinary ketones.

METHOTREXATE

Other names. Amethopterin, MTX, Mexate, Trexall.

Mechanism of action. Inhibition of dihydrofolate reductase, which results in a block of the reduction of dihydrofolate to tetrahydrofolate. This blockage in turn inhibits the formation of thymidylate and purines and arrests DNA (predominantly), RNA, and protein synthesis.

Primary indications.
1. Breast, head and neck, gastrointestinal, lung, and gestational trophoblastic carcinomas.
2. Osteosarcomas (high-dose methotrexate).
3. Acute lymphocytic leukemia.
4. Meningeal leukemia or carcinomatosis.
5. Non-Hodgkin's lymphoma.

Usual dosage and schedule.
1. *Gestational trophoblastic carcinoma.* 15 to 30 mg PO or IM on days 1 to 5 every 2 weeks.
2. *Other carcinomas.* 40 to 80 mg/m^2 IV or PO two to four times monthly with a 7- to 14-day interval between doses.
3. *Acute lymphocytic leukemia.* 15 to 20 mg/m^2 PO or IV weekly (together with mercaptopurine).
4. *Osteogenic sarcoma.* Up to 12 g/m^2 with leucovorin rescue (high-dose methotrexate). This usage requires on-site monitoring of methotrexate levels and a high degree of expertise to administer safely.
5. *Intrathecally.* 12 mg/m^2 (not more than 20 mg) twice weekly.

Special precautions.
1. High-dose methotrexate (over 80 mg/m^2) should be administered only by individuals experienced in its use and at institutions where serum methotrexate levels can be readily measured.
2. Intrathecal methotrexate must be mixed in buffered physiologic solution containing no preservative.
3. Avoid aspirin, sulfonamides, tetracycline, phenytoin, and other protein-bound drugs that may displace methotrexate and cause an increase in free drug.
4. Oral anticoagulants, for example, warfarin, may be potentiated by methotrexate; therefore prothrombin times should be followed carefully.
5. Oral antibiotics may decrease methotrexate absorption; penicillin and nonsteroidal anti-inflammatory drugs decrease clearance of methotrexate.
6. Monitor use with theophylline.
7. In patients with renal insufficiency, it may be necessary to markedly reduce the dose or discontinue methotrexate therapy.
8. Do not give if patient has an effusion because of "reservoir" effect.

Toxicity.
1. *Myelosuppression and other hematologic effects.* Occurs commonly, with nadir at 6 to 10 days after a single IV dose. Recovery is rapid.
2. *Nausea, vomiting, and other gastrointestinal effects.* Occasional at standard doses.
3. *Mucocutaneous effects.*
   a. Mild stomatitis is common and a sign that maximum tolerated dose has been reached. Higher doses may result in confluent or hemorrhagic stomal ulcers and bloody diarrhea.

      b. Erythematous rashes, urticaria, and skin pigment changes are uncommon.

      c. Mild alopecia is frequent.

  4. *Miscellaneous effects.*

      a. Acute hepatocellular injury is uncommon at standard doses.

      b. Hepatic fibrosis is uncommon but seen at low chronic doses.

      c. Pneumonitis is rare.

      d. Polyserositis is rare.

      e. Renal tubular necrosis is rare at standard doses.

      f. Convulsions and a Guillain–Barré–like syndrome following intrathecal therapy are uncommon.

MITOMYCIN

Other names. Mitomycin C, Mutamycin.

Mechanism of action. Alkylation and cross-linking by mitomycin metabolites interfere with structure and function of DNA.

Primary indications. Bladder (intravesical), esophagus, stomach, anal, and pancreas carcinomas.

Usual dosage and schedule.

  1. 20 mg/m^2 IV on day 1 every 4 to 6 weeks *or*

  2. 2 mg/m^2 IV on days 1 to 5 and 8 to 12 every 4 to 6 weeks.

  3. 10 mg/m^2 IV on day 1 every 8 weeks in combination with fluorouracil and doxorubicin for stomach and pancreatic carcinomas.

  4. 30 to 40 mg instilled into the bladder weekly for 4 to 8 weeks, then monthly for 6 months.

Special precaution. Administer as slow push or rapid infusion through the sidearm of a rapidly running IV infusion, taking care to avoid extravasation.

Toxicity.

  1. *Myelosuppression and other hematologic effects.* Serious, cumulative, and dose limiting. Nadir is reached usually by 4 weeks but may be delayed. Recovery is often prolonged over many weeks, and occasionally the cytopenia never disappears.

  2. *Nausea, vomiting, and other gastrointestinal effects.* Nausea and vomiting are common at higher doses, but severity is usually mild to moderate.

  3. *Mucocutaneous effects.*

      a. Stomatitis and alopecia are common.

      b. Cellulitis at injection site if extravasation occurs is common.

  4. *Miscellaneous effects.*

      a. Renal toxicity is uncommon.

      b. Pulmonary toxicity is uncommon but may be severe.

      c. Fever is uncommon.

      d. Secondary neoplasia is possible.

      e. Hemolytic–uremic syndrome is rare.

MITOTANE

Other names. *o,p′*-DDD, Lysodren.

Mechanism of action. Suppresses adrenal steroid production, modifies peripheral steroid metabolism, and is cytotoxic to adrenal cortical cells.

Primary indication. Adrenocortical carcinoma.

Usual dosage and schedule. Begin with 2 to 6 g PO daily in three or four divided doses and build to a maximum tolerated daily dose that is usually 8 to 10 g, although it may range from 2 to 16 g. Glucocorticoid and mineralocorticoid replacements during mitotane therapy are necessary to prevent hypoadrenalism. Cortisone acetate (25 mg PO in the a.m. and 12.5 mg PO in the p.m.) and fludrocortisone acetate (0.1 mg PO in the a.m.) are recommended.

Special precautions. Patients who experience severe trauma, infection, or shock should be treated with supplemental corticosteroids. Because of the effect of mitotane on peripheral steroid metabolism, larger-than-usual replacement doses may be necessary.

Toxicity.
1. *Myelosuppression and other hematologic effects.* None.
2. *Nausea, vomiting, and other gastrointestinal effects.* Common and may be dose limiting.
3. *Mucocutaneous effects.* Skin rash occurs occasionally.
4. *CNS effects.* Lethargy, sedation, vertigo, or dizziness in up to 40% of patients; may be dose limiting.
5. *Miscellaneous effects.* Albuminuria, hemorrhagic cystitis, hypertension, orthostatic hypotension, and visual disturbances are uncommon.

MITOXANTRONE

Other names. Novantrone, dihydroxyanthracenedione, DHAD, DHAQ.

Mechanism of action. DNA strand breakage mediated by anthracenedione effects on topoisomerase II.

Primary indications.
1. Acute nonlymphocytic leukemia.
2. Carcinoma of the breast or ovary.
3. Non-Hodgkin's and Hodgkin's lymphoma.

Usual dosage and schedule.
1. 12 to 14 mg/m^2 IV as a 5- to 30-min infusion once every 3 weeks for solid tumors.
2. 12 mg/m^2 IV as a 5- to 30-min infusion daily for 3 days for acute nonlymphocytic leukemia.

Special precautions. Rarely causes extravasation injury if infiltrated. Cardiotoxicity probably less than with doxorubicin; but prior anthracycline, chest irradiation, or underlying cardiac disease increases the risk.

Toxicity.
1. *Myelosuppression and other hematologic effects.* Universal.
2. *Nausea, vomiting, and other gastrointestinal effects.* Nausea and vomiting are common but less frequent and less severe than with doxorubicin. Diarrhea is uncommon.
3. *Mucocutaneous effects.* Alopecia is common, but its frequency and severity are less than with doxorubicin. Mucositis is occasional.
4. *Cardiac toxicity.* Probably less than with doxorubicin; there is no clear maximum dose, though the risk appears to increase at 125-mg/m^2 cumulative dose.
5. *Miscellaneous effects.*
   a. Local erythema and swelling with transient blue discoloration if extravasated, but rarely leads to severe skin damage.

b. Green or blue discoloration of urine.
c. Phlebitis is uncommon.

NILUTAMIDE

Other name. Nilandron.
Mechanism of action. Competitive inhibitor of androgens at the cellular androgen receptor in prostate cancer cells. Complements surgical castration.
Primary indication. Metastatic carcinoma of the prostate, in combination with surgical castration or luteinizing hormone–releasing hormone agonist.
Usual dosage and schedule. 300 mg PO once daily for 30 days, followed by 150 mg PO once daily thereafter.
Special precautions.
1. Should be restricted to patients with normal liver function test values.
2. A routine chest radiograph should be obtained before therapy and any time that the patient reports new exertional dyspnea or worsening of pre-existing dyspnea.
3. Inhibits activity of liver cytochrome P-450 isoenzymes and may delay elimination of drugs such as warfarin, phenytoin, and theophylline.
Toxicity.
1. *Myelosuppression and other hematologic effects.* None.
2. *Nausea, vomiting, and other gastrointestinal effects.* Occasional nausea. Constipation is uncommon.
3. *Mucocutaneous effects.* Rash, dry skin, and sweating are uncommon.
4. *Miscellaneous effects.*
    a. Hepatitis is rare (1%).
    b. Interstitial pneumonitis with dyspnea is uncommon (2%). May be higher in patients with Asian ancestry.
    c. Inhibits activity of liver cytochrome P-450 isoenzymes and may delay elimination of drugs such as warfarin, phenytoin, and theophylline.
    d. Hot flashes are common.
    e. Increased liver function test values are uncommon.
    f. Impaired adaptation to dark is common.

OCTREOTIDE

Other names. Sandostatin, Sandostatin LAR Depot.
Mechanism of action. Somatostatin analog that inhibits release of polypeptide hormones, particularly in the pancreas and gut. Slows gastrointestinal transit time. Promotes water and electrolyte absorption, reflecting change from overall secretory to absorptive state.
Primary indications.
1. Carcinoid tumors.
2. Vasoactive intestinal peptide tumors and other amine precursor uptake and decarboxylation tumors.
3. Chemotherapy-induced diarrhea.
4. Acromegaly.

Usual dosage and schedule. 100 to 1,500 µg/day SC in two to four divided doses. Doses are usually started at the lower end and titrated upward to the best symptomatic improvement. If patients respond favorably to the rapid-acting SC injections, may be maintained on Sandostatin LAR Depot in a dose of 20 mg given IM intragluteally at 4-week intervals. Caution should be used in treating for more than 3 months.

Special precaution. Lower doses indicated if severe renal dysfunction (creatinine level under 5 mg/dL).

Toxicity.
1. *Myelosuppression and other hematologic effects.* None.
2. *Nausea, vomiting, and other gastrointestinal effects.* Nausea, abdominal discomfort, bloating, and diarrhea are common, particularly early in early therapy. Vomiting is only occasionally seen. Decreased gallbladder contractility and decreased bile secretion may result in biliary abnormalities. Gallstones develop in less than 2% if treatment is for 1 month or less but can be 25% if treatment is for 1 year or more. Ascending cholangitis and pancreatitis are uncommon to rare.
3. *Mucocutaneous effects.* Local site reactions are occasional; other effects are rare.
4. *Endocrine effects.* Hypoglycemia or hyperglycemia is uncommon; hypothalamic pituitary dysfunction is rare.
5. *Cardiovascular effects.* Bradycardia and other conduction abnormalities occur in up to 25% of patients with acromegaly who are treated with octreotide.

OPRELVEKIN

Other names. Neumega, Interleukin-11, IL-11.

Mechanism of action. Stimulates proliferation of hematopoietic stem cells and megakaryocyte progenitor cells and induces megakaryocyte maturation, resulting in increased platelet production.

Primary indication. Prevention of severe thrombocytopenia after chemotherapy in patients with nonmyeloid malignancies.

Usual dosage and schedule. 50 µg/kg SC once daily, starting 6 to 24 h after completion of chemotherapy. Continue until the postnadir count is greater than or equal to 50,000/µL. (Treatment for more than 21 days in a row is not recommended.) Next planned cycle of chemotherapy should begin at least 2 days after discontinuation of oprelvekin.

Special precaution. Use with caution in patients with history of atrial arrhythmia or congestive heart failure.

Toxicity.
1. *Myelosuppression and other hematologic effects.* None. Mild decrease in hemoglobin concentration, due predominantly to increase in plasma volume.
2. *Nausea, vomiting, and other gastrointestinal effects.* None.
3. *Mucocutaneous effects.* Occasional rash, particularly at injection site.
4. *Miscellaneous effects.*
    a. Atrial arrhythmia (flutter or fibrillation) and palpitations are occasional (about 10%) but usually tran-

sient. Syncope is occasional. Fluid retention with edema (renal sodium and water retention) or dyspnea on exertion is common but usually mild to moderate. Not associated with capillary leak syndrome.

b. Conjunctival injection and mild visual blurring are occasional. Papilledema is rare but may be more common in children. Caution should be exerted in patients with pre-existing papilledema or tumors of the CNS.

c. Asthenia is occasional.

OXALIPLATIN

Other name. Eloxatin.

Mechanism of action. Similar to alkylating agents with respect to binding and cross-linking strands of DNA, forming DNA adducts and thereby inhibiting DNA replication and transcription.

Primary indication. Carcinoma of the colon and rectum.

Usual dosage and schedule.

1. *Single agent.* 130 mg/m^2 as a 2-h infusion every 3 weeks or 85 mg/m^2 as a 3-h infusion every 2 weeks.
2. *Combination therapy.* 85 to 100 mg/m^2 as a 2-h infusion every 2 weeks in combination with fluorouracil (often as a continuous infusion).

Special precautions. Acute neurosensory and neuromotor symptoms may develop with the infusion. Laryngospasm may be minimized by avoiding cold drinks or food for a few days following treatment. Chronic neurosensory symptoms are dose limiting.

Toxicity.

1. *Myelosuppression and other hematologic effects.* Low-grade myelosuppression is common, but grade 3 or 4 granulocytopenia, thrombocytopenia, or anemia is uncommon (about 5%). Hemolytic anemia is rare.
2. *Nausea, vomiting, and other gastrointestinal effects.* Nausea, vomiting, and diarrhea are common but not commonly severe. May be worsening of cholinergic syndrome when given with irinotecan.
3. *Mucocutaneous effects.* Alopecia is uncommon. Stomatitis is increased when used with fluorouracil.
4. *Miscellaneous effects.*
    a. Neurotoxicity consisting of paresthesias and cold-induced dysesthesias in the stocking glove or perioral distribution is common as acute transient change that begins with the infusion and lasts for less than 1 week. Chronic sensory neuropathy, fine motor disturbance, and ataxia are occasional to common with cumulative dosing (cumulative dose dependent) and may last for months. It is occasionally grade 3 to 4.
    b. Laryngospasm may develop during or within 2 h of the infusion and can last up to 5 days. Cold temperatures may induce, and warm liquids or a hot pack may ameliorate.
    c. Nephrotoxicity is uncommon.
    d. Ototoxicity is rare.
    e. Anaphylaxis is rare.

PACLITAXEL

Other name. Taxol.

Mechanism of action. Enhanced formation and stabilization of microtubules. Antineoplastic effect may result from nonfunctional tubules or altered tubulin–microtubule equilibrium. Mitotic arrest is seen and is associated with accumulated polymerized microtubules.

Primary indications.
1. Carcinomas of the ovary, breast, lung, head and neck, bladder, and cervix.
2. Melanoma.
3. Kaposi's sarcoma, AIDS related.

Usual dosage and schedule.
1. 135 to 200 mg/m^2 as a 24-h infusion every 3 weeks.
2. 135 to 225 mg/m^2 as a 3-h infusion every 3 weeks.
3. 100 mg/m^2 as a 3-h infusion every 2 weeks for the treatment of AIDS-related Kaposi's sarcoma.
4. 80 to 100 mg/m^2 as a 1-h weekly infusion.
5. 200 mg/m^2 as a 1-h infusion every 3 weeks.

Special precautions. Anaphylactoid reactions with dyspnea, hypotension (or occasionally hypertension), bronchospasm, urticaria, and erythematous rashes may occur as a result of the paclitaxel itself or the Cremophor vehicle required to make paclitaxel water soluble. Such reaction is minimized but not totally prevented by pretreatment with antihistamines and corticosteroids and by prolonging the infusion rate (to 24 h). Paclitaxel must be filtered with a 0.2-μm in-line filter.

Standard pretreatment regimen.
1. Dexamethasone 20 mg IV for doses greater than 100 mg/m^2 and 10 mg IV for doses less than or equal to 100 mg/m^2 30 to 60 min prior to treatment.
2. Diphenhydramine 50 mg IV 30 to 60 min before treatment.
3. Histamine H$_2$-receptor antagonist IV 30 to 60 min before treatment. (e.g., cimetidine 300 mg).

Toxicity.
1. *Myelosuppression and other hematologic effects.* Granulocytopenia is universal and dose limiting; thrombocytopenia is common; anemia is occasional.
2. *Nausea, vomiting, and other gastrointestinal effects.* Common but usually not severe.
3. *Mucocutaneous effects.* Alopecia is universal; mucositis is occasional at recommended doses.
4. *Hypersensitivity reactions.* Dyspnea, hypotension (or occasionally hypertension), bronchospasm, urticaria, and erythematous rashes are occasionally seen, despite precautions.
5. *Miscellaneous effects.*
   a. Sensory neuropathy is common (30% to 35%) and may be progressively worse with time. Recovery may take months to years.
   b. Hepatic dysfunction is uncommon.
   c. Diarrhea is occasional and mild.
   d. Myalgias and arthralgias are common (25%).
   e. Seizures are rare.

f.   Abnormal electrocardiogram is occasional. If clinically significant bradycardia, stop drug. Restart at slower rate when stable.

PAMIDRONATE

Other name. Aredia.

Mechanism of action. A bisphosphonate that inhibits osteoclastic resorption of bone and calcium release induced by tumor cytokines.

Primary indications.
1.   Hypercalcemia associated with malignancy.
2.   Osteolytic bone metastases of breast cancer.
3.   Osteolytic and osteoporotic bone lesions of multiple myeloma.
4.   Paget's disease.

Usual dosage and schedule.
1.   *Multiple myeloma.* 90 mg IV as a 4-h infusion every month.
2.   *Breast cancer.* 90 mg IV as a 2-h infusion every 3 to 4 weeks.
3.   *Hypercalcemia of malignancy.* 60 to 90 mg IV as a 4- to 24-h infusion. May be repeated every 1 to 8 weeks, as needed.

Special precautions. Potential for renal tubular damage, particularly if infused more rapidly. Renal clearance parallels creatinine clearance, but adverse effects do not appear to be worse with decreased clearance when given on a monthly basis. Serum electrolytes and renal function should be monitored closely.

Toxicity.
1.   *Myelosuppression and other hematologic effects.* Rare.
2.   *Nausea, vomiting, and other gastrointestinal effects.* Abdominal pain, anorexia, constipation, nausea, and vomiting are uncommon to occasional.
3.   *Mucocutaneous effects.* Infusion site reaction is occasional.
4.   *Miscellaneous effects.*
     a.   Fatigue is occasional.
     b.   Laboratory abnormalities are occasional (hypocalcemia, hypokalemia, hypomagnesemia, and hypophosphatemia, particularly at the 90-mg dose).
     c.   Uveitis, iritis, scleritis, and episcleritis are rare.
     d.   Bone pain and generalized pain are occasional.
     e.   Renal tubular damage uncommon.

PEGFILGRASTIM

Other names. Neulasta, Pegylated G-CSF.

Mechanism of action. Pegfilgrastim is recombinant granulocyte-stimulating factor (G-CSF) that is conjugated to polyethylene glycol. This delays renal clearance and increases the serum half-life from about 3.5 to about 15 to 80 h after a single SC injection. Promotes growth and differentiation of myeloid progenitor cells. May improve survival and function of granulocytes.

Primary indications. Prophylaxis of granulocytopenia and associated infection in patients who are at high risk from chemotherapy for nonmyeloid malignancies.

Usual dosage and schedule. 6 mg SC once (usually on day 2) for each 21- or 28-day chemotherapy cycle. Should not be given between 14 days before and 24 h after each chemotherapy cycle.

Special precautions.
1. Use with caution in disorders of myeloid stem cells as it may promote growth of leukemic cells.
2. The fixed-dose formulation should not be used in infants, children, and others weighing less than 45 kg.

Toxicity.
1. *Myelosuppression and other hematologic effects.* None (leukocytosis).
2. *Nausea, vomiting, and other gastrointestinal effects.* Rare to uncommon.
3. *Mucocutaneous effects.* Exacerbation of pre-existing dermatologic conditions is occasional; pyoderma gangrenosum is possible.
4. *Miscellaneous effects.* Usually mild and short lived.
   a. Bone pain, musculoskeletal symptoms such as cramps, and back or leg pain are common.
   b. Splenomegaly with prolonged use is possible. Splenic rupture has been reported with the parent compound filgrastim.
   c. Exacerbation of pre-existing inflammatory or auto-immune disorders is rare.
   d. Mild elevation of lactate dehydrogenase and alkaline phosphatase.
   e. Allergic-type reactions may occur, as they have been seen with the parent compound filgrastim.
   f. Adult respiratory distress syndrome has been reported in neutropenic patients receiving filgrastim and is possible with pegfilgrastim.

PEMETREXED (INVESTIGATIONAL)

Other names. Multitargeted antifolate (MTA), LY231514, Alimta.
Mechanism of action. Inhibition of thymidylate synthase, dihydrofolate reductase, and glycinamide ribonucleotide formyltransferase through pemetrexed's polyglutamated metabolites.
Primary indications.
1. Mesothelioma.
2. Carcinomas of the head and neck, breast, colon, and pancreas and non–small cell lung cancer.

Usual dosage and schedule. 500 to 600 mg/m^2 IV over 10 min every 21 days.
Special precautions.
1. Sporadic life-threatening toxicity may be caused by functional folate deficiency. Administration of folic acid 0.35 to 1 mg PO daily prior to and during drug administration and vitamin B$_{12}$ 1,000 µg IM every 9 weeks during therapy is recommended to decrease the frequency of grade 3 and 4 hematologic and other toxicity (perhaps in part from increased homocysteine formation).
2. Skin toxicity may also be reduced by dexamethasone 4 mg PO b.i.d. on the day prior, the day of therapy, and the day after therapy.

Toxicity.
1. *Myelosuppression and other hematologic effects.* Neutropenia is common. Grade 1 or 2 anemia is common. Significant thrombocytopenia is occasional.

2. *Nausea, vomiting, and other gastrointestinal effects.* Nausea and vomiting are common (35%). Diarrhea is occasional.
3. *Mucocutaneous effects.* Grade 2 to 3 skin toxicities are common (reduced by dexamethasone). Alopecia is occasional. Grade 1 or 2 stomatitis is common.
4. *Miscellaneous effects.*
   a. Elevations of bilirubin or transaminases are common but only occasionally grade 3 or higher.
   b. Fatigue is common.
   c. Pericarditis is uncommon to occasional.

PENTOSTATIN

Other names. 2′-Deoxycoformycin, Nipent.

Mechanism of action. Inhibition of adenosine deaminase, particularly in the presence of adenosine or deoxyadenosine, leads to cytotoxicity. Is associated with block of DNA synthesis through inhibition of ribonucleotide reductase. Other effects that may contribute to cytotoxicity include inhibition of RNA synthesis and increased DNA damage.

Primary indications.
1. Hairy-cell leukemia.
2. Chronic lymphocytic leukemia.
3. Other lymphoid neoplasms.
4. Mycosis fungoides.

Usual dosage and schedule. 4 mg/m^2 IV push over 1 to 2 min or diluted in a larger volume over 20 to 30 min. Patients should be given hydration with 500 to 1,000 mL of 5% dextrose in 0.5 N saline or equivalent before pentostatin administration and 500 mL after the drug is given. Repeat every 2 weeks.

Special precautions.
1. Hydration required to ensure urine output of 2 L daily on the day pentostatin is administered. Patients often are hospitalized for their first drug administration. Allopurinol 300 mg b.i.d. is recommended in patients with a large tumor mass. Sedative and hypnotic drugs should be used with caution or not at all because CNS toxicity may be potentiated. Dose reduction or discontinuation needed for renal impairment (creatinine clearance under 50 mL/min).
2. Should not be used in combination with fludarabine because of a high probability of severe or fatal pulmonary toxicity.

Toxicity.
1. *Myelosuppression.* Common but severity variable.
2. *Nausea, vomiting, and other gastrointestinal effects.* Nausea and vomiting are common but usually not severe. Diarrhea is occasional. Hepatic dysfunction is occasional at recommended doses.
3. *Mucocutaneous effects.* Mucositis is rare; skin rashes and pruritus are occasional to common.
4. *Pulmonary effects.* Cough is common, and dyspnea is occasional. Higher doses or use in combination of fludarabine may lead to severe pulmonary toxicity.
5. *Miscellaneous effects.*
   a. Fatigue is common.
   b. Chills and fever are common.

    c. Infections, probably related both to myelosuppression and to lymphocytopenia, are occasional.

    d. Renal insufficiency is rare at usual doses.

    e. High doses may cause serious neurologic and psychiatric symptoms, including seizures, mental confusion, irritability, and coma.

PORFIMER

Other name. Photofrin.

Mechanism of action. Photosensitizing agent. Cellular damage occurs as a result of light-induced radical reactions, including superoxide and hydroxyl radicals.

Primary indications.

1. Obstructing esophageal cancers.
2. Completely or partially obstructing endobronchial non–small cell lung cancer.
3. Microinvasive endobronchial non–small cell lung cancer in patients for whom surgery and radiotherapy are not indicated.

Usual dosage and schedule. 2 mg/kg as a slow IV injection over 3 to 5 min. This is followed by illumination with laser light 40 to 50 h following injection of porfimer. A second course may be given after a minimum of 30 days.

Special precautions.

1. Contraindicated in patients with porphyria and tracheoesophageal or bronchoesophageal fistulas.
2. Contraindicated if tumor is eroding into a major blood vessel.
3. Patients must avoid exposure of skin and eyes to direct sunlight or bright indoor light for 30 days to minimize severe photosensitivity reactions. Sunscreens are of no value.

Toxicity.

1. *Myelosuppression and other hematologic effects.* No marrow suppression, but anemia is common.
2. *Nausea, vomiting, and other gastrointestinal effects.* Nausea and vomiting are occasional to common. Other gastrointestinal effects including abdominal pain and constipation are occasional.
3. *Cutaneous effects.* Photosensitivity reaction is occasional to common, particularly if extravasates at injection site. See Special Precautions above.
4. *Miscellaneous effects.*
   a. Atrial fibrillation is occasional. Hypertension, hypotension, and tachycardia are occasional.
   b. Occasional cough, dyspnea, pleural effusion, pneumonia, and respiratory insufficiency have been seen.
   c. Ocular discomfort may be seen, particularly from bright light.
   d. Anxiety, anorexia, confusion, and insomnia are occasional.
   e. Occasional asthenia, back pain, chest pain, and other pain. (Chest pain is probably from inflammatory response within area of treatment.)

PROCARBAZINE

Other name. Matulane.
Mechanism of action. Uncertain but appears to affect preformed DNA, RNA, and protein.
Primary indications.
1. Hodgkin's and non-Hodgkin's lymphomas.
2. Brain tumors.
3. Melanoma.

Usual dosage and schedule. 60 to 100 mg/m^2 PO daily for 7 to 14 days every 4 weeks (in combination with other drugs).
Special precautions. Many food and drug interactions are possible, although their clinical significance may be low.

Drug or food	Possible result
Ethanol	Disulfiram-like reactions: nausea, vomiting, visual disturbances, headache
Sympathomimetics, tricyclic antidepressants, tyramine-rich foods (cheese, wine, bananas)	Hypertensive crisis, tremors, excitation, angina, cardiac palpitations
CNS depressants	Additive depression

Toxicity.
1. *Myelosuppression and other hematologic effects.* Pancytopenia is dose limiting. Recovery may be delayed.
2. *Nausea, vomiting, and other gastrointestinal effects.* Nausea is frequent during first few days until tolerance develops. Diarrhea is uncommon but may be severe.
3. *Mucocutaneous effects.*
   a. Stomatitis is uncommon.
   b. Alopecia, pruritus, and drug rash are uncommon.
4. *CNS effects.* Paresthesias, neuropathies, headache, dizziness, depression, apprehension, nervousness, insomnia, nightmares, hallucinations, ataxia, confusion, convulsions, and coma have been reported with varying frequency.
5. *Miscellaneous effects.*
   a. Secondary neoplasia is possible. Acute leukemia and lung cancer have been reported. Risk for lung cancer is increased by smoking.
   b. Visual disturbances are rare.
   c. Postural hypotension is rare.
   d. Hypersensitivity reactions are rare.
   e. Teratogenesis is strong potential.

PROGESTINS

Other names. Medroxyprogesterone acetate (Provera, Depo-Provera), hydroxyprogesterone caproate (Delalutin), megestrol acetate (Megace).
Mechanism of action. Mechanisms of antitumor effects or for appetite stimulation are not clear.
Primary indications.
1. Appetite stimulation.
2. Endometrial and breast carcinomas.

Usual dosage and schedule.
1. *As appetite stimulant.* Megestrol acetate 160 to 800 mg PO daily.
2. *As antineoplastic.* Megestrol acetate 80 to 320 mg PO daily; medroxyprogesterone acetate 1,000 to 1,500 mg IM weekly or 400 to 800 mg PO twice weekly; hydroxyprogesterone caproate 1,000 to 1,500 mg IM weekly.

Special precautions.
1. Acute local hypersensitivity or dyspnea due to oil in IM preparations is uncommon.
2. Hypercalcemia with initial therapy is occasional, particularly in patients with bone metastasis.

Toxicity.
1. *Myelosuppression and other hematologic effects.* None.
2. *Nausea, vomiting, and other gastrointestinal effects.* Rare.
3. *Mucocutaneous effects.* Mild alopecia and skin rash are uncommon.
4. *Miscellaneous effects.*
   a. Mild fluid retention is occasional to common.
   b. Mild liver function abnormalities are occasional; intrahepatic cholestasis may occur.
   c. Menstrual irregularities are common.
   d. Improved appetite and weight gain are common.

RALOXIFENE

Other name. Evista.

Mechanism of action. A selective estrogen receptor modulator that inhibits estrogen effects by competing with estrogen for binding on the cytosol estrogen receptor protein in normal and cancer cells. The receptor–hormone complex ultimately controls the promoter region of genes that affect cell growth. Effects may manifest as estrogen agonistic or antagonistic, depending on the tissue and other modifying factors. Has estrogen-like effects on bone, increasing bone mineral density.

Primary indications.
1. Prevention of osteoporosis in postmenopausal women.
2. Breast cancer prevention in postmenopausal women.

Usual dosage and schedule. 60 mg PO daily.

Special precautions.
1. Not recommended as primary cancer preventive agent for most women except under auspices of a controlled clinical trial.
2. Contraindicated in women with active or past history of venous thromboembolic events including deep vein thrombosis, pulmonary embolism, and retinal vein thrombosis.
3. May cause fetal harm if administered to a pregnant woman.

Toxicity.
1. *Myelosuppression and other hematologic effects.* Uncommon and mild.
2. *Nausea, vomiting, and other gastrointestinal effects.* Uncommon.
3. *Mucocutaneous effects.* Rash, sweating, and vaginitis are uncommon.

4. *Miscellaneous effects.*
   a. Thromboembolic events including deep vein thrombosis, pulmonary embolism, and retinal vein thrombosis are rare.
   b. Leg cramps are uncommon to occasional.
   c. Hot flashes are common.
   d. Lowers total cholesterol and low-density lipoprotein cholesterol.
5. *Carcinogenesis.* No apparent endometrial proliferation or increase in endometrial cancer.

RALTITREXED (INVESTIGATIONAL)

Other name. Tomudex.
Mechanism of action. Raltitrexed is a quinazoline antifolate that is a direct specific inhibitor of thymidylate synthase and thus blocks the conversion of uridylate to thymidylate and consequent DNA synthesis.
Primary indication. Colorectal carcinoma.
Usual dosage and schedule. 3 mg/m^2 IV over 15 min every 3 weeks.
Special precautions. None.
Toxicity.
1. *Myelosuppression and other hematologic effects.* Common and severe or worse 20% to 25% of time.
2. *Nausea, vomiting, and other gastrointestinal effects.* Nausea and vomiting are common and occasionally severe. Diarrhea is occasional.
3. *Mucocutaneous effects.* Mucositis is occasional and rarely severe.
4. *Miscellaneous effects.* Elevation of liver transaminase levels is occasional.

RITUXIMAB

Other name. Rituxan.
Mechanism of action. Rituximab is a genetically engineered chimeric (murine and human) monoclonal antibody directed against the CD20 antigen found on the surface of normal cells and in high copy number on malignant B lymphocytes (but not stem cells). The F_{ab} domain of rituximab binds to the CD20 antigen on B lymphocytes and B-cell non-Hodgkin's lymphomas, and the F_c domain recruits immune effector functions to mediate B-cell lysis.
Primary indications.
1. Non-Hodgkin's B-cell lymphoma that is low grade or follicular, CD20 positive, and refractory to conventional therapy.
2. Non-Hodgkin's B-cell lymphoma other than low grade or follicular, often in combination or sequence with other therapy.
Usual dosage and schedule. 375 mg/m^2 given as a slow IV infusion, initially at a rate of 50 mg/h. If hypersensitivity or other infusion-related events do not occur, escalate in 50-mg/h increments to a maximum of 400 mg/h. Usually takes 4 to 6 h to infuse initial therapy. Interrupt or slow the infusion rate for infusion-related events. Repeat the dose once weekly for four to eight

doses. Premedication with acetaminophen and diphenhydramine may attenuate infusion-related symptoms. Corticosteroids should not be used for premedication.

Special precautions. An infusion-related set of symptoms consisting of fever and chills, with or without true rigors, occurs commonly during the first infusion. Other hypersensitivity symptoms including nausea, urticaria, fatigue, headache, pruritus, bronchospasm, dyspnea, sensation of tongue or throat swelling, rhinitis, vomiting, hypotension, flushing, and pain at disease sites may also be seen. Rarely infusion-related events result in a fatal outcome. Fatal reactions have followed a symptom complex that includes hypoxia, pulmonary infiltrates, acute respiratory distress syndrome, myocardial infarction, ventricular fibrillation, and cardiogenic shock. Hypersensitivity reactions generally start within 30 to 120 min of starting the infusion. Most will resolve with slowing or interruption of the infusion and with supportive care, including IV saline, diphenhydramine, and acetaminophen. Severe reactions will additionally require aggressive cardiorespiratory support including oxygen, epinephrine, vasopressors, corticosteroids, and bronchodilators and may preclude additional treatment with rituximab. The rate of infusion events decreases from 80% during the first infusion to 40% during subsequent infusions.

Toxicity.

1. *Myelosuppression and other hematologic effects.* Uncommon. However, B-cell depletion occurs in 70% to 80% of patients, with decreased immunoglobulins in a minority of patients. Infectious events occur in about 30% of patients treated with rituximab, but only uncommonly are they severe.

2. *Nausea, vomiting, and other gastrointestinal effects.* Nausea is common (23%) but rarely severe. Vomiting and diarrhea are occasional.

3. *Mucocutaneous effects.* Pruritus, rash, urticaria, and night sweats are occasional. Severe mucocutaneous reactions including Stevens–Johnson syndrome, lichenoid dermatitis, vesiculobullous dermatitis, and toxic epidermal necrolysis are rare but have been reported from 1 to 13 weeks following rituximab exposure.

4. *Miscellaneous effects.*

    a. Infusion-related hypersensitivity reaction (may include fever, chills, headache, myalgia, weakness, nausea, urticaria, pruritus, throat irritation, rhinitis, dizziness, and hypertension) is common but usually resolves with interrupting or slowing the rate of the infusion and administration of supportive therapy; see Special Precautions above.

    b. Myalgia and arthralgia are occasional. Rarely, a serum sickness-like reaction may be seen that requires corticosteroid therapy.

    c. Hypotension is occasional but rarely severe. Chest pain, bronchospasm, tachycardia, edema, and postural hypotension are uncommon. Severe angioedema, arrhythmia, and angina are rare.

    d. Renal failure, possibly requiring dialysis, has been seen, particularly in association with tumor lysis syndrome in patients with high tumor cell burden.

SARGRAMOSTIM

Other names. Granulocyte–macrophage colony-stimulating factor, GM-CSF, Leukine.

Mechanism of action. Promotes growth and differentiation of myeloid progenitor cells. May improve survival and function of granulocytes, eosinophils, monocytes, and macrophages. Induces release of secondary cytokines (interleukin-1 and tumor necrosis factor).

Primary indications.
1. Myeloid reconstitution after peripheral blood or bone marrow progenitor cell transplantation.
2. Neutrophil recovery following chemotherapy in acute myelogenous leukemia.
3. Mobilization of peripheral blood progenitor cells.
4. Granulocytopenia from primary marrow disorders such as myelodysplastic syndrome and aplastic anemia.
5. Granulocytopenia associated with AIDS and its therapy.

Usual dosage and schedule.
1. *Myeloid reconstitution after autologous stem cell transplantation.* 250 µg/m^2 IV daily as a 2-h infusion beginning 2 to 4 h after the autologous stem cell infusion and not less than 24 h after the last dose of chemotherapy or less than 12 h after the last dose of radiotherapy. Continue for 21 days or until the absolute neutrophil count reaches 20,000/µL.
2. *Bone marrow transplantation failure or engraftment delay.* 250 µg/m^2 daily for 14 days as 2-h IV infusion. If no marrow recovery, may be repeated in 7 days at same or higher dose (500 µg/m^2). Dose and duration are dependent on the response.
3. *Mobilization of peripheral blood progenitor cells.* The recommended dose is 250 µg/m^2/day administered IV over 24 h or SC once daily. Dosing should continue at the same dose through the period of peripheral blood progenitor cell collection.
4. *Neutrophil recovery following chemotherapy in acute myelogenous leukemia.* 250 µg/m^2/day administered IV over a 4-h period starting 4 days following the completion of induction chemotherapy and continuing until the absolute neutrophil count is greater than 1,500 cells/µL for 3 consecutive days or a maximum of 42 days.
5. *Aplastic anemia, myelodysplastic syndrome, and AIDS.* Doses may be much lower (50 to 100 µg/m^2 SC or IM daily).

Special precautions. Flushing, tachycardia, dyspnea, and nausea occur commonly with the first dose of IV therapy; do not infuse over less than 2 h; longer infusion may help.

Toxicity.
1. *Myelosuppression and other hematologic effects.* None (leukocytosis).
2. *Nausea, vomiting, and other gastrointestinal effects.* Occasional.
3. *Mucocutaneous effects.* Rash is uncommon; exacerbation of pre-existing dermatologic conditions is occasional; mild local reactions at injection site are common.
4. *Miscellaneous effects.* Usually mild and short lived at standard doses, but with increasing dose may be more severe.

a. Bone pain, musculoskeletal symptoms such as cramps, and back or leg pain are common.
b. Pericarditis, fluid retention, and venous thrombosis are dose related and uncommon at standard doses.
c. Flu-like symptoms (fever, chills, aches, headache) are occasional at standard doses and common at higher doses.

STREPTOZOCIN

Other names. Streptozotocin, Zanosar.
Mechanism of action. Inhibition of DNA synthesis, possibly by interference with pyridine nucleotide synthesis. Streptozocin appears to have some specificity for neoplastic pancreatic endocrine cells. Glucose moiety attached to nitrosourea appears to diminish myelotoxicity.
Primary indications.
1. Pancreatic islet cell and pancreatic exocrine carcinomas.
2. Carcinoid tumors.
Usual dosage and schedule.
1. 1.0 to 1.5 g/m^2 IV weekly for 6 weeks followed by 4 weeks of observation.
2. 1.0 g/m^2 IV days 1 and 8 in combination with fluorouracil and mitomycin. Repeat every 4 weeks.
3. 500 mg/m^2 IV on days 1 to 5 every 6 weeks.
Special precautions.
1. A 30- to 60-min infusion is recommended to reduce local pain and burning around the vein during treatment.
2. Avoid extravasation.
3. Have 50% glucose available to treat sudden hypoglycemia.
Toxicity.
1. *Myelosuppression and other hematologic effects.* Uncommon and mild.
2. *Nausea, vomiting, and other gastrointestinal effects.* Nausea and vomiting are common and severe. May become progressively worse over 5-day course of therapy.
3. *Mucocutaneous effects.* Uncommon.
4. *Nephrotoxicity.* Renal toxicity is common. Although it is not clearly dose related, it may limit continued drug use in individual patients. Proteinuria, glucosuria, azotemia, and hypophosphatemia, if persistent or severe, are indications to discontinue therapy. Hydration may ameliorate the problem.
5. *Miscellaneous effects.*
   a. In patients with insulinoma, hypoglycemia may be severe (although transient) owing to a burst of insulin release.
   b. Hyperglycemia is uncommon in normal or diabetic patients, as normal beta cells are usually insensitive to streptozocin's effect.
   c. Transient mild hepatotoxicity is occasional.
   d. Second malignancies are possible.

SURAMIN (INVESTIGATIONAL)

Other names. Antrypol, Bayer 205, Germanin, Moranyl, Naganol, Naphuride NA.
Mechanism of action. Glycosaminoglycan agonist–antagonist that blocks the binding of growth factors to their receptors. Growth

factors affected include platelet-derived growth factor, transforming growth factor-β, and heparin-binding growth factor-2 (also known as basic fibroblast growth factor). Inhibits DNA polymerases, reverse transcriptase, and other proteins. Inhibits glycosaminoglycan metabolism.

Primary indications.
1. Prostate carcinoma that is hormone refractory.
2. High-grade gliomas.

Usual dosage and schedule. A loading dose of 1,000 mg/m^2 is infused over 2 h on day 1. One-hour infusions of 400, 300, 250, and 200 mg/m^2 are given on days 2, 3, 4, and 5, respectively, followed by 275-mg/m^2 infusions twice a week for 2 weeks (days 8, 11, 15, and 19) and once weekly thereafter through week 12. This dosing regimen is designed to achieve a sustained suramin plasma concentration of 100 to 300 μg/mL. Various other schedules are used to achieve a similar plasma level.

Special precautions.
1. Measurement of plasma levels has been advocated in many studies to achieve the narrow concentration that is therapeutic and not prohibitively toxic. Therapy should be held if the plasma concentration exceeds 300 μg/mL.
2. Because of adrenal suppression, patients require hydrocortisone 25 mg in the morning and 15 mg at bedtime.
3. Prothrombin time should be followed closely as coagulopathy may develop.

Toxicity.
1. *Myelosuppression and other hematologic effects.* Common but usually not severe.
2. *Nausea, vomiting, and other gastrointestinal effects.* Uncommon.
3. *Mucocutaneous effects.* Transient erythematous rash is common.
4. *Adrenocortical insufficiency.* Common.
5. *Neurotoxicity.* Paresthesias are seen commonly and severe polyradiculopathy occasionally. Motor weakness may be seen following termination of therapy. The degree of toxicity appears to be related to the plasma suramin level, with acute serious reactions uncommon at plasma levels of less than 350 μg/mL.
6. *Miscellaneous effects.*
   a. Vortex keratopathy with photophobia, tearing, and blurred vision are common.
   b. Liver function abnormalities are common but reversible.
   c. Coagulopathy is occasional with elevations of the prothrombin time, partial thromboplastin time, and thrombin time, with increased risk of spontaneous bleeding.
   d. Proteinuria is common; decrease in creatinine clearance is occasional.
   e. Malaise, fatigue, and lethargy are common after 2 to 4 months of therapy.

TAMOXIFEN

Other name. Nolvadex.

Mechanism of action. Tamoxifen is a selective estrogen receptor modulator that inhibits estrogen effects by competing with estrogen for binding on the cytosol estrogen receptor protein in cancer cells. This complex is probably transported into the nucleus, where it affects nucleic acid function. It also has effects on cellular growth factors, epidermal growth factors, and transforming growth factors-α and -β.

Primary indications.

1. Breast carcinoma.
   a. Metastatic tumors in postmenopausal or premenopausal women with estrogen receptor–positive (or unknown) tumors.
   b. Adjuvant therapy in women with estrogen receptor–positive (or progesterone receptor–positive) tumors after primary therapy. Optimal duration of therapy for most women is probably limited to 5 years.
   c. Breast cancer prevention in very high-risk women.
2. Melanoma, in combination with other drugs (controversial).

Usual dosage and schedule.

1. 20 mg PO as single daily dose.
2. 10 mg PO twice daily.

Special precautions.

1. Hypercalcemia may be seen during initial therapy.
2. Not recommended as primary cancer preventive agent for most women except under auspices of a controlled clinical trial.

Toxicity.

1. *Myelosuppression and other hematologic effects.* Uncommon and mild.
2. *Nausea, vomiting, and other gastrointestinal effects.* Nausea occurs early in the course of therapy in up to 20% of patients but abates rapidly as therapy is continued. Diarrhea is occasional.
3. *Mucocutaneous effects.* Cataracts and other eye toxicities have been observed, but effects due to drug are uncommon. Skin rash and pruritus vulvae are uncommon. May cause increase or marked decrease in vaginal secretions and result in difficult or painful intercourse.
4. *Miscellaneous effects.*
   a. Hot flashes are common.
   b. Vaginal bleeding and menstrual irregularity are uncommon to occasional.
   c. Lassitude, headache, leg cramps, and dizziness are uncommon.
   d. Peripheral edema is occasional.
   e. Increased bone pain, tumor pain, and local disease flare (associated both with good tumor response as well as with tumor progression) are occasional.
   f. Slowed progression of osteoporosis.
   g. Reduction in serum cholesterol with favorable changes in lipid profile.
   h. Thromboembolic phenomena are rare.
   i. Liver function test abnormalities are occasional.
5. *Carcinogenesis.* Uterine carcinomas are rare (two to four times the predicted incidence in adjuvant trials). Uterine sarcomas are very rare.

TEMOZOLOMIDE

Other name. Temodar.

Mechanism of action. Undergoes rapid conversion to the reactive substituted imidazole carboxamide MTIC. This compound is believed to be active primarily through alkylation (methylation) of DNA at the O^6 and N^7 positions of guanine.

Primary indications.
1. Anaplastic astrocytoma that is refractory to nitrosoureas.
2. Other gliomas.
3. Metastatic carcinoma to the brain.

Usual dosage and schedule.
1. 150 to 200 mg/m² PO on an empty stomach daily for 5 days every 28 days.
2. 75 mg/m² PO on an empty stomach daily during radiation therapy for up to 7 weeks.

Special precautions. Contraindicated in patients with a hypersensitivity to dacarbazine (DTIC), because both drugs are metabolized to MTIC.

Toxicity.
1. *Myelosuppression and other hematologic effects.* Some myelosuppression is common, but only occasionally is it severe.
2. *Nausea, vomiting, and other gastrointestinal effects.* Nausea, vomiting, and constipation are common but only occasionally severe. Occasionally patients may also develop abdominal pain or anorexia.
3. *Mucocutaneous effects.* Rash and pruritus are occasional.
4. *Miscellaneous effects.*
   a. Headache, fatigue, asthenia, and fever are common (20% to 65%).
   b. Peripheral edema is occasional.
   c. Neurologic symptoms are common on temozolomide, but it is difficult to distinguish whether the symptoms are from the drug or from the disease. Common findings are convulsions, hemiparesis, dizziness, abnormal coordination, amnesia, and insomnia. Occasional findings are paresthesias, somnolence, paresis, incontinence, ataxia, dysphasia, gait abnormality, myalgias, and confusion. Diplopia or other visual abnormalities are occasional.
   d. Anxiety and depression are occasional.

TENIPOSIDE

Other names. VM-26, Vumon.

Mechanism of action. Topoisomerase II–mediated double-strand DNA breaks. Causes cell cycle transit delay through S phase and arrest at late S/G_2 phase.

Primary indications.
1. Acute lymphocytic leukemia.
2. Neuroblastoma.
3. Non-Hodgkin's lymphomas.

Usual dosage and schedule.
1. 165 mg/m² IV over 30 to 60 min twice weekly for eight to nine doses (with cytarabine).
2. 250 mg/m² IV over 30 to 60 min weekly for 4 to 8 weeks (with vincristine and prednisone).

Special precautions.
1. Hypersensitivity reactions usually resolve with interruption of the infusion and often can be prevented with diphenhydramine and hydrocortisone pretreatment. Hypotension is alleviated by prolonging the infusion time. It is a possible vesicant.
2. See package insert for IV preparation and administration equipment requirements.

Toxicity.
1. *Myelosuppression and other hematologic effects.* Common and dose limiting.
2. *Nausea, vomiting, and other gastrointestinal effects.* Nausea, vomiting, and diarrhea are common.
3. *Mucocutaneous effects.* Alopecia and mucositis are common.
4. *Miscellaneous effects.*
   a. Hepatic and renal dysfunction are rare.
   b. Hypersensitivity reactions with urticaria and flushing are occasional. Anaphylaxis is uncommon.
   c. Hypotension is related to drug infusion rate but should be seen only occasionally at the recommended dose schedules.
   d. Secondary leukemias are uncommon.
   e. Chemical phlebitis is uncommon.

THALIDOMIDE

Other name. Thalomid.
Mechanism of action. Multiple potential mechanisms, including inhibition of vascular endothelial growth factor, inhibition of tumor necrosis factor-α, direct inhibition of G_1 growth and promotion of apoptosis, and expansion of natural killer cells and co-stimulation of T cells.
Primary indications.
1. Multiple myeloma.
2. Myelodysplastic syndrome.

Usual dosage and schedule. A starting dose of 50 to 100 mg once daily in the evening. The dose is escalated weekly by 50 to 100 mg until the maximum dose specified, commonly up to 400 mg daily.
Special precautions. Severe and life-threatening birth defects, primarily phocomelia, can be caused by taking even a single 50-mg dose. For this reason, special precautions must be taken to ensure that female patients are not pregnant when the drug is started and that both female and male patients practice strict birth control measures.
Toxicity.
1. *Myelosuppression and other hematologic effects.* None to minimal myelosuppression. Occasional deep venous thrombosis.
2. *Nausea, vomiting, and other gastrointestinal effects.* Constipation is common.
3. *Mucocutaneous effects.* Macular rash, usually involving the trunk, is common. Alopecia is uncommon. Rare severe or life-threatening epidermal damage.
4. *Miscellaneous effects.*
   a. Dose-dependent somnolence and dizziness are common. Tolerance usually develops to the sedative effects.

Dizziness may be related to hypotension and can be minimized by adequate hydration and avoidance of rapid postural changes.
  b. Peripheral neuropathy is common (25%) with chronic therapy. Occasional patients develop myalgia, tremor, or muscle spasms.
  c. Fatigue is common.
  d. Headache is occasional.
  e. Edema is occasional to common.
  f. Hypothyroidism is occasional.
  g. Birth defects (see Special Precautions above).
  h. Hypercoagulability with deep venous thrombosis is occasional.

THIOGUANINE

Other names. 6-Thioguanine, 6-TG, Tabloid.
Mechanism of action. A purine antimetabolite that, when converted to the active nucleotide, substitutes for the normal guanine nucleotide in DNA synthesis. Thioguanine also inhibits purine synthesis and conversion reactions.
Primary indication. Acute nonlymphocytic leukemia.
Usual dosage and schedule.
  1. *Induction.* 100 mg/m^2 PO twice daily on days 1 to 5 (with other drugs).
  2. *Maintenance.* 100 mg/m^2 PO twice daily on days 1 to 5 every 4 weeks (with other drugs).
Special precautions. None (no dose reduction required for concurrent use of allopurinol).
Toxicity.
  1. *Myelosuppression and other hematologic effects.* Major dose-limiting toxicity.
  2. *Nausea, vomiting, and other gastrointestinal effects.* Nausea and vomiting are occasional but not severe. Diarrhea is uncommon.
  3. *Mucocutaneous effects.*
      a. Stomatitis that may necessitate reduction of the dose is uncommon.
      b. Drug rash is rare.
  4. *Miscellaneous effects.*
      a. Hepatotoxicity is rare.
      b. Hyperuricemia with rapid tumor cell lysis is common.

THIOTEPA

Other names. Triethylenethiophosphoramide, Thioplex.
Mechanism of action. Alkylating agent similar to mechlorethamine.
Primary indications.
  1. Superficial papillary carcinoma of urinary bladder.
  2. Malignant peritoneal, pleural, or pericardial effusions.
  3. Carcinoma of breast and ovary.
  4. Neoplastic meningeal infiltrates.

Usual dosage and schedule.
1. 12 mg/m^2 IV bolus every 3 weeks in combination with vinblastine and doxorubicin for breast cancer.
2. 30 to 60 mg in 40 to 50 mL of water instilled into the bladder and retained for 1 h. Dose is repeated weekly for 3 to 6 weeks, then every 3 weeks for five cycles.
3. 25 to 30 mg/m^2 in 50 to 100 mL of saline solution as a single intracavitary injection. Dose may be repeated as tolerated by blood counts.
4. 10 to 15 mg intrathecally.
5. High-dose therapy with 500 to 1,000 mg/m^2 over 3 days has been used followed by stem cell rescue (e.g., bone marrow transplantation).

Special precaution. Dose should be reduced in patients with impaired renal function, as the drug is excreted primarily in the urine.
Toxicity.
1. *Myelosuppression and other hematologic effects.* Dose-limiting. pancytopenia and sepsis may follow intravesical or intracavitary administration. Nadir counts are reached in 1 to 2 weeks; recovery by 4 weeks is usual.
2. *Nausea, vomiting, and other gastrointestinal effects.* Uncommon.
3. *Mucocutaneous effects.* Uncommon. Thiotepa is *not* a vesicant. Hyperpigmentation of skin occurs at high doses.
4. *Miscellaneous effects.*
    a. Local pain, dizziness, headache, and fever are uncommon.
    b. Secondary neoplasms are possible.
    c. Amenorrhea and azoospermia are common.
    d. CNS effects occur with high-dose therapy.

TOPOTECAN

Other name. Hycamptin.
Mechanism of action. Topotecan, a semisynthetic derivative of camptothecin, is a potent inhibitor of topoisomerase I, an enzyme essential for effective replication and transcription. It binds to the topoisomerase I–DNA cleavable complex, preventing religation after cleavage by topoisomerase I.
Primary indications.
1. Ovarian carcinoma.
2. Small cell and non–small cell carcinoma of the lung.
Usual dosage and schedule. 1.5 mg/m^2 IV as a 30-min infusion daily × 5 every 3 weeks.
Special precautions. None.
Toxicity.
1. *Myelosuppression and other hematologic effects.* Leukopenia is universal and dose limiting. Anemia and thrombocytopenia are common and occasionally severe.
2. *Nausea, vomiting, and other gastrointestinal effects.* Nausea, vomiting, and diarrhea are common but usually mild. Other gastrointestinal symptoms including constipation and abdominal pain occur occasionally.
3. *Mucocutaneous effects.* Alopecia is common; stomatitis is occasional but usually mild; skin rash is rare.

4.   *Miscellaneous effects.*
   a.   Fever, headache, fatigue, and weakness are common (15% to 25%) but rarely severe.
   b.   Microscopic hematuria is occasional.
   c.   Dyspnea occurs occasionally, but it is uncommon for it to be severe.
   d.   Infection as a consequence of severe leukopenia is common.

TOREMIFENE

Other name. Fareston.
Mechanism of action. A selective estrogen receptor modulator that inhibits estrogen effects by competing with estrogen for binding on the cytosol estrogen receptor protein in cancer cells. The receptor–hormone complex ultimately controls the promoter region of genes that affect cell growth.
Primary indication. Metastatic carcinoma of the breast in postmenopausal women with estrogen receptor–positive (or unknown) tumors.
Usual dosage and schedule. 60 mg PO daily.
Special precautions.
1.   Uncertain whether it has any carcinogenic effect on endometrium as has been observed with tamoxifen.
2.   May result in increased prothrombin time in patients taking warfarin (Coumadin).
3.   Cytochrome P-450 3A4 enzyme inhibitors such as phenobarbital, phenytoin, and carbamazepine increase the rate of toremifene metabolism, lowering the concentration in the serum.
Toxicity.
1.   *Myelosuppression and other hematologic effects.* Uncommon and mild.
2.   *Nausea, vomiting, and other gastrointestinal effects.* Minimal nausea is common early in treatment; vomiting is occasional.
3.   *Mucocutaneous effects.* Dry eyes and cataracts are rare. May cause an increase or decrease in vaginal secretions, which may result in difficult or painful intercourse.
4.   *Miscellaneous effects.*
   a.   Hot flashes are common.
   b.   Sweating is occasional.
   c.   Vaginal bleeding and menstrual irregularity are occasional.
   d.   Hypercalcemia is uncommon.
   e.   Thromboembolic phenomena are rare.

^{131}I-TOSITUMOMAB

Other name. Bexxar.
Mechanism of action. ^{131}I-Tositumomab is a murine IgG2a monoclonal anti-CD20 antibody radiolabeled with ^{131}I, an emitter of both beta and gamma radiation. The mechanism of action includes antibody-mediated cytotoxicity and cellularly targeted radiotherapy (radioimmunotherapy).

Primary indications. Non-Hodgkin's lymphoma, chemotherapy refractory, CD20 positive, low grade or transformed low grade.

Usual dosage and schedule. Before dosimetric and therapeutic doses, patients are premedicated with acetaminophen 650 mg and diphenhydramine 50 mg. A saturated solution of potassium iodide, 2 to 3 drops PO three times daily, is given beginning 24 h before the dosimetric dose and continuing for 14 days after the therapeutic dose to prevent uptake of ^{131}I by the thyroid.

1. *Dosimetric dose.* 450 mg of unlabeled tositumomab is given as a 1-h infusion followed by a 20-min infusion of 5 mCi (35 mg) of ^{131}I-tositumomab to determine the patient-specific activity (millicuries) of radiolabeled tositumomab to deliver a therapeutic dose of 65 to 75 cGy 7 to 15 days later.

2. *Therapeutic dose.* 450 mg of unlabeled tositumomab is given as a 1-h infusion followed by a 20-min infusion of patient-specific (in millicuries) activity labeled to 35 mg of tositumomab (median 90 mCi, range 50 to 200 mCi).

Special precautions.

1. Use with caution in patients over 25% marrow involvement with lymphoma, prior external beam radiotherapy to over 25% of the bone marrow, or a history of HAMAs or HACAs.

2. A saturated solution of potassium iodide, 2 to 3 drops PO three times daily, is given beginning 24 h before the dosimetric dose and continuing for 14 days after the therapeutic dose to prevent uptake of ^{131}I by the thyroid.

Toxicity.

1. *Myelosuppression and other hematologic effects.* Myelosuppression is universal, with about 20% of patients having grade 4 thrombocytopenia or neutropenia. The nadir counts occur at a median of 5 to 6 weeks, with recovery to baseline by 10 weeks.

2. *Nausea, vomiting, and other gastrointestinal effects.* Nausea is common; vomiting, abdominal pain, and anorexia are occasional.

3. *Mucocutaneous effects.* Pruritus and rash are occasional.

4. *Miscellaneous effects.*
   a. HAMAs or HACAs may develop (5% to 10%).
   b. Infusion-related fever, chills, dizziness, asthenia, wheezing or coughing, nasal congestion, headache, back pain, arthralgia, and hypotension are occasional to common, more with dosimetric than therapeutic dose. Most commonly these are self-limited and mild to moderate in severity.
   c. Fatigue or asthenia is common.
   d. Cough and edema are occasional; dyspnea is uncommon.
   e. Thyroid suppression is uncommon when prophylaxis with potassium iodide is used.
   f. Myelodysplasia is occasionally seen 20 to 40 months after treatment.

TRASTUZUMAB

Other names. Herceptin.

Mechanism of action. A recombinant humanized monoclonal antibody that targets the extracellular domain of the HER2 growth factor receptor.

Primary indications.
1. Carcinoma of the breast that has overexpression of HER2 (c-erbB-2).
2. Other carcinomas that exhibit overexpression of HER2.

Usual dosage and schedule. 4 mg/kg IV loading dose over 90 min, then 2 mg/kg IV over 30 min weekly.

Special precautions.
1. During the first infusion and occasionally during later infusions, a systemic symptom complex similar to that seen with other human monoclonal antibodies is common. Severe hypersensitivity reactions and pulmonary adverse events have been reported but are uncommon to rare. These events include anaphylaxis, angioedema, bronchospasm, hypotension, hypoxia, dyspnea, pulmonary infiltrates, pleural effusions, noncardiogenic pulmonary edema, and acute respiratory distress syndrome. A more common symptom complex consists of mild to moderate chills, fever, asthenia, pain, nausea, vomiting, and headache. These latter symptoms are generally well managed by temporary slowing or interruption of the infusion and administration of acetaminophen, diphenhydramine, and meperidine.
2. Cardiac dysfunction (cardiac symptoms or an asymptomatic decrease in ejection fraction of 10% or greater) occurs in about 7% of patients treated with trastuzumab alone but in 28% of patients treated with trastuzumab plus anthracycline and in 11% of patients treated with trastuzumab plus paclitaxel. In most cases, this improves with symptomatic therapy. Severe disability or death from cardiac dysfunction occurs in about 1% of patients. Extreme caution should be exercised in treating patients with pre-existing cardiac dysfunction.

Toxicity.
1. *Myelosuppression.* Uncommon.
2. *Nausea, vomiting, and other gastrointestinal effects.* Nausea and vomiting are occasional to common during first infusion. Diarrhea is also occasional to common.
3. *Mucocutaneous effects.* A rash is occasional to common and may be associated with urticaria or pruritus.
4. *Miscellaneous effects.*
   a. Mild to moderate chills, fever, asthenia, pain, and headache are common, primarily during the first infusion.
   b. Cardiac dysfunction occurs in about 7% of patients treated with trastuzumab alone but in 28% of patients treated with trastuzumab plus anthracycline and in 11% of patients treated with trastuzumab plus paclitaxel. In most cases, this improves with symptomatic therapy.
   c. Chest pain, back pain, dyspnea, and cough are occasional to common.
   d. Peripheral edema is occasional.

TRETINOIN

Other names. All-*trans*-retinoic acid, *t*-RNA, ATRA, Vesanoid, Retin-A.

Mechanism of action. Binds to cytoplasmic retinoic acid–binding proteins and is transported to the nucleus where it interacts with nuclear retinoic acid receptors. These then affect expression of the genes that control cell growth and differentiation. In acute promyelocytic leukemia, which characteristically has a chromosomal translocation, t(15:17), abnormal mRNA transcripts are seen for retinoic acid receptor-α, the gene for which is on chromosome 17.

Primary indication. Acute promyelocytic leukemia for induction of remission.

Usual dosage and schedule. 45 mg/m^2 PO daily (divided into two doses in the morning and 6 h later) until 30 days after complete remission is documented, up to a maximum of 90 days.

Special precautions.

1. Avoid use in pregnant women because of marked teratogenic potential. Advise patient to avoid pregnancy by using two reliable contraceptive methods simultaneously.

2. Retinoic acid acute promyelocytic syndrome (see below) may require mechanical ventilation and dexamethasone 10 mg every 12 h at the first signs of fever with respiratory distress until resolution of the acute symptoms (often several days). Continuation of retinoid therapy is controversial.

Toxicity.

1. *Myelosuppression and other hematologic effects.* Myelosuppression is rare. Forty percent of patients develop leukocytosis, which increases the risk of retinoic acid acute promyelocytic syndrome. Disseminated intravascular coagulation is common (26%).

2. *Nausea, vomiting, and other gastrointestinal effects.* Nausea and vomiting, abdominal pain, diarrhea, anorexia, and constipation are common but usually not severe. Gastrointestinal hemorrhage is occasional to common and may be severe. Inflammatory bowel disease is rare.

3. *Mucocutaneous effects.* Universal, particularly at doses at higher end of range. They include redness, dryness, and pruritus of the skin and mucous membranes, increased sweating, possible vesicle formation, peeling of the skin of the palms and soles, cheilitis, and conjunctivitis. There also may be increased skin photosensitivity (e.g., to sun), and the nails may become brittle. Alopecia is uncommon.

4. *Retinoic acid syndrome.* High fever, respiratory distress, weight gain, diffuse pulmonary infiltrates, pleural or pericardial effusions with the possibility of impaired myocardial contractility, and hypotension, with or without concomitant leukocytosis, are common in patients with acute promyelocytic leukemia (25%) (see Chapter 18).

5. *Miscellaneous effects.*
    a. Arrhythmias, flushing, hypotension, hypertension, and phlebitis are occasional. Cardiac failure, cardiac arrest, pulmonary hypertension, and other more severe cardiovascular problems are uncommon.
    b. Cataracts and corneal ulcerations or opacities are uncommon.
    c. Arthralgias, bone pain, and muscle aches are occasional to common; skeletal hyperostosis is common at higher doses (80 mg/m^2/day).
    d. Regarding hypertriglyceridemia, mild to moderate elevations are common; marked elevations (more than five

times normal) are uncommon; hypercholesterolemia occurs to lesser degree.
e. Headache is common; paresthesias, dizziness, and visual disturbances are occasional; lethargy, fatigue, and mental depression are uncommon; pseudotumor cerebri is rare.
f. Hepatotoxicity with increased lactate dehydrogenase, SGOT, SGPT, γ-glutamyl transpeptidase, and alkaline phosphatase is common.
g. Hyperhistaminemia with shock is rare.
h. Renal insufficiency is occasional.
i. Fever, malaise, shivering, and edema are common.

VALRUBICIN

Other name. Valstar.
Mechanism of action. Valrubicin, a semisynthetic analog of doxorubicin, penetrates into cells where its metabolites inhibit the incorporation of nucleosides into nucleic acids, cause chromosomal damage, and arrest the cell cycle in G_2. A principal mechanism of valrubicin metabolites is DNA strand breakage mediated by anthracycline effects on topoisomerase II.
Primary indications. Intravesical therapy of bacille Calmette Guérin–refractory carcinoma *in situ* of the urinary bladder in patients for whom immediate cystectomy would be associated with unacceptable morbidity or mortality.
Usual dosage and schedule. 800 mg, diluted in 75 mL of normal saline, intravesically once a week for 6 weeks. Retain in bladder for 2 h before voiding.
Special precautions. Should not be administered if there is any question about perforation of the bladder or integrity of bladder mucosa.
Toxicity.
1. *Myelosuppression and other hematologic effects.* Uncommon, unless bladder rupture or perforation occurs, in which case severe neutropenia can be expected 2 weeks after administration.
2. *Nausea, vomiting, and other gastrointestinal effects.* Uncommon.
3. *Mucocutaneous effects.* Rash is uncommon.
4. *Miscellaneous effects.*
    a. Common local reactions comprise frequency, dysuria, urgency, bladder spasm, hematuria, and bladder pain. Urinary incontinence and cystitis are occasional. Local burning symptoms associated with the procedure, urethral pain, pelvic pain, and gross hematuria are uncommon to rare.
    b. Abdominal pain, asthenia, back pain, chest pain, fever, headache, and malaise are uncommon.

VINBLASTINE

Other names. VLB, Velban, vincaleukoblastine sulfate.
Mechanism of action. Mitotic inhibition with reversible metaphase arrest due to action on microtubular and spindle contractile proteins.

Primary indications.
1.   Hodgkin's and non-Hodgkin's lymphomas.
2.   Testicular, gestational trophoblastic, kidney, and breast carcinomas.

Usual dosage and schedule.
1.   4 to 18 mg/m² IV weekly.
2.   6 mg/m² IV on days 1 and 15 in combination with doxorubicin, bleomycin, and dacarbazine for lymphomas.
3.   4.5 mg/m² IV on day 1 every 3 weeks in combination with doxorubicin and thiotepa for breast cancer.

Special precaution. Administer as a slow push, taking care to avoid extravasation.

Toxicity.
1.   *Myelosuppression and other hematologic effects.* Dose-related leukopenia occurs with a nadir at 4 to 10 days and recovery in 7 to 10 days. Severe thrombocytopenia is uncommon.
2.   *Nausea, vomiting, and other gastrointestinal effects.* Common but not usually severe.
3.   *Mucocutaneous effects.*
     a.   Extravasation may lead to severe inflammation, pain, and tissue damage. Local infiltration with 1 to 6 mL of hyaluronidase (150 U/mL) may help.
     b.   Mild alopecia is common.
     c.   Stomatitis is occasionally severe.
4.   *Miscellaneous effects.*
     a.   Neurotoxicity manifested by (1) constipation, adynamic ileus, and abdominal pain if very high doses are used; or (2) paresthesias, peripheral neuropathy, and jaw pain with lower doses. Neurotoxicity is less frequent with vinblastine than with vincristine.
     b.   Transient hepatitis is uncommon.
     c.   Depression, headache, convulsions, and orthostatic hypotension are rare.

VINCRISTINE

Other names. VCR, Oncovin, Vincasar
Mechanism of action. Mitotic inhibition with reversible metaphase arrest due to drug action on microtubular and spindle contractile proteins.

Primary indications.
1.   Hodgkin's and non-Hodgkin's lymphomas.
2.   Acute lymphocytic leukemia.
3.   Multiple myeloma.
4.   Wilms' tumor, neuroblastoma, rhabdomyosarcoma, and Ewing's sarcoma of childhood.
5.   Breast carcinoma.

Usual dosage and schedule.
1.   1 to 2 mg/m² (maximum 2.0 to 2.4 mg) IV weekly.
2.   0.4 mg/day as a continuous IV infusion on days 1 to 4.

Special precautions.
1.   Administer as a slow IV push, taking care to avoid extravasation.

2. Because neurotoxicity is cumulative, neurologic evaluation should be done before each dose and therapy withheld if severe paresthesias, motor weakness, or other severe abnormalities occur. Underlying neurologic problems accentuate vincristine's effect.
3. Reduce dose if liver disease is significant.
4. Stool softeners or high-fiber or bulk diets may avert severe constipation.

Toxicity.
1. *Myelosuppression and other hematologic effects.* Mild and rarely of clinical significance.
2. *Nausea, vomiting, and other gastrointestinal effects.* Nausea and vomiting are not seen unless paralytic ileus occurs. Constipation is common.
3. *Mucocutaneous effects.* Severe local inflammation if extravasation occurs. Alopecia is common.
4. *Neurotoxicity.* Dose dependent and dose limiting. Mild paresthesias and decreased deep tendon reflexes are to be expected. More extensive peripheral neuropathies, severe constipation, and ileus are indications to reduce or hold therapy. Autonomic dysfunction with orthostatic hypotension or urinary retention may be seen.
5. *Miscellaneous effects.*
    a. Uric acid nephropathy due to rapid tumor cell lysis and release of uric acid is always a potential problem when therapy is first given.
    b. Syndrome of inappropriate antidiuretic hormone is rare.
    c. Jaw pain is uncommon.

VINDESINE (INVESTIGATIONAL)

Other name. Eldisine, VDS.
Mechanism of action. Mitotic inhibition with reversible metaphase arrest due to action on microtubule and spindle contractile protein.
Primary indications.
1. Lung, breast, and esophageal carcinomas.
2. Hodgkin's and non-Hodgkin's lymphomas.
3. Melanoma.

Usual dosage and schedule. 2 to 3 mg/m^2 IV bolus (2 to 3 min) weekly for induction, then every 2 weeks.
Special precautions. Take care to avoid extravasation.
Toxicity.
1. *Myelosuppression and other hematologic effects.* Leukopenia is common but not usually severe.
2. *Nausea, vomiting, and other gastrointestinal effects.* Occasional.
3. *Mucocutaneous effects.* Alopecia is common.
4. *Neurotoxicity.* Dose dependent and cumulative, consisting in constipation, paralytic ileus, paresthesia, myalgias, and weakness. Severity is intermediate between vincristine and vinblastine.
5. *Miscellaneous effects.*
    a. Chills and fever are occasional.
    b. Phlebitis is occasional.
    c. Confusion and lethargy are rare.

VINORELBINE

Other name. Navelbine.
Mechanism of action. Binds to tubulin; depolymerizes micro-tubules, causing mitotic inhibition, similar to other vinca alka-loids. Lower affinity for axonal microtubules associated with lower neurotoxicity.
Primary indications.
   1. Non–small cell carcinoma of the lung.
   2. Metastatic carcinoma of the breast.
Usual dosage and schedule.
   1. 30 mg/m^2 IV as 6- to 10-min rapid infusion weekly when used with a single agent or with cisplatin.
   2. 20 to 25 mg/m^2 IV as a 6- to 10-min rapid infusion in various schedules, when used with other myelotoxic agents.
Special precautions.
   1. Administer infusion through the sidearm of a freely flowing IV line, taking care to avoid extravasation.
   2. Reduce dose by 50% for serum bilirubin levels of 2.1 to 3 mg/dL and by 75% for bilirubin levels of over 3 mg/dL.
Toxicity.
   1. *Myelosuppression and other hematologic effects.* Granulo-cytopenia is common and dose limiting, with nadir at 7 to 10 days. Thrombocytopenia is uncommon. Anemia is occa-sional to common.
   2. *Nausea, vomiting, and other gastrointestinal effects.* Nausea and vomiting are common but usually mild to moderate. Diarrhea occurs occasionally.
   3. *Mucocutaneous effects.* Alopecia, mild diarrhea, and stom-atitis are occasional. Severe local inflammation can occur with extravasation.
   4. *Miscellaneous effects.*
      a. Regarding neurotoxicity, cumulative but reversible constipation and decreased deep tendon reflexes are oc-casional; paresthesias are uncommon.
      b. Erythema, pain, and skin discoloration at injection site are common; phlebitis at injection site is occasional.

ZOLEDRONIC ACID

Other name. Zometa.
Mechanism of action. A bisphosphonate that inhibits osteo-clastic resorption of bone and calcium release induced by tumor cytokines.
Primary indications.
   1. Hypercalcemia associated with malignancy.
   2. Bone metastases from breast cancer, prostate cancer (after progression on hormonal therapy), and other solid tumors in conjunction with standard antineoplastic therapy.
   3. Osteolytic and osteoporotic bone lesions of multiple myeloma.
Usual dosage and schedule.
   1. *Hypercalcemia of malignancy.* 4 mg IV as a 15-min infusion. May be repeated every 1 to 8 weeks, as needed.
   2. *Multiple myeloma or metastatic bone lesions.* 4 mg IV as a 15-min infusion every 3 to 4 weeks.

Special precautions. Do not infuse for less than 15 min. Potential for renal tubular damage, particularly if infused more rapidly. Serum creatinine should be measured prior to each dose. The risk of adverse reactions, particularly renal adverse reactions, may be greater in patients with impaired renal function. Dose adjustments are not necessary so long as initial serum creatinine is under 4.5 mg/dL. Withhold if there is deterioration in renal function (creatinine increase of 0.5 mg/dL in patients with normal baseline creatinine or 1 mg/dL in patients with abnormal baseline creatinine). Use caution when administered concurrently with aminoglycosides. Serum electrolytes and renal function should be monitored closely.

Toxicity.

1. *Myelosuppression and other hematologic effects.* Rare.
2. *Nausea, vomiting, and other gastrointestinal effects.* Abdominal pain, anorexia, constipation, nausea, and vomiting are uncommon to occasional.
3. *Mucocutaneous effects.* Infusion site reaction is occasional.
4. *Miscellaneous effects.*
   a. Flu-like syndrome with fever, chills, skeletal aches and pains is occasional.
   b. Hypocalcemia and hypomagnesemia are occasional, but grade 3 or 4 abnormalities are uncommon to rare.
   c. Increase of the serum creatinine of 0.5 mg/dL above baseline is occasional, but elevation to more than three times the upper limit of normal is uncommon.
   d. Hypophosphatemia to under 2 mg/dL is occasional to common but does not appear to have serious consequences or require treatment.
   e. Conjunctivitis and other ocular abnormalities are rare.
   f. Bronchoconstriction in aspirin-sensitive patients is potential.

SELECTED READINGS

Chabner B, Longo DL. *Cancer chemotherapy and biotherapy: principles and practice.* 3rd ed. Philadelphia: Lippincott Williams & Wilkins, 2001:1140.

Dorr RT, Van Hoff DD, eds. *Cancer chemotherapy handbook.* Norwalk: Appleton & Lange, 1994:1020.

Micromedex Inc. *USPDI oncology drug information.* Rockville: Association of Community Cancer Centers, 2000:525.

National Cancer Institute Cancer Therapy Evaluation Program. *Common Toxicity Criteria document* (***http://ctep.cancer.gov/reporting/ctc.html***). 1999.

Perry MC. *The cancer chemotherapy source book.* Philadelphia: Lippincott Williams & Wilkins, 2001:1003.

Tannock IF, Hill RP, eds. *The basic science of oncology.* New York: McGraw-Hill, 1998:539.

High-Dose Chemotherapy with Hematopoietic Progenitor Cell and Cytokine Support

Chatchada Karanes

Even though the first successful allogeneic hematopoietic stem cell transplantation (HSCT) occurred in 1959, the clinical practice of bone marrow transplantation was not widely used in the United States until the early 1970s. Recently, concepts for the transplantation of hematopoietic stem cells have changed dramatically. High-dose myeloablative conditioning regimens are in the process of being replaced by immunosuppressive regimens, ablating host myelopoiesis and neoplastic cells by the co-transplanted donor lymphocytes. Furthermore, the presence of stem cells in the bone marrow, capable of differentiating into a variety of nonhematopoietic tissues, as well as the presence of cells in other organs capable of differentiating into hematopoietic cells have led to the novel concept of the plasticity of stem cells derived from different tissues. It is anticipated that these remarkable studies will also lead to novel therapeutic strategies.

During the last 30 years, the number of transplants performed has grown exponentially. According to the International Bone Marrow Transplant Registry (IBMTR), more than 500 institutions worldwide are known to have active transplantation programs, performing more than 17,700 transplantations in 2000. There have been significant changing trends in the practice of stem cell transplantation (SCT) in the last 5 years. The introduction of nonmyeloablative allogeneic SCTs makes it safer for older patients to undergo allogeneic SCT. Renal cell carcinoma is now a frequent indication for allogenic SCT. In allogeneic SCT, there has been a shift to using peripheral blood stem cells (PBSCs) and umbilical cord blood (UCB) as stem cell sources in addition to bone marrow. The successful treatment of chronic myelogenous leukemia (CML) with Gleevec has significantly decreased the numbers of patients receiving unrelated donor transplants for this disease. For the first time in the last decade, the autologous transplant rate has declined. The recently published negative randomized trials in breast cancer have also reduced the autologous SCTs for this disease from 7,000/year in 1998 to 1,500 in 2000. PBSCs now account for 90% of the stem cell source used for autologous transplants in the last few years. With improved supportive care and decreasing costs, the indications for transplantation continue to increase. Select patients can receive high-dose therapy with HSCT as outpatients.

Clinical trials during the last 30 years have demonstrated that high-dose chemotherapy with or without the addition of radiation therapy can result in improved response and overall survival rates for patients with various malignant and nonmalignant diseases. High-dose chemotherapy enables the clinician to exploit the steep dose–response curves observed with many chemotherapeutic agents. The line representing log kill of malignant cells remains linear or slightly curvilinear for many chemotherapeutic agents, particularly for the alkylating agents. Most of the alkylating agents can be dose-escalated 4- to 10-fold; some alkylators such as thiotepa can be escalated 30-fold when supported with HSCT. Most non-alkylating agents cannot be dose-escalated more than twofold; some exceptions include cytarabine (cytosine arabinoside, ara-C), etoposide, mitoxantrone, and paclitaxel (Taxol). Improved supportive modalities including antibiotics, antiemetics, and hematopoietic cytokines and the availability of a variety of blood products have improved the safety of high-dose therapy. However, hematopoietic stem cells derived from bone marrow, peripheral blood, or cord blood or by newer *ex vivo* expansion technologies are required to rescue the patient from myeloablative therapy. Thus, the clinician can continue to escalate the doses of chemotherapy or radiation therapy beyond marrow toxicity to the next level of toxicity, the nonhematologic dose-limiting toxicity.

Although dose escalation is possible with hematopoietic stem cell rescue, not all malignancies can be cured with this treatment modality. In some diseases, the doses necessary to achieve complete tumor cell kill exceed the nonmarrow lethal doses of chemotherapy or radiation therapy. In other malignancies, dose escalation beyond the marrow lethal dose results in only modest increases in cell kill. Metastatic melanoma, non–small cell lung cancer, and colon cancer are examples of malignancies that high-dose therapy with hematopoietic stem cell rescue cannot cure.

Even with dose intensification, many patients ultimately experience disease relapse, which probably results from either failure to eradicate residual tumor cells or, in the case of autotransplantation, the reinfusion of hematopoietic stem cells containing contaminating tumor cells. With use of molecular techniques, the latter has been proven to be the case in some hematologic diseases such as acute myelogenous leukemia (AML) and low-grade lymphoma. In autologous transplant, which is the predominant modality, newer strategies are being developed to improve outcomes using posttransplantation immunotherapeutic approaches to eradicate minimal residual disease and to decrease potential tumor cell contamination by either positive (stem cell selection) or negative (purging) techniques. These approaches are discussed later.

Allogeneic transplantation provides a source of hematopoietic stem cells that is devoid of contaminating tumor cells. Growing clinical experience supports an immunotherapeutic (graft-versus-tumor) effect of the donor immune system to eradicate minimal residual disease after transplant. This immunoreactivity can be exploited following nonmyeloablative SCT for residual disease or at the time of disease relapse by donor lymphocyte infusions (DLIs), inducing complete remission in many hematologic malignancies. Unfortunately, transplant-related morbidity and mortality remain problematic because of graft-versus-host disease (GVHD) and prolonged immunosuppression.

I.   Scientific background
A.   High-dose therapy rationale. The cytocidal effect of chemotherapy in cell culture and animal models follows first-order kinetics. Each treatment kills a set fraction of cancer cells, irrespective of the starting number. The degree of kill in these

experimental systems is dose dependent: Tumor cell viability decreases in a logarithmic manner with a linear increase in drug dose. A modest escalation in the dose may result in a much higher fractional kill of tumor cells. Sublethal chemotherapy selects for and encourages development of resistant cells. The use of several chemotherapeutic agents in combination with different mechanisms of action inhibits the development of resistance. In addition, combinations of agents selected for nonoverlapping extramedullary dose-limiting toxicities should be used in maximal doses. Thus, the optimal approach uses the highest possible doses of non–cross-resistant agents with steep dose–response curves as early as possible in the patient's disease course to achieve the highest tumor cell kill and reduce the development of drug resistance. Eradication of tumor (cure) usually requires an 8- to 12-log kill of cancer cells. A complete clinical remission can be obtained with as little as a 4-log cell kill and a partial remission (50% tumor cytoreduction) with as little as a 1- or 2-log kill. Complete remissions are the surrogate short-term markers of potentially successful therapy.

The dosages of many active agents are limited by myelosuppression, even with the use of hematopoietic growth factors. The use of hematopoietic stem cell support allows for increased dosage and combination therapy with agents that would normally produce an unacceptable degree of myelosuppression.

B. Graft-versus-tumor effect. The eradication of leukemia after allogeneic HSCT results both from the cytotoxic chemoradiotherapy administered prior to transplant and the immunologic mechanisms. Two important clinical developments have evolved from identification of this immune-mediated graft-versus-leukemia (GVL) effect. The first is the use of DLI to treat patients with posttransplant leukemic relapse. With DLI, the majority of patients with recurrent CML after HSCT achieve a complete remission, and a smaller but significant fraction of patients with other malignancies respond to therapy. The second is the development of allogeneic HSCT using less toxic nonmyeloablative conditioning regimens. With this approach, low doses of irradiation and chemotherapy, which alone are not sufficient to eradicate tumors, are administered to facilitate graft acceptance, and tumor regression is induced by donor immune cells. Nonmyeloablative transplants have significant activity for patients with CML, chronic lymphocytic leukemia (CLL), myeloma, lymphoma, and renal cell carcinoma. The potent antitumor effects observed after DLI and allogeneic HSCT in a variety of advanced malignancies represent a remarkable demonstration of the curative potential of immunotherapy in contrast to the difficulty of eliciting effective autologous antitumor immune responses to tumor-associated antigens by vaccination or cellular therapy. However, with current approaches to allogeneic HSCT, it has not been possible to separate the beneficial GVL (or graft-versus-cancer) effect from deleterious GVHD. The association of GVL activity with GVHD has implicated donor T cells reacting with minor histocompatibility antigens expressed by recipient cells as major contributors to the GVL effect. The first clinical demonstration of GVL activity was observed after allogeneic HSCT for advanced leukemia, in which the probability of leukemic relapse was found to be significantly lower in those patients who developed acute and/or chronic GVHD. Analysis of patients with leukemia treated with either allogeneic unmodified HSCT, allogeneic T cell–depleted HSCT, or syngeneic HSCT showed that the risk of relapse was lowest for patients who received allogeneic unmodified HSCT and developed acute and/or chronic GVHD. Transplantation with syngeneic or T cell–depleted allogeneic marrow to avoid GVHD was associated with a higher risk of relapse unless the conditioning regimen was intensified. However, GVHD is not a prerequisite for GVL activity. A reduction in relapse was evident in the subset of CML and AML patients who received allogeneic unmodified HSCT but did not develop GVHD, and remissions have been observed after DLI in the absence of significant GVHD. This suggested that there may be antigenic determinants recognized by T cells that would permit the separation of GVL responses from GVHD. Other effector mechanisms such as natural killer cells may also contribute to GVL activity either directly or as a consequence of inflammation induced by allogeneic T cells.

II.   Indications for high-dose therapy with hematopoietic stem cell transplantation. The current indications for SCT have extended to include elderly patients undergoing allogeneic minitransplants, and tumor eradication has been improved by better conditioning regimens such as radioimmunoconjugates and methods to induce the GVL effect, such as DLIs and allogeneic minitransplants applied after autologous transplants.

A.   Disease. During the last 15 years, the indications for high-dose therapy and HSCT have changed markedly. The most common indications for allogeneic and autologous transplants differ (Fig. 5.1). For acute and chronic leukemias, myelodysplastic syndromes (MDSs), and nonmalignant diseases (aplastic anemia, immune deficiencies, inherited metabolic disorders), allogeneic transplantation is the predominant approach. Autotransplants are generally used for breast, ovarian, and other solid malignancies as well as Hodgkin's disease and non-Hodgkin's lymphoma (NHL) and multiple myeloma. Fifteen years ago, autologous transplants were performed almost exclusively for NHL and Hodgkin's disease. In the last 5 years leading up to 2000, breast cancer was the most common indication for autologous transplant. The recent negative results of several randomized trials in breast cancer have significantly decreased the numbers of autologous transplants performed for breast cancers since late 2000. In 2000, NHL was the most common indication for autologous transplant, followed by multiple myeloma and breast cancer. In addition, a growing number of transplants are being performed for other solid tumors including ovarian cancer, germ cell cancer, and neuroblastoma. The number of allogeneic transplants for nonmalignant diseases has also increased, including primary immunodeficiencies (severe combined immunodeficiency and Wiskott–Aldrich syndrome), thalassemia major, sickle cell anemia, and autoimmune disorders. In the hematologic malignancies, transplantations for multiple myeloma and MDSs are showing the most rapid rise compared with a decade ago. Although most allogeneic transplantations continue to be performed for acute and chronic

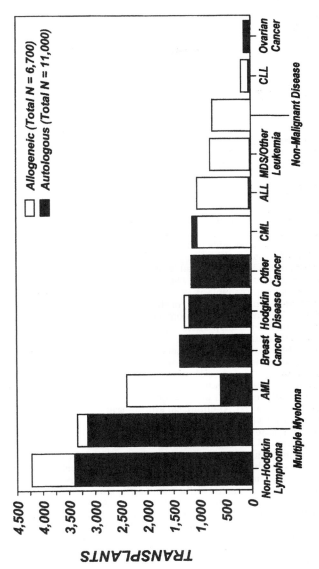

Fig. 5-1. Indications for blood and marrow transplantation in North America, 2000.

leukemias, there has been a recent increase in allogeneic transplantations for immunodeficiency disorders, inherited disorders of metabolism, and inherited erythrocyte abnormalities.

B.   Stem cell sources. Bone marrow was used as the only source of stem cells until the mid-1980s. The introduction of hematopoietic growth factors has made it possible to mobilize the stem cells from the bone marrow into the peripheral blood, resulting in the ability to collect large numbers of stem cells via apheresis and accelerate the engraftment. Currently, PBSCs are the major stem cell source, accounting for 90% of all autologous transplants. The remainder use bone marrow or a combination of bone marrow and blood stem cells. Most allogeneic transplants use bone marrow grafts. There has been a steady increase in the use of allogeneic PBSCs, from 20% in 1995 to 40% in 2000 in adult recipients, although PBSC use occurs in only 20% of the pediatric population (IBMTR data). In addition to differences in their stem cell content, transplants from the three sources differ in the composition and state of activation of immune cells. As a consequence, bone marrow, UCB, and PBSC transplants have different kinetics of hematologic recovery, the most rapid engraftment being observed with PBSCs and the slowest with UCB. Stem cell source also confers different risks for developing GVHD. PBSC transplants show similar incidence of acute and a possible increase in chronic GVHD compared with bone marrow. UCB transplants have a favorably low risk of GVHD even in mismatched transplants. Stem cell dose is an independent factor in transplants from any source, determining engraftment, transplant-related mortality, and risk of leukemic relapse. An understanding of the impact of stem cell source and dose is essential to obtain optimum conditions for a successful outcome after transplant.

III.   Patient eligibility

A.   Host factors. Autologous transplants can be conducted safely in patients up to 75 years of age if they have adequate performance status, physiologic organ function, and hematopoietic stem cells. For allogeneic transplantation, the usual upper age limit is 55 years, although some centers perform human leukocyte antigen (HLA)–identical sibling transplants in select patients up to 60 to 65 years old. For unrelated or mismatched related donors, the usual age limitation is 55 years and up to 75 years old for nonmyeloablative allogeneic HSCT. For both autologous and allogeneic transplants, patients must meet a minimum physiologic organ function. Common criteria include pulmonary function tests (forced vital capacity, forced expiratory volume, and corrected diffusing capacity) over 50% of predicted, cardiac function with a left ventricular ejection fraction over 40% to 45%, no active infections, liver function tests less than two to four times normal, performance status more than 60% on the Karnofsky scale or less than 2 on the Eastern Cooperative Oncology Group scale, and serum creatinine level of less than 2 mg/dL. In select diseases, patients with impaired renal function can also be considered for autotransplantation (e.g., multiple myeloma patients treated with high-dose melphalan).

B.   Disease factors. In general, patients with malignant disease should show at least a partial response to standard-dose chemotherapy before being considered for high-dose therapy with HSCT. Some exceptions to this generalization are patients with hematologic malignancies that are refractory to primary chemotherapy and who proceed early in their disease course to transplantation. For example, about 15% to 20% of patients with NHL refractory to induction therapy can achieve durable remissions with transplantation.

C.   Chemotherapeutic agents for dose-intensive strategies. Agents are chosen for dose intensification based on the steepness and linearity of their dose–response curve, the absence of nonhematologic toxicity that prevents dose escalation (preferably allowing a 5- to 10-fold dose escalation over conventional doses), and, when combined with other agents, a synergistic antitumor effect with a minimum of overlapping nonhematologic toxicity. The doses of alkylating agents are often reduced 20% to 40% when combined as compared with use as a single agent in high-dose conditioning regimens. There are few randomized trials comparing different preparative regimens. Indeed, in a retrospective study of more than 3,500 women with breast cancer undergoing high-dose therapy and autotransplant, more than 20 different preparative regimens were evaluated by multivariate analysis without identification of a statistically superior regimen. Thus, the choice of chemotherapeutic agents is arbitrary, based largely on anecdotal data and a matter of personal experience and preference. Extramedullary toxicities of the most commonly used conditioning agents are listed in Table 5.1. In most cases, drug doses are limited by gastrointestinal toxicity (mucositis, diarrhea) or major organ toxicity (e.g., heart, lung, kidney, or central nervous system [CNS]). When combining drugs in a conditioning regimen, particular attention must be given to overlapping toxicities. Pre-existing renal or hepatic insufficiency or both may seriously reduce drug clearance. This can result in higher drug levels and further end-organ toxicity.

IV.   Alkylating agents

A.   BCNU (carmustine) is a nitrosourea with clinical activity against a number of tumors. It is formulated in a 10% alcohol solution, which may account for the hypotension seen during or shortly after administration. BCNU, which undergoes spontaneous hydrolysis, should be protected from light and is usually administered as a 2-h infusion. At high dose, pulmonary and hepatic toxicity are dose limiting. Nonhematologic toxicities are delayed and cumulative. BCNU doses exceeding 300 mg/m^2 are associated with acute or late pneumonitis in at least 20% of patients. Patients should be informed to monitor exercise tolerance; if tolerance diminishes, further evaluation should be performed (chest radiograph, arterial blood gas, pulmonary diffusion capacity). If drug-induced pneumonitis is confirmed, prednisone should be started with a taper over 2 to 3 months. BCNU is also occasionally associated with an increased incidence of veno-occlusive disease.

B.   Busulfan (Myeleran [PO], Busulfex [IV]) has a more marked effect on myeloid cells than lymphoid cells and can cause prolonged aplasia. The major nonhematologic toxicities are veno-occlusive disease of the liver, pneumonitis, and mucositis. Busulfan rapidly enters the CNS and may cause seizures. Patients

Table 5.1.   Toxicity of common chemotherapeutic agents

Drug (dose)	Extramedullary dose-limiting toxicity	Other toxicities
BCNU (carmustine) (300–600 mg/m^2)	Interstitial pneumonitis	Renal insufficiency encephalopathy, N/V, VOD
Busulfan (12–16 mg/kg)	Mucositis, VOD	Seizures, rash, N/V, hyperpigmentation, pneumonitis
Cyclophosphamide (120–200 mg/kg)	Cardiomyopathy	Hemorrhagic cystitis, SIADH, N/V, interstitial pneumonitis
Cytarabine (ara-C) (4–36 g/m^2)	CNS ataxia, mucositis	Pulmonary edema, conjunctivitis rash, fever, hepatitis
Cisplatin (150–180 mg/m^2)	Renal insufficiency, peripheral neuropathy	Renal tubular acidosis, hypomagnesemia, hypokalemia, ototoxicity
Carboplatin (600–1,500 mg/m^2)	Ototoxicity, renal insufficiency	Hepatitis, hypomagnesemia, hypokalemia, peripheral neuropathy
Etoposide (600–2,400 mg/m^2)	Mucositis	N/V, hepatitis, fever, pneumonia
Ifosfamide (12–16 g/m^2)	Encephalopathy, renal insufficiency	Hemorrhagic cystitis
Melphalan (140–200 mg/m^2)	Mucositis	N/V, hepatitis, SIADH, pneumonitis
Mitoxantrone (30–75 mg/m^2)	Cardiomyopathy	Mucositis
Paclitaxel (Taxol) (500–775 mg/m^2)	CNS, ataxia, peripheral neuropathy	Anaphylaxis, mucositis
Thiotepa (500–800 mg/m^2)	Mucositis	Intertriginous rash, N/V, hyperpigmentation
Fludarabine (90–180 mg/m^2)	CNS visual disturbances peripheral neuropathy	N/V, tumor lysis syndromes immunosuppression

N/V, nausea/vomiting; VOD, veno-occlusive disease; SIADH, syndrome of inappropriate antidiuretic hormone; CNS, central nervous system.

should receive prophylactic phenytoin (with doses sufficient to achieve therapeutic levels) before initiation of high-dose busulfan, and the phenytoin should be continued for 24 h after the final dose. Busulfan is available in oral and recently in IV formulation. The IV formulation is dissolved in polyethylene glycol and N, N-dimethylacetamide to a final concentration of 6 mg/mL. The usual adult dose of Busulfex is 0.8 mg/kg of ideal body weight or adjusted body weight, whichever is lower, administered via a 2-h infusion through a central venous catheter every 6 h for 4 days. Ninety-three percent of patients achieve an area under the curve (AUC) below the target of 1,500 µmol/L/min with no dosage adjustments. If vomiting occurs within 30 min of an oral administration or if pill fragments are present in the emesis, most institutions repeat the dose. Busulfan is well absorbed after oral administration, exhibits low protein binding, and is metabolized through conjugation with glutathione to form a thiophenium ion. At a given dose, there is considerable variability in the systemic exposure of oral busulfan, typically expressed as AUC or average concentration at steady state. Relative to that in adolescents and adults, patients younger than 4 years have an increased apparent oral clearance of busulfan and a higher conjugation rate of busulfan with glutathione in the enterocyte. An increased risk of serious hepatic veno-occlusive disease has been reported when the AUC level exceeds 1,500 µmol/L/min. Busulfan administration via the IV route ensures complete bioavailability and reliable systemic drug exposure with more predictable blood levels and less veno-occlusive disease.

C. Cyclophosphamide (Cytoxan) is probably the most widely used chemotherapeutic agent for dose intensification. Cyclophosphamide requires activation in the liver, but there is no evidence that the P-450 system necessary for that activation is saturated at the doses used in intensification. Clearance of cyclophosphamide increases quickly after the first dose, and there is considerable interpatient variability in plasma concentrations with repeated dosing. Total doses as high as 5,000 to 7,000 mg/m^2 divided over 1 to 4 days can be safely administered as 1- to 2-h infusions each day. Aggressive hydration (hyperhydration) and diuresis or administration of mesna (Na 2-mercaptoethanesulfonate) as an uroprotectant is necessary to prevent hemorrhagic cystitis (also used for ifosfamide). The dose-limiting toxicities are cardiac and pulmonary. The cardiac effect, some degree of which occurs in up to 25% of patients, is a potentially fatal hemorrhagic myocarditis that may occur acutely or within days or may manifest as heart failure or pericardial effusions as long as 3 to 4 weeks after completion of treatment. The risk of cardiac toxicity is not cumulative, and repeated doses are tolerated in the patients who recover. This toxicity occurs most often in patients who receive more than 200 mg/kg (over 7,500 mg/m^2), are older than 50 years, and have a previous history of congestive heart failure. The pulmonary toxicity of cyclophosphamide consists of proliferation of atypical type II pneumocytes with fibrosis. It usually manifests clinically within 4 to 6 weeks of therapy as progressive dyspnea, nonproductive cough, hypoxia, and interstitial radiographic changes. Even at high doses, cyclophosphamide is not myeloablative, and its antitumor effect as a single agent is limited. In autologous transplant, cyclophosphamide, alone or in combination with hematopoietic growth factors, is often used for PBSC mobilization. In allogeneic transplantation, cyclophosphamide is included predominantly as an immunosuppressive agent owing to its lymphocytotoxic effects.

D.   Ifosfamide, a closely related analog of cyclophosphamide, is also a prodrug that must undergo hepatic metabolism. As with cyclophosphamide, hyperhydration and protection with mesna are required to prevent hemorrhagic cystitis. Unlike cyclophosphamide, the dose-limiting toxicity of ifosfamide is toxic encephalopathy manifested as lethargy, confusion, seizures, or stupor. Renal toxicity may also manifest as metabolic acidosis due to accumulation of metabolic by-products resulting in proximal renal tubular acidosis. No definite antitumor advantage of ifosfamide over cyclophosphamide has yet been established.

E.   Melphalan alkylates target tissues after spontaneous formation of a (nitrogen) mustard-type reactive intermediate *in vivo*. It is administered rapidly in two daily doses of 70 to 100 mg/m^2 or one dose of 140 to 200 mg/m^2. Because less than 15% of the intact drug is excreted renally, melphalan can be administered safely in patients with renal insufficiency. The dose-limiting toxicities are gastrointestinal toxicity (mucositis, diarrhea) and, less commonly, hepatitis and pneumonitis.

F.   Platinum compounds (cisplatin, carboplatin) covalently bind to deoxyribonucleic acid (DNA) bases and disrupt DNA function. Cisplatin can be escalated only two- to threefold owing to renal and neurologic toxicity. Cisplatin must be reconstituted in a chloride-containing solution to minimize spontaneous hydrolysis. Aggressive hydration and diuresis with normal saline loading and maintenance of good urine output are required to avoid renal tubular toxicity. Magnesium wasting commonly leads to hypocalcemia and hypokalemia. Peripheral neuropathy and high-frequency hearing loss are potential long-term side effects. Carboplatin has less renal and neurologic toxicities; myelosuppression and hepatic and gastrointestinal (mucositis and diarrhea) toxicities are more common with carboplatin. Some clinicians use the AUC (Calvert formula) of 20 to 28 for target drug dosing of carboplatin in high-dose preparative regimens.

G.   Thiotepa has one of the steepest dose–response curves of all the alkylating agents and is not cross-resistant with cyclophosphamide. It therefore has been included in many different dose-intensity regimens. Thiotepa penetrates the blood–brain barrier better than most alkylating agents. Mucositis is the dose-limiting toxicity, with CNS toxicity observed only at very high doses. It may increase the risk of hepatic veno-occlusive disease when used with other agents known to have that toxicity.

V.   Nonalkylating and less commonly used agents

A.   Cytarabine (ara-C) is an analog of deoxycytidine and has multiple effects on DNA synthesis. It is used in high doses for the treatment of leukemia and in some regimens for NHL. At high dose, cytarabine causes neurologic toxicity, manifested by cerebral and cerebellar dysfunction. Renal dysfunction increases the risk of neurotoxicity substantially. This toxicity may present as dysarthria, gait disturbances, dementia, and coma. These toxicities are usually reversible but may be fatal. If neurologic symptoms develop, the cytarabine should be stopped immediately. Another rare but life-threatening complication is noncardiogenic pulmonary edema. Pulmonary symptoms, when they develop, are often fatal. Cytarabine conjunctivitis is responsive to topical steroids, which should be used prophylactically.

B.   Etoposide is a topoisomerase II inhibitor that shows synergism with platinum compounds. It has high–single-agent activity in the treatment of leukemia, lymphomas, and testicular cancer. Its primary nonhematologic toxicities are mucositis, liver toxicity, and hypotension from the lipid formulation if administered rapidly.

C.   Mitoxantrone is an anthracenedione compound that induces breakage of DNA strands, perhaps through an effect on topoisomerase II. It can be escalated five- to eightfold above conventional dose. Mucositis and cardiotoxicity are the dose-limiting toxicities, although the latter is minimal compared with the structurally similar anthracyclines daunorubicin and doxorubicin.

D.   Paclitaxel (Taxol) is a taxane, which stabilizes microtubules leading to mitotic arrest. It has activity against breast and ovarian cancers. One Phase I study reported a maximum tolerated dose of 725 mg/m^2. At higher doses, unacceptable CNS, renal, mucosal, and pulmonary toxicities were observed. Peripheral neuropathy was tolerable and not associated with motor weakness. Because paclitaxel is eliminated through hepatic metabolism, hepatic insufficiency can prolong elimination and increase toxicity.

E.   Fludarabine phosphate (Fludara) is a nucleotide analog of adenine arabinoside and inhibits DNA synthesis by inhibiting DNA polymerase-α, ribonucleotide reductase, and DNA primase. The drug is converted rapidly to the active metabolite 2-fluoroara-A when given IV. The half-life is about 10 h. The drug is eliminated via the kidneys; 23% of the active drug is excreted unchanged in the urine. Therefore, it should be administered cautiously in patients with renal insufficiency. It produces lymphocytopenia and substantial immunosuppression and is approved for the treatment of B-cell CLL. Owing to its immunosuppression, it is used in combination with alkylating agents or low-dose total-body irradiation (TBI) to enhance engraftment of allogeneic hematopoietic progenitors. At this time, it is available only in IV formulation; the oral form is in clinical trials. The dose recommended for CLL is 25 mg/m^2/day IV over 30 min for 5 days; however, the dosage used for conditioning in nonmyeloablative HSCT varies from 25 to 50 mg/m^2 over 30 min once a day for 3 to 5 days. Once reconstituted, the drug should be used in 8 h owing to a lack of antimicrobial preservative. The dose-dependent toxicities include myelosuppression and immunosuppression. Visual disturbances and CNS symptoms have been reported at very high doses.

F.   Total-body irradiation. TBI is an integral component of several conditioning regimens, particularly for hematologic malignancies requiring allogeneic or autologous transplantation. It has been used since the earliest days of bone marrow transplantation for both immunosuppression (prevention of allograft rejection) and antitumor effect. However, the therapeutic ratio of TBI is small. The usual dosage of TBI is 10 to 14 Gy given in twice- or thrice-daily doses over 3 to 4 days (e.g., 2 Gy b.i.d. for 3 days). Fractionation (and hyperfractionation) substantially reduce the risk of both interstitial pneumonitis and veno-occlusive disease of the liver. Above that dose, pulmonary, hepatic, and gastrointestinal toxicities become limiting and life threatening with little therapeutic gain. Acute and chronic toxicities with TBI are summarized in Table 5.2.

VI.   Preparative regimens. During the last 25 years, a large number of intensive preparative (conditioning) regimens requiring hematopoietic stem cell support have been developed. The regimens used for dose intensification are largely empiric, and few have been compared in randomized trials. Important issues such as optimum combination or doses, the benefit of an "induction" regimen immediately preceding intensification, and the benefit of repeated cycles of dose intensity have not been rigorously addressed.

A.   Allogeneic transplant. Preparative regimens must provide effective antitumor activity and suppress host immunity to prevent graft rejection. Commonly used cytotoxic agents include TBI, cyclophosphamide, busulfan, cytarabine, and etoposide. Immunosuppressant agents to reduce the risk of GVHD include steroids, cyclosporine (and cyclosporine analogs such as tacrolimus), methotrexate, and antithymocyte globulin. Another modality is T-cell depletion of the transplanted cells by monoclonal antibodies, immunoaffinity columns, or immunomagnetic beads. After transplantation of a product that has undergone T-cell depletion, however, patients have an increased risk of graft failure and disease relapse. Therefore, more aggressive regimens are often used in T cell–depleted patients, including higher doses of TBI, antithymocyte globulin, or a second myeloablative agent (e.g., thiotepa, cytarabine) in addition to cyclophosphamide. Examples of commonly employed preparative regimens using TBI are shown in Table 5.3.

B.   Reduced-intensity (nonmyeloablative) allogeneic transplant. The conventional preparative regimen for allogeneic transplant is characterized by high-intensity conditioning, the requirement of prolonged and expensive hospital treatment, and treatment-related mortality of 10% to 30% depending on diagnosis, disease stage, patient age, and donor type. Increasing recognition of the role of graft-versus-tumor effect has shifted the emphasis from delivery of myeloablative therapy aiming at maximum tumor destruction to optimizing engraftment, thus providing the platform for further adoptive immunotherapy with DLI. This has resulted in the emergence of new concepts and procedures that allow replacement of the patient bone marrow and immune system with that of the donor by a transplant procedure with markedly reduced intensity of the preparative regimen. This type of transplant is sometimes referred to as mini–bone marrow, nonmyeloablative, or reduced-intensity transplant. The preparative regimen used in this type of transplant consists of low-dose TBI of 200 cGy alone or in combination with fludarabine. Others have used fludarabine with cyclophosphamide, melphalan, or lower-dose busulfan. This type of preparative regimen provides sufficient immunosuppression to allow engraftment of allogeneic blood progenitor cells without causing profound neutropenia and severe organ toxicity of myeloablative radio-

Table 5.2. Total body irradiation–associated acute and chronic toxicities

System	Acute symptoms and signs	Acute onset	Chronic symptoms and signs	Onset and incidence
Gastrointestinal	Nausea and vomiting, diarrhea	24–48 h	—	—
Hepatic	Veno-occlusive disease	6–21 d		
Mucosal tissues	Parotitis, decreased lacrimation, sore throat, mucositis	24–48 h	Sicca syndrome, cataracts	20% with fractionation at 0.5 to 3–4 yr
Endocrine	Acute pancreatitis, steroid-induced hyperglycemia	7–21 d	Gonadal failure Hypothyroidism Delayed bone growth	>90% 40%–50%
Pulmonary, renal	Pneumonitis	1–3 mo	Pulmonary fibrosis Bone marrow transplantation nephropathy	Uncommon
Skin, second malignancies	Erythema, alopecia	5–10 d	Secondary leukemia Solid tumors	5%–10% 2% at 10 yr, 7% at 15 yr

Table 5.3.   Common preparative regimens for high-dose therapy with total-body irradiation

Drug	Total dose	Daily dose	Schedule (day)[a]	Indications	Autologous or allogeneic
Single–cytotoxic drug regimens					
Cytoxan	120 mg/kg	60 mg/kg	−5, −4	Leukemia, lymphoma, aplastic anemia	Both
TBI	1,200 cGy	200 cGy b.i.d.	−3, −2, −1		
Etoposide	60 mg/kg	60 mg/kg	−3	Leukemia, lymphoma	Allogeneic
TBI	1,320 cGy	120 cGy t.i.d.	−7, −6, −5, −4		
Cytarabine (ara-C)	36 g/m²	3 g/m² b.i.d.	−9, −8, −7, −6, −5, −4	Leukemia, lymphoma	Allogeneic
TBI	1,200 cGy	200 cGy b.i.d.	−3, −2, −1		
Melphalan	140 mg/m²	140 mg/m²	−4	Leukemia, multiple myeloma	Both
TBI	1,200 cGy	200 cGy b.i.d.	−3, −2, −1		
Combination–cytotoxic drug regimens					
Cytarabine (ara-C)	18 g/m²	3 g/m² b.i.d.	−8, −7, −6	Leukemia, lymphoma	Allogeneic
Cytoxan	90 mg/kg	45 mg/kg	−5, −4		
TBI	1,200 cGy	200 cGy b.i.d.	−3, −2, −1		
Etoposide	60 mg/kg	60 mg/kg	−4	Leukemia, lymphoma	Both
Cytoxan	120 mg/kg	60 mg/kg	−3, −2		
TBI	1,320 cGy	120 cGy t.i.d.	−8, −7, −6, −5[b]		
Thiotepa	10 mg/kg	5 mg/kg	−5, −4	Leukemia, lymphoma	Allogeneic
Cytoxan	120 mg/kg	60 mg/kg	−3, −2		
ATG	120 mg/kg	30 mg/kg	−5, −4, −3, −2		
TBI	1,375 cGy	125 cGy t.i.d.	−9, −8, −7, −6[b]		
Fludarabine	90 mg/m²	30 mg/m²	−4, −3, −2	Leukemia, lymphoma	Allogeneic reduced intensity
TBI	200 cGy	200 cGy once	−1		

TBI, total-body irradiation; ATG, antithymocyte globulin.
[a] Day 0 is day of transplantation, day −5 is 5 days before transplantation, etc.
[b] TBI given twice on this day.

chemotherapy. To maintain the continued presence of donor cells following nonmyeloablative transplant, it is frequently necessary to give the recipient posttreatment infusions of additional donor cells. This is referred to as DLI. However, DLI also carries a significant risk of GVHD development. There are several approaches to improving the safety of DLI, including selective removal of the alloreactive T cells and/or induction of tolerance in the donor lymphocytes to the recipient tissues to prevent GVHD. Such an approach would be used in the follow-up phase of treatment for patients who need DLI to further consolidate/maintain the presence of the donor hematopoietic cells. Immunosuppressive agents used in this type of transplant are combinations of oral cyclosporine or tacrolimus with mycophenolate mofetil, avoiding the debilitating oral mucositis from the use of methotrexate as in conventional SCT. This approach reduces the toxicity of the transplant procedure and makes it possible to treat debilitated patients and possibly extend the use of transplantation to older patients (55 to 70 years old) who are not presently eligible for SCT procedures. Other possible indications include treatment of nonmalignant disorders and induction of tolerance for solid organ transplantation. The procedure can be performed in an outpatient setting. Although a potentially lower level of inflammatory cytokines may be present after nonmyeloablative therapies, fatal GVHD still occurs.

C.   Autologous transplant. In autologous transplant, non–cross-resistant cytotoxic agents with nonoverlapping extramedullary toxicities are often combined. Combination regimens of two or more agents are generally more effective than single-agent regimens; many of the newer regimens rely on the synergistic effect of alkylating agents with agents such as topoisomerase inhibitors. Immunosuppression is not required. Although TBI is used by some centers as part of the preparative regimen for hematologic malignancies (e.g., lymphoma, multiple myeloma), it is avoided in the treatment of solid tumors (e.g., breast, ovary, testicle) because effective tumoricidal doses exceed extramedullary dose-limiting toxicity. Examples of commonly employed preparative regimens using combination chemotherapy are shown in Table 5.4.

VII.   Hematopoietic stem cells. Hematopoietic progenitor cells (HPCs) are primitive pluripotent stem cells capable of self-renewal and maturation into any of the hematopoietic lineages and the committed and lineage-restricted progenitor cells. The first observations that lethally irradiated mice could survive after injection of spleen or marrow cells occurred more than 40 years ago. In humans, the first attempts at HPC transplantation began in the late 1960s and early 1970s in recipients of HLA-identical sibling marrow allografts. These initial allogeneic transplants were compromised by severe GVHD. During the subsequent decades, efforts in allogeneic transplantation have been directed toward reducing transplant-related toxicity, decreasing the risk and severity of GVHD, treating relapse with donor lymphocytes, and recently use of "nonmyeloablative transplant." Because technology now permits molecular tagging and tracking of both normal and malignant cells in the blood and marrow, evolving issues in autologous transplant relate to the use of marrow or peripheral blood as a source of HPCs

Table 5.4.   Common preparative regimens for high-dose therapy without total-body irradiation

Drug	Total dose	Daily dose	Schedule (day)	Indications	Autologous or allogeneic
"Big" BU/CY					
Busulfan	16 mg/kg	1 mg/kg q.i.d.	−9, −8, −7, −6	Leukemia, lymphoma	Allogeneic
Cytoxan	200 mg/kg	50 mg/kg	−5, −4, −3, −2		
"Little" BU/CY					
Busulfan	16 mg/kg	1 mg/kg q.i.d.	−7, −6, −5, −4	Leukemia, lymphoma, myeloma, breast cancer	Both
Cytoxan	120 mg/kg	60 mg/kg	−3, −2		
CPB "STAMP I"					
Cisplatin	165 mg/m^2	55 mg/m^2	−6, −5, −4	Breast cancer	Autologous
Cytoxan	5,625 mg/m^2	1,875 mg/m^2	−6, −5, −4		
BCNU	600 mg/m^2	600 mg/m^2	−3		
TC					
Thiotepa	500 mg/m^2	125 mg/m^2	−7, −6, −5, −4	Breast cancer	Autologous
Cytoxan	6 g/m^2	1.5 g/m^2	−7, −6, −5, −4		
CBV					
BCNU	300–600 mg/m^2	300–600 mg/m^2	−6	Hodgkin's disease	Autologous
Etoposide	900–2,400 mg/m^2	300–800 mg/m^2	−6, −5, −4		
Cytoxan	6–7.2 g/m^2	1.5–1.8 g/m^2	−6, −5, −4, −3		
BEAM					
BCNU	300 mg/m^2	300 mg/m^2	−6	Hodgkin's disease, lymphoma	Autologous
Etoposide	800 mg/m^2	200 mg/m^2	−5, −4, −3, −2		
Cytarabine	800–1,600 mg/m^2	200–400 mg/m^2	−5, −4, −3, −2		
Melphalan	140 mg/m^2	140 mg/m^2	−1		

Regimen / Drug	Total dose	Dose	Days	Indication	Transplant type
ICE					
Ifosfamide	16 g/m²	4 g/m²	−6, −5, −4, −3	Lymphoma, testicular cancer	Autologous
Carboplatin	1.8 g/m²	600 mg/m²	−6, −5, −4		
Etoposide	1.5 g/m²	500 mg/m² b.i.d.	−6, −5, −4		
BEAC					
BCNU	300 mg/m²	300 mg/m²	−6	Lymphoma, Hodgkin's disease	Autologous
Etoposide	800 mg/m²	200 mg/m²	−5, −4, −3, −2		
Cytarabine	800 mg/m²	200 mg/m²	−5, −4, −3, −2		
Cytoxan	140 mg/kg	35 mg/kg	−5, −4, −3, −2		
MEL					
Melphalan	200 mg/m²	100 mg/m²	−3, −2	Multiple myeloma	Autologous
MCC					
Mitoxantrone	75 mg/m²	25 mg/m²	−8, −6, −4	Ovarian cancer	Autologous
Carboplatin	AUC 28	1/5 total dose	−8, −7, −6, −5, −4		
Cytoxan	120 mg/m²	40 mg/m²	−8, −6, −4		
CBDA/VP					
Carboplatin	2.25 g/m²	750 mg/m²	−6, −5, −4	Testicular cancer	Autologous
Etoposide	2.1 g/m²	700 mg/m²	−6, −5, −4		
Fludarabine	90 mg/m²	30 mg/m²		Lymphoma	Allogeneic, reduced intensity
Cyclophosphamide	2,250 mg/m²	750 mg/m²			
Fludarabine	150 mg/m²	30 mg/m²	−6, −5, −4, −3, −2	Leukemia	Allogeneic, reduced intensity
Melphalan	140 mg/m²	70 mg/m²	−3, −2		
Fludarabine	180 mg/m²	30 mg/m²	−10, −9, −8, −7, −6, −5	Leukemia	Allogeneic, reduced intensity
Busulfan	8 mg/kg	4 mg/kg	−6, −5	Lymphoma	Allogeneic, reduced intensity
ATG	40 mg/kg	10 mg/kg	−4, −3, −2, −1	MDS	Allogeneic, reduced intensity

ATG, antithymocyte globulin.

and contamination of HPCs by malignant cells. The HPCs have now been characterized in humans to the extent that they can be isolated and expanded *in vitro.*

Hematopoietic recovery after transplantation (termed *engraftment*) is believed to occur in two waves: committed progenitor cells repopulating the marrow within the first month and the true pluripotent stem cells responsible for the delayed but durable component of hematologic recovery. Quantitation of the number of HPCs necessary to provide hematopoietic reconstitution has evolved during the last 25 years. Flow cytometry has become the gold standard since the surface marker CD34+ was identified in the late 1980s as being present on HPCs. Patients receiving more than 5×10^6 CD34+ cells/kg of recipient weight have prompt, predictable, and sustained engraftment. There is a growing consensus that more than 2.5×10^6 CD34+ cells/kg of recipient weight is the minimum number of HPCs associated with granulocyte and platelet recovery (absolute neutrophil count over 500, platelet count over 20,000) within 14 days after transplantation. More recently, subsets of CD34+ cells have been identified on the basis of other cell surface markers, including CD33, CD38, HLA-DR, Thy-1, and Lin, and also the ability to stain with the dye rhodamine. The most primitive HPCs can be identified as CD34+, Thy-1+, Lin–, CD33–, CD38–, HLA-DR–, and rhodamine–. Only 1% of a bone marrow harvest consists of CD34+ cells, with this more primitive pluripotent CD34+ subset comprising less than 0.01%. The most recent advances in stem cell technology use *ex vivo* expansion techniques, primarily through cytokine supplementation, to increase the number of hematopoietic stem cells for transplantation. Although promising results have been obtained with bone marrow and cord blood, it is becoming clear that novel methods must be developed before cellular therapies using these stem cells can become routine.

Recently, human pluripotent cell lines have been developed from the inner cell mass of human embryos at the blastocyst stage and fetal tissue obtained from terminated pregnancies. These embryonic stem cells can differentiate to all cell lineages *in vivo* and can be induced to differentiate to most cell types *in vitro.* Although embryonic stem cells have been isolated from humans, their use in research as well as therapeutics is encumbered by ethical considerations. Other investigators have also demonstrated a surprising plasticity of the human mesenchymal stem cells isolated from marrow aspirates. These adult mesenchymal stem cells could be induced to differentiate to lineages of mesenchymal cell tissues, including adipoblasts, chondroblasts, osteoblasts, and endothelial cells. Individual stem cells were identified that, when expanded to colonies, retained their multilineage potential. Like mesenchymal stem cells, embryonic stem cells can differentiate into all mesodermal cell types and may have an even greater proliferation potential. However, mesenchymal stem cells, but not embryonic stem cells, can be derived from bone marrow from most healthy donors irrespective of age, providing for an autologous source of stem cells. Thus, because mesenchymal stem cells can be selected and expanded under conditions that should be readily adaptable to production by good clinical manufacturing processes and are easily transduced with retroviral vectors, they may be an ideal source of cells for therapy of degenerative or traumatic disorders of mesodermal cells or for therapy of single-gene disorders.

A. Allogeneic transplant is used mostly for the treatment of leukemia and other hematologic malignancies. Less than 5% of allogeneic transplants are used for nonmalignant diseases such as aplastic anemia, immunodeficiency syndromes, or hemoglobinopathies. Although most allogeneic transplants consist of bone marrow donation from an HLA-identical sibling, there is a growing use of PBSCs, unrelated bone marrow donors, mismatched family donors, and UCB. Until recently, donors were identified by serologic phenotype testing for class I and class II major histocompatibility complex molecules HLA-A, -B, and -DR on lymphocytes. Mendelian inheritance predicts a 25% likelihood of identifying an HLA-identical sibling donor within a family; another 5% of patients have a one-antigen–mismatched family donor. Through the efforts of the National Marrow Donor Program (NMDP), which has HLA typing on more than 4.5 million volunteers, an HLA-compatible unrelated donor can be identified for many patients. Because of HLA polymorphism, most transplant centers now perform high-resolution HLA typing that includes HLA-C, -DRB1, and -DQ; occasionally, HLA sequence–based typing is required to confirm compatibility for both class I and class II HLA antigens. This is particularly important in evaluating potential unrelated donors. With use of this technology, an acceptable match can be identified in more than 60% of Caucasian patients in the NMDP. In contrast, minorities are still greatly underrepresented in the NMDP in spite of their significant growth in the registry in the last 5 years. Therefore, the likelihood of identifying an acceptable match for these patients is considerably lower. Transplant-related mortality rates range from 20% to 30% in HLA-identical sibling transplant recipients and are significantly higher in recipients of mismatched unrelated grafts and haploidentical grafts (40% to 45%) compared with recipients of matched unrelated marrow grafts (23%). Therefore, patients who lack a closely matched family donor should be offered a phenotypically matched unrelated donor if available. There is no apparent advantage to using a mismatched unrelated versus a haplo-identical family donor.

GVHD is the most common cause of treatment-related mortality, with significant acute GVHD (first 100 days after transplantation) occurring in 10% to 40% of HLA-identical sibling transplant recipients and in more than 40% to 80% of unrelated and mismatched marrow recipients. Chronic GVHD (occurring more than 100 days after transplantation) occurs in about 50% of HLA-identical sibling transplant recipients; the incidence is higher with unrelated donors and mismatched donors. GVHD prophylaxis requires immunosuppression of the donor immune system. A number of modalities are available, usually in combination, including antithymocyte globulin, methotrexate, cyclosporine and cyclosporine analogs such as tacrolimus, corticosteroids, T-cell depletion of allografts, and monoclonal antibodies (i.e., OKT3). Although the incidence of severe acute and chronic GVHD is lower with T-cell depletion techniques (5% to 20%), there is an increase in graft failure and disease relapse. Recent advances in GVHD prophylaxis have extended the potential donor pool to include partially mismatched donors and haplo-identical donors.

Another potential donor source is UCB. Transplantation of UCB was successfully performed for the first time in 1988 to treat a boy with Fanconi's anemia. By early 2002, 2,000 UCB transplantations had been reported worldwide, including 500 adult recipients (Netcord data). In allogeneic recipients under 20 years of age without matched sibling donors, the use of UCB increased from less than 5% in 1995 to 15% in 2000. The advantages of cord blood as a source of hematopoietic stem cells for transplantation are due to its superior proliferative capacity and lower risk of GVHD. A 100-mL unit of cord blood contains one-tenth the number of nucleated cells and progenitor cells (CD34+ cells) present in 1,000 mL of marrow, but because they proliferate rapidly, the stem cells in a single unit of cord blood can reconstitute the entire hematopoietic system. The immaturity of lymphocytes in cord blood dampens the GVHD reaction. A joint European study showed that recipients of cord blood from HLA-identical siblings had a lower risk of acute or chronic GVHD than marrow recipients from HLA-identical siblings. Children with acute leukemia who received HLA-mismatched cord blood from an unrelated donor also had a lower risk of GVHD than recipients of HLA-mismatched marrow from an unrelated donor. Most studies in children with malignant or nonmalignant hematologic diseases have shown that long-term survival after transplantation of cord blood is similar or superior to survival after transplantation of marrow when the donor is a sibling. Multicenter trials of cord blood transplants in adults reported 90% neutrophil engraftment and low GVHD rate despite HLA mismatches. Transplantation-related mortality was related to the number of nucleated cells in the graft and degree of HLA disparity. Patients who received no more than 1×10^7 nucleated cells/kg had a 75% probability of death, whereas recipients of at least 3×10^7 nucleated cells/kg had a 30% probability of death. Three or more HLA mismatches result in a 50% mortality rate in adults. An advantage of cord blood over adult marrow for allogeneic transplantation is that the cells are readily available in cord-blood banks, are routinely typed for HLA antigens and ABO blood groups, and are tested for infectious agents. This reduces the time required to search for and identify a suitable donor, which is crucial for patients in desperate need of a transplant. The age and weight of the recipient are not obstacles, as long as the unit of cord blood contains more than 2×10^7 nucleated cells/kg of the recipient's weight at the time of collection. A simultaneous search of registries of bone marrow donors and cord-blood banks for appropriate matches and adequate cell numbers should be initiated for patients without related family donors. In the United States, the NMDP provides a single point for both unrelated donor as well as cord blood unit search. Currently, 17,000 cord blood units are available for search through the NMDP. The final choice of the source of stem cells must take into account the degree of HLA identity, the availability of the donor, the urgency of transplantation, and the number of cells in the unit of cord blood.

A recent trend in allogeneic transplantation is to use hematopoietic growth factor–primed PBSCs. Sufficient numbers of HPCs can usually be collected in one or two aphereses. For allogeneic PBSC transplant, most centers prefer the minimum cell dose to be 5×10^6. The use of PBSCs negates the need for a bone marrow harvest and provides a 3- to 4-fold higher number of CD34+ cells and an approximately 10-fold higher total number of lymphoid subsets when mobilized with granulocyte colony-stimulating factor (G-CSF) than that obtained from bone marrow. This allows for more rapid engraftment. Even though PBSCs contain a log or more T cells than does bone marrow, the incidence of acute GVHD does not appear to be increased. The incidence of chronic GVHD remains unsettled: It was found to be higher after PBSC transplantation in the prospective and retrospective registry analyses but to be similar in two large prospective studies. Different cytokine and GVHD prophylaxis regimens may contribute to this discrepancy. In two major studies (prospective randomized and retrospective registry data), the disease-free survival rates were higher after PBSC transplantation, especially in patients with advanced-stage disease. Data on immune reconstitution are in favor of PBSC transplantation but discrepant for natural killer cell reconstitution. The significantly lower incidence of molecular and cytogenetic relapse in patients with CML is indicative of a more pronounced GVL effect after PBSC transplantation. Whether this beneficial GVL effect holds up in more aggressive disease categories remains to be shown. The megadose concept of CD34+ cells, including veto cells, contained in PBSC allografts allows the crossing of major HLA barriers. It has been proposed that G-CSF–primed bone marrow allografts combine fast cellular reconstitution with an incidence of GVHD similar to that of steady-state bone marrow transplantation, but the available data are inconclusive.

B. Autologous transplants and the number of centers performing them are increasing at a striking rate. Currently, most centers use autologous PBSCs as the source of HPCs to support high-dose therapy. With the advent of PBSCs and hematopoietic growth factors, the duration of marrow aplasia has been significantly shortened compared with that of autologous bone marrow transplants. Randomized trials have demonstrated that the use of PBSCs has resulted in fewer infectious complications, shorter hospitalizations, and lower costs. Many centers are performing autologous transplants in the outpatient setting.

PBSCs are collected by a process called leukapheresis. This is usually coordinated with the transplantation center's blood bank. Patients require insertion of a large-bore central venous catheter before initiation of apheresis. PBSCs can be collected in the steady state or after mobilization by hematopoietic growth factors (e.g., G-CSF or granulocyte–macrophage colony-stimulating factor [GM-CSF]) with or without chemotherapy (Table 5.5).

Although cyclophosphamide (1.5 to 7 g/m^2) is the most common single chemotherapeutic agent reported in stem cell mobilization regimens, a number of other agents have been used either alone or in combination with cyclophosphamide or with other agents. Several investigators have found that the infusion of at least 2.5×10^6 CD34+ cells/kg resulted in timely hematopoietic recovery. In addition, more recently it was observed that the infusion of at least 5.0×10^6 CD34+ cells/kg was consistently associated

Table 5.5. Relative increase in peripheral blood stem cells using different mobilization regimens

Modality	-Fold increase
Steady state	1
Chemotherapy	10–20
Growth factor alone (G-CSF most common)	10
Chemotherapy plus growth factor (G-CSF or GM-CSF)	100–1,000

G-CSF, granulocyte colony-stimulating factor; GM-CSF, granulocyte–macrophage colony-stimulating factor.

with more predictable and rapid recovery, particularly of platelets. Most patients reach their target CD34+ cell goal within two to five collections. However, in heavily pretreated patients, this minimum requirement is often difficult to achieve. Recent pilot trials indicate that some of the newer hematopoietic growth factors (stem cell factor, daniplestim, flt-3 ligand), either alone or in combination with other growth factors, increase the yield of CD34+ cells.

PBSC mobilization techniques may also increase the number of tumor cells in the peripheral blood. For example, tumor cells are commonly present in the bone marrow of patients with advanced breast cancer—and may be present even in those with stage I disease. About one-fourth of patients with advanced breast cancer have detectable cells in the peripheral circulation; during stem cell mobilization, significantly higher percentages of patients may have detectable tumor cells. Similar findings but with lower rates of contamination have been reported for lymphoma. Essentially all PBSC collections from patients with multiple myeloma contain contaminating tumor cells. The study of AML with neomycin resistance gene marking convincingly demonstrates that malignant cells within the autograft can survive and grow within a patient after reinfusion.

Efforts to reduce the number of contaminating tumor cells in PBSC autografts have used techniques based on physical, immunologic, and pharmacologic methods. Pharmacologic methods are generally aimed at removing tumor cells from the autograft (purging, negative selection) rather than by enrichment of HPCs. The most common pharmacologic agent is 4-hydroperoxycyclophosphamide. Although promising in pilot trials, the U.S. Food and Drug Administration has removed this drug from clinical trials. Physical methods (e.g., density gradients, counterflow centrifugal elutriation) are used less commonly; they use cell size, shape, and density to separate cell populations. The most commonly employed separation techniques use immunologic methodology, most often positive selection for CD34+ cells. An anti-CD34+ cell antibody is bound to a solid phase (e.g., immunoaffinity column, immunomagnetic beads), which binds cells, and then the cells are later released. This results in a 2- to 4-log depletion of contaminating tumor cells. One of the most recent advances in positive selection is the use of sequential columns (anti-CD2 followed by anti-CD34) and a combination of immunologic and physical methods (immunoaffinity columns followed by high-speed flow cytometry). The latter method has been reported to result in a 5- to 7-log depletion of tumor cells.

A new technology to reduce contaminating tumor cells uses *in vitro* culture. Small numbers of HPCs can be expanded 3- to 20-fold *ex vivo* with combinations of cytokines (e.g., interleukin [IL]-3, IL-6, G-CSF, SCF, flt-3, GM-CSF, GM-CSF/IL-3) in large-volume cultures or bioreactors. Preliminary results indicate that these expanded cells are capable of complete hematopoietic reconstitution after high-dose therapy. A similar technique using long-term culture permits growth of HPCs while malignant tumor cells are eliminated, allowing for potential autografts in patients with hematologic malignancies such as CML, who may not be candidates for allogeneic transplantation.

VIII.   Hematopoietic growth factors and cytokines. More than 20 different cytokines and growth factors are approved or under investigation for use in HSCT. CSFs shorten the time to bone marrow or PBSC engraftment after high-dose chemotherapy. They act by binding to specific cell surface receptors, stimulating proliferation, differentiation, commitment, and selected end-cell functions. Two commercially available hematopoietic growth factors are G-CSF (filgrastim) and GM-CSF (sargramostim). The most common dosages and indications for these growth factors are listed in Table 5.6. For HPC mobilization with growth factors alone, most clinicians start the growth factor on day 1, with initiation of apheresis on day 5. For chemotherapy plus growth factor mobilization, the growth factor is started on the day after completion of the chemotherapy, and apheresis commences when the white blood cell count

Table 5.6.   Hematopoietic growth factors: common doses and indications

Growth factor	Clinical indication	Dose
G-CSF[a]	Peripheral blood HPC mobilization	
	With chemotherapy	5–10 µg/kg SC
	Without chemotherapy	10–16 µg/kg SC
	Hematopoietic recovery after transplantation	
GM-CSF[b]	Peripheral blood HPC mobilization	
	With chemotherapy	250 µg/m² SC
	Hematopoietic recovery after transplantation	
Epoetin	Red blood cell recovery after transplantation	150–300 µg/kg SC 3×/wk

G-CSF, granulocyte colony-stimulating factor; HPC, hematopoietic progenitor cell; GM-CSF, granulocyte–macrophage colony-stimulating factor.
[a] Often rounded off to standard vial size of 300 or 480 µg; a common approach is 300 µg for patients who weight <60 kg and 480 µg for patients who weigh >60 kg.
[b] Often rounded off to standard vial size of 500 µg.

is more than 1,000. After transplantation, the growth factors are usually started the same day (day 0) or on day 1; growth factor support is continued daily until the absolute neutrophil count is more than 2,000 for a minimum of 1 day.

Several new hematopoietic growth factors are in clinical trials. These growth factors are designed to improve platelet recovery (IL-11, thrombopoietin, megakaryocyte-derived growth factor), to improve stem cell mobilization in patients who are predicted to be poor mobilizers with G-CSF or GM-CSF (IL-3, daniplestim, stem cell factor), or to enhance dendritic cell proliferation (flt-3 ligand, stem cell factor) as part of immunotherapeutic approaches.

Other cytokines under development or in clinical trials in HSCT are shown in Table 5.7. Many of these have multiple functions.

IX.   Toxicities. Toxicities of dose-intensive regimens can be formidable and life threatening. They vary considerably with the different preparative regimens, type of transplant (autologous versus allogeneic, related versus unrelated versus mismatched), and the patient's physiologic organ function and performance status. Some of the toxicities associated with transplant preparative regimens are outlined in Tables 5.1 and 5.2. As indicated, some of the toxicities are acute, whereas others are chronic. Stomatitis, esophagitis, and diarrhea can be severe with some regimens. Hepatic, renal, or pulmonary toxicities can occur in 20% to 30% of patients. Most patients require blood product support in the peritransplant period. Central venous catheter infections or thrombosis can be problematic. Most centers use prophylactic antibiotics to prevent bacterial, viral, and fungal infections. One of the most devastating late toxicities is the development of secondary malignancies: Allogeneic transplant recipients had a 8.3 times higher risk of new solid cancers than expected among those who survived 10 or more years after transplantation. The cumulative incidence

Table 5.7.   Cytokines in hematopoietic stem cell transplantation

Cytokine	Clinical application	Proposed mechanism
Interferon-α	Immune modulation after transplantation for CML, myeloma, lymphoma	Unknown
Interleukin-2	Immune modulation to prevent post-transplantation relapse	Activates T and natural killer cells
Interleukin-12	Immune modulation after transplantation	Increases Th1 helper T cells
GM-CSF, M-CSF	Treatment of fungal infections after transplantation	Enhances macrophage activity

CML, chronic myelogenous leukemia; GM-CSF, granulocyte–macrophage colony-stimulating factor; M-CSF, macrophage colony-stimulating factor.

rate was 2.2% at 10 years and 6.7% at 15 years. In multivariate analyses, higher doses of TBI were associated with a higher risk of solid cancers. Chronic GVHD and male gender were strongly linked with an excess risk of squamous cell cancers of the buccal cavity and skin. Long-term survivors of bone marrow transplant for childhood leukemia have an increased risk of solid cancers and posttransplant lymphoproliferative disorders related to both transplant therapy and treatment given before the transplant. Cumulative risk of solid cancers increased sharply to 11.0% at 15 years and was highest among children younger than 5 years at transplantation. Thyroid and brain cancers accounted for most of the strong age trend; many of these patients received cranial irradiation before bone marrow transplantation. Multivariate analyses showed increased solid tumor risks associated with high-dose TBI and younger age at transplantation, whereas chronic GVHD was associated with a decreased risk. Risk factors for posttransplant lymphoproliferative disorders included chronic GVHD, unrelated or HLA-disparate related donor, T cell–depleted graft, and antithymocyte globulin therapy. Hematologic disorders, including MDS, lymphoma, and secondary leukemias, have been variously reported in 5% to 15% of long-term survivors.

   X. Response and long-term outcomes. With a few exceptions, the goal of high-dose therapy with HSCT is to cure or substantially prolong good-quality survival. The short-term surrogate marker for improved survival or cure is complete remission. Partial remission rarely translates into important increases in survival and represents only a 1- to 3-log kill of malignant cells. Therefore, partial remission rates have little meaning in dose-intensive regimens. Less than half of patients with advanced malignancy obtain durable remissions with current dose-intensive regimens, stimulating major research efforts to eradicate minimal residual disease after transplantation.

   A. Leukemia
   1. Acute myelogenous leukemia is curable in 15% to 45% of patients with standard chemotherapy. The bone marrow karyotype at diagnosis is associated not only with the response to induction chemotherapy for adult AML but also with outcomes of postremission therapy. After first relapse, AML is incurable with standard therapy. Cytogenetic analysis is critical for determining which patients are candidates for transplantation as consolidation versus consideration at the time of relapse. Patients with favorable AML subtypes have a greater than 80% or 90% complete remission rate and a 50% to 65% 5-year survival rate with standard induction and consolidation therapy. These patients are usually considered for transplantation only at the time of disease relapse, although the U.S. intergroup trial suggests that autologous bone marrow transplantation may be useful in favorable AML. In contrast, patients with intermediate cytogenetic risk are often considered for transplantation in the first complete remission. If there is an HLA-matched sibling, allogeneic SCT should be recommended for patients in this group up to age 55 to 65 years. Allogeneic SCT provides the best antileukemic effect owing to a low relapse rate of 18% and 3-year survival rate of 65%, although the advantage of allogeneic SCT was not observed in

the U.S. intergroup study. Among intermediate-risk patients without a matched family donor, the 5-year survival after receiving either autologous transplant or high-dose cytarabine is 56% and 48%, respectively. However, the relapse rate is lower after autologous transplants. It is generally assumed that those patients going on to autologous SCT should receive prior intensive chemotherapy as the best method of *in vivo* purging. Preliminary reports using PBSCs collected after consolidation therapy for autologous transplants indicate a very low mortality rate and faster engraftment. Several cooperative groups are evaluating the role of gemtuzumab ozogamicin given along with high-dose cytarabine or prior to autologous transplants. For patients with unfavorable cytogenetic risk, allogeneic SCT from either a family matched donor or an unrelated donor is recommended. The probability of leukemia-free survival is 60% in the first complete remission, 40% in the second or later complete remission, and 20% in relapse using HLA-identical sibling donors (IBMTR data); lower rates are observed with matched unrelated donors or mismatched related donors, usually owing to the increased incidence of GVHD. Data from the Fred Hutchinson Cancer Research Center in Seattle indicate that similar results are obtained in patients undergoing transplant during an untreated early relapse and those undergoing transplantation in a second complete remission. About 10% to 20% of patients who fail induction therapy achieve long-term leukemia-free survival with allogeneic transplant.

2.   Acute lymphoblastic leukemia (ALL) is curable in 60% to 75% of affected children but in only 20% to 30% of adults. Even in high-risk patients, there are no clinical trials proving that early transplant is beneficial if complete remission is achieved with standard induction therapy. Because of the rarity of ALL in adults, few institutions have enough patients for randomized trials properly analyzed according to risk factors (e.g., CNS leukemia, high white blood cell count at presentation, male gender, hepatosplenomegaly, Philadelphia chromosome–positive [Ph+] cytogenetics, immunophenotype). Most clinicians agree, even without substantial clinical trial data, that patients with Ph+-positive ALL should proceed to transplant in the first complete remission. Patients who undergo transplant as consolidation of the first complete remission have a 50% leukemia-free survival rate compared with 40% in more than the second complete remission and 20% in relapse using HLA-identical sibling donors; again, lower rates are observed with alternative donors. The outcome of autologous transplantation in ALL is inferior to that of allogeneic transplants.

3.   Chronic myelogenous leukemia is no longer the most common indication for allogeneic transplantation since the demonstration that imatinib mesylate (STI-571, Gleevec) results in major cytogenetic responses in 60% of CML patients in chronic phase who have failed interferon. In spite of its encouraging response, whether this treatment can produce cure remains unanswered. Interferon, the previous best nontransplant therapy, results in major cytogenetic responses in 25%

to 40% of patients, with a median duration of survival of more than 7 years; however, no cures are achieved with interferon. The ability of allogeneic SCT to produce long-term remission and cure is well established. Cure rates approach 70% in patients with CML in the chronic phase who receive an HLA-identical sibling transplant within the first year of the disease. Waiting until the development of the accelerated phase or blast phase reduces the leukemia-free survival to 35% and 15%, respectively. In the setting of matched unrelated transplant, about 40% of patients are cured when transplantation is performed in the chronic phase within the first year. A report from Seattle indicates that the use of interferon for more than 6 months results in an increased incidence of acute GVHD in recipients of matched unrelated donor transplants and subsequently in lower survival rates than those seen in patients who did not receive interferon therapy. However, recent reports by the French group as well as IBMTR/NMDP show no adverse effect of interferon pretreatment on the outcome of subsequent SCT. Patients who relapse after transplant may enter a durable molecular remission with infusion of donor lymphocytes in 80% of patients. Escalated dose of DLI starting at CD3+ cells/kg of 1×10^7 for matched sibling transplant and 10^6 for matched unrelated donor results in less incidence of GVHD compared with a single large dose of lymphocytes. In an attempt to avoid GVHD from DLI, several centers have initiated DLI trials in which the infused lymphocytes carry a suicide gene, herpes simplex thymidine kinase, which confers sensitivity to ganciclovir. In the event of severe GVHD, administration of ganciclovir should terminate or ameliorate GVHD. There is no evidence that autografts in CML patients prolong survival. The reduced-intensity regimen is being investigated. The decision on how best to treat newly diagnosed CML patients and when to offer allogenic SCT remains controversial while we are waiting for the long term survival results of a randomized trial comparing imatinib mesolate and interferon in these patients. Many transplant physicians continue to recommend conventional allogeneic SCT within the first year of diagnosis to patients younger than 35 years who have HLA-matched sibling donors or molecularly HLA-matched unrelated donors.

4. Chronic lymphocytic leukemia is one of the more recent indications for high-dose therapy with HSCT. The overall survival of CLL patients under 60 years old who receive conventional treatment is 12 years. Patients with advanced disease (Binet C or Rai stage 3 and 4) have median survival of 3 years; only 10% can expect to live 10 years unless they achieve complete remission. Poor cytogenetic finding such as 11q deletion and disease transformation also imply poor prognosis. Both autologous and allogeneic SCT produces 40% to 60% overall survival at 4 years. In spite of lower transplant-related mortality of less than 10% in autologous SCT, a majority of patients receiving autologous SCT relapse. In most instances, the harvested stem cells are contaminated with residual CLL cells. This has prompted the investigation of several *in vitro* purging methods including an *in vivo* purging with monoclonal antibody such as Campath-1H and Rituximab. With allogeneic SCT, a survival plateau is seen at 57%, suggesting that these patients may be cured. This confirms a strong graft-versus-CLL effect in allogeneic stem cell recipients. Moreover, allogeneic SCT can induce sustained complete responses in patients refractory to treatment. Persistent minimal residual disease following allogeneic SCT does not necessarily correlate with leukemia relapse, although it predicts relapse in most autologous recipients. The sensitivity of the disease to treatment, disease status before transplantation, younger age, performance status, use of peripheral blood as a source of stem cells, normal cytogenetics, and prior therapy with fludarabine have been associated with better outcome. Owing to the advanced age of most CLL patients, the high transplant-related mortality associated with allotransplantation, and the important role of the graft-versus-CLL effect in eradicating disease, several investigators are exploring the use of reduced-intensity regimens with DLI. Preliminary results are encouraging, with a treatment-related mortality of 19% at 1 year. The event-free survival and overall survival at 1 year were 69% and 80%, respectively, with a median follow-up of 8 months. The long-term outcome of these patients needs to be established.

B. Lymphoma
  1. Hodgkin's disease is curable with conventional therapy in most patients. Transplantation is an effective modality for primary treatment failure and high-risk patients (e.g., stage IVB), as consolidation, and for patients with disease relapse; long-term disease-free survival is observed in 20% to 30%, 60% to 70%, and 40% to 50%, respectively, for each of these three disease subgroups (Autologous Blood and Marrow Transplant Registry [ABMTR] data). A variety of preparative regimens have been reported; the BEAM, CBV, and BEAC regimens listed in Table 5.4 are the most commonly employed. In patients receiving nitrosoureas (e.g., BCNU), the clinician must pay particular attention to respiratory symptoms (dry cough, shortness of breath, hypoxia, and interstitial infiltrates on chest radiograph) 4 to 12 weeks after transplant because these symptoms are suggestive of BCNU pulmonary toxicity, a potentially fatal complication that can be reversed with prompt initiation of corticosteroids. A long-term follow-up from the Johns Hopkins Oncology Center suggests a lower relapse rate of 34% in chemosensitive patients receiving allogeneic transplants versus 51% for autologous transplants, suggesting a graft-versus-Hodgkin's-disease effect. There was a continuing risk of relapse or secondary AML and MDS for 12 years after autologous bone marrow transplant, whereas there were no cases of secondary AML/MDS or relapses beyond 3 years after allogeneic bone marrow transplant. The allogeneic SCT is usually considered only in the setting of excessive bone marrow involvement or inability to collect sufficient PBSCs for autologous transplant.
  2. Non-Hodgkin's lymphoma is curable with conventional therapy in only 30% to 40% of patients. Less than 10% of relapsed patients achieve long-term survival with conventional

salvage therapy. The early transplant trials were conducted in patients with intermediate-grade lymphoma with disease relapse or disease that was refractory to secondary salvage therapy. In this setting, the survival rate was only about 20%. Cure rates of 30% to 50% were reported in patients who received high-dose therapy with autotransplant earlier in the disease course. A randomized trial comparing high-dose therapy with autologous transplant with standard salvage therapy (DHAP) in patients with chemotherapy-sensitive first relapse proved conclusively that high-dose therapy was the superior treatment (46% versus 12% 5-year event-free survival rate). Relapse within 12 months from diagnosis, elevated lactate dehydrogenase level, advanced stage, and poor performance status were independent adverse factors for survival and progression-free survival. About 30% of patients with primary refractory disease achieve durable remission with high-dose therapy. When transplantation was used as consolidation therapy, a randomized French trial of patients with aggressive NHL did not show significant differences in 3-year or disease-free survivals. However, when the data were retrospectively analyzed focusing on high-risk patients (Group 2 or 3 in the International Prognostic Index), high-dose chemotherapy with transplant was significantly superior to sequential chemotherapy, with 8-year disease-free survival rates of 55% and 39%, respectively. The Italian study also showed superior outcome of high-dose chemotherapy with transplant in untreated high-risk International Prognostic Index patients. Allogeneic transplantation does not appear to be superior to autologous transplantation in treating intermediate-grade lymphomas. Although fewer relapses are observed after allogeneic transplant, presumably because of a graft-versus-lymphoma effect, the transplant-related mortality offsets the lower relapse rate. The use of reduced-intensity regimen in NHL has increased the 1-year overall survival rate after allogeneic HSCT from 23% to 67% in one study.

Low-grade NHL accounts for about one-third of all lymphomas. These lymphomas are usually extensive at diagnosis and follow an indolent clinical course of 5 to 10 years with or without aggressive therapy. Some centers are treating patients in the first complete remission with high-dose therapy and autologous transplant. The most favorable results have been observed in patients with minimal disease at the time of transplant whose hematopoietic stem cells are polymerase chain reaction negative for *bcl-2*. This is usually accomplished by *in vitro* bone marrow purging with monoclonal antibody cocktails. However, because of the brevity of the follow-up in most of these reports, the benefit of high-dose therapy with autologous transplant remains uncertain. Most centers now use mobilized PBSCs rather than bone marrow in low-grade lymphoma not only to hasten hematologic engraftment but also because these stem cells are thought to be less contaminated with tumor. Several investigators have begun to explore the use of monoclonal antibodies in SCT for patients with lymphoma. These approaches include the development of new high-dose regimens with radiolabeled antibodies, *in vivo* purging techniques with the unlabeled antibodies, and posttransplant adjuvant immunotherapy. More recently, several reports of small numbers of patients from single centers suggest that durable remission can be obtained after allogeneic SCT in low-grade lymphomas. This approach has the advantage of the absence of contaminating tumor cells and a graft-versus-lymphoma effect. Results from the registry data demonstrate that allogeneic bone marrow transplantation is associated with high morbidity and mortality, attributable largely to GVHD. In this patient population, however, the probability of relapse appears low, with 50% disease-free survival rate 3 years after transplant.

One area of controversy is mantle cell lymphomas. These are aggressive intermediate-grade lymphomas with a median survival of about 2 years using conventional therapy. There is currently no definite evidence of a survival advantage using autologous or allogeneic transplant for primary refractory disease, relapsed disease, or after the second complete remission. Few single-institution data reported event-free survival of 36% to 48% at 3 to 4 years. Blastic morphology and heavily pretreated patients are associated with worse prognosis. Few investigators reported encouraging results with the use of rituximab after autologous SCT or using an intensive-chemotherapy regimen, hyper-CVAD, cytarabine, and methotrexate to induce molecular remission followed by allogeneic SCT.

Because most patients with NHL relapse even after high-dose therapy, current emphasis is focused on posttransplant immunotherapy to eradicate minimal residual disease. This includes low-dose IL-2, interferons, idiotype-specific vaccines, and dendritic cell vaccines.

C. Plasma cell dyscrasias

1. Multiple myeloma is an incurable B-cell malignancy that constitutes 10% of all hematologic malignancies. With standard therapy, the median survival is 30 to 36 months. A randomized trial comparing high-dose therapy plus autologous transplant with standard chemotherapy demonstrated a superior event-free survival and overall survival in the high-dose therapy arm (7-year event-free survivals of 16% versus 8% and overall survival time of 57 versus 44 months). More patients in the high-dose arm achieved complete or very good partial response (38% versus 10%); however, there was no plateau of the survival curve. To improve the outcome, a subsequent randomized study comparing melphalan 200 mg/m^2 and melphalan 140 mg/m^2 plus TBI was initiated. The melphalan 200 mg/m^2 regimen was significantly less toxic with shorter neutropenia and thrombocytopenia. The melphalan-alone group had better overall survival, even though the event-free survival and response rate were the same. Others have shown that tandem SCTs in newly diagnosed patients were safe and increased the complete response rate from 24% after the first transplant to 43% after two transplants. However, the impact of the tandem transplant on the event-free survival and overall survival needs further evaluation. In the French randomized trial, double transplant with PBSCs appears to be superior to double transplant with marrow and single–high-dose therapy in terms of immediate response, event-free survival, and overall survival. Therefore, the recommended preparative regimen is melphalan 200 mg/m^2, and the preferred source of stem cells is PBSCs. The absence of survival improvement with CD34+ selection in randomized studies in spite of a lower tumor load in the graft confirmed the persistence of the malignant cells in the patients after high-dose therapy. Interferon-α maintenance appears to prolong event-free survival and overall survival for patients responding to high-dose therapy in a retrospective study; a randomized trial in the United States is ongoing. Allogeneic transplant, in contrast, may be curative in 20% to 25% of patients but is associated with extremely high transplantation-related mortality rates, approaching 40% to 50% in most reports. There is no advantage of allogeneic SCT compared with autologous SCT. However, if undergoing transplantation early, about one-third of patients achieving complete remission after allogeneic SCT remain free of disease 6 years later. Several reports have confirmed the durable graft-versus-myeloma effect of DLIs in relapsed patients after allogeneic SCT. Several ongoing trials are evaluating the role of allogeneic nonmyeloablative SCT alone or following a tumor reduction by autologous SCT.

2.   Primary amyloidosis is a plasma cell dyscrasia associated with light-chain deposition in one or more organ systems. With standard therapy, the median survival time is 18 to 24 months, but less than 1 year for patients with cardiac amyloidosis. Recent reports from Boston University and the Mayo Clinic indicate that high-dose therapy with autotransplantation can effect high remission rates and improve survival rates. An Eastern Cooperative Oncology Group trial is now open to evaluate this modality.

D.   Myelodysplastic syndrome. MDS is a clonal disorder of HPCs. There is no effective standard therapy for this disorder. Allogeneic transplantation can produce long-term disease-free survivors: about 40% of patients younger than 40 years but only 15% to 20% of patients older than 40 years. The analysis of MDS transplants reported to the European Group for Blood and Marrow Transplantation showed the estimated disease-free survival and risk at 3 years to be both 36% for patients transplanted with stem cells from matched siblings. Age and stage of disease had independent prognostic significance for disease-free survival, survival, and treatment-related mortality. Patients transplanted at an early stage of disease had a significantly lower risk of relapse than patients transplanted at more advanced stages. The estimated disease-free survival at 3 years was 25% for patients with voluntary unrelated donors, 28% for patients with alternative family donors, and 33% for patients autografted in first complete remission. The relapse rate is lowest for nonidentical related donor and highest in autologous recipients. For patients younger than 55 years with MDS, allogeneic SCT offer the best effective treatment. The data using a reduced-intensity regimen are encouraging but need long-term follow-up.

E.   Myelofibrosis. With conventional therapies being often ineffective, with a median survival of 3 to 5 years, myelofibrosis has the worst prognosis of all the chronic myeloproliferative diseases. Recently, a report on 55 patients younger than 55 years with myelofibrosis who underwent allogeneic HSCT indicated that 48% of the recipients of an HLA-identical transplant survived event-free at 5 years. Nevertheless, the 1-year treatment-related mortality in this study was 27% in spite of the relatively young age (median 42 years) of the patients receiving transplants. Further, a recent follow-up from this same group of investigators noted only a 14% 5-year overall survival in a subgroup of transplant recipients older than 45 years compared with 62% for younger patients.

F.   Solid tumors. High-dose chemotherapy with autologous hematopoietic reconstitution is an accepted modality for the treatment of various solid tumors that show a steep dose–response curve. The optimal patient population, timing of high-dose therapy, and drug regimens are under investigation.

1.   Breast cancer remains a controversial disease in terms of the value of high-dose chemotherapy with autologous transplantation. An early Phase II study showed that 15% to 20% of patients with chemosensitive metastatic breast cancer were rendered free of disease long term by high-dose chemotherapy with transplant, which appeared to be substantially higher than the expected long-term disease-free survival of 0% to 3% using conventional chemotherapy. Therefore, several randomized trials have been conducted in both the metastatic and the high-risk primary disease settings. Thorough analysis of these studies indicates an evaluable improvement in favor of high-dose chemotherapy and PBSC transplant in three of the four randomized studies performed in metastatic breast cancer and two of the four high-risk primary studies. For metastatic breast cancer, the largest study, a National Cancer Institute (NCI)–sponsored randomized intergroup trial (PBT-101), shows no advantage of the high-dose arm. The other three showed survival advantage of the high-dose chemotherapy. One of the studies is now being audited owing to concerns about the methodology and the extent of dose intensity in both arms. The conflicting results may be due to the differences in study design and drug regimen used. A recent retrospective study that compared 1,079 women with metastatic breast cancer, aged 65 years or younger, and with chemosensitive disease registered in four cancer leukemia Group B trials with those receiving autotransplants reported to the ABMTR indicates a small but statistically significant survival difference after treatment with high-dose chemotherapy and autologous SCT versus standard-dose chemotherapy. This difference is not evident until approximately 3 years after treatment. Additionally, the hazards of death indicate a consistent advantage for high-dose chemotherapy for each 6-month interval between years 1 and 4 after treatment. In this report, the median survival for both groups is 1.8 to 1.9 years with a 5-year probability of survival of 22% in the high-dose chemotherapy and 13% in the standard-dose group. Of the women who achieved partial remission in response to induction chemotherapy, 43% achieved complete remission after high-dose chemotherapy. In general, patients who demonstrate chemotherapy-sensitive disease (partial or complete remission) after four to six cycles of salvage therapy are considered candidates for high-dose therapy as consolidation. Favorable prognostic features include chemotherapy-sensitive disease, smaller metastatic foci (under 2 cm), no prior adjuvant chemotherapy, hormone receptor positive, long interval between primary disease and recurrence (over 2 years), and nonvisceral metastasis. The survival after high-dose chemotherapy is the best in patients with stage IV oligometastatic breast cancer characterized by small-volume disease amenable to effective local control. At median follow-up of 5 years, the relapse-free survival and overall survival rates of oligometastatic patients enrolled in the high-dose chemotherapy study were 51.6% and 62.6%, respectively. Median relapse-free survival and overall survival times were 52 and 80 months, respectively. Local therapy, capable of controlling sites of detectable tumor, seems a major contributor to this multimodal approach. Evaluation of more than 20 different preparative regimens in a multivariate analysis failed to identify a single superior regimen; the most common regimens were STAMP I and STAMP V (see Table 5.4).

The other group of patients that may benefit from high-dose therapy are those considered high risk owing to the presence of four or more positive lymph nodes at the time of mastectomy or inflammatory breast cancer. The most rapidly growing indication for high-dose therapy with autotransplant is high-risk breast cancer. Peters and colleagues (1993) first reported the superior outcome of high-dose therapy with autotransplant, compared with historical control patients treated with conventional therapy, in patients with 10 or more positive (cancer-involved) axillary lymph nodes. In the initial report, a 72% disease-free survival was reported at 3.3 years (71% at 5 years in a follow-up report) in the transplant group compared with 25% to 35% in historical control subjects treated with standard therapy. Four large randomized adjuvant trials in breast cancer have now been completed to accrual, and four others are ongoing. Preliminary results showed a lower relapse rate in the high-dose therapy arm but similar overall survival in one study. Two studies clearly demonstrated a benefit of high-dose chemotherapy in the adjuvant setting; unfortunately, one is being discredited. The other large randomized adjuvant study followed patients for a median of 4.5 years shows statistically significant differences in favor of the transplantation arm with 77% disease-free survival and 89% overall survival. The transplantation arm has an improved outcome in subgroups with both 4 to 9 and more than 10 positive lymph nodes. Importantly, only after 2.5 to 3 years of follow-up did the disease-free survival and overall survival curves of both groups start to separate, which may help to interpret the early results of other trials. The mortality from high-dose chemotherapy is 0% to 2.5%. Even fewer data are available to evaluate the efficacy of high-dose therapy and autologous transplant in patients with four to nine involved lymph nodes. Historical control data indicate a 5-year disease-free survival rate ranging from 40% to 50%. Data from the ABMTR indicate a 3-year disease-free survival rate of about 60% in patients with stage II or III breast cancer. The disease-free survival rate approaches 70% in patients with hormone receptor–positive disease who receive posttransplant tamoxifen and radiation therapy to the chest wall and axilla. An NCI-sponsored randomized trial comparing intensive sequential chemotherapy with high-dose therapy for patients with four to nine involved lymph nodes is still open for accrual at this writing. Several new strategies are being actively pursued using high-dose chemotherapy in breast cancer. These include the development of new high-dose chemotherapy with transplant regimens, tandem or multiple transplantations, and combination of high-dose chemotherapy with transplant plus treatments with novel mechanisms of action targeting posttransplantation minimal residual disease.

2.   Ovarian cancer, like breast cancer, is sensitive to conventional-dose chemotherapy. Therefore, trials of dose-escalated chemotherapy with hematopoietic stem cell rescue have been pursued. The ABMTR reported the results of 421 patients with ovarian cancer completing high-dose therapy with autologous transplant; the 2-year progression-free survival and overall survival were 12% and 35%, respectively. Favorable prognostic factors included younger age, Karnofsky Performance Scale score of at least 90%, non–clear cell disease, remission at transplantation, and platinum sensitivity, which were associated with better outcomes. Progression-free and overall survivals were 22% and 55%, respectively, for women with a high Karnofsky score and non–clear cell, platinum-sensitive tumors. When debulking surgery and platinum-based chemotherapy followed by second-look operation were used prior to high-dose chemotherapy with a melphalan-based regimen, an improvement of the 5-year progression-free survival and overall survival (29% and 45%) was observed after a median follow-up of 60 months. Survival is dependent on the residual tumor at second-look surgery. Better outcomes were obtained in women with a complete pathologic response at second-look operation with 43% 5-year progression-free survival and 75% 5-year overall survival compared with 7% survival at 5 years in those with a partial response.

Two pilot trials evaluating high-dose therapy with autologous transplant as consolidation therapy for previously untreated advanced-stage ovarian cancer have demonstrated promising results. One trial reported 5-year progression-free survival and overall survival rates of 51% and 60%, respectively; the other reported 5-year values of 24% and 60%, respectively, with a median survival of 30 months. This compares favorably with historical control data showing a 20% to 30% 5-year survival rate with conventional therapy. The NCI is currently sponsoring a Phase II clinical trial evaluating high-dose therapy as initial therapy in patients with optimal debulked stage III ovarian cancer (GOG 9903). The European Bone Marrow Transplant Group is conducting a Phase III randomized trial comparing high-dose sequential therapy with standard chemotherapy in optimally debulked stage III and IV ovarian cancer. Another randomized trial is being planned at Loyola University in Chicago, and ABMTR, comparing conventional chemotherapy for two cycles after a clinical complete remission with high-dose chemotherapy and SCT using negative second-look surgery as the primary endpoint. The goal is to show a 20% improvement in negative second-look surgery.

3. Germ cell cancers are chemotherapy-sensitive malignancies that afflict young people. Patients with advanced-stage disease who fail to achieve complete remission in response to initial platinum-based standard therapy have a poor prognosis: Their long-term disease-free survival rate is less than 5%. High-dose therapy with autotransplantation in heavily pretreated patients results in a disease-free survival rate of 15% to 20%. A second group of patients who are potential candidates for transplantation includes the 10% of patients who relapse after achieving complete remission. Although salvage therapy with vinblastine, ifosfamide, and cisplatin (VeIP) produces a more than 50% response rate, only 20% to 30% of these patients achieve durable remissions. High-dose therapy with autotransplantation results in a 30% to 50% long-term disease-free survival rate for patients with responsive relapse. For resistant relapse, the long-term disease-free survival rate after autotransplant is 5% to 20%. A recent updated experience with 65 patients treated with tandem transplant as initial salvage therapy for testicular germ cell neoplasm reported 57% of patients were continuously disease-free after the median follow-up of 39 months. Patients in the intermediate- and poor-prognosis categories tend to do less well. Seventy percent of patients who achieved complete remission after high-dose chemotherapy or after surgery become long-term survivors.

4. Small cell lung cancer is a chemosensitive malignancy with a long-term disease-free survival rate of about 20% at 2 years in patients with limited disease. Autotransplants in advanced disease or early small lung cancer are associated with 6% to 10% transplant-related mortality. The response duration is short: Only 15% of patients survive disease-free for at least 2 years when transplants are performed early. Several trials used autotransplants to intensify therapy in small cell lung cancer patients responding to conventional therapy. Two-year survival was 13%, and less than 10% remained disease-free at more than 2 years. The results suggest that there is no advantage of high-dose chemotherapy with transplant over standard treatment.

5. Other diseases in which high-dose therapy with transplantation has reported efficacy include aplastic anemia and MDSs. Aplastic anemia has a guarded prognosis because of the risk of infection and fatal hemorrhage. The 1-year survival rate for severe aplastic anemia is less than 20%. Allogeneic transplantation results in a long-term survival rate ranging from 50% to 90%. Favorable prognostic factors are younger age (under 16 years), no prior transfusions, short interval from diagnosis to transplant, and no evidence of infection. The preparative regimen consists of immunosuppressive agents: cyclophosphamide alone or with antithymocyte globulin or with TBI. Patients who do not have a compatible sibling donor may be considered for a matched unrelated donor transplantation. About 15% to 30% of patients survive with engraftment.

One of the newest areas of clinical interest is autoimmune diseases. Although published predominantly in case reports, there appears to be clinical improvement or stabilization in disease parameters after high-dose therapy with autologous transplant for multiple sclerosis, systemic lupus erythematosus, scleroderma, and rheumatoid arthritis. Preparative regimens focus on immunosuppression with cyclophosphamide with TBI or antithymocyte globulin.

XI.   Future directions. The field of high-dose therapy is evolving into *ex vivo* HPC expansion, gene therapy, improved CD34+ selection techniques, minitransplants, improved GVHD prophylaxis and treatment, improvement in safety of matched unrelated and mismatched donor transplants, DNA and idiotype vaccines, dendritic cell recruitment and transplantation, novel hematopoietic growth factors, and posttransplant immunotherapy to eradicate minimal residual disease.

SELECTED READINGS

Ahpek G, Ambinder RF, Piantadosi S, et al. Long-term results of blood and marrow transplantation for Hodgkin's lymphoma. *J Clin Oncol* 2001;19:4314–4321.

Armitage JO, Antman KH, eds. *High-dose cancer therapy: pharmacology, hematopoietins, stem cells.* 3rd ed. Baltimore: Lippincott Williams & Wilkins, 1999.

Attal M, Harousseau JL, Stoppa AM, et al. A prospective, randomized trial of autologous bone marrow transplantation and chemotherapy in multiple myeloma. *N Engl J Med* 1996;335:91–97.

Berry BA, Broadwater G, Klein JP, et al. High-dose versus standard chemotherapy in metastatic breast cancer: comparison of cancer and leukemia group B trials with data from the Autologous Blood and Marrow Transplant Registry. *J Clin Oncol* 2002;20:743–750.

Brenner MK, Rill DR, Moen RC, et al. Gene-marking to trace origin of relapse after autologous bone-marrow transplantation. *Lancet* 1993;341:85–86.

Collins RH Jr, Shpilberg O, Drobyski WR, et al. Donor leukocyte infusions in 140 patients with relapsed malignancy after allogeneic bone marrow transplantation. *J Clin Oncol* 1997;15:433–444.

Curtis RE, Rowlings PA, Deeg HJ, et al. Solid cancers after bone marrow transplantation. *N Engl J Med* 1997;336:897–904.

De Witte T, Hermans J, Vossen J, et al. Haematopoietic stem cell transplantation for patients with myelodysplastic syndromes and secondary leukaemias: a report on behalf of the Chronic Leukaemia Working Party of the European Group for Blood and Marrow Transplantation. *Br J Haematol* 2000;110:620–630.

Ferme C, Mounier N, Divine M, et al. Intensive salvage therapy with high-dose chemotherapy for patients with advanced Hodgkin's disease in relapse or failure after initial chemotherapy: results of the Groupe d'Etudes des Lymphomes de l'Adulte H89 Trial. *J Clin Oncol* 2002;15:467–475.

Filipovich AH, Stone JV, Tomany SC, et al. Impact of donor type on outcome of bone marrow transplantation for Wiskott—Aldrich syndrome: collaborative study of the International Bone Marrow Transplant Registry and the National Marrow Donor Program. *Blood* 2001;97:1598–1603.

Forman SJ, Blume KG, Thomas ED, eds. *Bone marrow transplantation.* Boston: Blackwell Scientific, 1999.

Freedman AS, Gribben JG, Neuberg D, et al. High dose therapy and autologous bone marrow transplantation in patients with follicular lymphoma during first remission. *Blood* 1996;88:2780–2786.

Gianni AM, Bregni M, Siena S, et al. High-dose chemotherapy and autologous bone marrow transplantation compared with MACOP-B in aggressive B-cell lymphoma. *N Engl J Med* 1997;336:1290–1297.

Giralt S, Estey E, Albitar M, et al. Engraftment of allogeneic hematopoietic progenitor cells with purine analog-containing chemotherapy: harnessing graft-versus-leukemia without myeloablative therapy. *Blood* 1997;89:4531–4536.

Gluckman E. Hematopoietic stem-cell transplants using umbilical-cord blood. *N Engl J Med* 2001;344:1860–1861.

Goldman J. Implications of imatinib mesylate for hematopoietic stem cell transplantation. *Semin Hematol* 2001;38(suppl 8):28–34.

Guardiola P, Anderson JE, Bandini G, et al. Allogeneic stem cell transplantation for agnogenic myeloid metaplasia: a European Group for Blood and Marrow Transplantation, Societe Francaise de Greffe de Moelle, Gruppo Italiano per il Trapianto del Midollo Osseo, and Fred Hutchinson Cancer Research Center Collaborative Study. *Blood* 1999;93:2831–2838.

Hahn T, Wolff S, Czuczman M, et al. The role of cytotoxic therapy with hematopoietic stem cell transplantation in the therapy of diffuse large cell B-cell non-Hodgkin's lymphoma: an evidence-based review. *Biol Blood Marrow Transplant* 2001;7:308–331.

Kernan NA, Bartsch G, Ash RC, et al. Retrospective analysis of 462 unrelated marrow transplants facilitated by the National Marrow Donor Program (NMDP) for treatment of acquired and congenital disorders of the lymphohematopoietic system and congenital metabolic disorders. *N Engl J Med* 1993;328:593–602.

Körbling M, Anderlini P. Peripheral blood stem cell versus bone marrow allotransplantation: does the source of hematopoietic stem cells matter? *Blood* 2001;98:2900–2908.

McCune JS, Gibbs JP, Slattery JT. Plasma concentration monitoring of busulfan: does it improve clinical outcome? *Clin Pharmacokinet* 2000;39:155–165.

Nieto Y, Champlin RE, Wingard JR, et al. Status of high-dose chemotherapy for breast cancer: a review. *Biol Blood Marrow Transplant* 2000;6:476–495.

Peters WP, Ross M, Vredenburgh JJ, et al. High-dose chemotherapy and autologous bone marrow support as consolidation after standard-dose adjuvant therapy for high-risk primary breast cancer. *J Clin Oncol* 1993;11:1132–1143.

Philip T, Guglielmi C, Hagenbeek A, et al. Autologous bone marrow transplantation as compared with salvage chemotherapy in relapses of chemotherapy-sensitive non-Hodgkin's lymphoma. *N Engl J Med* 1995;333:1540–1545.

Rocha V, Cornish J, Sievers EL, et al. Comparison of outcomes of unrelated bone marrow and umbilical cord blood transplants in children with acute leukemia. *Blood* 2001;97:2962–2971.

Rowe JM, Ciobann N, Ascensao J, et al. Recommended guidelines for the management of autologous and allogeneic bone marrow transplantation. *Ann Intern Med* 1994;120:143–158.

Schmitz N, Dreger P, Zander A, et al. Results of a randomized, controlled, multicentre study of recombinant human granulocyte colony-stimulating factor (filgrastim) in patients with Hodgkin's disease and non-Hodgkin's lymphoma undergoing autologous bone marrow transplantation. *Bone Marrow Transplant* 1995;15:261–266.

Socie G, Curtis RE, Deeg HJ, et al. New malignant diseases after allogeneic marrow transplantation for childhood acute leukemia. *J Clin Oncol* 2000;18:348–357.

Stiff PJ, Veum-Stone J, Lazarus HM, et al. High-dose chemotherapy and autologous stem-cell transplantation for ovarian cancer: an Autologous Blood and Marrow Transplant Registry report. *Ann Intern Med* 2000;133:504–515.

Thomas ED, Clift TA. Indications for marrow transplantation in chronic myelogenous leukemia. *Blood* 1989;73:861–864.

Van Besien K, Sobocinski KA, Rowlings PA, et al: Allogeneic bone marrow transplantation for low-grade lymphoma. *Blood* 1998;92:1832–1836.

Zittoun RA, Mandelli F, Willemze R, et al. Autologous or allogeneic bone marrow transplantation compared with intensive chemotherapy in acute myelogenous leukemia. *N Engl J Med* 1995;332:217–223.

Chemotherapy of
Human Cancer

6

Carcinomas of the Head and Neck

Ronald C. DeConti

Achievement of a management plan resulting in long-term control or cure for many patients with carcinomas of the head and neck remains an elusive, only partially realized goal for head and neck surgeons, radiation oncologists, and medical oncologists. Important gains in understanding the natural history of these neoplasms have been made, and the individual achievements of irradiation, surgical techniques, and chemotherapy have been stressed. However, only recently have these modalities been combined to form new treatment plans, and any increased benefit to the patient that might result from this multidisciplinary effort is now being explored.

This discussion focuses on the squamous cell carcinomas of the lining of the upper aerodigestive tract, which extends from the lip to the esophagus. These tumors account for about 5% of the new cancer cases seen in the United States each year. Excluded from this discussion are the melanomas, lymphomas, and sarcomas (which also occur in this area) as well as carcinomas of the thyroid, esophagus, and salivary glands. A cross-sectional view of the anatomic regions and the relative frequency of cancer occurring in each area are shown in Fig. 6-1. The large number of potential tumor sites and some difficulty in determining the exact site of origin have led to broad use of these larger subdivision terms in an attempt to avoid confusion and to group the related sites. Table 6.1 lists major sites within each of these anatomic subdivisions.

I. **Common and divergent characteristics.** Carcinomas of the head and neck are frequently considered together by students, generalists, and medical oncologists as though they represent a single therapeutic problem. A number of factors promote this concept:

A. **Similarities.** In the United States, more than 90% of all lesions are squamous cell carcinomas, and these lesions occur predominantly in men (three-to-one ratio). Most patients share common demographic and epidemiologic risk factors. The incidence of head and neck cancer increases with the use of alcohol and tobacco and with advancing age. Head and neck cancers occur in continuity, one with another, and it is occasionally difficult to determine the precise site of origin in the close confines of the complicated interrelated structures comprising the oral cavity, pharynx, larynx, and sinuses. Furthermore, patterns of spread are similar, with local failure, local recurrence, and regional node failures predominating. For carcinomas originating at most sites, spread below the clavicle is unusual, occurring in only a few patients, usually as pulmonary involvement. Bone lesions, usually the result of local extension involving the mandible or floor of the skull, are not uncommon, although

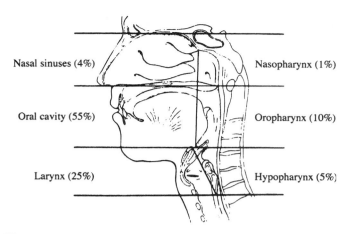

Fig. 6-1.   Anatomic divisions of the head and neck. Percentages indicate the relative frequencies of carcinoma in these regions.

Table 6.1.   Upper aerodigestive tract sites

Region	Area	Site
Oral cavity	—	Lip
		Buccal mucosa
		Lower alveolar ridge
		Upper alveolar ridge
		Retromolar trigone
		Floor of mouth
		Hard palate
		Oral tongue
Pharynx	Nasopharynx	Posterior wall
		Lateral wall
	Oropharynx	Faucial arch
		Tonsillar fossa and tonsil
		Base of tongue
		Pharyngeal wall
	Hypopharynx	Piriform fossa
		Postcricoid area
		Posterior wall
Larynx	Supraglottis	Ventricular band
		Arytenoid
		Epiglottis
	Glottis	True vocal cords
	Subglottis	Subglottis
Paranasal sinuses	—	Antrum
		Nasal cavity
		Ethmoid
		Sphenoid
		Frontal

widespread bone metastases are unusual. A few patients develop hepatic metastases. Inanition, oral ulceration, fistula formation, respiratory difficulty, and aspiration characterize the late course of the disease. Recurrence after primary treatment usually occurs within 18 months, and patients who are not cured usually die within 3 years of diagnosis.

B. **Differences.** For the surgeon or radiation oncologist, the differences among carcinomas at different sites may be more significant than the similarities. Certainly, presenting signs and symptoms differ markedly. For example, patients with an anterior tongue lesion may describe pain, sensation of mass, and limited motion of the tongue. Hoarseness, dysphagia, or sore throat may predominate in patients with carcinoma of the larynx. More importantly, differences in location influence the frequency of nodal spread and the chances for contralateral node involvement. These factors frequently determine the optimal treatment plan.

II. **Primary treatment.** A discussion of the specific variations in primary treatment choices for the multitude of sites where head and neck carcinomas occur is beyond the scope of this chapter. In general, early lesions in most locations are suitable for treatment by surgery or irradiation, and the therapeutic choice is usually made by considering the complications of each treatment, that is, the deformities of definitive surgery or the complications of irradiation. With increasing failure rates and the likelihood of pathologic, if not clinical, lymph node involvement as tumor bulk increases, clinicians have begun to investigate combined-modality approaches. Radiation can be used electively before operation or postoperatively after a microscopic assessment of regional nodes provides the opportunity for postsurgical pathologic staging. Many studies now report improved local and regional node control after such multimodality approaches. Although substantial progress has been made in improving end results for early-stage lesions at many sites and in decreasing the morbidity and deformity from the treatment, the outcome for tumors in advanced stages remains poor: For stage III disease, the 3- to 5-year survival rate is 25% to 60%. For stage IV disease, long-term survival rates of 10% to 30% have been reported.

III. **Staging.** Any consideration of outcome in relation to treatment relies heavily on detailed pretreatment assessment of the extent of the tumor.

A. **TNM classification.** A complex site-specific staging system has been devised by the American Joint Committee on Cancer. This system incorporates a TNM classification to identify, clinically and pathologically, the size of the primary tumor (T), the presence and extent of regional node metastases (N), and the presence of distant metastases (M). Table 6.2 outlines the TNM system for carcinoma of the oral cavity. For lesions of the nasopharynx, hypopharynx, and larynx, fixation or anatomic extensions are substituted for tumor size when determining the extent of the primary lesion.

B. **Stages.** The stage grouping for head and neck cancers is shown in Table 6.3. Stages I and II are determined by the size of the tumor in the absence of nodal involvement or distant metastases. Stage III includes both large tumors and tumors of

Table 6.2.   TNM staging system for carcinomas of the oral cavity

Primary tumor
TX	No available information on primary tumor
T0	No evidence of primary tumor
Tis	Carcinoma *in situ*
T1	Greatest diameter of tumor ≤2 cm
T2	Greatest diameter of tumor >2–4 cm
T3	Greatest diameter of tumor >4 cm
T4	Invasion to adjacent structures such as antrum, pterygoid muscles, base of tongue, or skin of neck

Regional nodal status
NX	Nodes cannot be assessed
N0	No clinically positive node
N1	Single clinically positive ipsilateral node ≤3 cm in diameter
N2	Single clinically positive ipsilateral node >3–6 cm; or multiple clinically positive nodes, none >6 cm; or bilateral or contralateral nodes, none >6 cm
N3	Metastasis in a lymph node >6 cm in greatest dimension

Distant metastasis
MX	Not assessed
M0	No (known) distant metastasis
M1	Distant metastasis present

any size with early regional node involvement. Stage IV lesions may be huge with local extension or may be of any size with distant metastatic disease. This stage grouping has been uniformly applied to each tumor site to demonstrate gradations in prognosis.

IV.   Chemotherapy

A.   Prognostic factors. Whether chemotherapy is considered for the treatment of advanced recurrent head and neck cancer or for preoperative induction treatment, a number of similar, single prognostic variables have now been clearly identified (Table 6.4).

Table 6.3.   Stage grouping for carcinomas of the oral cavity, pharynx, larynx, and paranasal sinuses

Stage	Groups
I	T1, N0, M0
II	T2, N0, M0
III	T3, N0, M0
	T1 or T2 or T3, N1, M0
IV	T4, N0 or N1, M0
	Any T, N2 or N3, M0
	Any T, any N, M1

Table 6.4. Factors prognostic for response to chemotherapy

Favorable	Unfavorable
Stage III	Stage IV
No metastasis	Pulmonary metastasis
ECOG performance status 0–1	ECOG performance status 2–3
No weight loss	Weight loss
Normal immune mechanism	Impaired delayed hypersensitivity
Prior surgery	Prior irradiation
Long disease-free interval	Short disease-free interval
No prior chemotherapy	Prior chemotherapy
Combination chemotherapy	Single-agent chemotherapy
Poorly differentiated tumor	Well-differentiated tumor
Nasopharynx	Other sites

ECOG, Eastern Cooperative Oncology Group.

1. Stage of carcinoma. Small lesions with minimal regional node involvement respond better than the massive tumors of stage IV. Patients with stage IV disease due to bulky lymph nodes commonly get little benefit from treatment. Response rates are lowest for stage IV disease with pulmonary or visceral metastases. Because patients with head and neck cancers have an increased risk of developing second primary neoplasms, the finding of distant metastases in the absence of primary or regional node recurrence suggests this possibility.

2. State of health. Both poor Eastern Cooperative Oncology Group (ECOG) performance status (see Table 2.2) and weight loss of more than 5% have been found to affect prognosis adversely. It is still unclear whether aggressive attempts to improve nutrition or restore cellular immunity with hyperalimentation result in gains in the response and survival rates.

3. Prior treatment. Many studies have reported the adverse effect of prior radiation therapy on response to chemotherapy. This effect has usually been attributed to an impaired tumor blood supply, a large tumor burden, and poor patient performance status. The failure to respond to irradiation and a rapid relapse after radiation therapy have also been shown to affect response rates adversely.

B. Pretreatment assessment. The extent of evaluation required to determine the suitability of a patient for chemotherapy depends, to a considerable degree, on the intent of therapy and type of program to be employed. The major organ systems affected by the antineoplastic drugs under consideration are bone marrow, lungs, and kidneys. Any pretreatment assessment should consider not only careful evaluation of the size and extent of tumor but also the presence of co-morbid disease processes involving these organ systems. A careful history, review of systems, physical assessment, and routine laboratory data may provide clues in these areas.

   1.   **Bone marrow function.** Chronic alcoholism and malnutrition or the effect of the tumor on glutition and appetite
may contribute to the high incidence of folate deficiency
seen in this population. Because of the additive effect of
this deficiency and the inhibition of folate metabolism by
methotrexate, there is often increased sensitivity to even
small doses of methotrexate, which manifests as marked
clinical toxicity.
   2.   **Pulmonary function.** Chronic obstructive pulmonary
disease is common in this group of patients. Moderate to severe pretreatment reductions in timed forced expiratory volumes may be reduced further with treatment with bleomycin.
If clinical assessment suggests impaired pulmonary reserve
and bleomycin is to be part of the treatment program, pretreatment pulmonary function studies should be performed.
   3.   **Renal function.** Both cisplatin and methotrexate affect
renal function. The major cumulative toxicity of cisplatin is
renal. Unfortunately, there may be considerable impairment
of renal function before the serum creatinine concentration
rises; cisplatin doses of 80 to 120 mg/m^2 require serial determination of creatinine clearance to assess the cumulative
effects of the drug on renal function.
   Limited renal excretion of methotrexate prolongs the duration of a high serum concentration, which in turn extends the
duration of impaired DNA synthesis for normal as well as
neoplastic tissues. Weekly IV methotrexate is usually given
to patients with advanced disease after it is established that
the serum creatinine level is normal. A careful clinical assessment at the time of each subsequent dose is probably a
more reliable indicator of actual and potential methotrexate
toxicity than are serial determinations of creatinine in this
situation. Most episodes of serious methotrexate toxicity relate to a failure to appreciate intercurrent events that limit
excretion of these relatively low doses of the drug. The most
common of these toxicities is probably dehydration, which is
related to progressive disease, increasingly poor oral intake,
nausea and vomiting, or mucositis that may have been caused
by prior drug treatment. Third-space reservoirs created by
pleural effusions or ascites may lead to delayed clearance, prolonged serum drug levels, and increased toxicity. The addition
of any drug that further alters renal clearance of methotrexate may tip the balance toward serious toxicity. Aspirin and
other nonsteroidal anti-inflammatory agents, probenecid,
sulfonamides, phenytoin, cefoxitin, and gentamicin may decrease methotrexate clearance and increase toxicity. Careful
patient assessment at intervals with these considerations in
mind helps to avoid these pitfalls.
C.   Single-agent responses. Methotrexate, bleomycin, fluorouracil, cisplatin, carboplatin, and doxorubicin (Adriamycin)
have been studied extensively as individual agents for head
and neck carcinomas. More recently, ifosfamide and the taxanes have been shown to have significant activity. Most combinations derive from these agents.
   1.   **Methotrexate.** In efforts to improve its therapeutic
index, methotrexate has been more extensively investigated

for the management of head and neck cancer than any other solid tumor.

    a.   Intravenous methotrexate in doses of 40 to 60 mg/m^2 weekly is probably the most widely accepted conventional single-agent treatment for this group of tumors. Treatment with methotrexate results in objective response in 25% to 50% of patients, 7% to 10% of which are complete responses. Responses may occur after 1 to 2 weeks but usually require 4 to 6 weeks to become evident. Median response durations range from 2 to 6 months. Responders survive significantly longer than nonresponders. Treatment is usually given on an outpatient basis, and drug-related mortality is less than 4%.

    b.   Intra-arterial infusions of methotrexate either alone or with systemic leucovorin have been used in an attempt to improve drug concentrations in tumor tissue and to improve the therapeutic index of treatment. Although these techniques have resulted in marginally superior response rates, the lack of a single predominant blood supply to most tumors, the technical difficulties of the procedure, and the morbidity of problems with clot, embolus, and infection have precluded widespread adoption of this approach; it is not recommended for general use.

2.   Bleomycin. Bleomycin attracted interest for treatment of head and neck cancers because of its generally mild myelosuppressive effects and the potential for its application in combination with myelosuppressive chemotherapy. Bleomycin 10 to 30 U/m^2 is usually given weekly, biweekly, or on a 5-day/month schedule by IM and IV injections. These approaches are convenient for outpatient use. Tumor response rarely occurs at cumulative doses of less than 200 U/m^2, and response most often requires a total dose of 300 U/m^2. These doses usually produce significant mucosal toxicity. Response rates range between 15% and 25% and are generally inferior in duration to those achieved with methotrexate. The mucosal toxicity that accompanies the use of bleomycin is generally more frequent and severe than that produced with the use of a weekly methotrexate schedule. These difficulties as well as the likelihood of developing drug-induced pneumonitis limit its use today as other drugs have become available.

3.   Cisplatin. Cisplatin 40 to 60 mg/m^2 IV is given on an every-3-week schedule. Higher doses result in an increased risk of renal toxicity unless special precautions are taken. Doses of 80 to 120 mg/m^2 may be tolerated if preceded by hydration and accompanied by mannitol administration (with or without furosemide) for diuresis to protect renal function (see Chapter 4). The effectiveness of the selective serotonin receptor antagonists (ondansetron [Zofran] and granisetron [Kytril]) in control of nausea and vomiting in the first 24 h after therapy has increased patients' tolerance to cisplatin and has made it considerably easier to administer an intermediate dose of this drug on an outpatient basis. Cisplatin produces objective tumor responses in about 25% of patients, many of whom were treated previously with other antineoplastic drugs. Occasionally, dramatic tumor responses occur, although the frequency of complete remission is still low. Its major side effects are severe nausea and vomiting (which may be more of a problem after 24 h than in the first 24 h, during which serotonin receptor antagonists offer better protection), tinnitus, occasional high-tone deafness, peripheral neuropathy, and, most significantly, renal toxicity (with progressive loss in creatinine clearance in some patients).

4.   Carboplatin. An analog of cisplatin that produces minimal renal toxicity, little peripheral neuropathy, and less emesis, carboplatin has a favorable toxicity profile that gives it considerable practical utility in head and neck cancer. Doses of 360 to 400 mg/m^2, usually divided in three daily doses and repeated at 4-week intervals, have resulted in response rates approaching those of cisplatin. Its ease of administration and favorable therapeutic index recommend its use for palliation. Prolonged thrombocytopenia can be dose limiting. Adoption of the Calvert formula (area under the curve [AUC]) to determine dose may improve both tolerance and efficacy.

5.   5-Fluorouracil. 5-Fluorouracil (5-FU) may be of somewhat greater value for oral cavity lesions than other agents; it has an overall 15% response rate. Use by prolonged infusion was popularized by a small Phase II study demonstrating a much higher response rate, which has not been duplicated. However, most combinations with 5-FU have used the drug this way. Attempts to improve response rates using leucovorin in conjunction with 5-FU have not yet demonstrated long-term value. Oral formulations of 5-FU (capecitabine, Zeloda) administered daily for 2 to 3 weeks have not been evaluated.

6.   Ifosfamide. Phase II studies have shown encouraging response rates of 20% to 42% for ifosfamide, with mesna used as a uroprotector in both bolus and infusion schedules.

7.   Taxanes. Both paclitaxel and docetaxel have shown high response rates in Phase II trials.

   a.   Paclitaxel, 250 mg/m^2 every 3 weeks with granulocyte colony-stimulating factor (G-CSF) support, achieved responses of 40% of advanced head and neck cancers in an ECOG Phase II trial. Other schedules and doses are under investigation; a 3-h infusion every 3 weeks has been found to be tolerable and convenient for outpatient therapy.

   b.   Docetaxel has been shown to produce response rates of 32% to 50% in small Phase II trials. A dose of 100 mg/m^2 IV administered over 1 h every 3 weeks was used to achieve these results.

8.   Other drugs

   a.   Anthracyclines appear to be of little overall value except in nasopharyngeal cancer, in which both doxorubicin and mitoxantrone have shown responses in about 25% of patients.

   b.   Vinca alkaloids such as vincristine and vinblastine achieve low response rates. Vinorelbine has little activity (8% to 16%) in single-agent trials.

   c.   Gemcitabine has shown modest activity (13% response rate) in one Phase II trial to date. Its value in combination therapy is under evaluation.

   d.   Topoisomerase inhibitors have shown little activity.

    e.   Retinoids have not yet been shown to be effective in advanced disease.

    f.   Numerous **biologic response modifiers** have been studied but have not demonstrated any value in clinical practice.

    g.   New directions. Encouraging data suggest that epidermal growth factor receptor antagonists (C225 [cetuximab], ZD1839 [gefitinib Iressa]), cyclin-dependent kinase inhibitors, and replication-competent adenoviruses may be useful, but their use remains investigational.

D.   Combination-chemotherapy responses. Multiple attempts have been made to improve single-agent response rates with combination chemotherapy. A number of studies using methotrexate, bleomycin, fluorouracil, cisplatin, and carboplatin in a variety of schedules have been reported. More recently, Phase II combination investigations include the taxanes, gemcitabine, and ifosfamide.

The ECOG, in a comparison of methotrexate, bleomycin, and cisplatin versus weekly methotrexate, demonstrated a clear-cut advantage for combination chemotherapy. Forty-eight percent of patients with advanced disease responded to an outpatient program using methotrexate, bleomycin, and cisplatin compared with 35% using methotrexate alone. Complete remissions were achieved in 16% of patients receiving combination chemotherapy and in 8% treated with methotrexate alone. The median duration of response was the same in both treatment groups, and no survival advantage was demonstrated for the combination treatment. Although neither response rate is exceptional, the careful randomization and stratification procedures used lend weight to the result.

Combinations of cisplatin or carboplatin with fluorouracil or bleomycin demonstrate like outcomes: improved response rates but no overall gain in survival. Phase II studies with newer agents, usually combined with cisplatin, suggest similar results. Comparative assessments of the quality-of-life or of symptom scores have rarely been performed. Phase III studies commonly compare other platinum combinations with cisplatin and fluorouracil.

E.   Combined-modality treatment. Attempts to increase tumor destruction with drugs before definitive therapy or together with radiation therapy are not new, although developments in combination chemotherapy reawakened enthusiasm for this approach.

    1.   Drugs before irradiation or surgery (neoadjuvant therapy)

        a.   Methotrexate. In several small single-institution studies, methotrexate in moderate and high doses with leucovorin rescue was given for several doses or cycles before irradiation or surgery. These schedules produced response rates of about 75% and avoided the problems of oral mucositis and ulceration reported by the older studies of concomitant chemotherapy with radiotherapy. No data are available to permit comparisons of these rescue programs with weekly methotrexate schedules.

        b.   Combination chemotherapy. A number of combination drug therapy programs have been developed as initial treatment for advanced locoregional disease. These programs were intended either to reduce tumor bulk and allow more effective radiotherapy or to improve resectability of advanced lesions. In general, the programs use high-dose cisplatin in conjunction with hydration and diuretics (see Chapter 4) combined with either bleomycin or fluorouracil and administered by IV infusion for 3 to 5 days. Vincristine is frequently included, and methotrexate is usually omitted. These programs produce high response rates (67% to 94%). Complete clinical disappearance of tumor is achieved in 19% to 28% of patients, and partial response is achieved in 48% to 74%. After one to three cycles of drug treatment, surgery, irradiation, or both follow. The number of patients with advanced locoregional disease who were made disease-free was higher than expected based on pretreatment staging expectations. Improvement in survival is limited to those patients who achieved complete response. The achievements and limitations of this plan of therapy are outlined in Table 6.5.

In general, neoadjuvant therapy best remains in the context of a clinical investigation. The most important demonstration of the value of neoadjuvant or induction chemotherapy relates to organ preservation. Trials stimulated by the high response rates achieved by these treatments have shown the ability to preserve the larynx and voice. The best-known trial (VA 268) showed that laryngeal preservation was possible in 64% of patients who received induction chemotherapy followed by radiation therapy, with survival rates comparable with those for

Table 6.5.   Achievements of induction or neoadjuvant chemotherapy for patients with head and neck cancers

Major tumor regressions occur in 60%–90% of patients with locally advanced disease.

Complete clinical regression occurs in 20%–50%.

Response rates increase with the number of cycles given, up to three.

Pathologic complete regressions are confirmed in 25%–60% of patients with clinical complete responses.

Treatment does not adversely affect surgical or radiation therapy complications.

Drug response appears to predict response to irradiation.

Complete responders may achieve locoregional disease control with radiation therapy and avoid surgery.

Quality of life may be improved for patients with tumors in some sites by organ preservation.

Frequency of distant metastasis as cause of treatment failure is reduced.

Complete responders have longer survival.

Overall survival is unchanged.

patients treated with laryngectomy and radiation therapy. Survival was not compromised in patients who received chemotherapy. Long-term survival was the same,
with evidence of preservation of voice and presumed maintenance of quality of life.

2.   Concurrent chemotherapy and radiotherapy. Bleomycin, fluorouracil, methotrexate, cisplatin, and the taxanes
have been administered synchronously with radiation therapy in attempts to demonstrate synergistic effects. Most uncontrolled studies suggested improved tumor responses and
some gain in survival for patients with unresectable disease. Two early studies demonstrated benefit for oral cavity
primary lesions with concurrent bleomycin or fluorouracil.
Enhanced mucositis has been a common limitation of combined treatment.

Cisplatin appears attractive as an agent for concurrent
therapy because of its radiosensitizing properties, established activity, and paucity of mucosal toxicity. Weekly dosing of cisplatin during radiotherapy resulted in higher
response rates but no overall difference in complete response
or survival rate compared with radiotherapy alone. When
cisplatin was given as a 100-mg/m^2 bolus every 3 weeks with
concurrent radiation therapy in a Radiation Therapy Oncology
Group trial, improvement in the number of complete responders and 4-year survival rates was suggested. A recent
intergroup trial has confirmed a significant survival advantage compared with standard fractionated radiotherapy
alone; multiagent chemotherapy did not compensate for the
decreased efficacy of split-course radiation therapy in that
study.

In nasopharyngeal carcinoma, a randomized intergroup trial
has demonstrated improved survival with that same schedule
of cisplatin together with radiation therapy compared with
radiation therapy alone. After radiation therapy, patients
also received two cycles of cisplatin and 5-FU.

Because combination chemotherapy has been demonstrated to be more effective than single-agent therapy, studies are now focusing on combination chemotherapy together
with radiation therapy. Because of the more severe local and
systemic toxicities that can be associated with these regimens, attempts have been made to modify radiation therapy
scheduling to facilitate the administration of combined-
modality therapy while avoiding intolerable toxicity. Several
randomized trials as well as meta-analyses have now demonstrated a survival advantage for concurrent chemoradiation
with platinum and 5-FU compared with radiation therapy
alone despite increased toxicity. Though a distinctly superior
drug regimen is not yet established, it seems clear that **concurrent chemoradiation is established as the new standard of care in advanced unresectable head and neck
cancer.** In contrast, if radiotherapy is used postoperatively in
patients with high risk of recurrence (two or more involved
nodes, extracapsular disease, or microscopically involved
margins), there does not appear to be any advantage to the
addition of concurrent cisplatin to radiotherapy. This subject

continues as an active and promising area of clinical investigation, exploring the taxanes and other new agents. Patients should be encouraged to participate in these trials.

3.   Drugs as posttreatment adjuvants. Whereas the most recent emphasis in head and neck cancer has been on achieving gains in early tumor control, little attention has been paid to the potential of postoperative or postirradiation adjuvant drug therapy studies. Suggestive Phase II data have not been confirmed in larger, randomized Phase III comparisons. Reasons for negative results include small sample size, inadequate therapy, poor patient compliance, and statistical analysis based on intention to treat. Posttreatment adjuvant therapy remains investigational. Current trials attempt to select postsurgical patients with poor prognostic pathologic features. These include multiple positive nodes, extracapsular spread, close or positive surgical margins, and *in situ* carcinoma at the margins.

F.   Selected treatment plans. Three types of drug treatment programs are displayed in Table 6.6.

1.   Cytoreductive induction treatment

a.   Selection of patients. This treatment is designed to reduce tumor bulk before surgery or radiation therapy in patients with advanced-stage disease and no prior therapy. The induction treatment regimen is intended primarily for patients with laryngeal carcinoma after assessment of the extent of the tumor and an evaluation to exclude co-morbid disease processes that might unacceptably increase the risks of treatment.

b.   Administration of cisplatin plus 5-fluorouracil. Oral hydration may be begun the evening before treatment. On the morning of treatment, an IV infusion of 5% dextrose in 0.5 N saline with potassium chloride 20 mEq/L and magnesium sulfate 1 g/L is begun at a rate of 500 mL/h. One of a number of intensive regimens to alleviate nausea and vomiting should be begun (see Chapter 26). Furosemide 40 mg IV and mannitol 12.5 g IV are given after the first liter. Immediately thereafter, if the patient is voiding freely, cisplatin 100 mg/m^2 is added to a calibrated solution set and infused IV over a 30-min period. An additional liter of fluid is given over a 2-h period. A continuous infusion of 5-FU 1,000 mg/m^2/day is begun and maintained for 5 days, usually with an infusion pump. The necessity for additional diuretics is judged by the extent of nausea and vomiting, the urinary volume, and evidence of congestive heart failure. If adequate oral intake is not ensured, additional IV fluids may be given. An interim clinic visit before a second induction course is recommended as a safeguard. A second course of treatment is planned on day 22 but should be administered only after hematologic values and serum creatinine levels are normal. If tumor regression is continuing on day 43 after two cycles of treatment, a third cycle may be considered, although the cumulative risks of renal and pulmonary toxicity increase with continued treatment. At this point, irradiation, surgery, or both should be considered once again.

Table 6.6. Selected drug treatment programs in head and neck cancer

Intent	Suitability	Scheme
Cytoreductive induction treatment	Advanced stage, no prior treatment	CF Cisplatin 100 mg/m² IV on d 1 with induced diuresis *and* Fluorouracil 1,000 mg/m²/d as 24-h infusion on d 1–5 Cycle repeats in 3–4 wk
Concurrent radiotherapy	Advanced stage, no prior treatment	Daily radiation therapy together with either: Cisplatin 100 mg/m² IV on d 1 with induced diuresis, repeat d 22, 43, or Carboplatin 70 mg/m² on d 1–4 *and* Fluorouracil 600 mg/m² on d 1–4 by ambulatory infusion pump; repeat days 23, 43 Split-course radiation therapy Cisplatin 75 mg/m² IV on d 1 with induced diuresis *and* Fluorouracil 1,000 mg/m² as 24-h infusion on d 1–4 Cycle repeats in 4 wk Radiotherapy 30 Gy/15 fractions begun on d 1 Evaluate at wk 9: CR or unresectable—repeat third chemotherapy cycle with 30 Gy/15 fractions; PR, stable, and resectable—have surgery with third cycle of chemotherapy and radiotherapy (30 Gy/15 fractions) 2–6 wk after operation

continued

Table 6.6. *Continued*

Intent	Suitability	Scheme
Palliation	Any prior treatment	Either cisplatin 20 mg/m^2 IV on d 1–5 *or* Carboplatin AUC 6 on d 1 *and* Fluorouracil 800 mg/m^2 on d 1–5 by ambulatory infusion pump Cycle repeats in 3–4 wk
		Paclitaxel (Taxol) 175 mg/m^2 as 3-h infusion on d 1 with steroid premedication and carboplatin AUC 6 on d 1 Cycle repeats in 4 wk
	Prior treatment and contra-indications to combination drugs	Methotrexate 40–60 mg/m^2 IV weekly *or* Paclitaxel (Taxol) 175–200 mg/m^2 IV every 3 wk with steroid premedication, *or* Docetaxel 60–100 mg/m^2 over 1 h with steroid premedication every 3 wk

CR, complete response; PR, partial response.

2. Concurrent chemotherapy

   a. Conventional-fraction radiation therapy

   (1) Cisplatin 100 mg/m^2 is given with appropriate hydration, diuresis, and antiemetics on days 1, 22, and 43 of radiation therapy, with attention to the cautions of cisplatin therapy. This is a relatively straightforward plan with no added mucosal toxicity.

   (2) Carboplatin is given at a dose of 70 mg/m^2/day for 4 days beginning on days 1, 22, and 43. 5-FU 600 mg/m^2/day over each 4-day period is given by continuous infusion. Added mucosal toxicity may necessitate nutritional support; the third cycle is frequently abbreviated owing to toxicity.

   b. Split-course radiotherapy. With this program, the dose of cisplatin is reduced to 75 mg/m^2 and the fluorouracil infusion duration is limited to 4 days. The plan of therapy is outlined in Table 6.6. Treatment is administered with hydration and antiemetics as described previously. Careful attention to fluid and nutritional support during possible periods of intense mucositis is necessary. In potentially operable patients, a decision for surgery is usually made after two courses of chemotherapy.

3. Combination chemotherapy for advanced recurrent disease. The approach to advanced recurrent disease is based on prior treatment and the perceived ability of the patient to tolerate intensive chemotherapy.

   a. Cisplatin plus 5-fluorouracil. With advanced recurrent disease, two courses of treatment with cisplatin plus 5-FU (see Section IV.F.1 and Table 6.6) may be elected, followed by an intermittent program with lower doses of drug.

   b. Ambulatory infusion. Alternative treatment choices use three to five daily doses of cisplatin or one dose of carboplatin together with continuous-infusion 5-FU administered using an ambulatory infusion pump. Either cisplatin 20 mg/m^2/day IV for 5 days or carboplatin AUC 6 on day 1 only as a short infusion can be combined with 5-FU 800 mg/m^2/day for 5 days as a continuous infusion. Dividing the dosage of cisplatin eliminates the need for aggressive hydration, shortens and simplifies the chemotherapy procedures, and promotes outpatient usage of these regimens.

   c. Carboplatin and paclitaxel (Taxol). Carboplatin, AUC 6 and paclitaxel (Taxol) 175 mg/m^2 are administered as a 3-h infusion in 500 to 1,000 mL of D5W or 0.9% sodium chloride after premedication with steroids (see Chapter 4) to avoid possibilities of shock. Thirty to 60 min before treatment, the patient is premedicated with diphenhydramine 50 mg IV and cimetidine 300 mg IV. Less aggressive rates of hydration may be necessary in older patients to prevent the development of congestive heart failure and pulmonary edema. Antiemetics are given as described previously.

4. Methotrexate alone for advanced disease

   a. Selection of patients. With a number of increased response rates reported for drug combinations compared with methotrexate alone, single-agent methotrexate should prob-ably be reserved for the following selected patients:

- Patients in relapse after induction treatment programs without methotrexate
- Patients who refuse treatment with cisplatin or pa-clitaxel
- Patients whose neuropathy excludes a cisplatin treat-ment program
- Patients whose reliability and follow-up opportunities are poor

b.   Treatment plan. The usual starting dose of methotrex-ate is 40 mg/m^2; if advanced age, nutritional status, ane-mia, borderline renal function, or other factors suggest sensitivity of normal tissues to methotrexate might be increased, the initial dose may be reduced to as low as 20 mg/m^2. Blood cell counts are done weekly, and if there is no evidence of mucositis or myelosuppression, the dose is escalated to a maximum of 60 mg/m^2. Most patients tol-erate this treatment with minimal nausea and vomiting. A few require antiemetics. Careful attention to oral hydra-tion may be helpful for preventing or reducing the severity of mucositis (see Chapter 26). Candidiasis is common and, if present, should be treated with nystatin (Mycostatin) or another antifungal agent. If mucositis or myelosuppression occurs, treatments are delayed until they clear and blood cell counts are normal. Six to 8 weeks of therapy may be necessary to achieve a response.

V.   Problems in supportive care
A.   Support systems. The population of patients with head and neck cancer includes many elderly men—often social repro-bates, recluses, heavy smokers and drinkers, and occasionally frank derelicts. They are frequently divorced or separated from their families, and many live alone, often in reduced circum-stances. Lack of family, friends, resources, and initiative are often impediments to adequate care, especially in advanced-disease situations in which close follow-up, regular clinic visits, and adherence to treatment schedules are important. These pa-tients desperately need a primary caregiver to be in the home or closely allied with the home to promote their well-being and optimal use of medical care and to derive advantage from the health care delivery system. Social service, ministerial help, American Cancer Society patient programs (such as I Can Cope), patient support groups, Alcoholics Anonymous, and other social care groups should be enlisted to help the patient cope with ill-ness. Smoking cessation programs may be appropriate for those with early cancers that may be cured.

B.   Nutrition. Gradual, progressive weight loss and inanition are common factors in the relentless illness of many patients. Their nutrition is generally inadequate, and repetitive efforts at reinforcing the need for a high-calorie diet, as free of alcohol as possible, must be given. Depending on the location of the tumor and the particular problems with swallowing, efforts need to be extended on a regular basis to ensure adequate pa-tient nutrition. Many patients or their families need to be instructed in the use of blended foods, high-protein supplements, or both. Some patients benefit from the use of a pediatric feeding tube when deformities in the anatomy prevent adequate swallowing. In selected patients, feeding by a gastrostomy tube may be appropriate, especially early in the patient's clinical course when it is hoped that it may be only a temporary expedient. Most patients benefit from any attempts at oral hyperalimentation. The role of IV hyperalimentation is not clear and needs to be considered early in the management course during the perioperative or radiation therapy period when induction treatment is taking place. Its role for patients with an advanced disease state is still unclear. Efforts to maintain nutrition must be reinforced at every opportunity with the family, the caregiver, and the patient. Dietary advice or consultation with a dietetic department should be sought.

C.   Mouth care. An important problem for some patients with head and neck cancer is mouth care. Many patients have difficulty with secretions. Xerostomia may be produced by radiation therapy and may require treatment with artificial saliva. An additional agent that may be helpful is pilocarpine 5 to 10 mg given orally three times daily with water. At the opposite extreme, patients with posterior tongue lesions may have edema and swelling that preclude adequate swallowing, and the pooling of secretions and subsequent aspiration become a problem. These patients may benefit from the use of suction to drain their secretions. Cleansing mouthwash may be appropriate (see Chapter 26), and efforts at dental hygiene need to be maintained. Radiation-induced bone necrosis or fistulas need to be cleaned or debrided and occasionally packed with toothpaste or other material to promote comfort. Dental consultation is helpful in many patients, particularly before radiation therapy.

D.   Granulocytopenia and infection. There is always an urgent need to identify pulmonary and other infections quickly in the presence of drug-induced granulocytopenia. The mortality due to pneumonia and sepsis is high in this situation. Appropriate cultures are needed in an effort to document infection and help distinguish the problem from aspiration. Fever in a granulocytopenic patient should be treated promptly with broad-spectrum antibiotics without awaiting results of blood or sputum cultures (see Chapter 27). In selected situations, the use of G-CSF may reduce the duration of granulocytopenia and ameliorate infections.

E.   Anemia. Fatigue, tachycardia, shortness of breath, and edema may result from or be exacerbated by anemia induced by chemotherapy, especially cisplatin. These symptoms can be ameliorated and transfusions reduced by the use of epoetin (Procrit).

F.   Hypothyroidism. Weakness, apathy, listlessness, and weight loss may develop insidiously in patients subjected to thyroid irradiation or resection. Such symptoms may mistakenly be construed as suggesting disease relapse.

G.   Hypercalcemia. Hypercalcemia is common in patients with epidermoid carcinoma of the head and neck. As many as 23% of patients with advanced recurrent head and neck cancers may experience hypercalcemia before their death. In general, this phenomenon accompanies late-stage recurrent tumor, often with little evidence of bone involvement. Dehydration, all too common in these patients, may be a precipitating factor; in many patients, hypercalcemia is mild and easily controlled with hydration, saline diuresis, or both. Although hydration, saline diuresis, or reduction in tumor (achieved with irradiation, drug therapy, or surgery) frequently reverses this phenomenon, a few patients require pamidronate for adequate treatment (see Chapter 29). If patients have advanced disease without the hope of substantial palliation, consideration can also be given to withholding treatment for hypercalcemia and allowing the patient to die a natural, more comfortable death than might occur if the hypercalcemia were treated and the patient were obligated to die of locally progressive disease.

H.   Aspiration pneumonia. The anatomic deformities induced by surgery, recurrent tumor, or both make patients with head and neck cancer highly susceptible to aspiration of pooled secretions. Fever, tachycardia, tachypnea, rales, and infiltrates in the lung are usual findings and are often confused with primary bacterial pneumonia. Knowledge of the aspiration or observation of the event may be the only decisive method of proving the diagnosis. Immediate recognition of aspiration should be followed by treatment with steroids, antibiotics, or both.

VI.   Cancer prevention. No discussion of treatment of head and neck cancer would be complete without mention of efforts in cancer prevention. Clearly, alcohol and tobacco use are synergistic epidemiologic factors in the development of these neoplasms, and all patients should be encouraged in behavior modification and other cessation programs.

Recent evidence suggests that isotretinoin (13-*cis*-retinoic acid) can both clinically improve and histologically mature oral leukoplakia and erythroplakia. Further, the incidence of second head and neck cancers and second primary lung cancers appears to be reduced by this treatment. Although the optimal dose is not yet established, 5.6 mg/m^2/day given orally appears to be a relatively safe and probably effective dosage. This represents a new and challenging area for research.

SELECTED READINGS

Adelstein DJ, Adams GL, Li Y, et al. A phase III comparison of standard radiation therapy (RT) versus RT plus concurrent cisplatin (DDP) versus split-course RT plus concurrent DDP and 5-fluorouracil (5FU) in patients with unresectable squamous cell head and neck cancer: an intergroup study. *Proc ASCO* 2000;19: 1624(abst).

Al-Kourainy K, Kish J, Ensley J, et al. Achievement of superior survival for histologically negative versus histologically positive clinically complete responders to cisplatin combination in patients with locally advanced head and neck cancer. *Cancer* 1987;59:233.

Al-Sarraf M, LeBlanc M, Giri PG, et al. Chemoradiotherapy vs. radiotherapy in patients with advanced nasopharyngeal cancer: phase III randomized intergroup study 0099. *J Clin Oncol* 1998;16: 1310–1317.

American Joint Committee on Cancer. *AJCC cancer staging manual.* 6th ed. New York: Springer, 2002:17–19.

Calais G, Alfonsi M, Bardet E, et al. Randomized trial of radiation therapy versus concomitant chemotherapy and radiation therapy for advanced-stage oropharynx carcinoma. *JNCI* 1999;91:2081–2086.

Department of Veterans Affairs Laryngeal Cancer Study Group. Induction chemotherapy plus radiation compared with surgery plus radiation in patients with advanced laryngeal cancer. *N Engl J Med* 1991;324:1685–1690.

Forastiere AA, Kock W, Trotti A, et al. Head and neck cancer. *N Engl J Med* 2001;345:1890–1900.

Forastiere AA, Trotti A. Radiotherapy and concurrent chemotherapy: a strategy that improves locoregional control and survival in oropharyngeal cancer [Editorial]. *JNCI* 1999;91:2065–2066.

Khuri FR, Shin DM, Glisson BS, et al. Treatment of patients with recurrent or metastatic squamous cell carcinoma of the head and neck: current status and future directions. *Semin Oncol* 2000;27 (suppl 8):25–33.

7

Carcinoma of the Lung

Tien Hoang and Joan H. Schiller

Carcinoma of the lung is responsible for more than 165,000 deaths each year in the United States. This represents one-third of all deaths due to cancer and more than the number of deaths due to breast, colon, and prostate cancers combined. The incidence of the disease continues to rise, particularly in women and blacks, and thus is likely to present a significant public health problem for years to come. Lung cancer consists of four major histologic types: adenocarcinoma, squamous cell carcinoma, large cell carcinoma, and small cell carcinoma. Because of the unique biologic features of small cell lung cancer (SCLC), its staging and treatment differ radically from those of the other three types of lung cancer, which collectively are called non–small cell lung cancer (NSCLC). Thus, these two groups are addressed in two separate sections.

   I. Etiology. Lung cancer is predominantly a disease of smokers. Eighty percent of lung cancer occurs in active or former smokers, and an additional 5% of cases are estimated to occur as a consequence of passive exposure to tobacco smoke. Tobacco smoke causes an increased incidence of all four histologic types of lung cancer, although adenocarcinoma (particularly the bronchoalveolar variant) is also found in nonsmokers. Other risk factors for lung cancer include exposure to asbestos or radon. Familial factors such as activity of carcinogen-metabolizing hepatic enzyme systems (e.g., 4-debrisoquine hydroxylase) may also play a role in determining an individual's propensity to develop lung cancer.
   II. Molecular biology. Numerous genetic changes have been associated with lung tumors. Most common among these include activation or overexpression of the *myc* family of oncogenes in SCLC and NSCLC and of the *K-ras* oncogene in NSCLC, particularly adenocarcinoma. Inactivation or deletion of the *p53* and retinoblastoma tumor suppressor genes and a recently identified tumor suppressor gene on chromosome 3p (the *FHIT* gene) have been found in 50% to 90% of patients with SCLC. Abnormalities of *p53* and 3p have been associated with 50% to 70% of cases of NSCLC. The clinical significance of *p53* mutations is unclear; early studies suggested that *p53* mutations imparted a negative prognosis, but subsequent studies have refuted this and even suggested the contrary. The *K-ras* mutation is more frequently found in smokers, those with adenocarcinoma, and those with poorly differentiated tumors. It is also associated with poor prognosis.
   III. Screening. Three U.S. randomized screening studies in the 1980s failed to detect an impact on mortality of screening high-risk patients with chest radiography or sputum cytology, although earlier-stage cancers were detected in the screened groups. Since then, however, low-dose spiral computed tomography (CT) has emerged as a possible new tool for lung cancer

screening. Spiral CT is CT imaging in which only the pulmonary parenchyma is scanned, thus negating the use of IV contrast medium and the necessity of a physician having to be present. This type of scan can usually be done quickly (within one breath) and involves low doses of radiation. In a nonrandomized controlled study from the Early Lung Cancer Action Project, low-dose CT was shown to be more sensitive than chest radiography in detecting lung nodules and lung cancer at early stage. However, despite these promising results, it is unclear whether screening with spiral CT will result in a reduction in lung cancer mortality. Concerns include issues related to lead-time bias, length time bias, and "overdiagnosis." In addition, in some parts of the country such as the Midwest, the incidence of benign nodules is extremely high, making the cost of the test with subsequent follow-up testing very expensive. To resolve the issue, the National Cancer Institute is conducting a large randomized controlled trial (the Lung Screening Study), which will involve at least 15,000 participants over several years.

IV. Non–small cell lung cancer. The prognosis and treatment of NSCLC are dependent primarily on stage of disease at the time of diagnosis. Although histologic differences (adenocarcinoma versus large cell carcinoma versus squamous cell carcinoma) among the NSCLCs affect their natural history and presentation, these differences are of relatively little importance in determining patient management.

A.   Staging. The current TNM staging classification is shown in Table 7.1. The stage grouping (Table 7.2) was updated in 1997 to reflect a need for greater specificity in staging and greater homogeneity of outcome within stages. The major differences in the new stage grouping are that (a) stages I and II are divided into IA and IB and IIA and IIB, respectively; (b) stage T3, N0, M0 is moved to IIB; and (c) satellite pulmonary nodules within the same lobe of the primary tumor are classified as T4 (nodules within another lobe on the ipsilateral side are M1).

B.   Pretreatment evaluation. The diagnosis of lung cancer is usually made by bronchial biopsy or percutaneous needle biopsy. Although the disease is usually discovered on chest radiographs, a CT scan of the chest is necessary to evaluate the extent of the primary disease, mediastinal extension or lymphadenopathy, and the presence or absence of other parenchymal nodules in patients in whom surgical resection is a consideration. CT of the upper abdomen is performed to look for asymptomatic hepatic or adrenal metastases. (The latter should be distinguished from benign adrenal adenomas.) Bone scans should be obtained for the patient with bone pain, chest pain, or an elevated calcium or alkaline phosphatase level. Head CT or magnetic resonance imaging is not routinely done in the absence of central nervous system (CNS) signs or symptoms.

Mediastinal nodal metastasis is a critical factor in determining tumor resectability. Mediastinoscopy has long been considered the gold standard for mediastinal staging and has been recommended for mediastinal lymph nodes greater than 1 cm on CT scan. Recently, however, positron emission tomography (PET), a metabolic imaging scan using [18F]fluorodeoxyglucose,

Table 7.1.   TNM definitions

Primary tumor (T)

TX	Tumor proven by the presence of malignant cells in bronchopulmonary secretions but not visualized roentgenographically or bronchoscopically or any tumor that cannot be assessed as in a retreatment staging
T0	No evidence of primary tumor
Tis	Carcinoma *in situ*
T1	A tumor that is ≤3 cm in greatest dimension, surrounded by lung or visceral pleura and without evidence of invasion proximal to a lobar bronchus at bronchoscopy
T2	A tumor >3 cm in greatest dimension or a tumor of any size that either invades the visceral pleura or has associated atelectasis or obstructive pneumonitis extending to the hilar region. At bronchoscopy, the proximal extent of demonstrable tumor must be within a lobar bronchus or at least 2 cm distal to the carina. Any associated atelectasis or obstructive pneumonitis must involve less than an entire lung
T3	A tumor of any size with direct extension into the chest wall (including superior sulcus tumors), diaphragm, or the mediastinal pleura or pericardium without involving the heart, great vessels, trachea, esophagus, or vertebral body or a tumor in the main bronchus within 2 cm of the carina without involving the carina
T4	A tumor of any size with invasion of the mediastinum or involving the heart, great vessels, trachea, esophagus, vertebral body, or carina, or presence of malignant pleural effusion; a satellite nodule within the same lobe

Nodal involvement (N)

N0	No demonstrable metastasis to regional lymph nodes
N1	Metastasis to lymph nodes in the peribronchial or the ipsilateral hilar region or both, including direct extension
N2	Metastasis to ipsilateral mediastinal lymph nodes or subcarinal lymph nodes or both
N3	Metastasis to contralateral mediastinal lymph nodes, contralateral hilar lymph nodes, ipsilateral or contralateral scalene or supraclavicular lymph nodes

Distant metastasis (M)

MX	Cannot be assessed
M0	No distant metastasis
M1	Distant metastasis, including pulmonary nodule not in the same lobe as the primary tumor

Table 7.2.   1997 revisions to the International Staging Classification for Lung Cancer

Stage	TNM subset	5-yr survival rate (%)	
		Clinical stage	Pathologic stage
IA	T1, N0, M0	61	67
IB	T2, N0, M0	38	57
IIA	T1, N1, M0	34	55
IIB	T2, N1, M0	24	39
	T3, N0, M0		
IIIA	T3, N1, M0	9	25
	T1–3, N2, M0		
IIIB	T4, any N, M0	13	23
	Any T, N3, M0		
IV	Any T, any N, M1	1	—

From Mountain CF. *Chest* 1997; 111:1710–1717.

has been developed as a useful complementary tool for staging. PET scans are more sensitive and specific than CT scans and could thus potentially save patients with advanced disease, either within or outside of the chest, from unnecessary invasive procedures. However, it is not yet clear as to whether PET scanning can replace mediastinoscopy, as the scan can be falsely positive in inflammatory processes and falsely negative in lung tumors with low metabolic activity such as bronchoalveolar carcinoma or carcinoid tumors.

Pulmonary function testing is necessary before definitive surgery. Increased postoperative morbidity is associated with a predicted postoperative 1-s forced expiratory volume of less than 800 to 1,000 mL, a preoperative maximum voluntary ventilation less than 35% of predicted, a carbon monoxide diffusing capacity less than 60% of predicted, and an arterial oxygen pressure (Po_2) of less than 60 mm Hg or a carbon dioxide pressure (Pco_2) of more than 45 mm Hg.

C. Management

1. Stage I disease. Lobectomy is the treatment of choice for stage I NSCLC, with cure rates of 60% to 80% reported. Within stage I, patients with T2, N0 disease do not fare as well as those with T1, N0 cancers. In patients with medical contraindications to surgery but with adequate pulmonary function, high-dose radiotherapy results in cure in about 20% of patients. No role for adjuvant (postoperative) chemotherapy for stage I NSCLC has been identified, although neoadjuvant (preoperative) chemotherapy is actively being investigated. Patients with a resected stage I NSCLC are at high risk for the development of second lung cancers (about 2% to 3%/year). Neither vitamin A nor its derivatives, β-carotene or *cis*-retinoic acid, have been found to have any benefit in chemoprevention, contrary to predictions, and may even be deleterious. Other agents are under investigation.

2.   Stage II disease. Treatment of stage II NSCLC is surgical resection. The subset of T3, N0 disease has a natural history and treatment strategy different from those of stage III N2 disease and thus has been moved to stage II. Patients with peripheral chest wall invasion should undergo resection of the involved ribs and underlying lung. Chest wall defects are then repaired with chest wall musculature or Marlex mesh and methylmethacrylate. Postoperative radiotherapy is often given. Five-year survival rates as high as 50% have been reported.

3.   Locally advanced (stage IIIA and IIIB) disease. Treatment of locally advanced NSCLC is one of the most controversial issues in the management of lung cancer. Treatment options include surgery for less advanced disease or radiotherapy, either of which has been given with or without chemotherapy for control of micrometastases. Interpretation of the results of clinical trials involving patients with locally advanced disease has been clouded by a number of issues including changing diagnostic techniques, different staging systems, and heterogeneous patient populations that may have disease that ranges from "nonbulky" stage IIIA (clinical N1 nodes, with N2 nodes discovered only at the time of surgery or mediastinoscopy) to "bulky" N2 nodes (enlarged adenopathy clearly visible on chest radiographs or multiple nodal level involvement) to clearly inoperable stage IIIB disease.

   a.   "Nonbulky" stage IIIA disease. The primary treatment of stage II and early stage IIIA (clinical N0) disease is surgical resection. However, even with a complete resection, the cure rate is disappointing, prompting investigation of adjuvant chemotherapy and radiotherapy. However, a meta-analysis published in 1995 failed to show a statistically significant survival benefit with surgery and chemotherapy compared with surgery alone. Three recent randomized studies, published in 2000 or later, also demonstrated no statistically significant survival advantage from the addition of more "modern" postoperative chemotherapy regimens for stage II and stage IIIA (N2) disease. Therefore, adjuvant chemotherapy for stage II and IIIA disease cannot be routinely recommended. Postoperative radiotherapy has been shown to reduce local recurrences after resection of stage II or III squamous cell carcinoma of the lung but does not prolong survival.

   b.   Pancoast tumors. Pancoast tumors are upper-lobe tumors that adjoin the brachial plexus and are frequently associated with Horner's syndrome or shoulder and arm pain; the latter is due to rib destruction, involvement of the C8 or T1 nerve roots, or both. Treatment consists of a combined-modality approach with radiotherapy and surgery. Five-year survival rates range from 25% to 50%. Combined preoperative chemotherapy and radiotherapy is being studied.

   c.   "Bulky" stage IIIA (N2) and stage IIIB with no pleural effusion. The optimal treatment for "bulky" stage IIIA and stage IIIB disease is also controversial. Current investigational efforts are directed at identifying the optimal combined-modality approach, involving treatments directed at local control of the disease (surgery or radiotherapy) and micrometastatic disease (chemotherapy). Possibilities for bulky stage IIIA include preoperative chemotherapy plus surgery or chemotherapy plus radiotherapy. Stage IIIB is generally considered unresectable, with the treatment consisting of combined chemoradiation or, in the case of IIIB with malignant pleural effusion, chemotherapy alone.

(1) Preoperative chemotherapy plus surgery. There have been two small positive randomized studies involving more than 40 patients, comparing surgery with or without preoperative chemotherapy in this patient population. In a European study, preoperative chemotherapy (mitomycin, ifosfamide, and cisplatin for three courses) followed by surgery was compared with surgery without preoperative chemotherapy in patients with stage IIIA disease. All patients also received postoperative mediastinal radiotherapy after surgery. The median survival time was 26 months for 30 patients receiving preoperative chemotherapy plus surgery compared with 8 months for 30 patients treated with surgery alone.

Investigators at the M.D. Anderson Cancer Center randomized patients to surgery or three cycles of cyclophosphamide, etoposide, and cisplatin followed by surgery and three cycles of postoperative chemotherapy. The median survival time of the 32 patients randomized to the surgery-alone group was 14 months compared with 21 months in the 28 patients randomized to the combined-modality arm.

In a larger randomized trial, French investigators compared preoperative mitomycin, ifosfamide, and cisplatin plus surgery with surgery alone in 355 patients with resectable stage I (except T1, N0), stage II, and stage IIIA (including N2 disease). The difference in median survival between two arms was not statistically significant (37 versus 26 months; $p = 0.15$). However, subset analysis suggested a survival advantage of neoadjuvant chemotherapy for N0 to N1 but not N2 disease.

Trimodality therapy is also being explored in a randomized intergroup trial, where patients with advanced IIIA disease receive 45 Gy of induction radiotherapy plus two cycles of cisplatin and etoposide and are subsequently randomized to surgery or boost radiotherapy plus an additional two cycles of chemotherapy. This study has recently completed accrual.

(2) Chemotherapy plus radiation therapy. Chemotherapy plus radiotherapy is the treatment of choice for patients with "bulky" or inoperable stage IIIA or IIIB disease without pleural effusion. Two randomized studies have demonstrated an improvement in median and long-term survival with chemotherapy (cisplatin and vinblastine) followed by radiation therapy versus radiotherapy alone. Active areas of investigation include proper sequencing of thoracic radiation therapy and chemotherapy (concurrent versus sequential), choice of chemotherapy, fractionation, and treatment fields.

A randomized Japanese trial reported a 3-month survival advantage with concurrent chemoradiation over a sequential approach. Initial reports from a confirmatory randomized Radiation Therapy Oncology Group trial also showed a trend in favor of concurrent cisplatin and vinblastine with radiation over sequential chemoradiation.

Chemotherapy can be given in full "systemic" doses with radiotherapy, in weekly "radiosensitizing" doses, or a combination of both. One of the most commonly used chemotherapy regimens for stage III NSCLC is carboplatin in combination with paclitaxel, which can be given in "standard" doses (e.g., paclitaxel 225 mg/m^2 and carboplatin area under the curve [AUC] 6) concurrently or sequentially with radiation therapy. Although single-agent weekly carboplatin has not resulted in a survival benefit when given with radiotherapy, preliminary results of weekly doses of paclitaxel 50 mg/m^2 and carboplatin AUC 2 with concurrent radiation have proved promising in Phase I/II studies. Paclitaxel appears to provide radiosensitization to the cancer but also increases the risk for radiation pneumonitis to the adjacent normal lung. Other agents such as gemcitabine, vinorelbine, and irinotecan are also being explored with platinum. Other areas of investigation include the role of "standard" systemic doses of chemotherapy either before or after concurrent weekly doses with radiotherapy.

4. **Stage IV disease**

    a. **Issues regarding treatment.** Chemotherapy improves survival in patients with metastatic NSCLC (about 10% 1-year survival rate in untreated patients versus 35% to 40% 1-year survival rate with treatment). It reduces symptoms, and a study on cost effectiveness demonstrated a cost benefit for chemotherapy compared with supportive care. However, median survival is still poor (9 to 10 months), and thus a discussion must ensue with the patient regarding possible benefits, chance of response, and quality of life with treatment as they relate to the patient's goals for therapy. Because chemotherapy is not curative, goals for treatment should include palliation of symptoms and a modest improvement in survival.

    The principal factors predicting response to chemotherapy and survival are performance status and extent of disease. Patients with a poor performance status (Eastern Cooperative Oncology Group [ECOG] performance status of 2 to 4) are less likely to respond to treatment and they tolerate the therapy poorly; thus, they probably should not be treated with standard combination-chemotherapy regimens. Favorable prognostic factors include no weight loss, female sex, normal serum lactic dehydrogenase level, and no bone or liver metastases.

b.   First-line chemotherapy. Chemotherapy for metastatic NSCLC should be a platinum-based regimen. A meta-analysis of large randomized trials indicated that there is a small but significant survival advantage with platinum-based therapy compared with best supportive care. Although a direct comparison of cisplatin-based therapies and carboplatin-based therapies is limited, most of the data suggest that cisplatin and carboplatin may have comparable efficacy. Although the benefits are modest, cisplatin-based chemotherapy has been shown to result in a statistically significant improvement in survival compared with supportive care alone. Whereas "best supportive care" resulted in median survival rates of 4 to 5 months and 1-year survival rates of 5% to 10%, current third-generation regimens with paclitaxel and docetaxel, gemcitabine, vinorelbine, and irinotecan have yielded median survivals of 8 to 9 months and 1-year survivals of 35% to 40%. Although these differences could be explained by other factors such as stage migration, most investigators and clinicians believe the prolongation of survival with treatment is real and clinically relevant. In addition, randomized studies have shown an improvement in symptoms and quality of life compared with patients treated with "best supportive care."

However, numerous randomized studies have failed to show an advantage of one new doublet regimen over another. In a recent ECOG trial, patients with advanced disease were randomly assigned to one of four regimens: cisplatin and paclitaxel (reference regimen), cisplatin and gemcitabine, cisplatin and docetaxel, or carboplatin and paclitaxel. There were no significant differences in overall survival, although there was a difference in toxicity and a slight difference in time to progression. A Southwest Oncology Group trial also failed to show a survival benefit to carboplatin and paclitaxel compared with cisplatin and vinorelbine, although, again, there were differences in cost and toxicities. The common chemotherapy regimens for NSCLC are shown in Table 7.3.

c.   Second-line chemotherapy. There have been two randomized trials evaluating second-line docetaxel in patients who have failed first-line therapy. Docetaxel at a dose of 75 mg/m^2 significantly prolongs survival in comparison with best supportive care and, in comparison with either vinorelbine or ifosfamide, improves time to progression and 1-year survival. Moreover, it also improves quality of life. It was noted that previous paclitaxel exposure did not affect patients' response to docetaxel, suggesting no cross-resistance between the two taxane agents.

d.   Duration of therapy. Three randomized studies failed to show a survival difference with "prolonged" (more than six) cycles of chemotherapy compared with a fewer (four to six) number of cycles. Thus, continuing chemotherapy until progression cannot be routinely recommended.

e.   "Doublets" versus "triplets." Although numerous Phase I/II studies have demonstrated the feasibility of

**Table 7.3.   Common chemotherapy regimens
for metastatic non–small cell lung cancer**

Cisplatin plus vinorelbine	
Cisplatin	100 mg/m² IV on d 1
Vinorelbine	25 mg/m² weekly
	Repeat cycle every 4 wk
Carboplatin plus paclitaxel	
Carboplatin	Area under the curve (AUC) of 6, d 1
Paclitaxel	225 mg/m² IV on d 1 over 3 h
	Repeat cycle every 3 wk
Cisplatin plus gemcitabine	
Cisplatin	100 mg/m² IV on d 1
Gemcitabine	1,000 mg/m² IV on d 1, 8, and 15
	Repeat each cycle every 4 wk
or	
Cisplatin	80 mg/m² IV on d 1
Gemcitabine	1,250 mg/m² IV on d 1 and 8
	Repeat each cycle every 3 wk
Cisplatin plus docetaxel	
Cisplatin	75 mg/m² IV on d 1
Docetaxel	75 mg/m² IV on d 1
	Repeat each cycle every 3 wk

triplet combinations, with promising 1-year survivals of 42% to 53%, most randomized trials have failed to demonstrate a survival advantage and have been at the expense of enhanced toxicity. Thus, three drug regimens cannot be routinely recommended from a clinical trial.

f.   Non-platin-based regimens. Given the toxicities associated with cisplatin, there is considerable interest in combining two non-platin drugs. However, the majority of recent randomized trials have failed to show an improvement in survival with non-platin regimens compared with platin-based regimens, and some of them report trends toward an inferior survival.

g.   Isolated brain metastases. In patients with controlled disease outside of the brain who have an isolated cerebral metastasis in a resectable area, resection followed by whole-brain radiotherapy is superior to whole-brain radiotherapy alone.

V.   Small cell carcinoma. SCLC differs from NSCLC in a number of important ways. First, it has a more rapid clinical course and natural history, with the rapid development of metastases, symptoms, and death. Untreated, the median survival time for patients with local disease is typically 12 to 15 weeks and for those with advanced disease 6 to 9 weeks. Second, it exhibits features of neuroendocrine differentiation in many patients (which may be distinguishable histopathologically) and is associated with paraneoplastic syndromes. Third, unlike NSCLC, SCLC is exquisitely sensitive to both chemotherapy and radiotherapy, although resistant disease often develops. Because of the rapid development of distant disease and its extreme sensitivity to the cytotoxic effects of chemotherapy, this mode of therapy forms the backbone of treatment for this disease, irrespective of stage.

A. Staging. Although SCLC has a propensity to metastasize quickly and micrometastatic disease is presumed to be present in all patients at the time of diagnosis, this disease is usually classified into either a local or an extensive stage. Local disease is typically defined as disease that can be encompassed within one radiation port, usually considered limited to the hemithorax and to regional nodes, including mediastinal and ipsilateral supraclavicular nodes. Extensive-stage disease is usually defined as disease that has spread outside those areas.

B. Pretreatment evaluation. Common sites of metastases for SCLC include the brain, liver, bone marrow, bone, and CNS. For this reason, a complete staging work-up consists of a complete blood cell count; liver function tests; CT of the brain, chest, and abdomen; a bone scan; and bone marrow aspiration and biopsy. However, this complete staging work-up should not be undertaken unless the patient is a candidate for combined-modality treatment with chest radiation and chemotherapy, the patient is being evaluated for a clinical study, or the information is helpful for prognostic reasons. If the patient is not a candidate for combined-modality treatment or a clinical study, stopping the staging at the first evidence of extensive-stage disease is usually appropriate.

C. Prognostic factors. As in NSCLC, the major pretreatment prognostic factors are stage, performance status, and bulky disease. Hepatic metastases also confer a poorer prognosis. If the patient's initial poor performance status is due to the underlying malignancy, these symptoms often disappear quickly with treatment, resulting in a net improvement in quality of life. However, major organ dysfunction from nonmalignant causes often results in an inability of the patient to tolerate chemotherapy.

D. Therapy. A number of combination chemotherapeutic regimens are available for SCLC (Table 7.4). Until recently, no clear survival advantage has been demonstrated for any one regimen over another. With these chemotherapy regimens, overall response rates of 75% to 90% and complete response rates of 50% for localized disease can be anticipated. For extensive-stage disease, overall response rates of about 75% and complete response rates of 25% are common. Despite these high response rates, however, the median survival time remains about 14 months for limited-stage disease and 7 to 9 months for extensive-stage disease. Less than 5% of patients with extensive-stage disease survive more than 2 years.

Until recently, either cisplatin or carboplatin together with etoposide have been the standard of care in North America for the treatment of SCLC. However, in a randomized Phase III study from Japan, four cycles of irinotecan/cisplatin were compared with four cycles of etoposide/cisplatin. The enrollment was stopped early because of an interim analysis showing a clear survival benefit in the investigational arm, with a median survival of 12.8 months for the irinotecan/cisplatin group versus 9.4 months for the etoposide/cisplatin group. The 1- and 2-year

Table 7.4.   Chemotherapy regimens for small cell lung cancer

Cisplatin based	
EP	
Etoposide	120 mg/m² IV on d 1–3 *or*
	120 mg/m² PO b.i.d. on d 1–3
Cisplatin	60 mg/m² IV on d 1
or	
Cisplatin	25 mg/m² IV on d 1–3
Etoposide	100 mg/m² IV on d 1–3
	Repeat cycle every 3 wk
Carboplatin based	
Carboplatin	300 mg/m² IV on d 1
Etoposide	100 mg/m² IV on d 1–3
or	
Carboplatin	100 mg/m² IV on d 1–3
Etoposide	120 mg/m² IV on d 1–3
	Repeat cycle every 4 wk
Irinotecan plus cisplatin	
Irinotecan	60 mg/m² IV on d 1, 8, and 15
Cisplatin	60 mg/m² IV on d 1
	Repeat cycle every 4 wk

survival for the two groups were 58% and 19.5% versus 38% and 5%. Two randomized trials are ongoing in the United States to confirm these results.

1. **Dose intensity.** A dose intensity meta-analysis of chemotherapy in SCLC, which evaluated doses not requiring bone marrow transplantation support, showed no consistent correlation between dose intensity and outcome. There have been several Phase I and II clinical trials evaluating the role of marrow-ablative doses of chemotherapy with subsequent progenitor cell replacement (e.g., autologous bone marrow transplantation) with disappointing survival results. In a randomized Phase III study, when compared with conventional-dose chemotherapy, high-dose regimen with stem cell support prolonged relapse-free but not overall survival.

2. **Duration of therapy.** Most randomized studies do not show a survival benefit for prolonged administration of chemotherapy. Several studies have demonstrated no survival benefit of prolonged first-line treatment over treatment on relapse. The optimal duration of treatment for SCLC is 4 to 6 months.

3. **Second-line therapy.** No curative regimens for patients with recurrent disease have been identified. The only drug approved for second-line therapy of SCLC is topotecan, which has a 20% to 40% response rate in patients with *sensitive* SCLC (those patients who relapsed 2 to 3 or more months after their first-line therapy), with a median survival of 22 to 27 weeks. For patients with *refractory* disease (progressed through or within 3 months of completion of first-line therapy), the response rate in Phase II studies is only be-

tween 3% and 11%. Median survival is about 20 weeks. Other agents including oral etoposide and the combination of cyclophosphamide, doxorubicin, and vincristine have been used with low response rates.

E. Chemotherapy plus chest irradiation. Numerous studies have been done with chemotherapy and thoracic radiotherapy for patients with limited-stage SCLC. Conflicting results have been attributed to differences in chemotherapy regimens and different schedules integrating chemotherapy and thoracic radiation (concurrent, sequential, and "sandwich" approach). Two meta-analyses concluded that thoracic irradiation does result in a small but significant improvement in survival and major control of the disease in the chest, although no conclusions could be made regarding the optimal sequencing of chemotherapy and thoracic radiation. In one randomized study, twice-daily hyperfractionated radiation was compared with a once-daily schedule; both were given concurrently with four cycles of cisplatin and etoposide. Survival was significantly higher with the twice-daily regimen (median survival of 23 versus 19 months, 5-year survival of 26% versus 16%), albeit at the expense of more grade 3 esophagitis. In another randomized trial, early administration of thoracic irradiation in the combined-modality therapy of limited-stage SCLC was superior to late or consolidative thoracic irradiation. These data suggest that patients with good performance status and with limited disease should receive concurrent chemoradiation, preferably with twice-daily hyperfractionation.

F. Prophylactic cranial irradiation. Numerous individual trials failed to show that prophylactic brain irradiation enhanced survival but did demonstrate a decrease in the risk of brain metastases without a decrease in mental function. However, in a recent meta-analysis of seven randomized trials, prophylactic cranial irradiation was shown to significantly increase 3-year survival with a net gain of 5.4%. It also increased disease-free survival and decreased the risk of developing brain metastasis.

VI. Palliation

A. Radiotherapy. Palliative radiotherapy is often helpful in controlling the pain of bone metastases or neurologic function in patients with brain metastases. Chest radiotherapy may help control hemoptysis, superior vena cava syndrome, airway obstruction, laryngeal nerve compression, and other local complications.

B. Pleural effusions. Common sclerosing agents include doxycycline, talc, and bleomycin. The disadvantage of bleomycin is its cost; talc, although effective, had the disadvantage of requiring a thoracoscopy and general anesthesia for insufflation. Comparative randomized trials are ongoing.

C. Brachytherapy. For patients with bronchial obstruction who have received maximum external-beam radiotherapy, the use of high-dose endobronchial irradiation may be of temporary benefit.

D. Cachexia. Megestrol acetate 160 to 800 mg daily may improve the appetite of some patients.

E.   Chemotherapy. In randomized trials involving both NSCLC and SCLC patients, chemotherapy has been shown to reduce the incidence of cancer-related symptoms such as pain, cough, hemoptysis, and shortness of breath.

F.   Colony-stimulating factors. Filgrastim (granulocyte colony-stimulating factor) decreases the incidence of neutropenic fevers, the median duration of neutropenia, days of hospitalization, and days of antibiotic treatment in patients with extensive-stage SCLC. However, the clinical benefit of maintaining a dose-intense approach in the treatment of SCLC patients has not been established.

Caution must be exercised when using colony-stimulating factors in patients receiving combined-modality treatment with both chemotherapy and thoracic irradiation. A randomized study by the Southwest Oncology Group found that patients receiving sargramostim (granulocyte–macrophage colony-stimulating factor) and chemotherapy with concurrent thoracic irradiation had a significant increase in thrombocytopenia over patients receiving concurrent chemotherapy and radiation therapy without growth factor.

VII.   Possible future treatments for lung cancer: molecularly targeted therapy? Despite the modest improvements in survival for lung cancer patients, prognosis remains dismal; the 1-year survival of metastatic NSCLC is 35%, and almost all extensive-stage SCLC cases are doomed to failure. The expanding knowledge of tumor biology has opened a new door for management of this disease: molecularly targeted agents. These drugs are aimed at well-defined pathways that are abnormal specifically in cancer cells, hence minimizing adverse effects on normal tissues.

Although there are a number of different pathways that are being targeted (e.g., COX2 inhibition, farnesyl transferase inhibition), two in particular deserve mention. One of the most exciting areas of research involves the epidermal growth factor receptor (EGFR), which is frequently expressed or overexpressed in NSCLC tumors. Binding of ligand to the EGFR causes dimerization of the receptor, which in turn activates tyrosine kinase on the intracellular domain of the receptor. Autophosphorylation of the receptor induces a cascade of intracellular events leading to cell proliferation, inhibition of apoptosis, angiogenesis, and invasion, all resulting in tumor growth and spread. Inhibition of the EGFR pathway leads to apoptosis and tumor regression in preclinical models. Hence, the EGFR, ligands, and signaling pathway have become active targets for anticancer therapy. Agents targeting this pathway include EGFR tyrosine kinase inhibitors such as gefitinib (ZD1839 Iressa) and OSI-774 (Tarceva); monoclonal antibodies to EGFR, which block ligand binding to EGFR; and antisense oligonucleotides, which inhibit the expression of EGFR by base-pair hybridization with its messenger ribonucleic acid. Phase I and II trials with these agents have shown promising results.

Iressa monotherapy has been investigated in two Phase II multicenter trials: one conducted in the U.S.A. and the other conducted primarily in Japan and Europe. Both studies included advanced NSCLC patients who failed at least one chemotherapy regimen.

In the European/Japanese study, 210 patients who had primarily one prior chemotherapy were randomly assigned to receive 250 or 500 mg PO of Iressa daily. The overall response rate was 18.7%, with no difference between the two doses. In a U.S. study involving patients with two prior chemotherapy regimens, including docetaxel, the response rate was 11%. Two large randomized controlled Phase III studies (gemcitabine plus cisplatin with Iressa or placebo or paclitaxel plus carboplatin plus Iressa or placebo) have recently completed accrual. Results of these studies showed advantage by adding Iressa.

Antiangiogenesis is another concept that is being intensively studied, based on the observations that neovascularization occurs in tumor tissues and rarely in other physiologic processes except wound healing. Theoretical advantages for targeting angiogenesis include the fact that endothelial cells are diploid, nonmutated cells and thus less likely to be able to develop resistance to drugs. Vascular endothelial growth factor (VEGF) is a potent stimulator for formation of new blood vessels. Through binding to its receptor (VEGFR) on endothelial cells, VEGF initiates biologic pathways leading to different events including endothelial cell proliferation and migration, remodeling of extracellular matrix, and tumor vascularization. Several antiangiogenesis agents have been investigated, such as VEGFR tyrosine kinase inhibitors and anti-VEGF monoclonal antibodies (e.g., bevacizumab). Bevacizumab is being evaluated in a randomized ECOG trial in combination with chemotherapy for advanced NSCLC. Other antiangiogenic drugs that inhibit the endothelial cell directly include endostatin and thalidomide, which is currently being investigated in a Phase III study in combination with chemoradiation for locally advanced NSCLC.

SELECTED READINGS

Dillman RO, Herndon J, Seagren SL, et al. Improved survival in stage III non–small cell lung cancer: seven-year follow-up of CALGB 8433. *JNCI* 1996;88:1210.

Eddy DM. Screening for lung cancer. *Ann Intern Med* 1989;111:232.

Furuse K, Fukuoka M, Kawahara M, et al. Phase III study of concurrent versus sequential thoracic radiotherapy in combination with mitomycin, vindesine, and cisplatin in unresectable stage III non–small cell lung cancer. *J Clin Oncol* 17;1999;2692–2699.

Giaccone G, Dalesio O, McVie GJ, et al. Maintenance chemotherapy in small cell lung cancer: long-term results of a randomized trial. *J Clin Oncol* 1993;11:1230–1240.

Henschke CI, McCauley DI, Yankelevitz DF, et al. Early Lung Cancer Action Project: a summary of the findings on baseline screening. *Oncologist* 2001;6:147–152.

Keller SM, Adak S, Wagner H, et al. A randomized trial of postoperative adjuvant therapy in patients with completely resected stage II or IIIA non–small cell lung cancer. *N Engl J Med* 2000; 343:1217–1222.

Kelly K, Crowley J, Bunn PA, et al. Randomized phase III trial of paclitaxel plus carboplatin versus vinorelbine plus cisplatin in the treatment of patients with advanced non–small cell lung cancer: a Southwest Oncology Group trial. *J Clin Oncol* 2001;19: 3210–3218.

Klasa R, Murray N, Coldman A. Dose-intensity meta-analysis of chemotherapy regimens in small-cell carcinoma of the lung. *J Clin Oncol* 1991;9:499.

Mountain CF. Revisions in the International System for Staging Lung Cancer. *Chest* 1997;111:1710–1717.

Murray N, Coy P, Pater J, et al. Importance of timing for thoracic irradiation in the combined modality treatment of limited-stage small-cell lung cancer. *J Clin Oncol* 1993;11:336.

Neal CR, Amdur RJ, Mendenhall WM, et al. Pancoast tumor: radiation therapy alone vs. preoperative radiation and surgery. *Int J Radiat Oncol Biol Phys* 1991;21:651–660.

Noda K, Nishiwaki Y, Kawahara M, et al. Irinotecan plus cisplatin compared with etoposide plus cisplatin for extensive small cell lung cancer. *N Engl J Med* 2002;346:85–91.

Non–Small Cell Lung Cancer Collaborative Group. Chemotherapy in non–small cell lung cancer: a meta-analysis using updated data on individual patients from 52 randomized clinical trials. *Br Med J* 1995;311:899.

Pignon JP, Arriagada R, Ihde DC, et al. A meta-analysis of thoracic radiotherapy for small-cell lung cancer. *N Engl J Med* 1992; 327:1618–1624.

Rosell R, Gomez-Codina J, Camps C, et al. A randomized trial comparing preoperative chemotherapy plus surgery with surgery alone in patients with non–small-cell lung cancer. *N Engl J Med* 1994;330:153–158.

Sause W, Scott C, Taylor S, et al., for the Radiation Therapy Oncology Group (RTOG) 88-08 and ECOG 3488. Preliminary results of a phase III trial in regionally advanced, unresectable non–small cell lung cancer. *JNCI* 1995;87:198.

Schiller JH, Harrington D, Belani C, et al. Comparison of four chemotherapy regimens for advanced non–small cell lung cancer. *N Engl J Med* 2002;346:92–98.

Turrisi AT, Kim K, Blum R, et al. Twice-daily compared with once-daily thoracic radiotherapy in limited small-cell lung cancer treated concurrently with cisplatin and etoposide. *N Engl J Med* 1999;340:265–271.

Von Pawel J, Schiller JH, Shepherd FA, et al. Topotecan versus cyclophosphamide, doxorubicin, and vincristine for the treatment of recurrent small-cell lung cancer. *J Clin Oncol* 1999;2:658.

Warde P, Payne D. Does thoracic irradiation improve survival and local control in limited-stage small-cell carcinoma of the lung? A meta-analysis. *J Clin Oncol* 1992;10:890.

screening. Spiral CT is CT imaging in which only the pulmonary parenchyma is scanned, thus negating the use of IV contrast medium and the necessity of a physician having to be present. This type of scan can usually be done quickly (within one breath) and involves low doses of radiation. In a nonrandomized controlled study from the Early Lung Cancer Action Project, low-dose CT was shown to be more sensitive than chest radiography in detecting lung nodules and lung cancer at early stage. However, despite these promising results, it is unclear whether screening with spiral CT will result in a reduction in lung cancer mortality. Concerns include issues related to lead-time bias, length time bias, and "overdiagnosis." In addition, in some parts of the country such as the Midwest, the incidence of benign nodules is extremely high, making the cost of the test with subsequent follow-up testing very expensive. To resolve the issue, the National Cancer Institute is conducting a large randomized controlled trial (the Lung Screening Study), which will involve at least 15,000 participants over several years.

IV. Non–small cell lung cancer. The prognosis and treatment of NSCLC are dependent primarily on stage of disease at the time of diagnosis. Although histologic differences (adenocarcinoma versus large cell carcinoma versus squamous cell carcinoma) among the NSCLCs affect their natural history and presentation, these differences are of relatively little importance in determining patient management.

   A. Staging. The current TNM staging classification is shown in Table 7.1. The stage grouping (Table 7.2) was updated in 1997 to reflect a need for greater specificity in staging and greater homogeneity of outcome within stages. The major differences in the new stage grouping are that (a) stages I and II are divided into IA and IB and IIA and IIB, respectively; (b) stage T3, N0, M0 is moved to IIB; and (c) satellite pulmonary nodules within the same lobe of the primary tumor are classified as T4 (nodules within another lobe on the ipsilateral side are M1).

   B. Pretreatment evaluation. The diagnosis of lung cancer is usually made by bronchial biopsy or percutaneous needle biopsy. Although the disease is usually discovered on chest radiographs, a CT scan of the chest is necessary to evaluate the extent of the primary disease, mediastinal extension or lymphadenopathy, and the presence or absence of other parenchymal nodules in patients in whom surgical resection is a consideration. CT of the upper abdomen is performed to look for asymptomatic hepatic or adrenal metastases. (The latter should be distinguished from benign adrenal adenomas.) Bone scans should be obtained for the patient with bone pain, chest pain, or an elevated calcium or alkaline phosphatase level. Head CT or magnetic resonance imaging is not routinely done in the absence of central nervous system (CNS) signs or symptoms.

   Mediastinal nodal metastasis is a critical factor in determining tumor resectability. Mediastinoscopy has long been considered the gold standard for mediastinal staging and has been recommended for mediastinal lymph nodes greater than 1 cm on CT scan. Recently, however, positron emission tomography (PET), a metabolic imaging scan using [^{18}F]fluorodeoxyglucose,

Table 7.1.   TNM definitions

Primary tumor (T)

TX   Tumor proven by the presence of malignant cells in bronchopulmonary secretions but not visualized roentgenographically or bronchoscopically or any tumor that cannot be assessed as in a retreatment staging

T0   No evidence of primary tumor

Tis   Carcinoma *in situ*

T1   A tumor that is ≤3 cm in greatest dimension, surrounded by lung or visceral pleura and without evidence of invasion proximal to a lobar bronchus at bronchoscopy

T2   A tumor >3 cm in greatest dimension or a tumor of any size that either invades the visceral pleura or has associated atelectasis or obstructive pneumonitis extending to the hilar region. At bronchoscopy, the proximal extent of demonstrable tumor must be within a lobar bronchus or at least 2 cm distal to the carina. Any associated atelectasis or obstructive pneumonitis must involve less than an entire lung

T3   A tumor of any size with direct extension into the chest wall (including superior sulcus tumors), diaphragm, or the mediastinal pleura or pericardium without involving the heart, great vessels, trachea, esophagus, or vertebral body or a tumor in the main bronchus within 2 cm of the carina without involving the carina

T4   A tumor of any size with invasion of the mediastinum or involving the heart, great vessels, trachea, esophagus, vertebral body, or carina, or presence of malignant pleural effusion; a satellite nodule within the same lobe

Nodal involvement (N)

N0   No demonstrable metastasis to regional lymph nodes

N1   Metastasis to lymph nodes in the peribronchial or the ipsilateral hilar region or both, including direct extension

N2   Metastasis to ipsilateral mediastinal lymph nodes or subcarinal lymph nodes or both

N3   Metastasis to contralateral mediastinal lymph nodes, contralateral hilar lymph nodes, ipsilateral or contralateral scalene or supraclavicular lymph nodes

Distant metastasis (M)

MX   Cannot be assessed

M0   No distant metastasis

M1   Distant metastasis, including pulmonary nodule not in the same lobe as the primary tumor

8

Carcinomas of the Gastrointestinal Tract

Al B. Benson III

Cancers of the gastrointestinal (GI) tract (esophagus, stomach, small and large intestines, and anus) account for nearly 13% of all cases of cancer in the United States and for about 15% of cancer deaths. Colon cancer is by far the most common of these malignancies, with cancer of the rectum, stomach, esophagus, small intestine, and anus occurring with decreasing frequency. Surgery continues to be the principal curative modality, but irradiation and chemotherapy have increasingly important roles and, in certain adjuvant situations, improve the cure rate produced by surgery. Select patients with isolated, resectable metastatic colorectal cancer lesions also may be cured with surgical resection. Chemotherapy alone is not curative in patients with overt metastatic disease. Drugs produce objective responses in only 15% to 40% of patients, with increasing numbers of individuals obtaining stabilization of their disease. There is little question that meaningful palliation and an increase in survival can be achieved in patients who respond to chemotherapy or achieve disease stabilization. Controlled clinical trials, often by cooperative groups, have been useful in defining the natural history and therapeutic benefit of various treatment modalities. Participation in such clinical trials should be encouraged.

I. **Carcinoma of the esophagus**
A. **General considerations and aims of therapy**
  1. **Epidemiology.** Cancer of the esophagus has been predominantly of the squamous cell (epidermoid) histology and represents about 1% of the cases of cancers in the United States. Risk factors include heavy tobacco and alcohol use. It is more common in men than women and occurs more often in blacks than in whites. The average patient is in his or her sixties at presentation. In certain parts of China, epidermoid esophageal cancer is the most common kind of cancer, which is thought to be related to dietary habits of the region and perhaps a consequence of fungal contamination of pickled vegetables. Other predisposing factors for esophageal cancer include achalasia, a history of lye burns of the esophagus, and prior epidermoid carcinomas of the aerodigestive tract.
  In recent years, the incidence of adenocarcinoma of the esophagus (along with adenocarcinoma of the proximal stomach) has increased greatly. By the mid-1980s, it accounted for about one-third of all esophageal cancer cases among white men and in some institutions is approaching 60% of newly diagnosed cancers of the esophagus. Adenocarcinoma is predominantly a disease of middle-aged white men, is less strongly linked with alcohol and tobacco use, and is frequently associated with Barrett's esophagus (epithelial metaplasia of

the lower esophagus), which is sometimes seen with reflux esophagitis. The rate of increase of adenocarcinomas of the esophagus and gastric cardia during the 1970s and 1980s exceeded that of any other cancer, including lung cancer, non-Hodgkin's lymphoma, and melanoma. The cause of this impressive increase is not known, although recent epidemiologic studies have implicated obesity, which has been increasing in the U.S. population during the last few decades. This may in turn be associated with epithelial metaplasia in the esophagus (Barrett's esophagus). Adenocarcinomas of the esophagus tend to involve the lower third of that organ, whereas the middle third is the most common site for the epidermoid subtype. Optimal chemotherapy for the two histologic types of esophageal cancer is not known to be different, with little or no difference in response rate in most series. It has been suggested, however, that a lower expression of thymidylate synthase in squamous cell carcinoma than in adenocarcinoma may make the former more sensitive to fluorouracil-based chemotherapy. Other predictive molecular markers or laboratory correlates are under investigation.

2. Clinical manifestations and pretreatment evaluation. Carcinoma of the esophagus is usually associated with progressive and persistent dysphagia. Pain, hoarseness, weight loss, and chronic cough are unfavorable manifestations that indicate spread to regional structures (e.g., mediastinal nodes), recurrent laryngeal nerve, or fistula formation between the esophagus and the airway. The most common sites of metastasis are regional lymph nodes (which may include cervical, supraclavicular, intrathoracic, diaphragmatic, celiac axis, or periaortic), the liver, and the lungs.

Diagnosis is usually made by barium swallow, endoscopy, and biopsy or lavage cytology. Staging should be based on chest radiographic appearance, computed tomography (CT) scan of the abdomen and chest, and careful physical examination of the cervical and supraclavicular nodes. Endoscopic esophageal ultrasound may be useful in assessing the depth of tumor invasion. The preoperative staging of esophageal cancer is still inadequate, owing to the inability to evaluate lymph nodes accurately. Bronchoscopy should be done for upper- and middle-third tumors, and a bone scan is useful in patients with bone pain or tenderness. Recent studies investigating positron emission tomography scanning suggest improved nodal evaluation compared with endoscopic esophageal ultrasound and CT. In addition, a Cancer and Leukemia Group B (CALGB) trial demonstrated that thoracoscopy and laparoscopy also may refine staging accuracy. Survival is related to pathologic stage, which only can be defined surgically (Table 8.1).

3. Treatment and prognosis. The primary treatment of stage I and II carcinoma of the esophagus is surgical resection. About half of esophageal cancers are operable, and half of these are resectable. Patients with more advanced disease (stage III) are best treated, at least initially, with nonsurgical means, usually a combination of radiation therapy and chemotherapy. In patients who respond to such treatment, the carcinoma may subsequently be operable, whereas pa-

Table 8.1.   TNM stages for carcinoma of the esophagus

Primary tumor
Tis	Carcinoma *in situ*
T1	Invades lamina propria or submucosa
T2	Invades muscularis propria
T3	Invades adventitia
T4	Invades adjacent structures

Regional lymph nodes
N0	No nodal metastasis
N1	Regional node metastasis

Distant metastasis
M0	None
M1	Present

Stage grouping
0	Tis, N0, M0
I	T1, N0, M0
IIA	T2 or T3, N0, M0
IIB	T1 or T2, N1, M0
III	T3, N1, M0
	T4, any N, M0
IV	Any T, any N, M1

Modified from American Joint Committee on Cancer. *AJCC staging manual.* 6th ed. New York: Springer, 2002.

tients with metastatic disease to the liver, lung, or bone are best treated with systemic therapy. Palliative feeding procedures such as with a jejunostomy or gastrostomy tube may be useful if subsequent surgical resection is not to be done. The overall median survival time is less than 1 year, and the overall 5-year survival rate is 5% to 10%. The prognosis is related to the size of the lesion, the depth of penetration of the esophagus, and nodal involvement. Current controlled clinical trials are helping to evaluate the relative roles of chemotherapy, radiation, and surgery in all stages of the two predominant histologic types. Most emphasis has been on preoperative ("neoadjuvant") combined-modality treatment, with few supporting data available for postoperative treatment, although the concept is being evaluated as more patients survive initial combined-modality therapy. This is important because many patients who achieve good local control have disease recurrence in distant sites subsequent to surgery. Recent randomized clinical trials, however, have produced conflicting results with respect to the long-term survival benefits of neoadjuvant therapy.

B.   Treatment of advanced (metastatic) disease. Various agents with modest activity when used alone are available. These include cisplatin, carboplatin, fluorouracil, bleomycin, paclitaxel, methotrexate, mitomycin, vinorelbine, and doxorubicin. Response rates range from 15% to 30% and are usually brief. Most data are for epidermoid carcinoma, the exception being paclitaxel, which appears equally effective in both histologic types. The most active drugs appear to be cisplatin, paclitaxel, and fluorouracil. Patients with no history of prior chemotherapy are more likely to respond than those who have had previous treatment. Single agents are less helpful than combination chemotherapy because of their lower response rates and brief duration of response. Cisplatin-based regimens have been most extensively tested. Among the most active are the following:

  1. **Cisplatin + fluorouracil**
     a. Cisplatin 75 to 100 mg/m^2 IV on day 1.
     b. Fluorouracil 1,000 mg/m^2/day as a continuous IV infusion on days 1 to 5. Repeat every 28 days.
  2. **Paclitaxel + cisplatin**
     a. Paclitaxel 175 mg/m^2 IV.
     b. Cisplatin 75 mg/m^2 IV. Repeat every 21 days.
  3. **Carboplatin + paclitaxel**
     a. Carboplatin area under the curve (AUC) 5 IV.
     b. Paclitaxel 150 mg/m^2 IV. Repeat every 21 days.
  4. **Paclitaxel + cisplatin + 5-fluorouracil**
     a. Paclitaxel 175 mg/m^2 IV over 3 h on day 1.
     b. Cisplatin 20 mg/m^2/day IV on days 1 to 5.
     c. 5-Fluorouracil (5-FU) 750 mg/m^2/day continuous IV on days 1 to 5. Repeat every 28 days.
  5. **Second-line therapy** may be chosen from the following single agents: methotrexate 40 mg/m^2 IV weekly; bleomycin 15 U/m^2 IV twice weekly; vinorelbine 25 mg/m^2 IV weekly; or mitomycin 20 mg/m^2 IV every 4 to 6 weeks.

C. **Combined-modality treatment for potentially curable patients.** The poor results with immediate surgery, due in part to inadequate staging techniques, have focused attention for some years on preoperative combined-modality treatment with radiation therapy, chemotherapy, or both, followed by surgery (or, in some instances, not followed by surgery). This approach is controversial because of uncertainty of staging and conflicting results from randomized clinical trials. When this approach is used, aggressive staging including endoscopic ultrasound, CT scanning, and laparoscopy is needed and is often combined with jejunostomy feeding tube placement for nutritional support. Despite conflicting results from randomized trials, patients with stage II and III disease are often treated in this fashion.

  1. **Preoperative chemotherapy.** The National Cancer Institute Gastrointestinal Intergroup has reported a randomized trial of 440 patients with either adenocarcinoma or epidermoid cancer of the esophagus, which compared preoperative chemotherapy (cisplatin and fluorouracil for three cycles) versus surgery alone. After a median follow-up of 55.4 months, there were no median, 1-year, or 2-year survival differences between the two groups. These results differ compared with recent data from the Medical Research Council Clinical Trials Unit in the United Kingdom, which included 802 patients randomized to receive either two cycles of preoperative cisplatin and fluorouracil followed by surgery versus surgery alone. Approximately 66% of patients had adenocarcinoma. In this study, the median survival was 17.2 months for the preoperative chemotherapy patients compared with 13.3 months for the patients treated

with surgery alone, a statistically significant difference. The 2-year survival rates were 43% and 34%, respectively. Different proportions of the two different histologies contribute to the difficulties in interpretation of these trials.

2. Radiation therapy with surgery, chemotherapy, or both. Radiation therapy, as either a preoperative or a postoperative adjunct to surgery, has not improved overall survival in most series. Radiation therapy alone has 5-year survival rates ranging from 0% to 10%. Combined-modality treatment of radiotherapy with chemotherapy has been superior. In a randomized trial comparing radiotherapy alone with radiotherapy plus chemotherapy in 121 patients, 88% of whom had squamous cell cancer, the Radiation Therapy Oncology Group reported a 5-year survival rate of 27% for the combined-modality group and 0% for the radiation therapy alone group. Median survival times were 14.1 and 9.3 months, respectively. Most patients had stage T2 disease and were node negative by CT scanning. The Eastern Cooperative Oncology Group performed a similar trial of 135 patients with stage I or II squamous cell cancer of the esophagus. Patients were randomized to receive 4,000 cGy versus radiation with a 96-h continuous infusion of 5-FU plus mitomycin. Median survival was improved for patients treated with chemoradiation (14.8 months) compared with those receiving radiation therapy alone (9.2 months). Combined chemotherapy and radiotherapy is therefore a reasonable approach for patients who refuse surgery or whose disease is unresectable for anatomic or physiologic reasons, particularly those with epidermoid carcinoma.

  a. Radiation therapy + fluorouracil + cisplatin

  (1) Radiation therapy 180 to 200 cGy/day for 3 weeks, 5 days weekly, then 2 additional weeks to the boost field for a total of 5,040 cGy, *and*

  (2) Fluorouracil 1,000 mg/m^2/day by continuous infusion for 4 days on weeks 1, 5, 8, and 11, with cisplatin 75 mg/m^2 IV at 1 mg/min on the first day of each course. Reduce fluorouracil for severe diarrhea or stomatitis and cisplatin for severe neutropenia or thrombocytopenia.

  (3) Surgery, when it can be done, is probably appropriate because most patients treated with chemotherapy and radiotherapy still have residual tumor. Even though a high proportion, 25% in many series, have complete pathologic responses at surgery, the preoperative identification of these patients is not accurate.

  A recent randomized trial from Ireland of 113 patients with adenocarcinoma of the esophagus has shown a 3-year survival rate of 32% for patients treated with preoperative chemotherapy with fluorouracil and cisplatin and with radiotherapy followed by surgery compared with 6% for patients treated with surgery alone. Similarly, a recent study from the University of Michigan of 100 patients (68% adenocarcinoma) has shown a 3-year survival rate of 30% for combined-modality treatment compared with 16% for surgery alone, with a reduction in local recurrence in the combined group (42% versus 19%). At a median follow-up of 8.2 years, there was no difference in survival between the two groups (17.6 and 16.9 months, respectively). Optimal results may involve all three major treatment modalities, with at least some of the chemotherapy being given concurrently with radiation therapy. Alternative preoperative treatments are being defined in Phase II trials, incorporating such agents as paclitaxel and irinotecan, and postoperative chemotherapy is also being evaluated. The following have been used in potentially resectable patients:

b.   Cisplatin + fluorouracil + radiotherapy (Dublin regimen)

   (1)   Fluorouracil 15 mg/kg (555 mg/m^2) IV over 16 h daily, days 1 to 5, *and*

   (2)   Cisplatin 75 mg/m^2 IV infused over 8 h on day 7 after 1 full day of hydration. Repeat both drugs at 6 weeks.

   (3)   Radiotherapy 40 Gy in 15 fractions over 3 weeks, beginning on the first day of chemotherapy.

   (4)   Surgery is done 8 weeks after beginning treatment, blood counts permitting.

c.   Fluorouracil + cisplatin + vinblastine + radiotherapy (Michigan regimen)

   (1)   Vinblastine 1 mg/m^2 IV on days 1 to 4 and 17 to 20 of radiotherapy, *and*

   (2)   Cisplatin 20 mg/m^2/day by continuous IV infusion on days 1 to 5 and 17 to 21 of radiotherapy, *and*

   (3)   Fluorouracil 300 mg/m^2/day by continuous IV infusion on days 1 to 21 of radiotherapy, *and*

   (4)   Radiotherapy 45 Gy in 15 fractions (300 cGy b.i.d.) for 3 weeks.

   (5)   Surgery is done at 6 weeks.

D.   Supportive care. Esophagitis during a combined-modality treatment program is nearly universal, and nutritional support frequently is required, preferably using alimentation by feeding tube placed by enterostomy. Peripheral alimentation is difficult with the continuous chemotherapy administration. Gastrostomy tubes are to be avoided because of the usual requirement for a gastric pull-up after resection of the esophageal tumor.

E.   Follow-up studies. For asymptomatic patients with potentially curative therapy, history and physical examination may be done every 4 months for 1 year, then every 6 months for 2 years. Chest radiographs, CT scans, endoscopy, chemistries, and complete blood count should be evaluated as clinically indicated.

II.   Gastric carcinoma

A.   General considerations and aims of therapy

   1.   Epidemiology. The incidence of stomach cancer has decreased dramatically in the United States since the beginning of the century, although it has stabilized in the last 20 years. The leading cause of cancer death in 1930; it now ranks 12th. No improvement has been seen, however, in 5-year survival rates, which range from 5% to 16%. A recent large randomized U.S. clinical trial, however, has shown improved survival for individuals treated with surgery followed by combined radiation and chemotherapy. The male-to-female ratio is nearly two to one. Stomach cancer is still the leading cause of cancer deaths among men in Japan and is also common in China, Finland, Poland, Peru, and Chile. A high rate of chronic gastritis and intestinal metaplasia of the stomach is associated with a high incidence of gastric cancer. *Helicobacter pylori* has been implicated in such changes and in gastric cancer, particularly the more distal "intestinal" type, as well as in peptic ulcer. Although the incidence in the United States has decreased, the location of gastric cancers has migrated proximally. Cancers in the fundus of the stomach have increased from 14% of gastric cancers in 1950 to 24% at present. Nearly half the stomach cancers occurring in white men are located proximally.

2. Clinical manifestations and evaluation. The most common symptoms are weight loss, abdominal pain, nausea, vomiting, changes in bowel habits, fatigue, anorexia, and dysphagia. The diagnosis generally is made by endoscopy and biopsy, although barium swallow is frequently helpful. Endoscopic ultrasonography is increasingly used; it is more accurate in gauging the depth of the cancer in the gastric wall than in determining nodal involvement. Metastases are to the liver, pancreas, omentum, esophagus, and bile ducts by direct extension and to regional and distant lymph nodes such as those in the left supraclavicular area. Pulmonary and bone metastases are a late finding. Staging of suspected gastric cancer should be based on CT scans of the chest, abdomen, and pelvis and on liver function tests. Tumor markers such as carcinoembryonic antigen (CEA), CA 19-9, and CA 72-4 may be useful for subsequent assessment of the response to therapy. Prognosis is reflected by accurate staging (Table 8.2). The revised staging method classifies patients according to the number of pathologically involved regional lymph nodes. The groupings are 1 to 6, 7 to 15, and more than 15 involved lymph nodes; surgically staged patients resected for cure have 5-year survival rates of 46%, 30%, and 10%, respectively.

3. Treatment and prognosis. Most stomach cancers are adenocarcinomas. Important prognostic factors include tumor grade and gross appearance. Diffusely infiltrating lesions are less likely to be cured than sharply circumscribed, nonulcerating lesions. The presence of regional lymph node involvement or involvement of contiguous organs in the surgical specimen indicates an increased likelihood of recurrence, as does the presence of dysphagia at the time of diagnosis. Patients with proximal lesions or lesions requiring total, rather than distal subtotal, gastrectomy are also at greater risk.

B. Treatment of advanced (metastatic, locally unresectable, or recurrent) disease

1. Single agents with activity include epirubicin, mitomycin, doxorubicin, cisplatin, etoposide, fluorouracil, irinotecan, hydroxyurea, the taxanes, and the nitrosoureas. Single agents have low response rates (15% to 30%), brief durations of response, and few complete responses, and they have little impact on survival.

Table 8.2.   **TNM stages for carcinoma of the stomach**

Primary tumor
  Tis   Carcinoma *in situ*
  T1   Invades lamina propria or submucosa
  T2   Invades muscularis propria or subserosa
  T3   Penetrates serosa (visceral peritoneum)
  T4   Invades adjacent structures
Regional lymph nodes
  N0   No nodal metastasis
  N1   Metastasis in 1–6 regional lymph nodes
  N2   Metastasis in 7–15 regional lymph nodes
  N3   Metastasis in > 15 regional lymph nodes
Distant metastasis
  M0   None
  M1   Present
Stage grouping
  0   Tis, N0, M0
  IA   T1, N0, M0
  IB   T1, N1, M0
          T2, N0, M0
  II   T1, N2, M0
          T2, N1, M0
          T3, N0, M0
  IIIA   T2, N2, M0
          T3, N1, M0
          T4, N0, M0
  IIIB   T3, N2, M0
  IV   T4, N1, M0
          T1, N3, M0
          T2, N3, M0
          T3, N3, M0
          T4, N2, M0
          T4, N3, M0
          Any T, any N, M1

Modified from American Joint Committee on Cancer. *AJCC staging manual.*
6th ed. New York: Springer, 2002.

2.   Combinations of drugs are more widely used than single agents, largely because of higher response rates, more frequent complete responses, and the theoretical potential of
longer survival. A controlled trial (1985) of fluorouracil alone
versus fluorouracil plus doxorubicin (Adriamycin) (FA) versus
fluorouracil, doxorubicin, and mitomycin (FAM), however,
failed to show a survival benefit for the combinations, which
were more costly and toxic. Response rates, which were measurable in only about half the patients, were higher with the
combinations. A European study compared methotrexate,
fluorouracil, and doxorubicin with etoposide, leucovorin, and
fluorouracil and with fluorouracil and cisplatin, showing no
significant difference among the combinations. New combi-

nations are continually being reported; however, initial response rates are generally higher than those found in subsequent confirmatory studies or randomized trials. Some epirubicin regimens from Europe appear to be active, but that agent is not routinely used in the United States because of reimbursement issues. The combination of cisplatin and irinotecan has been reported to be active, as have taxane combinations. Drug combination therapy has been shown to improve median survival by about 6 months in patients with metastatic disease compared with the best supportive care in four small, randomized trials.

   a.   ELF. The ELF (leucovorin, etoposide, and fluorouracil) regimen was designed to be less toxic than the regimen of etoposide, doxorubicin, and cisplatin (EAP), and in the hands of its originators, it appears to be as effective. Initial experience suggested a response rate of about 50%, with an 11-month median survival. The regimen is as follows:

   (1)   Leucovorin 300 mg/m^2 as a 10-min IV infusion, *followed by*
   (2)   Etoposide 120 mg/m^2 as a 50-min IV infusion, *followed by*
   (3)   Fluorouracil 500 mg/m^2 IV as a 10-min infusion.
   All agents are given on days 1, 2, and 3. The course is repeated in 21 to 28 days.

   b.   FAMTX. This regimen compared favorably with FAM in a large European clinical trial and with EAP in the United States. Response rates were 41% and 33% in the two studies, with median survival times of 10.5 and 7.3 months, respectively. The need for leucovorin "rescue" of methotrexate makes it rather cumbersome.

   Before methotrexate administration, hydrate with 1 L of isotonic sodium bicarbonate (1.4% bicarbonate; urine pH must be higher than 7.0). Infuse 2 L of an identical solution over 24 h after methotrexate is given. The regimen is as follows:

   (1)   Methotrexate 1.5 g/m^2 by IV bolus infusion after the hydration and urine alkalinization on day 1, *and*
   (2)   Fluorouracil 1.5 g/m^2 by IV bolus infusion starting 1 h after the end of the methotrexate infusion, *and*
   (3)   Leucovorin 15 mg/m^2 orally starting 24 h later on day 2, given every 6 h for 3 days or until the methotrexate level is less than $2 \times 10^{-8}\ M$. If the methotrexate level is more than $2.5 \times 10^{-6}\ M$ at 24 h, increase leucovorin dose to 30 mg/m^2 every 6 h for 96 h.
   (4)   Doxorubicin 30 mg/m^2 IV on day 15 if the white blood cell count is more than 3,000/μL or the absolute neutrophil count is more than 1,500/μL and the platelet count is more than 70,000/μL.
   The cycle is repeated every 4 weeks. Renal function must be normal and blood levels of methotrexate should be monitored with this regimen.

   c.   Hydroxyurea + leucovorin + fluorouracil + cisplatin. A large Phase II study of this regimen in France has reported a response rate of 62% and median survival time of 11 months. The regimen is as follows:

(1)   Hydroxyurea 1.5 to 2 g PO on days 0, 1, and 2, *and*
(2)   Leucovorin 200 mg/m² IV as a 2-h infusion on days 1 and 2, *before*
(3)   Fluorouracil 400 mg/m² IV bolus and 600 mg/m² by 22-h infusion on days 1 and 2, *then*
(4)   Cisplatin 80 mg/m² IV on day 3 every other cycle.
The cycle is repeated every 14 days.

d.   Irinotecan + cisplatin
(1)   Irinotecan 70 mg/m² IV over 90 min on days 1 and 15.
(2)   Cisplatin 80 mg/m² IV over 2 h on day 1.
The cycle is repeated every 28 days.

C.   Adjuvant chemotherapy. Despite numerous trials of postoperative chemotherapy following potentially curative gastric resection, its value is uncertain. Until benefit is shown, there is no specific role for adjuvant chemotherapy alone after surgery.

D.   Combined-modality therapy. The U.S. Gastrointestinal Intergroup recently has reported the results of a 556-patient randomized trial comparing surgery with or without postoperative chemotherapy (5-FU and leucovorin) and combined chemotherapy and radiation followed by two additional cycles of chemotherapy. Patients had resected stages IB through stage IV M0 adenocarcinoma of the stomach or gastroesophageal junction. Postoperative combined therapy produced a statistically significant median survival benefit (36 versus 27 months, respectively; $p = 0.005$). Although the study did not show any significant difference in relapse-free or overall survival according to the extent of lymph node dissection, 54% of patients had a D0 lymphadenectomy (surgery that did not remove all of the N1 nodes), 36% had a D1 dissection, and only 10% underwent a D2 dissection (includes perigastric, celiac, splenic, hepatic artery, and cardial lymph nodes). Major toxic effects (grade 3 or higher) in the chemoradiotherapy group were predominantly hematologic (54%) and gastrointestinal (33%).

The recommended postoperative adjuvant combined regimen from the intergroup trial includes the following:

1.   Chemotherapy. Leucovorin 20 mg/m² IV bolus days 1 to 5, fluorouracil 425 mg/m² IV bolus days 1 to 5 (cycle 1).
2.   Radiotherapy. 45 Gy at 180 cGY/day to the tumor (or tumor bed) and nodal chains daily for 5 days weekly × 5 weeks (begin 28 days after initial chemotherapy).
3.   Chemotherapy. Started on the first day of radiotherapy.
   a.   Leucovorin 20 mg/m² IV bolus on days 1 to 4 and during the last 3 days of radiation.
   b.   Fluorouracil 400 mg/m² IV bolus on days 1 to 4, each dose given after the leucovorin and during the last 3 days of radiation.
4.   Chemotherapy. One month after completing chemoradiation, begin two 5-day cycles of leucovorin and fluorouracil as given during cycle 1.

E.   Follow-up studies. Reasonable follow-up studies for patients in remission after surgery consist of history and physical examination every 4 months for 1 year, every 6 months for 2 years, and then annually. Complete blood cell count, chemistries, endoscopy, and radiologic imaging should be evaluated as clinically indicated. Vitamin B_{12} supplementation is recommended for patients who have had proximal resections or total gastrectomy.

The use of preoperative, or neoadjuvant, chemotherapy is somewhat in vogue at the present time, owing to some encouraging responses and apparent conversion of unresectable tumors to resectable ones by the administration of multidrug combinations. This approach is still under investigation.

F.   Complications. Hematologic and GI toxicities from the chemotherapy may be accentuated by concurrent radiotherapy. If the complications are sufficiently severe, chemotherapy, radiotherapy, or both should be withheld until improvement. Consideration is given to treating at reduced doses. Hematopoietic growth factors may be of benefit in preventing severe infections secondary to neutropenia, but their use has not yet resulted in improved survival.

G.   Treatment of refractory disease. If the patient's disease recurs or progresses with the recommended regimens, it is reasonable to consider combinations containing drugs not previously administered or any of the single agents mentioned in Section II.B.1.

III.   Cancer of the small intestine

A.   Carcinoid tumors. Carcinoid tumors are the most common tumors of the appendix and ileum. They may develop in other parts of the GI tract but much less commonly. The usual histologic criteria of malignancy are not always applicable. Invasion and evidence of distant spread are more useful prognostic features. In one series, the 60% of patients with intestinal carcinoids that were still confined to the wall of the gut had a 5-year survival rate of 85%, whereas those with tumors invading the serosa or beyond had a 5% survival rate at 5 years. Patients in the latter group were nearly always symptomatic, whereas patients in the former group were not. (Their tumors were discovered at surgery for appendicitis or other causes.) Tumors of the appendix are usually benign by these criteria, whereas those of the ileum are more often invasive. Surgical resection is the definitive therapy.

1.   Carcinoid syndrome. About 10% of patients with carcinoid tumors have the carcinoid syndrome, which includes diarrhea, abdominal cramps, malabsorption, and flushing. With tumors of intestinal origin, liver metastases are nearly always present. Serotonin is thought to be responsible for the abdominal symptoms. Its metabolite, 5-hydroxyindoleacetic acid (5-HIAA), is excreted in large quantities in the urine and is a useful marker of disease activity. Other markers include chromogranin A. The symptoms may respond to simple antidiarrheal therapy. The flushing caused by the syndrome has been attributed to bradykinin, formed by the interaction of kallikrein (produced by the tumor) with a plasma protein. If simple symptomatic measures do not suffice, the best treatment is the synthetic long-acting somatostatin analog octreotide acetate (Sandostatin). This agent, injected at a dose of 50 to 150 µg SC every 6 to 12 h or as the long-acting formulation (octreotide LAR depot) 20 to 30 mg IM every month, effectively decreases the secretion of serotonin and other gastroenteropancreatic peptides such as insulin or gastrin. It has been helpful in ameliorating the symptoms of carcinoid tumors (e.g., flushing and diarrhea). There are even modest objective antitumor effects. The excretion of 5-HIAA is reduced by octreotide.

2.   Treatment of advanced carcinoid tumors

a.   Effective agents. The chemotherapy agents doxorubicin, fluorouracil, mitomycin, cyclophosphamide, methotrexate, and streptozocin have been shown to have limited activity in this disease. Response rates for combinations of fluorouracil and streptozocin or for streptozocin and cyclophosphamide in treating carcinoids of various kinds are 25% to 35%, with response durations usually less than 9 months; the overall response rate for patients with tumors of intestinal origin is 41%. A median duration of response of 7 months may be expected, and patients with a good performance status have the greatest likelihood of response. Tumor response correlates well with reduction of 5-HIAA excretion. Some reports have indicated responses with interferon-α, including responses in combination with octreotide and in some patients previously treated with chemotherapy. When the disease is confined to the liver, it is sometimes possible to achieve good palliation with hepatic artery embolization or chemoembolization.

b.   Recommended regimens

(1)   Octreotide LAR 20 to 30 mg IM q21 to 28 days.

(2)   Interferon-α 3 to 6 × 10^6 U/day or 10 × 10^6 U three times per week.

c.   Precautions. Treatment of carcinoid tumors may precipitate or exacerbate the carcinoid syndrome during the first days of treatment, and the serotonin antagonists cyproheptadine and methysergide as well as octreotide should be available.

B.   Adenocarcinomas. Adenocarcinomas of the small intestine are so uncommon that there is no large chemotherapy experience to report. Survival of patients with small intestinal cancer is a function of stage (Table 8.3). Radiation and infusional 5-FU may be considered for patients with local recurrence or unresectable disease. The chemotherapy regimens employed for advanced colorectal cancer (e.g., irinotecan, 5-FU, and leucovorin) also are generally used to treat patients with small intestine adenocarcinoma.

IV.   Cancer of the large intestine

A.   General considerations and aims of therapy. Taken together, cancers of the colon and rectum are by far the most frequent malignancies of the GI tract, and they account for the most deaths. Approximately half of patients found to have large-bowel cancers are cured by surgery, which remains the only curative modality. Local recurrence is much more common for rectal cancer (40% to 50% in nonirradiated patients). About half of large-bowel cancer recurrences are in the liver.

1.   Staging. A commonly used staging system is the Dukes staging system including the Astler–Coller modifications. The TNM system for colorectal cancer is being used increasingly (Table 8.4) and is the recommended system. The many

Table 8.3. TNM stages for carcinoma of the small intestine

Primary tumor

Tis	Carcinoma *in situ*
T1	Invades lamina propria or submucosa
T2	Invades muscularis propria
T3	Invades through the muscularis propria into subserosa or into nonperitonealized perimuscular tissue with extension of ≤2 cm
T4	Perforates visceral peritoneum or directly invades other organs or structures

Regional lymph nodes

N0	No nodal metastasis
N1	Regional node metastasis

Distant metastasis

M0	None
M1	Present

Stage grouping

0	Tis, N0, M0
I	T1 or T2, N0, M0
II	T3 or T4, N0, M0
III	Any T, N1, M0
IV	Any T, any N, M1

Modified from American Joint Committee on Cancer. *AJCC staging manual.* 6th ed. New York: Springer, 2002.

Table 8.4. TNM stages for carcinoma of the colon and rectum

Primary tumor

Tis	Carcinoma *in situ* and intramucosal (within lamina propria)
T1	Invades through muscularis mucosa into submucosa
T2	Invades muscularis propria
T3	Invades through muscularis propria into subserosa or nonperitonealized pericolic or perirectal tissues
T4	Invades adjacent organs or structures or perforates visceral peritoneum

Regional lymph nodes

N0	No nodal metastasis
N1	Metastasis in 1–3 regional nodes
N2	Metastasis in ≥4 regional nodes

Distant metastasis

M0	None
M1	Present

Stage grouping		Dukes'
0	Tis, N0, M0	—
I	T1 or T2, N0, M0	A
II	T3 or T4, N0, M0	B
III	Any T, N1, N2, M0	C
IV	Any T, any N, MI	—

Modified from American Joint Committee on Cancer. *AJCC staging manual.* 6th ed. New York: Springer, 2002.

modifications of the Dukes system support the argument that TNM staging should be used to avoid confusion. These systems classify the tumor in terms of the extent to which it penetrates the bowel wall and involves regional lymph nodes. Dukes A lesions (stage I) are confined to the mucosa and submucosa. Dukes B1 lesions (stage I) penetrate the muscularis but do not reach the serosa. Stage I patient survival is more than 85%. Dukes B2 lesions (stage II) penetrate to the serosa or through it into the pericolic fat; patient survival approximates 75% to 80%. Dukes C lesions (stage III) indicate nodal involvement. If the serosa has not been penetrated (in the Astler–Coller modification of the Dukes system), it is called a C1 lesion; C2 lesions are through the serosa. Patients with stage III disease and who have received adjuvant therapy have a survival of approximately 60% to 65%. Dukes D lesions (stage IV) include distant metastases at the time of initial staging, with less than 7% 5-year survival rate. This pathologic staging method is helpful for selecting patients who are at sufficiently high risk to justify adjuvant therapy such as chemotherapy or irradiation. Staging is most accurately performed at the time of surgery. Abdominal, chest, and pelvic CT are helpful for preoperative assessment of extrabowel involvement, but the findings may be falsely negative when small peritoneal implants are present. Bone scans are seldom needed, except for assessment of bone pain, because bone metastases occur rather late in the course of the disease. Positron emission tomography scanning is considered to determine the presence of metastatic disease.

2. Serum carcinoembryonic antigen. CEA level may parallel disease activity, although it is not increased in all patients with colon cancer. It is worth measuring preoperatively and, if elevated, postoperatively because failure of an elevated value to return to normal may signify incomplete removal of the tumor. Likewise, a serial rise in CEA values after an initial fall to normal indicates recurrence. CEA values may also be an indicator of response during chemotherapy treatment. Patients who have a normal serum CEA level preoperatively may still demonstrate an elevated CEA value at the time of recurrence. A rising CEA level is an indication for careful re-evaluation with CT, positron emission tomography, and possibly laparoscopy because some patients may have isolated, resectable, and thus potentially curable metastases, particularly involving the liver.

B. Treatment of advanced disease

1. Effective agents and combinations. For more than 30 years, fluorouracil has been the standard agent in the treatment of advanced colorectal disease not amenable to surgical or radiotherapeutic control. Response rates have varied widely, but a generally agreed-on figure is 10% to 15%. Combinations of other agents with fluorouracil, including leucovorin, irinotecan (CPT-11) and oxaliplatin, have demonstrated improved response rates and survival.

Second-line treatment for metastatic colorectal cancer is of particular interest because of the benefits of single-agent irinotecan in this setting. Trials have demonstrated response rates of greater than 20%, with greater than 50% of patients achieving stable disease and with median survivals of approximately 12 months. In addition, a European study, which randomized metastatic colorectal cancer patients who had progressed within 6 months of treatment with fluorouracil to receive irinotecan versus supportive care, demonstrated a significant 1-year survival advantage (36.2% versus 13.8%; $p = 0.0001$) for those patients receiving irinotecan, including an improved pain-free survival.

First-line irinotecan trials for previously untreated patients with advanced colorectal cancer also have demonstrated response and survival benefits compared with 5-FU and leucovorin. For example, a U.S. trial comparing weekly CPT-11, 5-FU, and leucovorin with 5-FU and leucovorin and with CPT-11 alone revealed an overall response rate favoring the three-drug combination (39% versus 21% versus 18%, respectively) and a median survival advantage (14.8 versus 12.6 versus 12 months, respectively; $p = 0.04$). A European trial evaluating infusional 5-FU regimens with or without CPT-11 also confirmed a response advantage for the three drugs (49% versus 31%) and improved median survival (17.5% versus 14.1%; $p = 0.03$).

Capecitabine is the only oral fluoropyrimidine available for use in colorectal cancer. Two trials have demonstrated a better response with capecitabine than with 5-FU and leucovorin with similar median time to disease progression, median time to treatment failure, and median overall survival (approximately 13.3 months for 5-FU/leucovorin and 12.5 months for 5-FU/leucovorin in a U.S. study). Capecitabine is therefore available for first-line colorectal cancer patients, particularly those who may not be optimal candidates for a CPT-11 combination.

A number of new agents are also in development with promising results, including oxaliplatin, C225, rhuMAb–vascular endothelial growth factor, SU5416, and Iressa. A combination regimen with oxaliplatin appears to be at least as good as and possibly better than the weekly CPT-11, 5-FU, and leucovorin. Further follow-up will be necessary to determine whether longer time to treatment failure and improved survival results will hold up. The regimen is as follows:

    a. Oxaliplatin 85 mg/m^2 as a 120-min IV infusion in 500 mL of D5W on day 1 **only,** *and*

    b. Leucovorin 200 mg/m^2 as a 120-min IV infusion over 120 min, followed by fluorouracil 400 mg/m^2 IV bolus, then 600 mg/m^2 as an IV infusion over 22 h on day 1 and in an identical schedule on day 2.

    The cycle (Sections IV.B.1.a and b) is repeated every 14 days. Day 1 leucovorin may be given during the same 2-h period as the oxaliplatin, but because of the incompatibility of oxaliplatin with saline, both drugs must be in D5W.

2. Liver metastasis. A 2-week continuous infusion with floxuridine with or without leucovorin plus dexamethasone given every 28 days and administered by an implantable or portable infusion pump produces among the highest responses for metastatic colorectal cancer to the liver. The impact on survival, however, remains controversial, with no definitive survival benefit shown by the hepatic artery infusion. More recently, investigators have included systemic therapy alternating with the hepatic artery infusion. A recent trial evaluating hepatic artery infusion with fluorouracil versus systemic therapy failed to show any advantage for the fluorouracil hepatic infusion.

3.   Recommended regimens

a.   Fluorouracil + high-dose leucovorin. Leucovorin 500 mg/m^2 IV is given over 2 h with fluorouracil 500 mg/m^2 IV bolus injected 1 h after beginning the leucovorin infusion. The combination is administered weekly for 6 weeks followed by a 2-week rest. This regimen is now widely favored as the preferred fluorouracil + leucovorin combination.

b.   Fluorouracil + leucovorin. Leucovorin 20 mg/m^2 IV is followed by fluorouracil 425 mg/m^2 IV. The combination is given daily for 5 days. Courses are repeated every 4 weeks.

Significant numbers of patients require dose reductions, and therefore, the weekly regimen is now favored (see Section IV.B.3.a).

c.   Fluorouracil by 24-hour continuous infusion. Fluorouracil 2,600 mg/m^2 is given by 24-h continuous IV infusion weekly.

d.   Fluorouracil by protracted venous infusion. Fluorouracil 250 to 300 mg/m^2 over 24 h is given continuously until toxicity (e.g., erythrodysesthesia, mucositis, or diarrhea) or for 4 weeks continuously followed by a 1-week break.

e.   Irinotecan. Irinotecan 125 mg/m^2 as a 90-min IV infusion is given weekly for 4 weeks with a 2-week rest.

f.   Irinotecan + 5-fluorouracil + leucovorin. Irinotecan 125 mg/m^2 as a 90-min IV infusion with 5-FU 500 mg/m^2 and leucovorin 20 mg/m^2 administered weekly for 4 weeks with a 2-week rest. Recent toxicity data are such that many oncologists have begun using irinotecan 100 mg/m^2 and 5-FU 400 mg/m^2 with leucovorin 20 mg/m^2. Dose escalation to full dose is an option for patients with minimal toxicity.

g.   Capecitabine. Capecitabine 1,250 mg/m^2 administered twice daily orally days 1 to 14 every 3 weeks (2,500 mg/m^2/day). Many oncologists have begun patients on a lower dose of 1,000 mg/m^2 PO b.i.d. on days 1 to 14 every 3 weeks because of toxicity including erythrodysesthesia and mucositis in particular.

The following regimens are used less commonly:

h.   Irinotecan + infusional 5-fluorouracil + leucovorin. Irinotecan 80 mg/m^2 plus leucovorin 500 mg/m^2 with fluorouracil 2,300 mg/m^2 by 24-h infusion are administered weekly for 6 weeks with a 1-week break.

i.   Irinotecan + 5-fluorouracil + leucovorin. Irinotecan 180 mg/m^2 on day 1, leucovorin 200 mg/m^2 days 1 and 2, 5-FU 400 mg/m^2 IV bolus days 1 and 2, and 5-FU 600 mg/m^2 as a continuous infusion over 24 h on days 1 and 2, repeated every 2 weeks.

j.   FOLFIRI. Irinotecan 180 mg/m^2, 5-FU 400 mg/m^2 IV bolus, and leucovorin 200 mg/m^2 all on day 1 followed by 5-FU 2.4 to 3.0 g/m^2 as a continuous infusion over 24 h repeated every 2 weeks.

k.   Fluorouracil + methotrexate + leucovorin. Methotrexate 200 mg/m^2 IV is given over 30 min after hydration with 1,500 mL of 5% dextrose in 0.5 N saline. At 24 h, fluorouracil 600 mg/m^2 IV bolus is given, followed by leucovorin 10 mg/m^2 (to the nearest 5 mg) PO every 6 hours × 6. The regimen is repeated every 2 weeks.

l.   Hepatic artery infusion. Most patients are managed by an implantable pump. A preferred regimen includes floxuridine 0.25 mg/kg/day in heparinized saline (50,000 U of heparin) plus 20 mg of dexamethasone administered for 2 weeks, alternating with 2 weeks of heparinized saline without floxuridine. Some patients will need a dose reduction of floxuridine to 0.15 to 0.2 mg/kg. The dexamethasone has helped to prevent biliary sclerosis that sometimes accompanies such treatment. If leucovorin is added, the recommended dose of floxuridine is 0.18 mg/kg.

C.   Adjuvant chemotherapy

1.   Colon cancer. For patients with node-positive (stage III, Dukes C) resectable colon cancer, the combination of fluorouracil plus leucovorin given either by the 5-day or the weekly schedule for 6 months improves the disease-free as well as the overall survival of patients. It is equally effective as the older regimen of fluorouracil and levamisole given for 1 year. Most randomized clinical trials have not demonstrated a survival advantage for stage II patients who have been treated with adjuvant chemotherapy, and the current standard is observation. A current large stage II colon cancer intergroup trial is exploring the postoperative use of the murine monoclonal antibody 17-1A compared to observation. A future trial will define risk for stage II patients based on molecular markers including 18q allele deletion and microsatellite instability. In addition, the role of adjuvant chemotherapy with irinotecan and oxaliplatin-based regimens will be defined by the most recent intergroup adjuvant trials.

Although historical data support the use of postoperative radiotherapy for locally advanced colon cancer (Dukes B3 or C3 or any T4 lesion), a small intergroup trial did not confirm its efficacy. Chemotherapy with fluorouracil should probably be incorporated into the regimen and used for a total of 6 months after radiation therapy.

The recommended colon cancer adjuvant regimens for node-positive patients (stage III) are as follows:

a. Leucovorin 500 mg/m^2 over 2 h with fluorouracil 500 mg/m^2 IV given at 1 h after beginning the leucovorin infusion administered weekly × 6 with a 2-week break. A total of four cycles is given. Many physicians now favor this weekly regimen because of the toxicity noted with the 5-day schedule shown in Section IV.C.1.b below, *or*

b. Leucovorin 20 mg/m^2 IV and fluorouracil 425 mg/m^2 IV daily × 5 on weeks 1, 5, 9, 14, 19, and 24.

2.   Resected hepatic metastases. Past data have demonstrated that patients with resected hepatic metastases secondary to colorectal cancer have a survival of at least 25%. Two recently completed clinical trials evaluating hepatic artery infusion with floxuridine compared to surgery have demonstrated significant reduction in recurrence of hepatic metastases with a trend toward improved survival for the patients receiving the hepatic artery infusion.

3.   Rectal cancer

   a.   Preoperative irradiation. Several studies have shown that preoperative irradiation benefits patients with rectal cancer, although there are disadvantages in terms of accuracy of staging, delay before surgery, incomplete knowledge of the extent of tumor for treatment planning, and inappropriate administration of radiation to patients with early (Dukes A or B1) or advanced (Dukes D) lesions. Possible advantages include downstaging of tumor, improved sphincter preservation, improved resectability, and earlier initiation of systemic therapy. Better preoperative staging includes the use of magnetic resonance imaging and endorectal ultrasound. Clinical trials are ongoing.

   b.   Postoperative irradiation, with and without chemotherapy. Several controlled clinical trials have shown convincingly that radiation therapy alone reduces local recurrence but has little or no effect on overall survival. Fluorouracil-based chemotherapy added to radiation therapy is superior to either modality alone in terms of both local control and distant disease, thus improving overall survival. The optimal administration of fluorouracil during radiation therapy appears to be by protracted venous infusion, requiring a port and ambulatory pump, rather than by bolus. Whether the chemotherapy that does not accompany radiation therapy should be by bolus or protracted venous infusion, along with the role of leucovorin, is being addressed by recently completed clinical trials.

   The recommended postoperative adjuvant regimen for stage II or III rectal cancers is as follows:

   (1)   Fluorouracil 500 mg/m^2 IV bolus daily on days 1 to 5 and days 36 to 40.

   (2)   Radiation therapy 4,500 cGy in 180-cGy fractions over 5 weeks, with tumor boost of 540 to 900 cGy, beginning on day 64.

   (3)   Fluorouracil 225 mg/m^2/day by protracted venous infusion throughout the period of radiation therapy, days 64 to 105.

   (4)   Fluorouracil 500 mg/m^2 IV bolus daily, on days 134 to 138 and days 169 to 173.

   If leucovorin is added to the 5-FU schedule (without radiation), the dose of leucovorin is 20 mg/m^2 and the dose of 5-FU is 425 mg/m^2/day for 5 days before radiation. After radiation, 5-FU should be reduced to 380 mg/m^2/day with the leucovorin. Future planned intergroup trials will evaluate the use of capecitabine with radiation as a preoperative regimen, and another trial will explore irinotecan, 5-FU, and leucovorin versus 5-FU and leucovorin as a postoperative chemotherapy regimen.

D. Follow-up. In the asymptomatic patient, follow-up after treatment includes history, physical examination, and CEA every 3 months for 2 years, then every 6 months for 3 years. Colonoscopy often is performed 1 year after surgery and then every 3 years if no polyps are found. There is no evidence that additional testing, including CT scans, is helpful and it should not be done routinely except to evaluate symptoms or a rising CEA level, which can indicate recurrent but sometimes resectable disease.

E. Complications of therapy or disease. The complications of chemotherapy are those attributable to the individual drugs. Myelosuppression, nausea, vomiting, and diarrhea are common and may require dose modification and symptomatic treatment. Radiation complications are similar and also include dysuria, tenesmus, and rectal discharge of blood or mucus. Phenazopyridine (Pyridium) is useful in treating dysuria, and loperamide (Imodium) or diphenoxylate (Lomotil) is recommended for diarrhea. If toxicity is substantial (grade 3 or 4) during radiotherapy, a treatment delay of at least 1 week is warranted. During chemotherapy with fluorouracil-based regimens, mild diarrhea (grade 1) may be treated symptomatically. Moderate diarrhea (grade 2 or 3) is an indication for dose reduction by 50%, and severe diarrhea (grade 3 or 4) is an indication for stopping chemotherapy for 1 week or longer. Dehydration is a real risk with grade 3 or 4 diarrhea, and IV hydration may be necessary. Tincture of opium or octreotide 150 μg t.i.d. may help to alleviate severe diarrhea.

Recent recommendations for management of irinotecan toxicity include evaluation for a GI syndrome, which can encompass diarrhea, nausea, vomiting, anorexia, abdominal cramping, dehydration, neutropenia, fever, and electrolyte abnormalities. There is also a vascular syndrome, which can include myocardial infarction, pulmonary embolus, or cerebral vascular accident. Patients receiving irinotecan should undergo weekly assessment, at least during the first cycle, looking for concurrent toxicities. In addition to treating the diarrhea with loperamide, tincture of opium, or octreotide, oral fluoroquinolone should be initiated in any patient experiencing neutropenia even in the absence of fever or diarrhea or in any patient experiencing fever and diarrhea even in the absence of neutropenia. Antibiotics should be initiated in any hospitalized patient with prolonged diarrhea regardless of granulocyte count and should be continued until resolution of diarrhea. Any patient who experiences significant treatment-related diarrhea should not receive irinotecan until diarrhea-free or at baseline bowel function for at least 24 h without the use of antidiarrheal agents or antibiotics. In addition, abdominal cramping should be considered equivalent to diarrhea.

Oral mucositis can often be prevented on subsequent courses without dose reduction by holding ice in the mouth for 20 min before, during, and after the IV bolus of fluorouracil. Nausea is usually not severe with fluorouracil regimens and usually responds to prochlorperazine or dexamethasone. Hematopoietic growth factors are seldom warranted for the mild neutropenia that is observed with bolus fluorouracil therapy.

V.   Cancer of the anal canal. These cancers, constituting only 1% to 3% of all cases of large-bowel cancer, were historically treated by abdominoperineal resection with about a 50% cure rate. They have been seen more commonly in women. However, in recent years, there is an increase of these cancers in men, particularly homosexuals. The human papillomavirus has been implicated in some patients, and anal warts are sometimes seen as well. Patients infected with the human immunodeficiency virus also have an increased incidence of anal cancer.

A.   Local disease. It has been found that combined-modality treatment with chemotherapy and irradiation is curative in 75% to 80% of patients and thus allows avoidance of abdominoperineal resection with retention of anal function. The following regimen is recommended:

1.   Radiotherapy 4,500 cGy in 25 fractions (5 weeks), *and concurrently*

2.   Fluorouracil 1,000 mg/m^2 by continuous IV infusion daily × 4 days (days 1 to 4 and 29 to 32), *and*

3.   Mitomycin 10 mg/m^2 IV on days 1 and 29.

A large U.S. Gastrointestinal Intergroup trial is comparing this standard regimen with preradiation chemotherapy with cisplatin and 5-FU followed by cisplatin, 5-FU, and radiation. A biopsy should be done 8 weeks after radiation therapy only for a suspicious residual area of abnormality. If negative, no further treatment is needed. If positive, consider an additional 900 cGy (five fractions) and a 4-day course of fluorouracil 1,000 mg/m^2 by continuous IV infusion on days 1 to 4 and cisplatin 100 mg/m^2 IV on day 2. If the biopsy is persistently positive, an abdominoperineal resection is appropriate.

B.   Metastatic disease. For metastatic disease, the following regimen may be considered:

1.   Mitomycin 10 mg/m^2 IV every 4 weeks × 2, then every 10 weeks, *and*

2.   Doxorubicin 30 mg/m^2 IV every 4 weeks × 2, then every 5 weeks, *and*

3.   Cisplatin 60 mg/m^2 IV, every 4 weeks × 2, then every 5 weeks.

SELECTED READINGS

Al-Sarraf M, Martz K, Herskovic A, et al. Progress report of combined chemoradiotherapy versus radiotherapy alone in patients with esophageal cancer: an Intergroup study. *J Clin Oncol* 1997;15: 277–284.

American Joint Committee on Cancer. *AJCC staging manual.* 6th ed. New York: Springer, 2002, 89–125.

Benson AB III, Desch CE, Flynn PJ, et al. 2000 update of American Society of Clinical Oncology colorectal cancer surveillance guidelines. *J Clin Oncol* 2000;18:3586–3588.

Blot WJ, Devesa SS, Kneller RW, et al. Rising incidence of adenocarcinoma of the esophagus and gastric cardia. *JAMA* 1991;265: 1287–1289.

Boku N, Ohtsu A, Shimada Y, et al. Phase II study of a combination of CDDP and CPT-11 in metastatic gastric cancer: CPT-11 Study Group for Gastric Cancer. *Proc Am Soc Clin Oncol* 1997;16: 264(abst).

Camma C, Giunta M, Fiorica F, et al. Preoperative radiotherapy for resectable rectal cancer: a meta-analysis. *JAMA* 2000;284: 1008–1015.

Clark P. Surgical resection with or without pre-operative chemotherapy in oesophageal cancer: an updated analysis of a randomised controlled trial conducted by the UK Medical Research. Council Upper GI Tract Cancer Group. *Proc Am Soc Clin Oncol* 2001; 20:126a(abst 502).

Conti JA, Kemeny NE, Saltz LB, et al. Irinotecan is an active agent in untreated patients with metastatic colorectal cancer. *J Clin Oncol* 1996;14:709–715.

Costa F, Ilson D, Forastiere A, et al. Phase II study of paclitaxel and cisplatin in patients with advanced adenocarcinoma and squamous cell carcinoma of the esophagus. *Proc Am Soc Clin Oncol* 1997;16:262(abst).

Cunningham D, Pyrhonen S, James RD, et al. Randomised trial of irinotecan plus supportive care versus supportive care alone after fluorouracil failure for patients with metastatic colorectal cancer. *Lancet* 1998;352:1413–1418.

Desch CE, Benson AB III, Smith TJ, et al. Recommended colorectal cancer surveillance guidelines by the American Society of Clinical Oncology. *J Clin Oncol* 1999;17:1312–1321.

Douillard JY, Cunningham D, Roth AD, et al. Irinotecan combined with fluorouracil compared with fluorouracil alone as first-line treatment for metastatic colorectal cancer: a multicentre randomised trial. *Lancet* 2000;355:1041–1047.

Dunst J, Reese T, Frings S. Phase I study of capecitabine combined with standard radiotherapy in patients with rectal cancer. *Proc Am Soc Clin Oncol* 2000;19:256a(abst 995).

Fisher B, Wolmark N, Rockette H, et al. Postoperative adjuvant chemotherapy or radiation therapy for rectal cancer: results from NSABP protocol R-01. *JNCI* 1988;80:21–29.

Flam MS, John MJ, Mowry PA, et al. Definitive combined modality therapy of carcinoma of the anus: a report of 30 cases including results of salvage therapy in patients with residual disease. *Dis Colon Rectum* 1987;30:495–502.

Gastrointestinal Tumor Study Group. Prolongation of disease-free interval in surgically treated rectal cancer. *N Engl J Med* 1985;312: 1465–1472.

Grem JL, Danenberg KD, Behan K, et al. Thymidine kinase, thymidylate synthase, and dihydropyrimidine dehydrogenase profiles of cell lines of the National Cancer Institute's anticancer drug screen. *Clin Cancer Res* 2001;7:999–1099.

Haller DG, Catalano PJ, Macdonald JS, et al. Fluorouracil (FU), leucovorin (LV) and levamisole (LEV) adjuvant therapy for colon cancer: four-year results of INT-0089. *Proc Am Soc Clin Oncol* 1997; 16:265(abst).

Hoff PM, Ansari R, Batist G, et al. Comparison of oral capecitabine versus IV fluorouracil plus leucovorin as first-line treatment in 605 patients with metastatic colorectal cancer: results of a randomized phase III study. *J Clin Oncol* 2001;19:2282–2292.

International Multicentre Pooled Analysis of Colon Cancer Trials (IMPACT) Investigators. Efficacy of adjuvant fluorouracil and folinic acid in colon cancer. *Lancet* 1995;345:939–944.

Kapiteijn E, Marijnen AM, Nagtegaal ID, et al. Preoperative radiotherapy combined with total mesorectal excision for resectable rectal cancer. *N Engl J Med* 2001;345:638–646.

Kelsen DP. Postoperative adjuvant chemoradiation therapy for patients with resected gastric cancer: Intergroup 116. *J Clin Oncol* 2000;18:32S–34S.

Kelsen D, Atiq OT, Saltz L, et al. FAMTX versus etoposide, doxorubicin and cisplatin: a random assignment trial in gastric cancer. *J Clin Oncol* 1992;10:541–548.

Kelsen DP, Ginsberg R, Pajak TF, et al. Chemotherapy followed by surgery compared with surgery alone for localized esophageal cancer. *N Engl J Med* 1998;339:1979–1984.

Kemeny MM, Adak S, Gray B, et al. Combined modality treatment for resectable metastatic colorectal carcinoma to the liver: surgical resection of hepatic metastases in combination with continuous infusion of chemotherapy: an Intergroup study. *J Clin Oncol* 2002; 20:1499–1505.

Kemeny N, Huang Y, Cohen AM, et al. Hepatic arterial infusion of chemotherapy after resection of hepatic metastases from colorectal cancer. *N Engl J Med* 1999;341:2039–2048.

Leichman L, Nigro N, Vaitkevicius VK, et al. Cancer of the anal canal: model for preoperative adjuvant combined modality therapy. *Am J Med* 1985;78:211–215.

MacDonald JS, Smalley SR, Benedetti J, et al. Chemoradiotherapy after surgery compared with surgery alone for adenocarcinoma of the stomach or gastroesophageal junction. *N Engl J Med* 2001; 345:725–730.

Moertel CG, Hanley JA. Combination chemotherapy trials for metastatic carcinoid tumor and the malignant carcinoid syndrome. *Cancer Clin Trials* 1979;2:327–334.

Neugut AI, Marvin MR, Rella VA, Chabot JA. An overview of adenocarcinoma of the small intestine. *Oncology* 1997;11:529–536.

O'Connell MJ, Laurie JA, Kahn M, et al. Prospectively randomized trial of postoperative adjuvant chemotherapy in patients with high-risk colon cancer. *J Clin Oncol* 1998;16:295–300.

O'Connell MJ, Martenson JA, Wieand HS, et al. Improving adjuvant therapy for rectal cancer by combining protracted-infusion fluorouracil with radiation therapy after curative surgery. *N Engl J Med* 1994;331:502–507.

O'Connell MJ, Martenson JA, Wieand HS, et al. Improving adjuvant therapy for rectal cancer by combining protracted-infusion fluorouracil with radiation therapy after curative surgery. *N Engl J Med* 1994;331:502–507.

O'Dwyer PJ, Manola J, Valone FH, et al. Fluorouracil modulation in colorectal cancer: lack of improvement with *N*-phosphonoacetyl-L-aspartic acid or oral leucovorin or interferon, but enhanced therapeutic index with weekly 24-hour infusion schedule—an Eastern Cooperative Oncology Group/Cancer and Leukemia Group B study. *J Clin Oncol* 2001;19:2413–2421.

Poon MA, O'Connell MJ, Moertel CG, et al. Biochemical modulation of fluorouracil: evidence of significant improvement of survival and quality of life in patients with advanced colorectal carcinoma. *J Clin Oncol* 1989;7:1407–1418.

Reed ML, Vaitkevicius VK, Al-Sarraf M, et al. The practicality of chronic hepatic artery infusion therapy of primary and metastatic hepatic malignancies: ten-year results of 124 patients in a prospective protocol. *Cancer* 1981;47:402–409.

Roder JD, Bottcher K, Busch R, et al. Classification of regional lymph nodes metastasis from gastric carcinoma. *Cancer* 1998;82:621–631.

Rothenberg ML, Meropol NJ, Poplin EA, et al. Mortality associated with irinotecan plus bolus fluorouracil/leucovorin: summary findings of an independent panel. *J Clin Oncol* 2001;19:3801–3807.

Rougier P, Bugat R, Douilllard JY, et al. Phase II study of irinotecan in the treatment of advanced colorectal cancer in chemotherapy-naive patients and patients pretreated with fluorouracil-based chemotherapy. *J Clin Oncol* 1997;15:251–260.

Saltz LB, Cox JV, Blanke C, et al. Irinotecan plus fluorouracil and leucovorin for metastatic colorectal cancer. *N Engl J Med* 2000;343:905–914.

Sargent DJ, Goldberg RM, Jacobson SD, et al. A pooled analysis of adjuvant chemotherapy for resected colon cancer in elderly patients. *N Engl J Med* 2001;345:1091–1097.

Schrag D, Gelfand SE, Bach PB, et al. Who gets adjuvant treatment for stage II and III rectal cancer? Insight from surveillance, epidemiology, and end results—Medicare. *J Clin Oncol* 2001;19:3712–3718.

Shepard KV, Levin B, Karl RC, et al. Therapy for metastatic colorectal cancer with hepatic artery infusion chemotherapy using a subcutaneous implanted pump. *J Clin Oncol* 1985;3:161–169.

Smith TJ, Ryan LM, Douglass HO, et al. Combined chemoradiotherapy vs. radiotherapy alone for early stage squamous cell carcinoma of the esophagus: a study of the Eastern Cooperative Oncology Group. *Int J Radiat Oncol Biol Phys* 1998;42:269–276.

Tepper JE, O'Connell MJ, Niedzwiecki D, et al. Impact of number of nodes retrieved on outcome in patients with rectal cancer. *J Clin Oncol* 2001;19:157–163.

Tepper JE, O'Connell MJ, Petroni GR, et al. Adjuvant postoperative fluorouracil-modulated chemotherapy combined with pelvic radiation therapy for rectal cancer: initial results of Intergroup 0114. *J Clin Oncol* 1997;15:2030–2039.

Urba S, Orringer M, Turrisi A, et al. A randomized trial comparing surgery to preoperative concomitant chemoradiation plus surgery in patients with resectable esophageal cancer: updated analysis. *Proc Am Soc Clin Oncol* 1997;16:277(abst).

Urba SG, Orringer MB, Turrisi A, et al. Randomized trial of preoperative chemoradiation versus surgery alone in patients with locoregional esophageal carcinoma. *J Clin Oncol* 2001;19:305–313.

Van Cutsem E, Twelves C, Cassidy J, et al. Oral capecitabine compared with IV fluorouracil plus leucovorin in patients with metastatic colorectal cancer: results of a large phase III study. *J Clin Oncol* 2001;19:4097–4106.

Vaughn DJ, Haller DG. Adjuvant therapy for colorectal cancer: past accomplishments, future directions. *Cancer Invest* 1997;15:435–447.

Wadler S, Benson AB III, Engelking C, et al. Recommended guidelines for the treatment of chemotherapy-induced diarrhea. *J Clin Oncol* 1998;16:3169–3178.

Walsh TN, Noonan N, Hollywood D, et al. A comparison of multimodal therapy and surgery for esophageal adeno-carcinoma. *N Engl J Med* 1996;335:462–467.

Watanabe T, Tsung-Teh W, Catalano PJ, et al. Molecular predictors of survival after adjuvant chemotherapy for colon cancer. *N Engl J Med* 2001;344:1196–1206.

Wilke H, Preusser P, Fink U, et al. High dose folinic acid/etoposide/ 5-fluorouracil in advanced gastric cancer—a phase II study in elderly patients or patients with cardiac risk. *Invest New Drugs* 1990; 8:65–70.

Wolmark N, Wieand HS, Hyams DM, et al. Randomized trial of post-operative adjuvant chemotherapy with or without radiotherapy for carcinoma of the rectum: National Surgical Adjuvant Breast and Bowel Project protocol R-02. *JNCI* 2000;92:388–396.

9

Carcinomas of the Pancreas, Liver, Gallbladder, and Bile Ducts

Daniel Y. Danso

Carcinomas of the pancreas, liver, and biliary passages account for about 2% of all cases of cancer and for 5% of all cancer-related deaths in the United States. Virtually all patients with these cancers die from this disease. However, advances in molecular biology are expected to lead to earlier diagnosis and improved treatment.

I. Adenocarcinoma of the pancreas

A. Epidemiology and etiology. Pancreatic cancer occurred with increasing incidence during the last several decades and currently is the fifth leading cause of cancer-related deaths in the United States. In the year 2002, approximately 29,200 cases diagnosed, and 28,900 deaths were ascribed to this cancer. Risk factors for pancreatic cancer include age, male sex, race (Polynesians, blacks), and tobacco exposure. It is rare before 30 years of age, and the incidence rises throughout life, with peak occurrence during the seventh decade. Smokers have 1.6 to 3.9 times the risk of developing pancreatic cancer compared with nonsmokers. Pancreatitis is commonly associated with carcinoma of the pancreas in pathologic specimens. Whether patients with chronic pancreatitis are at greater risk for developing pancreatic cancer is uncertain. Patients with familial pancreatitis appear to have a greater risk. Diabetes mellitus is often discovered just before the diagnosis of pancreatic cancer, but patients with diabetes mellitus do not have a greater risk of pancreatic cancer. Hereditary pancreatic cancer has been observed in rare families with an autosomal site-specific pattern, in families with *BRCA2* mutations, and in hereditary nonpolyposis colorectal cancer families. Likewise, families with *p16* germline mutations may be at higher risk of developing pancreatic cancer. Greater than 80% of resected pancreatic cancers harbor either activating point mutations in *K-ras* or inactivating mutations of the tumor suppressor genes *p16, p53,* and *DPC4.*

B. Presenting signs and symptoms. Pain is the most common presenting symptom. It usually relates to localized invasion of peripancreatic structures. It occurs in three-fourths of patients with carcinoma of the head of the pancreas and in virtually all patients with carcinoma of the body or tail. Usually, the pain is a dull ache in the epigastrium that radiates to the right upper quadrant when the tumor is in the head of the pancreas or to the left upper quadrant when the tumor is in the body or tail. It may be an atypical sharp or intermittent epigastric pain, or it may be located in the lumbar region of the back. As many as one-fifth of patients present with nonspecific symptoms including weight loss, anorexia, nausea, vomiting, and constipation. The nonspecific, vague nature of these complaints may delay diagnosis for several months. Seventy percent of patients with carcinoma of the head of the pancreas have jaundice, whereas fewer than 15% of patients with carcinoma of the pancreatic body have jaundice. Physical findings are generally associated with advanced carcinomas and include weight loss, hepatomegaly, and abdominal mass. A palpable gallbladder in the absence of cholecystitis or cholangitis suggests malignant obstruction of the common bile duct (Courvoisier's sign), and it is present in about 25% of all pancreatic cancer patients. Other physical findings, which usually are indicative of distant metastases, include Trousseau's syndrome (migratory superficial phlebitis), ascites, Virchow's node (left supraclavicular lymph node), a periumbilical mass (Sister Mary Joseph's node), or a palpable pelvic shelf on rectal examination (Blumer's shelf).

C.   Diagnostic evaluation. Ultrasonography and computed tomography (CT) demonstrate masses in the pancreas or dilation of the pancreatic duct or the common bile duct. Sensitivity and specificity of CT are about 90%, whereas sensitivity and specificity of ultrasonography are somewhat less. Both tests detect relatively large mass lesions of the pancreas and usually miss 1- to 2-cm carcinomas. Endoscopic retrograde cholangiopancreatography demonstrates subtle ductal abnormalities; sensitivity and specificity are in excess of 90%. Endoscopy-directed biopsies of pancreatic ducts have diagnosed tumors smaller than 1 to 2 cm in diameter. Percutaneous transhepatic cholangiography may be performed if endoscopic retrograde cholangiopancreatography is unsuccessful and yields similar information. Percutaneous fine-needle aspiration of suspicious abnormalities identified on CT scan can confirm the diagnosis of pancreatic cancer, with 80% to 90% sensitivity and 100% specificity. A common histologic hallmark of pancreatic adenocarcinoma is an associated desmoplastic reaction that, in a given tumor mass, can vastly overestimate the malignant cell mass. Furthermore, pancreatic cancer may be associated with varying degrees of acute or chronic pancreatitis or cyst formation, which may make it difficult to make a diagnosis with needle aspiration and may lead to false-negative results.

D.   Laboratory tests. CA 19-9 is a cell surface glycoprotein associated with pancreatic cancer. Rising serum levels may be a useful early indicator of recurrent or progressive disease.

E.   Staging and preoperative evaluation

1.   Staging. The primary tumor, regional lymph nodes, and potential sites of metastatic disease must be carefully assessed (Table 9.1). CT of the abdomen assesses the primary site, regional lymph nodes, and liver. Chest radiographs screen for metastatic disease in the chest. Routine laboratory studies and physical examination screen for other sites of involvement.

2.   Preoperative evaluation. Preoperative evaluation should be performed stepwise from least invasive to most invasive as indicated by the clinical situation. Preoperative evaluation can be stopped when metastatic disease or defi-

Table 9.1. TNM staging for pancreatic cancer

Stage	Definition
I	T1 (tumor ≤ 2 cm), T2 (tumor >2 cm, confined to pancreas), N0, M0
IIA	T3 (tumor extends to duodenum, bile duct, or peripancreatic tissue), N0, M0
IIB	T1–3, N1, M0
III	T4 (tumor extends to stomach, spleen, colon, or adjacent large vessels), N0–1, M0
IV	T1–4, N0–1, M1

N1, any nodal metastases; M1, any distant metastases.
From American Joint Committee on Cancer. *AJCC staging manual.* 6th ed. New York: Springer, 2002.

nite evidence for unresectable locoregional spread is identified. All patients should undergo abdominal CT scanning. If no hepatic metastasis or major blood vessel involvement is identified, then arteriography can be performed to assess major blood vessel involvement and tumor blood supply. More recently, spiral CT has emerged as a preferred technique for increasing the accuracy of detecting pancreatic carcinoma in general and vessel encasement in particular. It permits rapid data acquisition and computer-generated three-dimensional images of the mesenteric arterial and venous tributaries in any plane. It is quicker and less expensive and uses less contrast medium than angiography. If no major blood vessel involvement is identified, then laparoscopy can be used to identify small metastases in the liver or peritoneum. Laparoscopy identifies metastatic disease in 40% of patients with pancreatic cancer who have had negative findings on CT and arteriogram. In one series, nearly 80% of cancers were resectable when all tests, including laparoscopy, were negative. After negative CT and arteriography alone, only 15% to 20% of pancreas cancers were resectable at laparotomy. The use of positron emission tomography with 2-[^{18}F]fluoro-2-deoxy-D-glucose in the evaluation of patients with pancreatic cancer is expanding. This imaging modality is useful in detecting small primaries and metastatic disease and in differentiating between cancer and pancreatitis.

F. Primary therapy

1. Surgery. Three-fourths of patients with pancreatic cancer are operative candidates, but only 15% to 20% have resectable tumors. Patients without evident metastatic cancer or major blood vessel involvement, whose performance status permits operative intervention, are candidates for curative surgery. Five to 10% of the patients resected for cure survive 5 years. Surgical bypass procedures may also palliate obstructive jaundice and gastric outlet obstruction. Endoscopic stent placement may palliate obstructive jaundice.

2. Radiation therapy. External-beam radiation therapy can palliate unresectable carcinomas. It may also be used as a surgical adjuvant in combination with chemotherapy. Great care and expertise must be exercised to plan the radiation fields. These fields must encompass known disease without excessive involvement of adjacent normal tissue. Surgical clips placed at laparotomy or laparoscopy can guide treatment. Intraoperative external-beam radiotherapy has been successful in placing a high dose on the local tumor while protecting the surrounding normal tissues but has not increased the cure rate of pancreas cancer.

3. Combined-modality therapy
  a. Resected carcinomas. On the basis of a randomized study by the Gastrointestinal Tumor Study Group (GITSG), postoperative combined-modality therapy is recommended for patients with resected carcinoma of the pancreas. The GITSG demonstrated that postoperative adjuvant radiotherapy (split course in their study) plus fluorouracil is better than adjuvant radiotherapy alone. On the basis of the demonstrated benefit of prolonged infusion of fluorouracil or fluorouracil modulated by leucovorin in colon and rectal carcinomas, both of these approaches have been safely combined with radiotherapy (40 to 50 Gy in standard fractionation) in pancreatic cancer. The recommended treatments have the advantage of avoiding split-course radiotherapy. Recommended regimens are as follows:

  (1) Fluorouracil 225 mg/m^2 by continuous IV infusion throughout radiation therapy or 300 mg/m^2 by continuous IV infusion 5 days/week during radiation therapy, *or*
  (2) Fluorouracil 425 mg/m^2 by IV push 1 h after leucovorin, 20 mg/m^2 by IV push daily for 4 days during the first week of radiation therapy and for 3 days during the fifth week of radiation therapy, *or*
  (3) Fluorouracil 500 mg/m^2 by IV push midway during a 2-h infusion of leucovorin, 500 mg/m^2 weekly for the first 6 weeks of radiation therapy.

  At the completion of combined-modality therapy, chemotherapy should be continued for 6 months using weekly IV push fluorouracil or a modulated fluorouracil regimen. Two-year and 5-year survival rates similar to the 43% and 25% rates seen in the combined-modality groups in the GITSG trials may be anticipated, although this has not yet been adequately tested.

  b. Localized unresectable carcinoma. A series of randomized trials conducted by the GITSG demonstrated superior survival of patients with localized but unresectable pancreatic cancer when treated with combined-modality therapy compared with patients treated with radiation therapy or chemotherapy alone. These clinical trials also used split-course radiation therapy. As discussed in Section I.F.3.a, current clinical trials do not support a specific combined-modality treatment program. However, 60 Gy of radiation should be delivered in a single course of external-beam radiation to gross tumor and 40 to 50 Gy to microscopic cancer. Chemotherapy may be given by any of the regimens noted in Section I.F.3.a. After completion of combined-modality therapy, chemotherapy should be continued for 6 months using bolus fluorouracil or a modulated fluorouracil regimen. More recently, gemcitabine has been used after the completion of the combined-modality phase. In the GITSG trials, the median survival time was 10 months in the combined-modality group compared with 5 months in the radiotherapy-alone group. Specialized modes of administration of the radiation therapy may be considered, including intraoperative radiotherapy to boost the dose to the gross tumor or conformational radiation therapy to minimize the dose to surrounding tissues while delivering maximum dose to the tumor. Quality-of-life studies have not been reported.

G. Chemotherapy of metastatic disease. Patients with pancreatic cancer are often poor candidates for chemotherapy because of severe weight loss, poor performance status, severe pain, lack of measurable or evaluable disease, and presence of jaundice or hepatic involvement, which may interfere with clearance of therapeutic agents. However, two recent randomized clinical trials demonstrated survival and quality-of-life benefits to chemotherapy in selected patients with advanced pancreatic cancer.

    1. Single agents. A number of single agents have demonstrated activity (Table 9.2), although no agent has demonstrated consistent complete and partial response rates of 20% or greater using CT to measure response. Gemcitabine has been accepted as first-line therapy for metastatic pancreatic cancer in patients with adequate performance status, based on two Phase II trials and one Phase III trial. These trials

Table 9.2.   Single-agent chemotherapy in pancreatic cancer

Drug	No. of patients	Complete plus partial response rate range (%)	Clinical benefit[a] range (%)
Gemcitabine	158	5.4–11	17.2–27
Fluorouracil	237	0–12.5[b]	5–50
Mitomycin	44	27[c]	NA
Streptozocin	27	11[c]	NA
Doxorubicin	28	8[c]	NA
Ifosfamide	113	6–22	NA
Irinotecan (CPT-11)	95	9–10	NA
Topotecan	62	0–10	NA
Docetaxol	30	20	NA

NA, not available.

[a] Sustained (=4-wk) improvement of one of the following parameters without worsening of any of the others: performance status, composite pain measurement (average pain intensity and narcotic analgesic use), or weight.

[b] Studies reported with response evaluation by computed tomography.

[c] Studies reported before routine use of computed tomography.

demonstrated modest antitumor activity (complete and partial response rates 5.4% to 11%), whereas "clinical benefit" was observed in about one-quarter of patients. Clinical benefit was defined as sustained (more than 4 weeks) improvement of one of the following parameters without worsening of any of the others: performance status, composite pain measurement (average pain intensity and narcotic analgesic use), and weight. Bolus fluorouracil had a 0% objective response rate and 5% clinical benefit rate in the randomized trial with gemcitabine. Although response rates with modulated fluorouracil regimens have been poor, responses in CT-monitored studies are better with modulated fluorouracil than with bolus fluorouracil.

   2.   Combination chemotherapy. Combination chemotherapy has been investigated (Table 9.3). The most commonly used regimens are fluorouracil + doxorubicin + mitomycin (FAM) and streptozocin + mitomycin + fluorouracil (SMF), with response rates reported between 13% and 43%. These and other combination regimens have not shown an advantage over single-agent therapy. A recent report of a Phase II study combined docetaxel and gemcitabine (GT) in unresectable pancreatic cancer with a reported response rate of 46%. Another study combined gemcitabine, docetaxel, and capecitabine (GTX) with a reported 50% partial response rate among 20 patients with liver metastases and complete response among 5 of 8 patients with no liver metastases but inoperable disease. Patients received gemcitabine 750 to 1,000 mg/m^2 IV and docetaxel (Taxotere) 90 mg/m^2 IV, each drug given every 3 weeks with the GT regimen, and a docetaxel (Taxotere) dose of 30 mg/m^2 and capecitabine (Xeloda) at 1,500 mg/m^2/day in two oral doses for days 1 to 14 for the GTX regimen.

   3.   Current recommendations. Single-agent therapy with gemcitabine 1,000 mg/m^2 IV weekly for 7 weeks followed by 1-week rest, then 4-week cycles of three weekly doses followed by 1-week rest, is recommended for patients with metastatic pancreatic cancer and with an Eastern Cooperative Oncology Group performance status of 0 to 2, who are not eligible for clinical trials. Toxicity is generally modest with

Table 9.3.   Combination chemotherapy for carcinoma of exocrine pancreas

Regimen	Dosages
SMF	Streptozocin 1 g/m^2 IV on d 1, 8, 29, and 36 Mitomycin 10 mg/m^2 IV on d 1 Fluorouracil 600 mg/m^2 IV on d 1, 8, 29, and 36 Repeat cycle every 8 wk
FAM	Fluorouracil 600 mg/m^2 IV on d 1, 8, 29, and 36 Doxorubicin (Adriamycin) 30 mg/m^2 IV on d 1 and 29 Mitomycin 10 mg/m^2 IV on d 1 Repeat cycle every 8 wk

moderate myelosuppression, with neutropenia and anemia, mild to moderate nausea, an influenza-like syndrome that includes low-grade fever and malaise, minimal alopecia, and occasional rash. If the tumor does not respond or progresses after initial response to gemcitabine, treatment with fluorouracil in a modulated or weekly bolus regimen or mitomycin 20 mg/m^2 IV on day 1 every 4 to 6 weeks may be considered. Because of the limited effectiveness of current therapy, participation in clinical trials should be encouraged, especially with Phase II trials of new agents or combinations. Novel therapies currently under development for advanced pancreatic cancer are farnesyl transferase inhibition, antisense oligonucleotides against the *ras* gene (ISIS 5132, an antisense oligonucleotide against c-raf kinase), and monoterpene inhibition of isoprenylation of guanosine triphosphate–binding proteins (perillyl alcohol in Phase II trials).

II. Malignant islet cell carcinomas

A. Epidemiology and natural history. Islet cell neoplasms occur in about 1 in 100,000 people per year. These tumors cover a spectrum of neoplasms, many, but not all, of which originate from the pancreatic islets of Langerhans. Eighty percent of these tumors secrete one or more hormones excessively: most commonly insulin or gastrin, less commonly glucagon, serotonin, or adrenocorticotropic hormone, and rarely vasoactive intestinal peptides (VIPs), growth hormone–releasing hormone, or somatostatin. Twenty percent are nonfunctional. Islet cell tumors may occur with the multiple endocrine neoplasia type I (MEN-I) syndrome. In families with this autosomal dominant syndrome, 80% of affected members develop islet cell tumors, most commonly gastrinoma (54%), insulinoma (21%), glucagonoma (3%), or VIPoma (1%). The gene for MEN-I has been localized to the long arm of chromosome 11 and was recently identified and named *MENIN*. Other endocrine manifestations of MEN-I include parathyroid hyperplasia, pituitary adenomas (often a prolactinoma), and occasionally adrenal or thyroid adenomas. About one-fourth of gastrinomas are associated with MEN-I. Eighty to 90% of gastrinomas occur in the head of the pancreas. Insulinomas are equally common in the head, body, and tail. Gastrinomas tend to be multiple small tumors, whereas insulinomas tend to be single tumors and glucagonomas and VIPomas single large tumors. The median age of patients is in the sixth decade. There are no sex or race associations.

Islet cell tumors generally present with symptoms caused by hormone hypersecretion, most commonly fasting hypoglycemia or the Zollinger–Ellison syndrome followed by others. VIPomas are associated with episodic severe secretory diarrhea with hypokalemia, hypochlorhydria, and metabolic acidosis. Classically, glucagonomas are associated with necrolytic migratory erythema, mild diabetes, severe muscle wasting, and marked hyperaminoaciduria.

Sixty percent of gastrinomas are malignant. Histologic appearance and tumor size do not predict malignancy; only the presence of metastatic disease confirms malignancy. Ninety percent of malignant gastrinomas have liver metastases. Other sites of spread include abdominal nodes, peritoneum, bone, and lung. Median survival from time of diagnosis of metastatic disease is about 2.5 years. Only 10% of insulinomas are malignant. They are usually larger than 2.5 cm, whereas benign insulinomas are generally smaller than 2.5 cm. Most glucagonomas and VIPomas are malignant (60% to 80%).

B.   Treatment of advanced disease

1.   Endocrine syndromes. The first goal of treatment must be to control endocrine syndromes.

   a.   Gastric acid suppression. The H^+, K^+-adenosine triphosphatase inhibitors omeprazole and lansoprazole successfully control gastric acid secretion in patients with gastrinoma. Optimal doses must be individualized and periodically re-evaluated. Gastric acid secretion in the hour preceding the next dose of omeprazole or lansoprazole should be less than 10 mEq in patients who have had no previous gastric surgery and less than 5 mEq in those who have had an acid-reducing procedure. The starting dose is 60 mg/day with both agents. Doses greater than 80 mg/day should be divided. Similar, newer agents in the same class of proton pump inhibitors are equally as efficacious.

   b.   Insulin suppression. Diazoxide, an insulin release inhibitor, when given at 3 to 8 mg/kg/day PO divided in three doses (e.g., 50 to 150 mg PO t.i.d.), is the therapy of choice for hypoglycemia associated with insulinoma when dietary measures fail. A diuretic should be given with diazoxide to prevent water retention.

   c.   Octreotide acetate (Sandostatin). Octreotide acetate is a somatostatin analog that inhibits gut hormone secretion. It is generally useful for carcinoid and VIPoma syndromes and is possibly useful for controlling symptoms in patients with glucagonomas, gonadotrophic hormone–releasing hormone tumors, and gastrinomas. In patients with unresectable insulinoma, it can reduce insulin secretion by 50% and return blood glucose levels to normal. However, it must be initiated cautiously in patients in the hospital because profound hypoglycemia may occur. The usual starting dose of octreotide is 50 μg SC b.i.d.; thereafter, the dose and frequency of injections can be increased to 100 μg t.i.d. More recently, a long-acting preparation (Octreotide LAR) has become available. It is designed to provide the convenience of once-a-month or twice-a-month injections once a stable dose of the shorter-acting preparation is established.

2.   Chemotherapy for advanced islet cell tumors. Streptozocin is the most active single agent, with a 50% response rate. It is a nonmyelosuppressive nitrosourea with diabetogenic effects in animals. Doxorubicin is also an active agent. The combination of streptozocin and doxorubicin was demonstrated to have a superior response rate (69%), time to tumor progression (20 months), and survival time (2.2 years) than the combination of streptozocin and fluorouracil or single-agent chlorozotocin in a North Central Cancer Treatment Group study. This combination is recommended as first-line chemotherapy.

   **a.   **Streptozocin 500 mg/m^2 IV on days 1 to 5 and doxorubicin 50 mg/m^2 IV, on days 1 and 22. Repeat every 6 weeks.

Renal impairment occurs in about 30% of patients receiving a streptozocin-based regimen; about one-third of those with renal insufficiency have creatinine levels higher than 2 mg/dL. Nausea and vomiting occur in about 60% of patients. Leukopenia occurs in about 75%, but only 10% have a white blood cell count of less than 1,000/µL. Stomatitis is uncommon. Liver function test abnormalities may also occur. Deaths caused by treatment are rare.

b. α-Interferon may diminish excess hormone secretion and induce shrinkage of tumors; some trials have reported 50% response rates. This agent can be used after chemotherapy failure.

III. Ampullary carcinomas. In up to 80% of people, the common bile duct and main pancreatic duct empty into a common channel, the ampulla of Vater. Periampullary carcinomas can be classified according to their site of origin. Type I tumors originate in the ampulla of Vater or the duodenal portion of the common bile duct. Type II carcinomas are duodenal tumors involving the ampulla of Vater. Type III are mixed ampullary–periampullary carcinomas, and type IV are pancreatic head carcinomas involving the ampulla. Type IV tumors carry a much worse prognosis and should be distinguished from the ampullary or periampullary carcinomas. Type I to III periampullary and ampullary carcinomas generally can be extirpated surgically. Large tumors require a Whipple resection, whereas local excision may be curative for small tumors. The overall 5-year survival rate is 40% to 50% for patients with type I to III carcinomas. The roles of irradiation and chemotherapy are uncertain. Tumors larger than 2 cm in diameter should be treated as adenocarcinoma of the pancreas.

IV. Carcinoma of the bile ducts (cholangiocarcinoma)

A. Epidemiology and natural history. The incidence of primary biliary tree carcinoma is about 2 per 100,000 population. Men are affected more commonly than women. Tumors occur most often in late-middle-aged and elderly patients. They are associated with cholelithiasis, ulcerative colitis, obesity, liver flukes, exposure to thorium oxide (Thorotrast), primary sclerosing cholangitis, and congenital anomalies of the pancreaticobiliary tree. Patients present with obstructive jaundice, except for the occasional patient with a carcinoma identified at laparotomy for cholelithiasis. About half of bile duct tumors are located proximally. Ten percent have multicentric involvement of the bile ducts. Local invasion is common. Liver involvement occurs in nearly half of these patients. Surgical cure is uncommon. Bypass procedures or intubation of the biliary tree may offer palliation to patients whose tumors cannot be resected. Radiation therapy may relieve proximal obstruction without intubation or a bypass procedure. Combined-modality therapy with radiation and fluorouracil should be considered in patients with an unresectable but localized cancer.

B. Chemotherapy for advanced disease. Few reports are available for this unusual tumor, but its response rate to fluorouracil, alone or in combination with streptozocin, is about 10%. Outside the context of a clinical trial, one of the following regimens is recommended:

1. Fluorouracil 500 mg/m^2 IV push on days 1 to 5 every 4 weeks or 500 mg/m^2 IV weekly, *or*

2.   Fluorouracil 400 mg/m^2 IV on days 1 to 5 and strepto-zocin 500 mg/m^2 IV on days 1 to 5. Repeat every 6 weeks.
3.   More recently, a combination of gemcitabine and fluorouracil has been used in young individuals with good performance status. In a Phase II North Central Cancer Treatment Group trial, gemcitabine 1,000 mg/m^2, fluorouracil 600 mg/m^2, leucovorin 20 mg/m^2 IV days 1, 8, and 15 every 4 weeks were used.

V.   Carcinoma of the gallbladder
A.   Epidemiology and natural history. Carcinomas of the gallbladder are seen predominantly in late-middle-aged and elderly women, with the highest incidence in Native Americans and the populations of Central and Eastern Europe and Israel. The areas of high frequency also report a high incidence of cholelithiasis. Patients with "porcelain" or calcified gallbladders identified on radiographs have a 12% to 62% risk of cancer. Carcinoma of the gallbladder most commonly presents with pain, nausea and vomiting, and weight loss. Jaundice occurs in only one-third of patients. Anorexia, abdominal distention, pruritus, and melena occur in some patients. One percent of patients undergoing cholecystectomy are found to have carcinoma of the gallbladder. Overall survival is poor; less than 5% of patients who undergo resection survive 5 years. When the tumor is histologically confined to the mucosa or submucosa, survival rates of 64% at 5 years and 44% at 10 years have been reported. Gallbladder carcinomas may invade locally into the bile ducts, liver, pancreas, stomach, or duodenum. They also may spread to regional lymph nodes and distantly to liver.
B.   Chemotherapy for advanced disease. Few reports are available for review. Seven (18%) of 40 patients responded to fluorouracil. Seven (28%) of 25 patients responded to mitomycin. Four (31%) of 14 patients treated with fluorouracil + doxorubicin + mitomycin responded. Choices of therapy are as follows:
1.   Fluorouracil 500 mg/m^2 IV on days 1 to 5 every 4 weeks or 500 to 600 mg/m^2 IV weekly, *or*
2.   FAM, a three-drug combination of fluorouracil 600 mg/m^2 IV on days 1, 8, 29, and 36 plus doxorubicin (Adriamycin) 30 mg/m^2 IV on days 1 and 29 plus mitomycin 10 mg/m^2 IV on day 1. Repeat every 8 weeks.
   Although there may be a slightly improved response rate with FAM, the toxicity is significant, and no survival or quality-of-life benefit has been demonstrated.
3.   Gemcitabine shows promise as a new agent in the treatment of biliary cancers. In a recent North Central Cancer Treatment Group trial, gemcitabine has been combined with fluorouracil and leucovorin:

Gemcitabine 1,000 mg/m^2 IV over 30 min
Leucovorin 25 mg/m^2 IV push, *and*
Fluorouracil 600 mg/m^2 IV push following the leucovorin
are each given weekly × 3, followed by a 1-week rest.

VI.   Primary carcinoma of the liver
A.   Epidemiology. Primary carcinoma of the liver is rare in the United States. There are fewer than 10,000 new patients

annually, accounting for less than 2% of all malignancies. However, it is the leading cause of cancer death in parts of Africa and Asia. Ninety percent of primary cancers of the liver are hepatocellular carcinomas or hepatoma; the remaining cancers include cholangiocarcinomas (about 7%), hepatoblastomas, angiosarcomas, and other sarcomas. Histologic subsets of hepatocellular carcinoma have been recognized. Fibrolamellar carcinomas occur in young patients and are more likely to be resectable and cured. Hepatocellular carcinomas are more common in men than women. The peak occurrence is during the sixth decade, with the highest incidence during the ninth decade.

There appear to be three major factors associated with hepatocellular carcinoma: viral hepatitis B and C, alcohol abuse, and aflatoxin exposure. Seventy-five percent of patients with hepatocellular carcinoma have concomitant cirrhosis, and 4% to 20% of patients with cirrhosis have hepatocellular carcinoma at autopsy, depending on the population studied. Among the patients with hepatocellular carcinoma, 15% to 80% have hepatitis B surface antigenemia. In China, the incidence of hepatocellular carcinoma parallels the incidence of hepatitis B infection. The introduction of an effective hepatitis B vaccine may reduce the risk of hepatocellular carcinoma in these areas. In Africa, the increased risk appears to be related to exposure to aflatoxin, which is produced by the fungi *Aspergillus flavus* and *A. parasiticus* during improper food storage. Three to 27% of patients with long-standing hemochromatosis develop hepatocellular carcinoma. Anabolic steroids have also been associated with hepatocellular carcinoma. Tumors induced by anabolic steroids may retain hormone dependence and regress after withdrawal of the steroid.

B. Presentation. Patients with primary carcinoma of the liver commonly complain of right upper quadrant pain, abdominal distention, or weight loss. The pain is usually dull or aching but may be acute and radiate to the right shoulder. Fatigue, loss of appetite, and unexplained fever may occur. Patients with underlying cirrhosis may present with hepatic decompensation: new ascites, variceal bleeding, jaundice, or encephalopathy. Rarely, patients present with paraneoplastic syndromes: Erythrocytosis is most common; hypercalcemia, hyperthyroidism, and carcinoid syndrome have been described. Physical findings include nodular hepatomegaly with an arterial bruit and hepatic rub. Extrahepatic spread occurs in about 50% of patients during the course of the illness. Twenty percent of patients have lung metastases.

C. Diagnostic evaluation and screening. α-Fetoprotein levels are elevated in 70% of patients and associated with a poor prognosis. Ultrasonography and CT have a high sensitivity when lesions are larger than 2 cm; however, small lesions are frequently missed. Magnetic resonance imaging is generally equivalent to CT but at a greater cost. Fine-needle aspiration with cytology or biopsy usually confirms the diagnosis. Serial α-fetoprotein measurements every 3 to 4 months and liver ultrasound every 4 to 6 months should be considered in high-risk patients with hepatitis B antigenemia or with hepatitis C and cirrhosis. Patients with hepatitis C without cirrhosis and patients with hemochromatosis should be considered for less intensive screening.

D. Staging. Staging procedures should include a chest radiograph, CT of the abdomen, a complete blood cell count, a blood chemistry profile, and an α-fetoprotein measurement (Table 9.4). If these do not disclose unresectable cancer or sites of metastatic cancer, then CT of the chest and arteriogram (upper abdominal and hepatic) should be performed to guide surgical intervention and further screening for extrahepatic involvement.

E. Primary therapy. At presentation, 25% of patients with hepatocellular carcinoma have potentially resectable lesions. At laparotomy, only 10% to 12% are resected. Operative mortality is 10% to 30%. Cirrhosis and advanced lesions are the factors limiting resection. Long-term survival is achieved in 15% to 30% of patients whose tumors are resected. Recurrences appear in liver, regional lymph nodes, lungs, and bone. Liver transplantation may permit resection of small tumors in patients with advanced cirrhosis, and survival is similar to or better than that seen after resection without transplantation. Percutaneous ethanol injection can also control selected patients' tumors.

F. Therapy of advanced hepatocellular carcinoma

1. Single agents. Numerous single agents have been tested in primary hepatocellular carcinoma: Alkylating agents, antimetabolites, plant alkaloids, and cisplatin have been ineffective. Doxorubicin 60 mg/m^2 IV every 21 days is recommended. This regimen results in a partial response rate of about 16%.

2. Combination chemotherapy and other modes of treatment. Combination chemotherapy has not had better success than single agents. Hepatic artery infusion has been studied and appears to have an increased response rate com-

Table 9.4. TNM staging for hepatocellular cancer

Stage	Definition
I	T1 (solitary tumor any size without vascular invasion), N0, M0
II	T2 (solitary tumor any size with vascular invasion; or multiple tumors, none greater than 5 cm, N0, M0
IIIA	T3 (multiple tumors 75 cm or tumor involving a major brance of the portal or hepatic vein[s], N0, M0), N0, M0
IIIB	T4 (direct invasion of adjacent organs other than gall bladder or with perforation of visceral peritonum.)
IIIC	Any T, NI, MO
IVB	Any T, any N, M1

Modified from American Joint Committee on Cancer. *AJCC staging manual.* 6th ed. New York: Springer, 2002.

pared with IV chemotherapy. Similarly, chemoembolization has been employed. To date, no survival advantage has been proved for intra-arterial therapy or chemoembolization. Immunotherapy has not shown promise in hepatocellular carcinoma. Irradiation has had a limited role in treating liver tumors because of hepatic intolerance to radiation. Cryotherapy has been used in tumors greater than 3 cm, but it requires laparotomy. Radiofrequency ablation is also being used in smaller lesions, and it can be done percutaneously.

SELECTED READINGS

Berlin JD, Rothenberg M. Chemotherapy for respectable and advanced pancreatic cancer. *Oncology (Huntingt)* 2001;15:1241–1254.

Burris HA, Moore MJ, Andersen J, et al. Improvements in survival and clinical benefit with gemcitabine as first-line therapy for patients with advanced pancreas cancer: a randomized trial. *J Clin Oncol* 1997;15:2403–2413.

Collier J, Sherman M. Screening for hepatocellular carcinoma. *Hepatology* 1998;27:273–278.

Figueras J, Jaurrieta E, Valls C, et al. Survival after liver transplantation in cirrhotic patients with and without hepatocellular carcinoma: a comparative study. *Hepatology* 1997;25:1485–1489.

Gastrointestinal Tumor Study Group. Further evidence of effective adjuvant combined radiation and chemotherapy following curative resection of pancreatic cancer. *Cancer* 1987;59:2006–2010.

Glimelius B, Hoffman K, Sjoden PO, et al. Chemotherapy improves survival and quality of life in advanced pancreatic and biliary cancer. *Ann Oncol* 1996;7:593–600.

Howard TJ. Pancreatic adenocarcinoma. *Curr Probl Cancer* 1996; 20:281–328.

Jadavar H, Fischman AJ. Evaluation of pancreatic carcinoma with FDG PET. *Abdom Imag* 2001;26:254–259.

Jensen RT, Fraker DL. Zollinger–Ellison syndrome: advances in treatment of gastric hypersecretion and the gastrinoma. *JAMA* 1994;271:1429–1435.

Kalser MH, Ellenberg SS. Pancreatic cancer: adjuvant combined radiation and chemotherapy following curative resection. *Arch Surg* 1985;120:899–903.

Lencioni R, Pinto F, Armillotta N, et al. Long-term results of percutaneous ethanol injection therapy for hepatocellular carcinoma in cirrhosis: a European experience. *Eur Radiol* 1997;7:514–519.

Moertel CG, Gunderson LL, Mailliard JA, et al. Early evaluation of combined fluorouracil and leucovorin as a radiation enhancer for locally unresectable, residual, or recurrent gastrointestinal carcinoma. *J Clin Oncol* 1994;12:21–27.

Moertel CG, Hahn RG, O'Connell MS. Therapy of locally unresectable pancreatic carcinoma: a randomized comparison of high dose (6000 rads) radiation alone, moderate dose radiation (4000 rads–5-fluorouracil), and high dose radiation–5-fluorouracil. Gastrointestinal Tumor Study Group. *Cancer* 1981;48:1705–1710.

Moertel CG, Lefkopoulo M, Lipsitz S, et al. Streptozocin–doxorubicin, streptozocin–fluorouracil, or chlorozotocin in the treatment of advanced islet-cell carcinoma. *N Engl J Med* 1992;326:519–523.

Palmer KR, Kerr M, Knowles G, et al. Chemotherapy prolongs survival in inoperable pancreatic carcinoma. *Br J Surg* 1994;81:882–885.

Schifeling DJ, Konski AA, Howard JM, et al. Radiation therapy and 5-fluorouracil modulated by leucovorin for adenocarcinoma of the pancreas. *Int J Pancreatol* 1992;12:239–243.

Schnall SF, Macdonald JS. Chemotherapy of adenocarcinoma of the pancreas. *Semin Oncol* 1996;23:220–228.

Sherman WH, Fine RL. Combination gemcitabine and docetaxel therapy in advanced adenocarcinoma of the pancreas. *Oncology* 2001; 60:316–321.

Shutze WP, Sack J, Aldrete JS. Long-term follow-up of 24 patients undergoing radical resection for ampullary carcinoma, 1953 to 1988. *Cancer* 1990;66:1717–1720.

Stabile BE. Islet cell tumors. *Gastroenterologist* 1997;5:213–232.

Tsukuma H, Hiyama T, Tanaka S, et al. Risk factors for hepatocellular carcinoma among patients with chronic liver disease. *N Engl J Med* 1993;328:1797–1801.

Warshaw AL, Gu ZY, Wittenberg J, et al. Preoperative staging and assessment of resectability of pancreatic cancer. *Arch Surg* 1990;125:230–233.

Wolff RA. Novel therapies for pancreatic cancer. *Cancer J* 2001; 7:349–358.

10

Carcinoma of the Breast

Iman Mohamed and Roland T. Skeel

I. **Natural history, evaluation, and modes of treatment**
A. **Epidemiology and etiology.** Carcinoma of the breast gave way to carcinoma of the lung as the most common cause of cancer deaths among women in the United States in 1986. Nonetheless, in 2002, more than 200,000 new cases of breast cancer were diagnosed, and there were nearly 40,000 women who died from this cancer. The incidence of breast cancer varies widely among different populations. Women in Western Europe and the United States have a higher incidence than women in most other parts of the world, possibly in part because of the high intake of animal protein and fat. Despite a slight increase in the incidence of breast cancer, the disease-specific mortality seems to be declining. This is due largely to more tumors being diagnosed at earlier stages as well as improvements in the efficacy of treatment with chemotherapy. Although discrete causes of breast cancer cannot be identified in individual women, many factors increase a womans risk of developing the disease. Among the strongest of the risk factors is family history, particularly if more than one family member has developed breast cancer at an early age. Genetic linkage analysis has led to the discovery of dominant germline mutations in two tumor-suppressor genes, *BRCA1* and *BRCA2,* localized to chromosomes 17 and 13, respectively, which are associated with a high risk of female breast cancer as well as ovarian cancer (*BRCA1* and *BRCA2*), male breast cancer (*BRCA2*), and other cancers. Although these mutations account for less than 10% of all cases of breast cancer, together they may account for over 70% of inherited cases in some high-risk populations. It is important to note, however, that most patients with a family history of breast cancer do not have a defined inherited mutation. However, if a woman with breast cancer is under the age of 50 and has any relative who developed breast cancer before she was 50, her chance of having a mutation in *BRCA1* or *BRCA2* rises to 25%. Other factors that increase her probability of a mutation include any relative with ovarian cancer or a personal history of bilateral breast cancer or ovarian cancer. Carriers of these mutations have up to a 70% lifetime risk of breast cancer, depending on familial history, perhaps the specific mutation, and other cellular genes that may modify penetrance. The 5-year survival rate of patients with either of the *BRCA* mutations is not significantly less than for other patients with breast cancer. Other less common or less well-defined genetic mutations may be present in other familial breast cancers. Additional factors that increase breast cancer risk are early menarche, late age at birth of first child, and prior benign breast disease (particularly if there is a high degree of benign epithelial atypia). Present use of birth control pills appears to have a small effect on the risk

of developing breast cancer (relative risk 1.24); risk from prior use diminishes over time. Although breast cancer may occur among men, such cases represent fewer than 1% of all breast cancers and are infrequently seen in most hospitals. Male carriers of *BRCA2* mutations have a 6% lifetime risk of breast cancer, significantly increasing their risk in comparison with the general population.

B. Detection, diagnosis, and pretreatment evaluation

1. Screening. Because more lives can be saved if breast cancer is diagnosed at an early stage, many programs have been designed to detect small, early cancers. Monthly breast self-examination for all women after puberty and yearly breast examinations by a physician or other trained professional after a woman is 30 years of age are recommended. Notwithstanding some skepticism in the literature, most breast cancer specialists and statistical analyses have concluded that mammography, when done on a regular basis, can reduce mortality due to breast cancer by 30% in women older than 50 years. The benefit for women aged 40 to 50 years has been more difficult to demonstrate. Mammography is recommended at age 40 years as a baseline, once every 1 to 2 years between the ages of 40 and 50 years (depending on risk factors and the recommending organization), and yearly after 50 years of age. An upper age of effectiveness is not established. Although each method for early detection can be of some help in finding early lesions that can be successfully removed before metastasis has occurred, mammography is capable of detecting the smallest and therefore the most curable lesions. Thus, despite the high cost of screening mammography ($75 to $140 in many areas of the United States), it is highly recommended that the above guidelines be followed. Mammography has clearly led to the discovery of many earlier cancers and sharply increased the discovery of preinvasive cancers (ductal carcinoma *in situ*). Screening breast ultrasound is commonly used in Europe. Its role in the United States remains limited to evaluation of palpable lesions, especially in premenopausal women where mammography has a high false-negative rate due to higher breast radiographic density.

2. Presenting signs and symptoms. Although an increasing number of nonpalpable cancers are found by mammography, breast cancer is still most often discovered by a woman herself as an isolated, painless lump in the breast. If the mass has gone unnoticed, ignored, or neglected for a time, there may be fixation to the skin or underlying chest wall, ulceration, pain, or inflammation. Some early lesions present with discharge or bleeding from the nipple. At times, the primary lesion is not discovered, and the woman presents with symptoms of metastatic disease such as pleural effusion, nodal disease, or bony metastases. About half of all lesions are in the upper outer quadrant of the breast (where most of the glandular tissue of the breast is). About 20% are central masses, and 10% are in each of the other quadrants. Up to one-quarter of all women with breast cancer have axillary node metastasis at the time of diagnosis, although this is less common when the primary tumor has been detected by screening mammography or other screening method.

3.   Staging. Carcinoma of the breast is staged according to the size and characteristics of the primary tumor (T), the involvement of regional lymph nodes (N), and the presence of metastatic disease (M). An abridged version of the commonly used TNM classification of breast cancer is shown in Table 10.1, and the stage grouping is outlined in Table 10.2. Although preliminary staging is commonly done before surgery, definitive staging that can be used for prognostic and further treatment planning purposes usually must await postsurgical pathologic evaluation when the primary tumor size and the histologic involvement of the lymph nodes are established. In up to 30% of patients with palpable breast

Table 10.1.   Abridged TNM classification of breast cancer

Primary tumor

Tis	Carcinoma *in situ:* intraductal carcinoma, lobular carcinoma *in situ,* or Paget's disease of the nipple with no tumor
T1	Tumor ≤2 cm
	T1mic ≤0.1 cm
	T1a >0.1–0.5 cm
	T1b >0.5–1 cm
	T1c >1–2 cm
T2	Tumor >2–5 cm
T3	Tumor >5 cm
T4	Any size with extension to chest wall or skin (chest wall includes ribs, intercostal muscles, and serratus anterior muscle, but not pectoral muscles)
	T4a Extension to chest wall
	T4b Edema, skin ulceration, or satellite skin nodules confined to same breast
	T4c Both (T4a and T4b) criteria
	T4d Inflammatory carcinoma

Nodal involvement: pathologic

pN0	No regional lymph node metastasis histologically
pN1mi	Micrometastasis >0.2 to 2 mm
pN1a	Metastasis to 1–3 nodes, any > 2 mm
pN2	Metastasis to 4–9 nodes or clinically apparent internal mammary lymph nodes without axillary lymph node metastasis
pN3	Metastasis to 10 or more axillary lymph nodes, or to infraclavicular lymph nodes, or ipsilateral supraclavicular lymph nodes, or clinically apparent mamary lymph nodes with axillary lymph node metastasis

Distant metastasis

M0	None known
M1	Metastases present, including to ipsilateral supraclavicular lymph nodes

Table 10.2.   Stage grouping of breast cancer[a]

Stage	Description
0	Tis, N0, M0
I	T1, N0, M0
IIA	T0–1, N1, M0
	T2, N0, M0
IIB	T2, N1, M0
	T3, N0, M0
IIIA	T0–2, N2, M0
	T3, N1–2, M0
IIIB	T4, any N, M0
IIIC	Any T, N3, M0
IV	Any T, any N, M1

[a] Patients are staged in the highest group possible for their composite TNM. For example, a patient with T1a, N2, M0 would have stage IIIA disease because of the N2 status.

masses (not found by mammography), but without clinical evidence of axillary lymph node involvement, the histologic evaluation of the nodes reveals cancer. In patients with negative nodes by routine histologic evaluation, serial sectioning may reveal microscopic cancer deposits in additional patients. Tumor cell detection using immunocytologic evaluation of the bone marrow, such as the presence of cytokeratin-positive cells, may also be of prognostic value. It is less certain whether there is prognostic value if cancer cells in nodes are detected by molecular markers. In a somewhat smaller number, nodes that clinically appear positive contain no cancer when examined histologically.

4.   **Diagnostic evaluation**

   a.   Before biopsy, the woman should have a careful **history,** during which attention should be paid to risk factors, and a **physical examination,** with a focus not only on the involved breast but also on the opposite breast, all regional lymph node areas, the lungs, bone, and liver. This examination should be followed by bilateral mammography to help assess the extent of involvement and to look for additional ipsilateral or contralateral disease.

   b.   Excisional or core needle biopsy of the primary lesion is performed, and the specimen is given intact (not in formalin) to the pathologist, who can divide the specimen for histologic examination, hormone receptor assays, overexpression of genes such as *HER2,* flow cytometric measurements of ploidy and the percentage of cells in the S phase, and other specialized tests.

   c.   After confirmation of the histology, the patient is evaluated for possible metastatic disease.

      (1)   Mandatory studies include a chest radiograph, complete blood count, blood chemistry profile, and estrogen and progesterone receptor assays on the primary breast carcinoma and grossly cancerous nodal tissues.

(2) **Other studies,** including radionuclide scan of the bones, skeletal survey (usually obtained only if the radionuclide scan is positive), and computed tomography scan of the liver (abdomen) are optional unless the history, physical examination, or blood studies suggest a poor prognosis or point to specific organ involvement. Additional studies that may impart clinically useful prognostic information include evaluation of the ploidy of the malignant cells and their deoxyribonucleic acid (DNA) synthesis rate (percentage in S phase) and the content of other markers such as the overexpression of *c-erbB-2* (*HER2*) oncogene (using fluorescence *in situ* hybridization [FISH]) or its growth factor receptor protein product (immunohistochemistry assay of cell surface membranes), *p53* mutations, or cathepsin D.

5. **Histology.** About 75% to 80% of all breast cancers are infiltrating ductal carcinomas and 10% are infiltrating lobular carcinomas; these two types have similar biologic behavior. The remainder of the histologic types of invasive breast carcinoma may have a somewhat better prognosis but are usually managed more according to the stage than to the histologic type.

C. **Approach to therapy**

1. **Prevention.** Until recently, it was unknown whether any preventive measures would be effective in reducing the incidence of breast cancer. Two trials using selective estrogen receptor modulators (SERMs) have demonstrated that 3 to 5 years of preventive treatment with these agents reduces the rate of cancer development over the short term. Women at increased risk because of family history, age, and other risk factors, who were treated with tamoxifen 20 mg/day, were found to have a 45% reduction in the rate of occurrence of invasive breast cancer compared with women treated with placebo. Noninvasive disease and preneoplastic breast lesions are also decreased. Raloxifene 60 or 120 mg/day also appears to reduce the risk of breast cancer in postmenopausal women (who had osteoporosis and a standard or reduced risk of breast cancer), with a relative risk of 0.26. Raloxifene appears to have a lower risk for the development of endometrial cancer than tamoxifen, which has been associated with a risk for endometrial cancer of two to four times that of untreated women. Effects on survival, when used in breast cancer prevention, have not yet been demonstrated for either agent. A trial under way is comparing these two agents in postmenopausal women.

The approach to management of women at very high risk because of family history or known suppressor gene mutations is in evolution. Increased surveillance such as increasing the frequency of mammography to every 6 months has been suggested as a reasonable conservative approach. In mutation carriers who are at risk for both breast and ovarian cancer, bilateral oophorectomy after child-bearing age has been recommended because of the inadequacy of screening tests for ovarian cancer. Prophylactic mastectomy may be preferred by some women. In a recent study from the Mayo

Clinic, bilateral simple mastectomy in mutation carriers was found to reduce their risk of breast cancer by 90%. A small risk of breast cancer in residual breast glandular tissue persists and the irreversible loss of nipple sensation may be distressing to some women. Bilateral oophorectomy in the premenopausal woman who has completed her family reduces her risk of breast cancer by about 50% and avoids the psychological trauma of bilateral mastectomy.

The role of SERMs in patients with these *BRCA1* and *BRCA2* mutations is evolving as well. Analysis of blood samples of women who participated in the Prevention Trial with tamoxifen showed that mutation carriers also had a 47% lower risk of breast cancer, suggesting a useful role for this group of drugs in mutation carriers.

2.   Surgery. Surgery has been and remains the most frequently used mode of primary therapy for most women with carcinoma of the breast. The role of surgery in the primary management of carcinoma of the breast has been evolving with a **trend to lesser surgery (e.g., wide local excision)** together with axillary node dissection. Complete axillary node dissection may become unnecessary when the reliability of **sentinel node identification,** removal, and histologic assessment is established with greater certainty. This technique may spare many women the additional surgical procedure of axillary node dissection and its attendant risk of arm edema and dysesthesias. The **lumpectomy and axillary node evaluation (or removal)** are followed by radiotherapy to control the microscopic cancer remaining in the breast. Depending on the stage of the cancer, additional radiotherapy may be used to treat upper internal mammary nodes. For most women, this therapy yields therapeutic results that are as good as **modified radical mastectomy** without the need for amputating the breast and its attendant physical deformity and psychological trauma.

Although many women and their physicians are opting for lesser surgery, some version of the modified radical mastectomy is still more commonly performed in many areas of the United States; in this operation, the breast, pectoralis fascia (with or without the pectoralis minor muscle), and lymph nodes are removed. There are wide geographic variations in the use of breast-conserving surgery throughout the United States. For most women, operations more extensive than the modified radical mastectomy are probably of no benefit, and lesser operations that are not combined with radiotherapy are insufficient in terms of providing important prognostic information regarding the status of the axillary lymph nodes and controlling the local disease (40% of women treated with excisional biopsy alone have recurrence in the ipsilateral breast).

For patients who have had mastectomy, reconstruction is being done with increasing frequency. It may be done at the time of mastectomy or delayed for a period (usually 1 to 2 years). Options include insertion of a silicone or saline implant or transposition of a muscle flap. Neither procedure has resulted in worsening of the prognosis from the breast cancer or a significant increase in the difficulty in detecting local recurrences.

3.   Radiotherapy. Radiotherapys role in the management of carcinoma of the breast has been expanded since the early 1970s. Radiotherapy is now commonly used in conjunction with excisional biopsy of varying degree as part of the primary therapy. In this circumstance, the radiotherapy is commonly delivered using external-beam therapy to the entire breast with a boost of therapy to the tumor bed using either external-beam therapy or implantation of radioactive substances. Radiotherapy may also be given after mastectomy in women who have a high likelihood of local recurrence, and it is highly effective in preventing the reappearance of disease in the treated fields. In some circumstances, it may also improve survival. Local recurrences and distant metastases also are frequently treated successfully with radiotherapy. This mode of treatment is particularly critical to the management of painful bony lesions or sites of impending pathologic fracture.

4.   Chemotherapy and endocrine therapy. Chemotherapy and endocrine therapy are used to reduce the likelihood of recurrence in early disease and to treat more advanced disease with or without distant metastasis. Endocrine therapy may consist in surgical, radiotherapeutic, or chemotherapeutic ablation or inhibition of the ovaries or adrenal glands; or it may consist of additive therapy with antiestrogens, aromatase inhibitors, progestins, androgens, or luteinizing hormone–releasing hormone (LRHR) agonists. Endocrine therapy is generally ineffective (as sole therapy) for the treatment of metastatic disease in patients with low levels of estrogen and progesterone receptors in the cancer cells and is increasingly effective as the level of receptors rises. The best responses can be expected in women in whom the estrogen receptor level is high and progesterone receptors are present. Chemotherapy is apparently equally effective regardless of the level of hormone receptors in the cancer cell. Other factors such as *HER2* expression may also affect responsiveness to hormonal therapy; patients overexpressing this gene have a lower response rate to tamoxifen but appear to retain responsiveness to aromatase inhibitors such as letrozole. There is no established role for hormonal therapy or chemotherapy for treating ductal carcinoma *in situ,* though there may be an emerging role for antiestrogen therapy in the prevention of invasive or new *in situ* disease.

5.   Multimodal therapy. Multimodal therapy has had a more beneficial impact on carcinoma of the breast than on any other common cancer affecting adults.

   a.   Postoperative chemotherapy or hormonal therapy (including ovarian ablation in premenopausal women) for women with a high risk of recurrence owing to positive axillary nodes (i.e., nodes containing cancer) is selected on the basis of the hormone receptor status of the tumor and also on the menopausal status and age of the woman. Most node-positive patients benefit from adjuvant therapy, with a decrease in the annual rates of recurrence by 25% to 40% and of death by 15% to 30%.

Studies have shown that many women with negative nodes also benefit from adjuvant chemotherapy or hormonal (tamoxifen) therapy. Although the percentage decrease in mortality is similar to that for node-positive women, the lower baseline mortality for node-negative women results in less absolute benefit per 100 women treated. Current clinical trials use tumor size, hormone receptor status, and other factors to aid in determining the patients, among those with negative nodes, who are most likely to relapse and thus most likely to benefit from adjuvant therapy. Equal consideration must be given to potential short- and long-term risks of treatment. Here the physiologic age of the patient and co-morbid conditions will become important considerations.

b. **Radiotherapy** to the breast and nodal areas after excisional biopsy or quadrantectomy of the breast cancer is as effective a treatment as mastectomy in terms of local recurrence and survival. For most patients, it is not only equivalent but preferable treatment because of the preservation of the breast.

c. **Consultation** with a surgeon, radiotherapist, and medical oncologist is critical once the diagnosis of carcinoma is highly suspected or histologically confirmed. It is important to have all of these oncology specialists see the patient before final decisions regarding therapy are made, so the primary physician and the patient can have opinions from several perspectives about optimal management. This is best achieved during multidisciplinary treatment planning conferences where opportunities arise to discuss treatment, identify patients who require psychosocial support, and identify patients that may benefit from genetic testing and those eligible for clinical trials.

It is critical to have the patient (and her family, if she desires) share in the therapy decisions after hearing the options, the relative advantages and disadvantages of each option, and the recommendations of the consultants. The patient should be given an opportunity to hear why the recommended treatment is thought by the physicians to be best and to decide whether that is acceptable to her.

D. **Prognosis.** There is a broad spectrum in the biologic behavior of breast carcinoma from aggressive, rapidly fatal, inflammatory carcinoma to relatively indolent disease with late-appearing metastasis and survival time of 10 to 15 years. The likelihoods of relapse and survival are influenced by the stage of the disease and the hormone receptor status at diagnosis, pathologic characteristics of the tumor, measures of proliferative activity of the cancer cell, oncogene and tumor suppressor gene (tumor) expression or amplification (*HER2, c-myc, p53*), and age and general health of the patient. Recent data suggests that the "genetic profile" of the cancer may be the strongest predictor of risk for relapse.

1. **Stage.** Axillary node involvement and the size of the primary tumor are major determinants of the likelihood of survival.

a. **Nodes.** In one large National Surgical Adjuvant Breast Project study, before the use of modern adjuvant therapy,

65% of all patients who underwent radical mastectomy survived 5 years and 45% survived 10 years. When no axillary nodes were positive, the 5-year survival rate was nearly 80% and the 10-year survival rate 65%. If any axillary nodes were positive, the 5-year survival rate was less than 50% and the 10-year survival rate 25%. If four or more nodes were positive, the 5-year survival rate was 30% and the 10-year survival rate less than 15%. Since that time (1975), there has been improvement, with 5-year survival rates of 87% for stage I, 75% for stage II, 45% for stage III, and 13% for stage IV breast cancer.

b. Primary tumor. Patients with large primary tumors do not do as well as patients with small tumors, irrespective of the nodal status, although patients with large primary tumors are more likely to have node involvement. Tumors that are fixed to the skin or to the chest wall do worse than those that are not. Patients with inflammatory carcinomas have a particularly poor prognosis, with a median survival time of less than 2 years and a 5-year survival rate of less than 10% in some series. Aggressive initial (neoadjuvant) chemotherapy may improve the outlook for some patients.

2. Estrogen and progesterone receptors. Patients without estrogen or progesterone receptors (or with very low levels) are twice as likely to relapse during the first 2 years after diagnosis as those who are receptor positive. This observation is true for both premenopausal and postmenopausal patients within each major node group (zero, one to three, and four or more).

3. *Her-2/neu* amplification. *Her-2/neu* amplification is associated with impaired survival in early-stage breast cancer. This is a cellular proto-oncogene that codes for a transmembrane receptor of the epidermal growth factor receptor family. Amplification (as is seen in 25% to 30% of early breast cancer) results in worse prognosis with earlier appearance of metastatic disease.

4. Other factors. Other prognostic factors are still under study as to whether they can provide information as independent prognostic factors, particularly for node-negative cancers. These include the percentage of cells in DNA synthesis (low percentage in S phase better than high percentage) and the ploidy of the breast cancer cells (diploid better than aneuploid). Additional tumor markers that may have predictive value include cathepsin D, *c-myc* oncogene amplification, and *p53* suppressor gene expression.

II. Chemotherapy and endocrine therapy

A. General considerations and aims of therapy. Carcinoma of the breast is responsive to many cytotoxic chemotherapeutic agents, hormonal agents, and other endocrine manipulations.

1. Endocrine therapy. Endocrine therapy is presumed to be effective because the breast cancer tissue retains some of the endocrine sensitivity of the normal breast tissue. In premenopausal women, if the breast cancer growth is supported by estrogen production from the ovary, antiestrogen therapy, removal of endogenous estrogen by oophorectomy, or suppression of estrogen production using an LHRH agonist logically results in regression of the cancer, at least those tumor cells that are dependent on the estrogen. (The dependent cells seem to be those that have the estrogen receptors.) Other mechanisms of action of the antiestrogen tamoxifen include inhibition of the epithelial growth factor transforming growth factor-α and stimulation of the epithelial inhibitory factor transforming growth factor-β. Complicating the anticipated interactions of SERMs further are the presence of different classes of estrogen receptors, different ligands, many receptor-interacting proteins, a host of transcription-activating factors, and several response elements.

2.   Chemotherapy. As with other cancers, the basis for the effectiveness of cytotoxic drugs in the treatment of carcinoma of the breast is not completely understood. It is clear, however, that combinations of drugs are considerably more effective than single agents (although how many is enough is not as certain), and nearly all treatment programs use the drugs in various combinations, at least during initial therapy. In addition to their cytotoxic effects, chemotherapeutic agents may induce menopause in premenopausal women, thus affecting estrogen production as well as killing cells directly. Recent studies suggest a trend toward a lower recurrence rate in women who develop chemotherapy-induced amenorrhea.

3.   Biologic therapy. With the development of the humanized anti-*HER2* antibody (trastuzumab, Herceptin) and *HER2* peptide vaccines, biologic therapy of breast cancer has become a reality. Although it appears that these modes of therapy now have a substantial role in the armamentarium of the oncologist, their optimal use and the degree to which biologic therapy will have an impact on survival and quality of life in patients with breast cancer are uncertain.

4.   Aims of therapy. Aims of therapy differ depending on the stage of disease being treated.

    a.   For early disease, the aim is to eradicate micrometastases to render the patient free of disease and prevent recurrence. If eradication of cancer cells cannot be achieved, long-term suppression is desirable. Coincident with this aim is the goal of avoiding unnecessarily excessive drug-induced toxicity, both short and long term. Of particular concern is the increased incidence of second cancers (myelodysplasia and leukemia in particular) arising years after the completion of chemotherapy. Thus, a goal of investigational studies has been to try to determine the minimum therapy that is effective for preventing the maximum number of recurrences in any given clinical situation. If micrometastases cannot be eradicated, long-term suppression is also a reasonable goal of therapy. This may, in fact, be what is accomplished by tamoxifen and other SERMs and the reason why chronic (5 years) therapy is needed.

    b.   For advanced disease, the aim is usually to reduce the tumor burden and the resultant disability in order to alleviate the patients symptoms, improve performance, and prolong meaningful survival. Whereas long-term toxicity is not usually of great import, short-term toxicity is a major area of concern for both physician and patient because the aim of therapy is to improve how the patient feels (quality of life) as well as to prolong survival time.

B.   Effective agents. Effective agents for treating carcinoma of the breast can be found among the alkylating agents, antimetabolites, natural products (antibiotics, vinca alkaloids, and taxanes), hormones, hormone antagonists, and biologic agents.

1.   Among the cytotoxic drugs, the most commonly used agents include doxorubicin, cyclophosphamide, methotrexate, fluorouracil, paclitaxel, docetaxel, gemcitabine, capecitabine, vinorelbine, mitoxantrone, thiotepa, and vincristine. Each of these agents has a response rate of 20% to 40% when used as a single agent. Because combinations are so much more effective (60% to 80% response rate) than single agents, these drugs are rarely used alone as initial therapy.

2.   Among the hormones and antihormones, the most commonly used agents are tamoxifen (the other SERMs toremifene and raloxifene are not as widely used) and one of the aromatase inhibitors (anastrozole, letrozole, and exemestane). Other hormonal agents including various progestins (e.g., megestrol acetate), aminoglutethimide, fluoxymesterone, the LHRH agonists (leuprolide and goserelin), and prednisone are used less commonly. These agents are most often used alone but may be used in combination with cytotoxic drugs or sequentially with cytotoxic drugs; prednisone is used less commonly than in previous years and is used only with cytotoxic agents.

3.   Biologic agents are new in the armamentarium of effective agents in breast cancer. Trastuzumab (Herceptin) has demonstrated efficacy, and the demonstration of the capability of *HER2* peptide vaccines to elicit T-cell immunity may presage an additional effective biologic therapy in breast cancer. Current data suggest that the addition of trastuzumab to chemotherapy in *HER2*-positive patients with advanced disease may improve their long-term outcome. There is concern, however, over cardiac toxicity especially when trastuzumab is combined with an anthracycline.

4.   Radiotherapy should generally be delayed until the completion of adjuvant chemotherapy to decrease the frequency of distant recurrence, particularly in women with positive nodes or other unfavorable prognostic indicators.

C.   Treatment of early disease. Standard treatment of early disease depends on primary tumor size, nodal status, menopausal status of the patient, hormone receptor status of the tumor, and other tumor characteristics. Because there is not yet optimal therapy for any subset of women with breast cancer, the patient and her physician should be encouraged to participate in clinical trials. If none is available or the patient declines, Table 10.3 can be used as a guide for assessing risk. Table 10.4 may be used as a guide to select the type of therapy, depending on stage of disease, menopausal state, age, receptor status, and other risk factors.

Table 10.3.   Prognostic factors for assessing risk of recurrence of breast cancer

Value	Parameter
Nodal status	Risk increases with presence of metastasis and numbers of nodes involved
Tumor size	Risk increases with tumor size independently of nodal status
Estrogen and progesterone receptors	Positive receptors confer better prognosis
Age	Complex factor. Women aged 45–49 yr have best prognosis, with increasing likelihood of deaths from their breast cancer in older and younger age groups
Morphology	Higher nuclear grade, higher histologic grade, tumor necrosis, peritumoral lymphatic vessel invasion, increased microvessel density tumors have worse prognosis
DNA content and proliferative capacity	Tumors that are diploid and have low S-phase fraction do better than those that are aneuploid or have a high S-phase fraction (by flow cytometry)
Oncogene expression	HER2 / neu (c-erbB-2) and c-myc amplification have association with earlier relapse and shorter survival
Tumor suppressor gene mutations	BRCA1 and BRCA2 mutations seem to have little effect on prognosis

Table 10.4.   Systemic adjuvant therapy for breast cancer: guidelines

Tumor category	Premenopausal women	Postmenopausal women[a] ≤80 yr	Postmenopausal women[a] >80 yr
Node-positive			
ER- and/or PR-positive	CT with TAM or oophorectomy	TAM with or without CT	TAM
ER- and PR-negative	CT	CT	None or CT
Node-negative			
ER- and PR-indeterminate because tumor too small	None	None	None
ER- and/or PR-positive			
≤2 cm			
Low risk[b]	None	None	None
High risk	CT plus TAM	TAM	TAM
>2 cm	CT plus TAM	TAM with or without CT	TAM
ER- and PR-negative	CT	CT	None

ER, estrogen receptor; PR, progesterone receptor; CT, chemotherapy: AC (doxorubicin [Adriamycin] plus cyclophosphamide) for four cycles; CAF, cyclophosphamide, doxorubicin, fluorouracil; CMF, cyclophosphamide, methotrexate, fluorouracil; CMFP (cyclophosphamide, methotrexate, fluorouracil, prednisone) for six cycles; other chemotherapy may be of equal or better efficacy (such as AC followed by paclitaxel); TAM, tamoxifen (for 5 yr, alone or after completion of chemotherapy).

[a] Co-morbid conditions may modify decision to treat and choice of therapy.

[b] Based on factors such as size of <1 cm, low histologic grade, or low percentage (<6%–10%) of cells in S phase (see Table 10.3).

1. Cytotoxic therapy Cytotoxic therapy is recommended for all premenopausal and most postmenopausal women with positive nodes, irrespective of hormone receptor status. It should also be used in higher-risk premenopausal and postmenopausal women with negative nodes, particularly if they have negative hormone receptors. We are less inclined to use cytotoxic therapy in the adjuvant treatment of older women (over 70 years of age with co-morbid conditions, over 80 years of age without co-morbid conditions), particularly if they are hormone receptor positive and are at lower risk. How much, if any, cytotoxic therapy adds to antiestrogen (tamoxifen) therapy in lower-risk node-negative, hormone receptor–positive patients is not established. We use AC (doxorubicin [Adriamycin] and cyclophosphamide) more commonly in women with a higher risk of recurrence and CMF (cyclophosphamide, methotrexate, and fluorouracil) more in those who have lesser risks (e.g., are node negative), who have co-morbid conditions, or in whom the cardiac risk of doxorubicin is deemed important. There may be a slight advantage to doxorubicin-based regimens (AC or CAF [cyclophosphamide, doxorubicin, and fluorouracil]) in terms of disease-free or overall survival, but the difference, if present, is small and the toxicity is greater. There may be advantage in some node-positive women to the sequential use of AC followed by a taxane (paclitaxel or docetaxel). Longer follow-up studies are needed to determine whether this should become standard for all women with node-positive disease. Moderate escalation of the doses of the standard chemotherapy regimens does not appear to be of benefit in improving survival and may increase the risk for treatment-related myelodysplasia and leukemia. Very high-dose chemotherapy with autologous bone marrow or peripheral blood progenitor cell reinfusion has not fulfilled the promise of improving the survival of women at very high risk of recurrence. After analysis of recently completed clinical trials, it has become clear that no single group of patients with advanced breast cancer, regardless of tumor factors or clinical features, demonstrated benefit from high-dose chemotherapy. The potential benefit for women with a large number of positive lymph nodes remains investigational.

    a. Commonly used regimens

        (1) AC

            Doxorubicin 60 mg/m^2 IV push through a rapidly running IV, *and*

            Cyclophosphamide 600 mg/m^2 IV.

            Repeat every 3 weeks for four cycles.

        (2) CAF

            Cyclophosphamide 100 mg/m^2/day PO on days 1 to 14 (given as a single daily dose), *and*

            Doxorubicin 30 mg/m^2 IV push on days 1 and 8, through the sidearm of a free-flowing IV infusion of normal saline, *and*

            Fluorouracil 500 mg/m^2 IV push on days 1 and 8.

            Repeat every 28 days for six cycles.

(3) CMF(P)

Cyclophosphamide 100 mg/m^2 PO on days 1 to 14, *and*

Methotrexate 40 mg/m^2 IV on days 1 and 8, *and*

Fluorouracil 600 mg/m^2 IV on days 1 and 8, *with or without*

Prednisone 40 mg/m^2 PO on days 1 to 14, during the first three cycles only.

Repeat cycle every 28 days for six cycles.

(4) Dose modifications are outlined in Table 10.5.

(5) A minimal effective dose and duration of drugs are required for therapy of micrometastases to be effective. If women are arbitrarily given less therapy than they can tolerate, their likelihood of remaining disease-free appears to be less than those who are given full doses of the drugs. This observation has led to the recommendation that if postoperative chemotherapy is to be given, doses should be as high as the patient can tolerate and should be continued for the entire planned period of therapy.

2. Tamoxifen. Tamoxifen 20 mg daily is recommended in hormone receptor–positive women with positive nodes. It should be continued for 5 years. Longer durations do not improve survival. It is also beneficial in hormone receptor–positive premenopausal and postmenopausal women with negative nodes who are not determined to be at low risk of recurrence. Although there were earlier suggestions that tamoxifen was of benefit to older (over 70 years) women irrespective of receptor status, this seems less likely now. In patients who are receptor positive and receive cytotoxic chemotherapy, tamoxifen appears to have an added benefit. It has a relatively low risk in the adjuvant setting, and our current recommendations generally include tamoxifen where it is indicated in addition to chemotherapy in Table 10.4.

3. Response to therapy. It is impossible to determine whether individual patients have responded to treatment for micrometastatic disease unless they relapse because there are no parameters to measure. The effectiveness of such treatment must therefore depend on population studies. Because breast cancer may have a long natural history and the disease may recur even beyond 10 years, it is critical to defer final conclusions regarding any study until at least 5 years and preferably 10 years have passed. It is possible to make some observations, however, regarding the benefits of this kind of multimodal therapy.

a. Chemotherapy improves both disease-free and overall survival by about 25% in all groups of patients. Although the proportional reduction in death rate is similar for both high- and low-risk patients (e.g., node positive and node negative), the absolute benefit is greater for those at higher risk of recurrence and death (e.g., younger patients with positive nodes).

b. Tamoxifen (and probably other SERMs) improves disease-free and overall survival in most estrogen receptor–

Table 10.5. Dose modification for chemotherapy of breast carcinoma

Dysfunction			Percentage of full dose to use			Percentage of full dose — Dose as percentage of immediately preceding cycle
Hematologic toxicity ANC (WBC)/µL on day of scheduled treatment[a]		Platelets/µL on day of scheduled treatment	M	T	Capecitabine	Others
≥1,800 (≥3,500)	and	≥100,000	100	100	100	100
1,500–1,800 (3,000–3,500)	or	75,000–100,000	50	75	75	75[a]
1,000–1,500 (2,500–3,000)	or	50,000–75,000	0	50	0	50
<1,000 (<2,500)	or	<50,000	0[b]	0[b]	0	0 (delay 1 wk)

Dysfunction	M	T	Capecitabine	Others
Renal dysfunction (serum creatinine, mg/dL)	A, VLB, VCR	C, M, F, T		
<1.5	100	100	100	100
1.5–2	50	100	? 100	100
2–3.5	25	100	[b]	100
>3.5	0[b]	0[b]	[b]	0[b]
Hepatic dysfunction (serum bilirubin, mg/dL)				
<1.5				
1.5–3				
3.1–5				
>5				

Hemorrhagic cystitis	Discontinue cyclophosphamide and substitute melphalan 4 mg/m² PO on d 1–5 of each cycle.
Gastrointestinal toxicity	For debilitating vomiting or diarrhea, reduce doses of C, M, F, and A by 25% for one cycle. For severe mucositis (ulcerations that inhibit eating), reduce subsequent F, M, capecitabine, and A by 50%. Re-escalate if possible.
Cardiotoxicity	Discontinue doxorubicin.
Hypercorticism	If side effects such as hypertension, severe insomnia, psychosis, or uncontrolled diabetes occur, reduce or stop prednisone.
Neurotoxicity	Reduce taxanes, vincristine, vinblastine, or vinorelbine dose by 50% for moderate paresthesias or severe constipation. Discontinue for severe paresthesias, decreased strength, difficulty walking, cranial nerve palsies, etc.
Hypersensitivity reactions	See guidelines for paclitaxel, docetaxel, and other individual drugs.
Hand–foot syndrome	Hold at first occurrence of grade 2 or greater toxicity; reduce by 25% for second episode of grade 2. Reduce by 25–50% for grade 3 toxicity.

ANC, absolute neutrophil count; WBC, white blood cell count; A, doxorubicin (Adriamycin); C, cyclophosphamide; F, fluorouracil; M, methotrexate; T, thiotepa; VCR, vincristine; VLB, vinblastine.

[a] ANC is the preferred parameter, if available. Some use 100% dosing for ANC 1,500–1,800. If counts are rising at the end of a treatment cycle, an alternative is to delay for a few days to a week and then treat at a higher dose according to the count on the day of actual treatment. If the nadir ANC is <1,000/µL and is associated with fever of >38.3°C (101°F) or the nadir platelet count is <40,000/µL, decrease dose by 25% in subsequent cycles. If the nadir WBC is >3,500/µL and the platelet count is >125,000/µL, increase the dose by 25%.

[b] Safe guidelines cannot be given, and expert evaluation is required before therapy is applied.

positive patients. Although the proportional reduction (about 25%) in death rate is similar for both high- and low-risk patients (e.g., node positive and node negative), the absolute benefit is greater for those at higher risk of recurrence and death.

c.   Chemotherapy plus tamoxifen is better than chemotherapy alone in many estrogen receptor–positive patients. Relative benefits depend on disease status, likelihood of recurrence, and perhaps other factors such as *HER2* (*c-erbB-2*) status (confers less benefit with tamoxifen alone).

d.   Aromatase inhibitors anastrozole and letrozole have greater response rates and time to progression in metastatic disease than tamoxifen, and early data suggest a lower recurrence rate for anastrozole-treated patients than those treated with tamoxifen or the combination of anastrozole and tamoxifen. The role of these agents must await maturation of data and results from additional trials.

D.   Treatment of advanced disease. Treatment of advanced disease is undergoing continuing evolution with the aim of improving the quality and duration of remissions and survival. In patients with bony metastasis or cerebral metastasis, radiotherapy usually is an important component in the management, and a radiation oncologist should participate in planning the patients treatment. Regardless of the role of radiotherapy, however, chemotherapy or endocrine therapy is generally indicated in patients who have advanced disease.

1.   Endocrine therapy is indicated in women who have had a positive test for estrogen or progesterone receptors in their tumor tissue. It is not generally recommended as the sole therapy for women who have low receptor levels or have previously been shown to be unresponsive to hormonal manipulation. It is also not appropriate therapy for women with brain metastasis, lymphangitic pulmonary metastasis, or other dire visceral disease such as extensive liver metastasis, in which a slow response could jeopardize survival. For **premenopausal women,** oophorectomy still may be the treatment of choice, but few women opt for this, given the effectiveness of medical therapies. The LHRH analogs goserelin and leuprolide can achieve the equivalent of a medical oophorectomy. This treatment may be combined with tamoxifen. For **postmenopausal women,** tamoxifen or another SERM is the initial hormonal therapy commonly used. Aromatase inhibitors have recently gained acceptance as first-line treatment for postmenopausal women with metastatic disease with receptor-positive primary tumors and may be become the "gold standard" within a few years. Adrenal suppression with aminoglutethimide is less commonly used because of greater side effects but is still effective.

a.   Commonly used regimens

Tamoxifen 20 mg PO daily (alternative: toremifene 60 mg PO daily).

Anastrozole 1 mg PO daily (alternative: letrozole 2.5 mg PO daily or exemestane 25 mg PO daily).

b. **Less commonly used regimens**

Fulvestrant 250 mg IM (into buttock) monthly as either a single 5-mL or two 2.5-mL injections.

Megestrol acetate 40 mg PO q.i.d.

Aminoglutethimide 250 mg PO q.i.d.; hydrocortisone 100 mg PO in divided doses daily for the first 2 weeks, then 40 mg PO in divided doses daily. Fludrocortisone 0.05 to 0.1 mg PO may be given daily or every other day if there is evidence of salt wasting.

Fluoxymesterone 10 mg PO b.i.d.

2.   Cytotoxic combination chemotherapy is used as the first treatment for advanced disease, in hormone receptor–negative patients, and at times in patients with several organs involved because the responses are more rapid and the rate of response is greater when drugs are used in combination than when endocrine therapy is used alone. For patients over 65 years of age, however, initiation of hormone therapy alone may be justified, with cytotoxic therapy being reserved for patients who have failed one or more hormonal treatments.

a.   **Primary therapy.** Although several regimens have been shown to be effective, AC, CAF, and CMF(P) are the most commonly used as initial therapy. With the discovery of the effectiveness of paclitaxel in the treatment of breast cancer, this drug is also included as first-line therapy, often with doxorubicin or carboplatin. If the patient has not failed adjuvant therapy within 6 months of receiving a doxorubicin-containing regimen, and it is not contraindicated because of recent myocardial infarction, congestive heart failure, or reduced left ventricular ejection fraction, doxorubicin is commonly employed in initial therapy. If doxorubicin cannot be used, then either paclitaxel or CMF is used.

(1)   **CAF**

Cyclophosphamide 100 mg/m^2 PO on days 1 to 14, *and*

Doxorubicin 30 mg/m^2 IV on days 1 and 8, *and*

Fluorouracil 500 mg/m^2 IV on days 1 and 8.

Repeat the cycle every 4 weeks.

(2)   **AC**

Doxorubicin 60 mg/m^2 IV push through a rapidly running IV, *and*

Cyclophosphamide 600 mg/m^2 IV.

Repeat every 3 weeks.

When the cumulative doxorubicin dose reaches 550 mg/m^2, substitute methotrexate 40 mg/m^2.

(3)   **CMFP**

Cyclophosphamide 100 mg/m^2 PO on days 1 to 14, *and*

Methotrexate 40 mg/m^2 IV on days 1 and 8, *and*

Fluorouracil 600 mg/m^2 IV on days 1 and 8, *and*

Prednisone 40 mg/m² PO on days 1 to 14, during the first three cycles only.

Repeat the cycle every 4 weeks.

(4)   Doxorubicin plus paclitaxel with or without filgrastim (Neupogen)

Doxorubicin 50 to 60 mg/m² IV, *followed in 4 h by*
Paclitaxel 150 mg/m² IV over 3 to 24 h, *and*
Filgrastim 300 µg/day SC starting 24 h after the end of chemotherapy for 10 days.

Limit the number of cycles of doxorubicin to six (300 to 360 mg/m²) to limit enhanced cardiotoxicity from the combination. Alternatively, paclitaxel administered over 3 h on day 2 may also limit cardiotoxicity. Left ventricular ejection fraction should be monitored when the doxorubicin dose reaches 300 mg/m².

b.   Secondary therapy. Secondary therapy depends on what treatment the patient has had previously. If the patient relapses while on CMF or CMFP treatment or within 6 months after finishing CMF treatment for micrometastatic disease, it is not likely that these drugs used in combination can be helpful in achieving a second remission. Because doxorubicin is among the most effective agents against breast carcinoma, it should be used in any combination in this situation. One of the regimens listed previously may be used. Additional choices include the following:

Paclitaxel 150 to 175 mg/m² IV over 3 h every 3 weeks, *or*

Docetaxel 60 to 100 mg/m² IV over 1 h every 3 weeks (premedication with oral corticosteroids such as dexamethasone 8 mg b.i.d. for 3 days starting 1 day prior to starting docetaxel is necessary to reduce the severity of fluid retention and hypersensitivity reactions), *or*

Vinorelbine 30 mg/m² IV over 6 to 10 min weekly.

Other agents with activity include mitomycin, gemcitabine, capecitabine, epirubicin, mitoxantrone, and vindesine. If fluorouracil has not been used in previous regimens, using it with leucovorin may be effective.

Most recently, taxotere combined with capecitabine has been shown to be an alternative regimen that is showing a slight survival advantage.

Capecitabine is given at a dose of 1,000 to 1,250 mg/m² IV b.i.d. on days 1 to 14.

Docetaxel is given at a dose of 75mg/m² IV on day 1 of a 3-week cycle.

c.   For patients who are *HER2* 3+ positive by immunohistochemistry or who are FISH positive, paclitaxel is often used in combination with trastuzumab either on a weekly or an every-3-weeks basis. Carboplatin is being used with the combination of paclitaxel and trastuzumab in various schedules with the hope of finding an active regimen without the cardiotoxicity of the doxorubicin–trastuzumab combination:

> **Trastuzumab** 4 mg/m² IV as an initial loading dose, followed by 2 mg/m² IV weekly, *and*
> **Paclitaxel** 200 mg/m² every 3 weeks, *either alone or in combination with*
> **Carboplatin** at an area under the curve (AUC) of 6 IV every 3 weeks for patients with advanced disease.

Alternative combinations combine trastuzumab as above with gemcitabine 1,200 mg/m² weekly for 2 weeks, followed by a week off, continuing so long as the absolute neutrophil count remains greater than 1,000/μL; or with vinorelbine 25 mg/m² IV push weekly until disease progression or undue toxicity.

3. **Dose modifications** are outlined in Table 10.5.
4. **Response to therapy**
   a. **Endocrine therapy.** Of patients who are estrogen receptor negative, fewer than 10% have a response to either additive or ablative endocrine therapy. Among estrogen receptor–positive patients, about 60% have a partial or better response to either additive or ablative endocrine therapy. Responses to endocrine therapy tend to last longer than responses to cytotoxic chemotherapy, frequently lasting 12 to 24 months.
   b. **Cytotoxic chemotherapy.** Cytotoxic chemotherapy produces responses in 60% to 80% of patients regardless of their estrogen receptor status. The responses to therapy at times are durable, but the median duration in most studies is less than 1 year. Clearly, improved survival is desirable. This is not achievable with most current regimens, with the exception of regimens that include trastuzumab. The benefits of trastuzumab (Herceptin) are limited to patients who are *HER2* 3+ positive by immunohistochemistry or who are FISH positive.

E. **Complications of therapy.** Acute toxicities are primarily hematologic and gastrointestinal. Subacute toxicities include alopecia, hemorrhagic cystitis, hypertension, edema, and psychoneurologic abnormalities. Chronic or long-term toxicities may be cardiac, neoplastic or psychoneurologic. Dose modifications for the more common problems are given in Table 10.5. These guidelines are designed to be helpful in selecting a course of therapy that will be effective with the least risk of life-threatening toxicity. Because of individual differences, toxicities that are worse than expected may occur, and the responsible physician must always be alert to special circumstances that dictate further attenuation of the drug doses. The drug data listed in Chapter 4 should be consulted for the individual toxicities, precautions, and toxicity prevention measures for each drug.

Adjuvant tamoxifen therapy also has consequences. These include a two- to fourfold increase in endometrial cancer, an increase in cataracts, and an increase in thromboembolic disease. Hot flashes are common but can be ameliorated in some women by venlafaxine 25 to 50 mg daily. While there is also reduction in the hot flashes from using a progestin such as megestrol 20 mg b.i.d., the effect of the progestin on the risk of recurrence is not known. Adverse effects on vaginal mucosa may be ameliorated with minimal systemic estrogen effect by the estradiol vaginal ring. Whereas fractures related to osteoporosis decrease with tamoxifen, there does not appear to be any reduction in cardiovascular events. Aromatase inhibitors, on the other hand, increase osteoporosis. Women with factor V–Leiden deficiency should not begin tamoxifen or other SERMs.

SELECTED READINGS

American Joint Committee on Cancer. *AJCC cancer staging manual.* 6th ed. New York: Springer, 2002:221.

Auquier A, Rutqvist LE, Host H, et al. Post-mastectomy megavoltage radiotherapy: the Oslo and Stockholm trials. *Eur J Cancer* 1992;28:433–437.

Benner SE, Clark GM, McGuire WL. Review: steroid receptors, cellular kinetics, and lymph node status as prognostic factors in breast cancer. *Am J Med Sci* 1988;296:59–66.

Bonadonna G, Valagussa P. Adjuvant systemic therapy for resectable breast cancer. *J Clin Oncol* 1985;3:259–275.

Buzdar AU, Hortobagyi GN, Frye D, et al. Bioequivalence of 20-mg once-daily tamoxifen relative to 10-mg twice-daily tamoxifen regimens for breast cancer. *J Clin Oncol* 1994;12:50–54.

Collaborative Group on Hormonal Factors in Breast Cancer. Breast cancer and hormonal contraceptives: collaborative reanalysis of individual data on 53,297 women with breast cancer and 100,239 women without breast cancer from 54 epidemiological studies. *Lancet* 1996;347:1713–1727.

Cummings SR, Norton L, Ekert D, et al. Raloxifene reduces the risk of breast cancer and may decrease the risk of endometrial cancer in post-menopausal women: two-year findings from the Multiple Outcomes of Raloxifene Evaluation (MORE) trial. *Proc Am Soc Clin Oncol* 1998;17:2a.

Early Breast Cancer Trialists Collaborative Group. I. Systemic treatment of early breast cancer by hormonal, cytotoxic, or immune therapy: 133 randomised trials involving 31,000 recurrences and 24,000 deaths among 75,000 women. *Lancet* 1992;339:1–15.

Early Breast Cancer Trialists Collaborative Group. II. Systemic treatment of early breast cancer by hormonal, cytotoxic, or immune therapy: 133 randomised trials involving 31,000 recurrences and 24,000 deaths among 75,000 women. *Lancet* 1992;339:71–85.

Early Breast Cancer Trialists Collaborative Group. Effects of radiotherapy and surgery in early breast cancer: an overview of the randomised trials. *N Engl J Med* 1995;333:1444–1455.

Early Breast Cancer Trialists Collaborative Group. Ovarian ablation in early breast cancer: overview of the randomised trials. *Lancet* 1996;348:1189–1196.

Early Breast Cancer Trialists Collaborative Group. Tamoxifen for early breast cancer: an overview of the randomised trials. *Lancet* 1998;351:1451–1467.

Early Breast Cancer Trialists Collaborative Group. Polychemotherapy for early breast cancer: an overview of the randomised trials. *Lancet* 1998;352:930–942.

Eddy DM. High-dose chemotherapy with autologous bone marrow transplantation for the treatment of metastatic breast cancer. *J Clin Oncol* 1992;10:657–670.

Fisher B, Costatino J, Redmond C, et al. A randomized trial evaluating tamoxifen in the treatment of patients with node-negative breast cancer who have estrogen-receptor positive-tumors. *N Engl J Med* 1989;320:479–484.

Fisher B, Costatino JP, Redmond CK, et al. Endometrial cancer in tamoxifen-treated breast cancer patients: findings from the National Surgical Adjuvant Breast and Bowel Project (NSABP) B-14. *JNCI* 1994;86:527–537.

Fisher B, Costantino JP, Wickerham DL, et al. Surgical Adjuvant Breast and Bowel Project P-1 study. *JNCI* 1998;90:1371–1388.

Fisher B, Dignam J, Bryant J, et al. Five versus more than five years of tamoxifen therapy for breast cancer patients with negative lymph nodes and estrogen receptor-positive tumors. *JNCI* 1996;88:1529–1542.

Fisher B, Dignam J, Mamounas EP, et al. Sequential methotrexate and fluorouracil for the treatment of node-negative breast cancer patients with estrogen receptor-negative tumors: eight-year results from National Surgical Adjuvant Breast and Bowel Project (NSABP) B-13 and first report of findings from NSABP B-19 comparing methotrexate and fluorouracil with conventional cyclophosphamide, methotrexate, and fluorouracil. *J Clin Oncol* 1996;14:1982–1992.

Fisher B, Redmond C, Fisher ER, et al. Relative worth of estrogen or progesterone receptor and pathologic characteristics of differentiation as indicators of prognosis in node-negative breast cancer. *J Clin Oncol* 1988;6:1076–1087.

Fisher B, Redmond C, Jimitrov NV, et al. A randomized clinical trial evaluating sequential methotrexate and fluorouracil in the treatment of node negative breast cancer who have estrogen negative tumor. *N Engl J Med* 1989;320:473–478.

Fisher B, Redmond C, Legault-Poisson S, et al. Postoperative chemotherapy and tamoxifen compared with tamoxifen alone in the treatment of positive-node breast cancer patients aged 50 years and older with tumors responsive to tamoxifen: results from the National Surgical Adjuvant Breast and Bowel Project B-16. *J Clin Oncol* 1990;8:1005–1018.

Fisher B, Redmond C, Poisson R, et al. Eight-year results of a randomized clinical trial comparing total mastectomy and lumpectomy with or without irradiation in the treatment of breast cancer. *N Engl J Med* 1989;320:822–828.

Fisher B, Slack N, Katrych D, et al. Ten year follow-up results of patients with carcinoma of the breast in a cooperative clinical trial evaluating surgical adjuvant chemotherapy. *Surg Gynecol Obstet* 1975;140:528–534.

Fowble BL, Solin LJ, Schultz DJ, et al. Ten year results of conservative surgery and irradiation for stage I and II breast cancer. *Int J Radiat Oncol Biol Phys* 1991;21:269–277.

Gail MH, Brinton LA, Byar DP, et al. Projecting individualized probabilities of developing breast cancer for white females who are being examined annually. *JNCI* 1989;81:1879–1886.

Gasparini G, Weidner N, Bevilacqua P, et al. Tumor microvessel density, p53 expression, tumor size, and peritumoral lymphatic vessel invasion are relevant prognostic markers in node-negative breast carcinoma. *J Clin Oncol* 1994;12:454–466.

Goldberg RM, Loprinzi CL, O'Fallon JR, et al. Transdermal clonidine for ameliorating tamoxifen-induced hot flashes. *J Clin Oncol* 1994;12:155–158.

Goldhirsch A, Glick JH, Gelber RD, et al: Meeting highlights: International Consensus Panel on the Treatment of Primary Breast Cancer. Seventh International Conference on Adjuvant Therapy of Primary Breast Cancer. *J Clin Oncol* 2001;19: 3817–3827.

Henderson IC, Berry D, Demetri G, et al. Improved disease-free and overall survival from the addition of sequential paclitaxel but not from the escalation of doxorubicin dose level in the adjuvant chemotherapy of patients with node-positive breast cancer. *Proc Am Soc Clin Oncol* 1998;17:101a.

Hudis C, Riccio L, Seidman A, et al. Lack of increased cardiac toxicity with sequential doxorubicin and paclitaxel. *Cancer Invest* 1998;16:67–71.

Ingle JN, Krook JE, Green SJ, et al. Randomized trial of bilateral oophorectomy versus tamoxifen in premenopausal women with metastatic breast cancer. *J Clin Oncol* 1986;4:178–185.

Mansour EG, Gray R, Shatila AH, et al. Survival advantage of adjuvant chemotherapy in high-risk node-negative breast cancer: ten-year analysis—an intergroup study. *J Clin Oncol* 1998;16: 3486–3492.

McGuire WL, Tandon AK, Allred DC, et al. How to use prognostic factors in axillary node-negative breast cancer patients. *JNCI* 1990;82:1006–1015.

Mouridsen H, Gershanovich M, Sun Y, et al. Superior efficacy of letrozole (Femara) versus tamoxifen as first-line therapy for postmenopausal women with advanced breast cancer: results of a phase III study of the International Letrozole Breast Cancer Group. *J Clin Oncol* 2001;19:2596–2606.

National Institutes of Health Consensus Development Panel. National Institutes of Health Consensus Development Conference Statement: Adjuvant Therapy for Breast Cancer, November 1–3, 2000. *JNCI* 2001;93:979–989.

Nattinger AB, Gottlieb MS, Veum J, et al. Geographic variation in the use of breast-conserving treatment for breast cancer. *N Engl J Med* 1992;326:1102–1107.

Osborne CK. Tamoxifen in the treatment of breast cancer. *N Engl J Med* 1998;339:1609–1618.

Peters WP, Ross M, Vredenburgh JJ, et al. High-dose chemotherapy and autologous bone marrow support as consolidation after standard-dose adjuvant therapy for high-risk primary breast cancer. *J Clin Oncol* 1993;11:1132–1143.

Phillips K-A, Andrulis IL, Goodwin PH. Breast carcinomas arising in carriers of mutations in BRCA1 or BRCA2: Are they prognostically different? *J Clin Oncol* 1999;17:3653–3663.

Pickle LW, Johnson KA. Estimating the long-term probability of developing breast cancer. *JNCI* 1989;81:1854–1855.

Pritchard KI, Paterson AH, Paul NA, et al. Increased thromboembolic complications with concurrent tamoxifen and chemotherapy in a randomized trial of adjuvant therapy for women with breast cancer. *J Clin Oncol* 1996;14:2731–2737.

Rivkin SE, Green S, Metch B, et al. Adjuvant CMFVP vs tamoxifen vs concurrent CMFVP and tamoxifen for postmenopausal, node-positive, and estrogen receptor-positive breast cancer patients: a Southwest Oncology Group study. *J Clin Oncol* 1994;12:2078–2085.

Rizzieri DA, Vredenbrugh JJ, Jones R, et al. Prognostic and predictive factors for patients with metastatic breast cancer undergoing aggressive induction therapy followed by high dose chemotherapy with autologous stem cell support. *J Clin Oncol* 1999;17:3064–3074.

Rosen PP, Groshen S, Kinne DW, et al. Factors influencing prognosis in node-negative breast carcinoma: analysis of 767 T1N0M0/T2N0M0 patients with long-term follow-up. *J Clin Oncol* 1993; 11:2090–2100.

Rosen PP, Groshen S, Saigo PE, et al. Pathological prognostic factors in stage I (T1 N0 M0) and stage II (T1 N1 M0) breast carcinoma: a study of 644 patients with median follow-up of 18 years. *J Clin Oncol* 1989;7:1239–1251.

Rutqvist LE, Mattsson A. Cardiac and thromboembolic morbidity among postmenopausal women with early-stage breast cancer in a randomized trial of adjuvant tamoxifen. *JNCI* 1993;85:1398.

Sigurdsson H, Baldetorp B, Borg A, et al. Indicators of prognosis in node-negative breast cancer. *N Engl J Med* 1990;322:1045–1053.

Slamon DJ, Godolphin W, Jones LA, et al. Studies of HER-2/neu proto-oncogene in human breast and ovarian cancer. *Science* 1989;244:707–712.

Slamon DJ, Leyland-Jones B, Shak S, et al. Use of chemotherapy plus a monoclonal antibody against HER2 for metastatic breast cancer that overexpresses HER2. *N Engl J Med* 2001;344:783–792.

Taylor SG IV, Gelman RS, Falkson G, et al. Combination chemotherapy compared to tamoxifen as initial therapy for stage IV breast cancer in elderly women. *Ann Intern Med* 1986;104:455–461.

Van Dam FSAM, Schagen SB, Muller MJ, et al. Impairment of cognitive function in women receiving adjuvant treatment for high-risk breast cancer: high-dose versus standard-dose chemotherapy. *JNCI* 1998;90:210–218.

Veronesi U, Saccozzi R, Del Vecchio M, et al. Comparing radical mastectomy with quadrantectomy, axillary dissection, and radiotherapy in patients with small cancers of the breast. *N Engl J Med* 1981;305:6–11.

Zujewski J, Liu ET. The 1998 St. Galens consensus conference: an assessment. *JNCI* 1998;90:1587–1589.

11

Gynecologic Cancer

C. O. Granai, Walter H. Gajewski, Robert D. Legare, and Mary Gordinier

The ability to help women with "gynecologic cancer," a designation today better thought of as cancers uniquely affecting women, has evolved considerably in the last several decades. Improvements have come consequent to scientific and medical advances as well as humanistic, societal, political, even cultural changes. Together they have made possible superior oncologic therapy, itself offered in environments dedicated to women and their special needs. Fulfilling this potential takes a committed, focused, genuinely expert multidisciplinary team, with shared ideals and human values.

As a first step, all women's cancers, indeed all cancers, should be reviewed by a prospective, multidisciplinary Tumor Board, whose core membership possess sincere expertise—in this case, expertise about women's cancers. Once the woman and her family understand the Tumor Board's recommendations and their rationales, along with the alternatives, it is for her to decide on how she wishes to proceed. Usually patients will follow the Tumor Board's recommendations, but either way, the oncology team must be prepared to be supportive and helpful.

To the extent possible, today's cancer treatment should be given in thoughtful environments dedicated to the specific constituents they wish to serve. Women receiving oncologic therapy appreciate and benefit from the deeper sense of caring conveyed by a total environment, where the clinical staff understands them and their specific type of malignancy and where the physical space, aesthetics, support services, and philosophy of the program are dedicated to them.

They achieve the sense of being truly cared for if they believe they are receiving the best evidence-based and technical care medicine has to offer. Opening dialogues that can lead to addressing questions about alternative medicine and providing complementary options (i.e., massage, art, poetry, acupuncture, pet companions) are as enhancing of care as of the relationship between patients, families, and the medical team. Patients rarely leave conventional care when their medical team is actively open to wide-ranging, nonjudgmental discussions and new ideas. Not infrequently, it turns out that some of those same ideas, if incorporated into the patient's overall treatment plan, serve to improve patient satisfaction, comfort, and quality of life by enhancing "the moment" relative to what would otherwise be.

I. Carcinoma of the cervix. Cervical cancer is the most common female malignancy worldwide but ranks only 10th in the United States. The 70% reduction in cervical cancer deaths in the United States in the last 30 years is largely the result of effective screening by Papanicolaou's (Pap) smear, which identifies disease while preinvasive. Nevertheless, there will be an estimated

13,700 new cases and 4,900 deaths from invasive cervical cancer in the United States in 2002. Cervical cancer correlates with sexual intercourse at an early age, multiple sex partners, high parity, human papilloma virus infection (particularly types 16 and 18), human immunodeficiency virus infection, and cigarette smoking. The established relationship with sexual and social behavior permits squamous cancer of the cervix to be categorized as a sexually or socially transmitted disease and thus is theoretically preventable.

  A. Pathology and patterns of spread

    1. Histology. More than 80% of cervical cancers are of the squamous cell histologic type. The remaining 20% are principally adenocarcinomas. Squamous cell cancer arises from the exocervix, whereas adenocarcinoma is from the columnar epithelium of the endocervix. Less common cervical malignancies also occur, each having unique biologic behaviors. For example, adenosquamous and adenoid cystic carcinomas are aggressive tumors and thus have a relatively poor prognosis. Adenoid basal and verrucous cancers behave in the opposite fashion. More virulent yet is the infrequent small cell cancer of neuroendocrine origin, which sometimes presents with confusing paraendocrine symptoms. Lymphomas, carcinomas, melanomas, and primary sarcomas (e.g., embryonal rhabdomyosarcomas, leiomyosarcomas, malignant mixed müllerian tumors) also develop on the cervix. Finally, not all neoplasms on the cervix are primary from that site. Metastasis to the cervix can arise from the uterus, breast, colon, and kidney. Discussed here are the management principles pertaining to squamous cell cancer only.

    2. The continuum of neoplasia. Cervical neoplasia is a disease continuum, spanning from mild dysplasia (cervical intraepithelial neoplasia type I) to invasive cancer. Not uncommonly, preinvasive neoplasia, particularly that of low grade, spontaneously stabilizes or resolves, but rapid, unpredictable progression to malignancy can also occur. The next step beyond the highest degree of preinvasive neoplasia is microinvasion. Expert opinions differ on what parameters best define this lesion. Fundamental to all concepts of microinvasion, however, is localized, readily resectable disease without or with very low risk of metastases.

    Unlike squamous neoplasia, in which there is a clear-cut histologic demarcation (the basement membrane) beyond which the invasion becomes obvious, there are no equivalent histologic boundaries within the cervical stroma by which to delineate degrees of glandular (*adeno*) neoplasia. This makes diagnostic distinctions between preinvasion, microinvasion, and true invasion more precarious with glandular histologies.

    3. Spread pattern. Expanding through the cervical stroma, the squamous cancer extends onto the vagina and uterus and laterally into the paracervical and parametrial soft tissues, ultimately to involve the pelvic sidewall and obstruct the ureters. Direct extension into the bladder or rectum is uncommon. While invading the stroma, the cancer can enter lymphatic vessel spaces. Consequent spread usually follows an orderly sequence, first to the obturator and iliac lymph nodes and then with subsequent ascension to the aortic and supraclavicular groups. Hematogenous dissemination is found in 10% of patients. Distant sites of metastases include the lungs, mediastinum, bone, and liver.

B.   Diagnosis and staging

1.   Clinical manifestations. Because of effective screening, many diagnoses of cervical cancer are made before the onset of symptoms. However, intermenstrual bleeding, postcoital bleeding (classic, but uncommon), postmenopausal bleeding, and vaginal discharge can result from friable, ulcerated, often necrotic cervical epithelium. Pelvic, lumbosacral, gluteal, and back pains are worrisome symptoms for advanced disease (e.g., nodal metastasis). Hematuria and rectal bleeding rarely occur but suggest organ involvement.

2.   Diagnosis. The diagnosis of cervical cancer can be proved only by biopsy, not by Pap smear. Although the correlation between Pap smear (cytology) and biopsy (histology) results is good (60% to 85%), cytology *per se* is insufficient for diagnosing any degree of cervical neoplasia, let alone malignancy. Practically, an abnormal Pap smear should be considered a "red flag," a warning of possible neoplasia, thus demanding further investigation (e.g., colposcopy and biopsy). Although most cervical neoplasia is identified through abnormal Pap smears, any gross cervical lesions should be sampled for biopsy.

3.   Staging. In contrast to ovarian and endometrial cancers, which are staged surgically, cervical cancer is staged clinically (Table 11.1). Surgically obtained information may be used for treatment planning and risk stratification, but it does not change clinical stage. The most important determinant of stage in cervical cancer is the clinical examination, with particular emphasis on the pelvic and rectal examination. Chest x-ray studies and evaluation of the ureters using computed tomography (CT) are also done. In clinically early disease, cystoscopy and proctoscopy are neither helpful nor cost effective.

C.   Treatment

1.   Early clinical disease

a.   Stage IA. Stage IA1 disease can be treated by either cone biopsy, simple total hysterectomy, or modified radical hysterectomy. Theoretically, the same option exists for stage IA2 disease, but the recurrence rate is higher after cone biopsy compared with radical surgery. To the extent that it exists, the extra risk inherent in pursuing a minimalistic treatment strategy (i.e., cone biopsy) must be assumed by the well-informed patient, who typically makes the choice because of the strong desire to preserve fertility.

b.   Stages IB and IIA. For stages IB and IIA disease, either a radical hysterectomy with pelvic lymphadenectomy or radical radiation therapy (whole pelvis plus brachytherapy), sometimes with sensitizing chemotherapy, whose full application remains to be better defined, can be used. Both approaches produce comparable 5-year survival rates. Surgery, however, offers certain advantages: less long-term morbidity, ovarian conservation, better posttreatment

Table 11.1. 1995 FIGO staging (Montreal) for carcinoma of the cervix uteri

Stage grouping	Definition
I	The carcinoma is strictly confined to the cervix (extension to the corpus should be disregarded).
IA	Invasive cancer identified only microscopically. All gross lesions even with superficial invasion are stage IB cancers. Invasion is limited to measured stromal invasion with maximum depth of 5 mm and no wider than 7 mm.
IA-1	Measured invasion of stroma no greater than 3 mm in depth and no wider than 7 mm.
IA-2	Measured invasion of stroma greater than 3 mm, no greater than 5 mm, and no wider than 7 mm. The depth of invasion should not be more than 5 mm, taken from the base of the epithelium, either surface or glandular, from which it originates. Preformed space involvement (vascular or lymphatic) should not alter the staging but should be specifically recorded to determine whether it should affect treatment decisions in the future.
IB	Clinical lesions confined to the cervix or preclinical lesions greater than those of stage IA.
IB-1	Clinical lesions no greater than 4 cm in size.
IB-2	Clinical lesions greater than 4 cm in size.
II	The carcinoma extends beyond the cervix but has not extended to the pelvic wall. The carcinoma involves the vagina but does not extend as far as the lower third.
IIA	No obvious parametrial involvement.
IIB	Obvious parametrial involvement.
III	The carcinoma has extended to the pelvic wall. On rectal examination, there is no cancer-free space between the tumor and the pelvic wall. The tumor involves the lower third of the vagina. All cases with hydronephrosis or nonfunctioning kidney are included unless they are known to be due to other causes.
IIIA	No extension to the pelvic wall.
IIIB	Extension to the pelvic wall and/or hydronephrosis or nonfunctioning kidney.
IV	The carcinoma has extended beyond the true pelvis or has clinically involved the mucosa of the bladder or rectum. A bullous edema as such does not permit a case to be allotted to stage IV.
IVA	Spread of the growth to adjacent organs.
IVB	Spread to distant organs.

sexual function, and surgicopathologic staging permitting risk stratification.

c.   Risk stratification. Nodal metastasis significantly worsens prognosis. In stage IB cervical cancer, factors correlating with pelvic node involvement are lesion size, tumor grade, vascular and lymphatic space invasion (VSI), parametrial extension, and depth of stromal invasion. Microvessel counts are also being investigated as risk predictors. High-risk patients identified by surgical staging are candidates for adjuvant treatment, preferably on protocol. Recent Gynecologic Oncology Group (GOG) trials showed decreased recurrence rates among patients with two or more high-risk factors who received postoperative radiotherapy with sensitizing chemotherapy. The matter still remains controversial, however.

d.   Special cases. The optimal therapy for the bulky cervical cancer (stage IB2) is controversial. Survival rates with either radical surgery or radiation therapy are substantially less than with smaller stage IB cancers. A recent GOG study showed a significant survival advantage when weekly infusions of cisplatin were added to pelvic radiotherapy followed by radical hysterectomy. Neoadjuvant (up-front) chemotherapy followed by either radical surgery or radiation therapy is being used by some as an alternative approach in managing these difficult lesions.

Other special cases of cervical cancer include cervical cancer and neoplasia occurring during pregnancy, carcinoma of the cervical stump after supracervical hysterectomy, the unexpected finding of cancer after "benign hysterectomy," cervical cancer and a coexisting pelvic mass or pelvic inflammatory disease, cervical cancer and ureteral obstruction, and cervical cancer and acquired immune deficiency syndrome. Each of these complex situations needs appropriate, often unique, interventions (or no intervention) in the context of the actual tumor biology, anatomic circumstances, and the specific patient.

2.   Advanced disease

a.   Stage IIB to IVA cervical cancers have, historically and by default, have been managed by radical radiation therapy. The modest 5-year survival rates reported vary with stage and institution but generally range from 20% to 60%. Recent results from five Phase III trials show an overall survival advantage for cisplatin-based therapy given concurrently with radiation therapy (cisplatin 40 mg/m^2 weekly or cisplatin 75 mg/m^2 plus 5-fluorouracil 4,000 mg/m^2 over 96 h every 3 weeks). Such treatment has become the new standard for stage IIB to IIIB disease. With stage IVA cervical cancer, barring evidence of distant or unresectable disease, cure is also occasionally possible using ultraradical surgery (i.e., primary pelvic exenteration).

b.   Stage IVB disease is essentially incurable. Accordingly, treatment is individualized and palliative.

c.   Chemotherapy in advanced disease, using either single agents or combinations, can produce short-term responses. Cisplatin has been considered the most active single agent; other drugs that demonstrate a response rate of 15% or more include vinorelbine, paclitaxel, irinotecan, carboplatin, bleomycin, vincristine, mitomycin, ifosfamide, fluorouracil, etoposide, and methotrexate. Combination chemotherapy such as cisplatin and ifosfamide with or without bleomycin or paclitaxel and carboplatin has been studied and may yield higher response rates. At present, however, the use of combination regimens is controversial because the role of chemotherapy in this setting is currently palliative, and a survival advantage of combination chemotherapy over single-agent chemotherapy has not been conclusively demonstrated. With recurrent squamous cancer, cisplatin produces a 20% to 30% response rate, 10% of cases being complete responses. No clear dose–response relation has been demonstrated, so cisplatin 50 mg/m^2 IV every 3 weeks is typically recommended.

   d.   New approaches to advanced disease. A recent randomized trial for stages IB2 to III, which included intent-to-treat analysis, has reported that especially for stages IB to IIB, there was a significant 5-year survival and progression-free survival advantage for the group receiving neoadjuvant chemotherapy and radical hysterectomy compared to radical radiation therapy. Use of neoadjuvant chemotherapy in certain clinical situations seems logical, and reports have been promising; but the result of five randomized trials comparing neoadjuvant chemotherapy followed by irradiation with irradiation alone have failed to show the hoped-for improvement in outcome when neoadjuvant chemotherapy was added to radical radiotherapy. This has been true despite the high response rates of locally advanced cancer to chemotherapy. Studies are continuing, however; and the concept is sometimes employed against local/regional, aggressive cancers where extraordinary therapies are the only hope for maximal outcome.

3.   Recurrent cervical cancer. The recurrence rate for all cervical cancer is 35%. In contrast, only 10% to 20% of patients with stage IB disease have recurrence. This rate increases to 45% to 60%, however, when lymph nodes contain metastasis. Recurrences generally develop within 2 to 3 years of primary treatment, and most of these patients die from disease. Recurrent cervical cancer must be treated within the constraints presented by the site of the recurrence and the type of treatment originally rendered (i.e., surgery, radiation therapy, or both). Sites of recurrence are categorized as local/central (resectable, thus potentially curable), regional (in the pelvis but unresectable), extending to the sidewall or to lymph nodes (rarely curable), and distant.

   Recurrence after primary surgery can be managed with radiation therapy (likely with sensitizing chemotherapy). Salvage rates as high as 25% to 50% are reported. A curative alternative for a true central recurrence, particularly in previously irradiated patients, is the select use of ultraradical surgery. Employed under ideal clinical circumstances, pelvic exenteration offers a 30% to 60% 5-year survival rate (i.e., if complete, negative-margin resection proves possible). Because of the high surgical complication rate and the risk of major long-term physical and psychological morbidity, exenterative surgery is indicated only with the intent of cure.

D.   Survival. The overall 5-year survival rate for cervical cancer is only 50%. Stage is the most significant predictor. The survival rate for stage IA is 98%, stages IB and IIA 75% to 85%, stage IIB 55%, stage III 10% to 50%, and stage IVB essentially none. Discouragingly, despite improvements in radiotherapy technology and better delineation of disease, survival rates have not improved in 30 years.

II.   Endometrial cancer. Endometrial cancer is the most common gynecologic pelvic malignancy in developed nations. There was an estimated 39,300 new cases and 6,600 deaths from endometrial cancer in the United States in 2002. Because endometrial cancer usually presents as postmenopausal bleeding, any amount of postmenopausal bleeding is suspect. Epidemiologic risk factors for endometrial cancer include obesity, nulliparity, diet, advancing age, and unopposed estrogen use. The use of oral contraception and, surprisingly, smoking are negatively correlated. The diagnosis is established by simple, cost-effective, endometrial biopsy performed in the office. The physical examination and Pap smear are not usually contributory to diagnosis.

A.   Pathology and patterns of spread

1.   Histology. The dominant histologic type of endometrial cancer is endometrioid. Together with the other less common adenocarcinomas of the endometrium (adenosquamous, papillary serous, and clear cell cancers), they constitute 90% of cases of "uterine cancer." Differentiating among the adenocarcinoma subtypes is important because each has its own biologic behavior and outcome, which in turn impact surgical management as well as the need for adjuvant therapies. For example, the patterns of spread and the 90% 5-year survival rate for early-stage endometrioid cancer differ greatly from those of papillary serous and clear cell carcinomas, which have 40% and 44% survival rates, respectively.

2.   Patterns of spread. Endometrioid carcinoma first invades the myometrium and then the vascular and lymphatic space. Metastases to the pelvic lymph nodes and periaortic lymph nodes follow. The vagina is another common site of lymphatic spread. Thus, metastases to the vagina usually represent only the "visible tip of the iceberg," rather than an innocuous, truly isolated lesion. The presence of simultaneous, but occult, lymphatic metastasis accounts for the high failure rate of treatment focused only on the obvious vaginal site. In another means of dissemination, malignant cells can exfoliate from endometrial primary tumor and implant throughout the peritoneal cavity, especially with serous or clear cell histologies. Hematogenous metastases to the lungs, liver, bone, and brain are usually late-occurring events. Concomitant endometrioid cancer found in both the endometrium and the ovaries is surprisingly frequent, up to 15%. Distinguishing whether the simultaneous involvement of organs represents metastasis, one site to the other, or two separate stage I primary tumors has therapeutic relevance.

B. Pretreatment evaluation

 1. Diagnostic tests. In clinically early-stage endometrial cancer, few preoperative tests are fruitful. Still, chest x-ray and CT studies are generally obtained to look for advanced disease. CA 125 levels are occasionally elevated in endometrial neoplasms and, if so, are useful in monitoring treatment response. Cystoscopy, sigmoidoscopy, and pelvic ultrasound invariably show negative results and hence should be avoided unless symptoms indicate otherwise. Magnetic resonance imaging is sensitive in determining the extent and depth of myometrial invasion but is expensive and rarely alters current treatment.

 2. Staging. Federation Internationale de Gynecologie et d'Obstetrique (FIGO) staging of endometrial cancer is surgical (Table 11.2). Stage according to disease distribution is further subcategorized by tumor grade. Because most endometrial cancers are heralded by abnormal bleeding, diagnosing the disease in a low stage is facilitated; consequently, 75% are stage I and 15% stage II at the time of diagnosis.

 3. Risk stratification. Risk factors in stage I endometrial cancers are tumor grade (G1, G2, G3), depth of myometrial invasion, VSI, age, hormonal receptor status, tumor histology, deoxyribonucleic acid (DNA) ploidy, and S-phase fraction. In a major GOG study of stage I endometrioid cancer, there was only a 3% risk of pelvic nodal involvement for G1 lesions compared with 18% for G3 lesions. Without myometrial invasion, the risk of nodal metastases was 1%. This risk increased to 25% with myometrial penetration to the outer third. Among patients with cancer showing no VSI, 7% had pelvic nodal metastases compared with 27% if there was VSI. The significance of finding malignant cells on cytology of abdominal and

Table 11.2. FIGO staging for carcinoma of the corpus uteri

Stage	Definition
I	Tumor confined to the uterine fundus
IA G123	Tumor limited to the endometrium
IB G123	Invasion to less than one-half of the myometrium
IC G123	Invasion to more than one-half of the myometrium
II	Tumor extends to the cervix
IIA G123	Endocervical glandular involvement only
IIB G123	Cervical stromal invasion
III	Regional tumor spread
IIIA G123	Tumor invades the serosa and/or adnexa and/or has positive peritoneal cytology
IIIB G123	Vaginal metastases
IIIC G123	Metastases to pelvic and/or periaortic lymph nodes
IV	Bulky pelvic disease or distant spread
IVA G123	Tumor invasion of the bladder and/or bowel mucosa
IVB	Distant metastases, including intra-abdominal and/or inguinal lymph nodes

pelvic washings in the absence of other risk factors is controversial. Still, it appears that "positive" washings are an independent marker for aggressive disease, thus carrying a worse prognosis (e.g., risk of occult, current, or later-developing extrapelvic disease). In recognition of this fact, FIGO has upstaged patients with malignant cytology to stage IIIA. (The best management for the situation is less clear, however.)

After surgery, the combined power of all the pathologically confirmed prognostic factors is used for risk stratification, and in that process, the need for adjuvant treatment is best determined.

C.   Management
1.   Surgery. The standard central treatment for endometrial cancer is surgery. Although historically, preoperative radiation therapy was widely used, for good reason, that practice has been abandoned.

Surgery for endometrial cancer consists of exploratory laparotomy, cytologic washings, extrafascial total hysterectomy, bilateral salpingo-oophorectomy, and staging. A selective approach is often taken to decide on the extent of staging. An intraoperative assessment is made of myometrial invasion and disease distribution; then, based on the presence or absence of those risk factors, pelvic and para-aortic lymph node sampling and other staging can be performed as suggested by FIGO. Specific adjustments in the operation are made according to histology, tumor grade, and intraoperative findings (e.g., if deep myometrial invasion exists).

2.   Rare inoperable cases. For the rare patient deemed absolutely inoperable for medical reasons, radiation therapy (external beam and intracavitary implants) as sole treatment becomes a not-so-unmorbid alternative. The cure rate achieved by radiation therapy alone, even with early-stage disease, is inferior to that of hysterectomy. Hormonal therapy as a medical alternative is rarely of sustained benefit.

3.   Postoperative management
  a.   Adjuvant treatment. Based on the surgical pathology, patients with a poor prognosis can be identified. Although proof of survival benefit is lacking, pelvic irradiation is nevertheless the most common type of adjuvant treatment given to patients considered at high risk for proven enhancement of local control. At Women and Infants Hospital/Brown University, adjuvant treatment protocols for stage I endometrioid cancer currently employ postoperative whole-pelvis irradiation if there is deep myometrial invasion, VSI, G3 lesions, or extension to the endocervix stroma—assuming the lymph nodes are negative for cancer. If the lymph nodes have metastasis, extrauterine disease is present, or abdominal or pelvic washings contain malignant cells, then the potential rationale of adjuvant radiation therapy is less obvious. Therefore, we view such patients as better candidates for advanced-disease treatment, preferably on protocols.

  b.   Advanced-disease treatment
    (1)   Radiotherapy. Effective treatment for advanced endometrial cancer remains elusive. Lacking other op-

tions, pelvic radiation therapy is often tried, even with high-risk or high-stage regional disease. In this setting, radiation may palliate vaginal bleeding and pain. The generally poor outcome is understandable because treating a simultaneously bulky and diffuse malignant process with necessarily constrained, nontumoricidal radiation doses is bound to fail.

(2) Systemic therapy. Hormonal therapy, though logical and once highly touted, has thus far proved largely ineffective in controlled studies. Occasionally, however, meaningful responses to high-dose progestins do occur, particularly with late-recurring grade 1 tumors, at sites outside the irradiated field. Similarly, there are individual responses to systemic chemotherapy, though larger studies have yet to identify a routine role for potentially toxic current drugs (especially administered to symptom-free patients). Despite a lack of compelling response data, doxorubicin, considered the most active single agent, and other single agents with notable responses, including paclitaxel, cisplatin, cyclophosphamide, and irinotecan, are also emerging as agents with activity in this disease. Combinations of these agents may be given for their short-term benefit.

c. Recurrent disease. In select patients with a presumably limited recurrence of endometrial cancer, surgical restaging can be helpful in the final decision-making process. When possible, complete resection of the recurrent tumor (e.g., upper vaginectomy) appears to enhance subsequent salvage therapy. In general, however, for advanced or recurrent endometrial cancer, surgery and radiation therapy are of limited local control value, and systemic therapies are briefly palliative. Because individual good responses can occur, thoughtful chemotherapy, surgery, and radiation therapy, especially in the protocol setting, are justified for the informed patient wishing to try.

4. Special cases. A variety of less common uterine neoplasms can also occur. These need to be managed according to their own unique biology, which differs from that of the endometrioid histology.

a. Papillary serous carcinoma. Papillary serous carcinoma (PSC) of the endometrium behaves biologically more like the histologically identical PSC of the ovary. In an ovarian-like fashion, the endometrial PSC spreads and recurs diffusely on peritoneal serosal surfaces throughout the entire abdomen. Compared with its ovarian counterpart, however, responses to adjuvant platinum-based chemotherapy have been less substantial. Although large randomized controlled trials are lacking, several studies have shown a significant response with paclitaxel. Given the biologic behavior of this disease, a combination of pelvic radiotherapy and systemic adjuvant therapy (commonly paclitaxel and carboplatin) seems appropriate, though that aggressive treatment will have accompanying toxicities.

b. Other uterine malignancies. About 5% of uterine malignancies are sarcomas, which can emanate from the myometrium or the endometrial stroma. The mixed müllerian mesodermal tumor, formally called carcinosarcoma, is the most common type, followed by leiomyosarcoma and then endometrial stromal sarcomas.

In general, the primary treatment of mixed müllerian mesodermal tumor and leiomyosarcomas is surgery: total abdominal hysterectomy and bilateral salpingo-oophorectomy and staging, followed by consideration of adjuvant treatment. Both lesions recur locoregionally and distally; thus, adjuvant pelvic irradiation may reduce local recurrence but has no overall survival benefit. Although there is a need, there is currently no proven role for adjuvant chemotherapy in the treatment of these malignancies. Ifosfamide as a single agent or in combination with other drugs has traditionally received the greatest interest for treating advanced disease. Data suggest that taxanes in combination with platinum may also be helpful. Appropriate regimens include the following:

Ifosfamide 1.2 to 1.5 g/m^2 IV days 1 to 4 with mesna protection, *or*

Ifosfamide 1.2 to 1.5 g/m^2 IV days 1 to 4 with mesna protection, *plus*

Cisplatin 20 mg/m^2/day IV for 4 days every 3 weeks for eight cycles, *or*

Paclitaxel 175 mg/m^2 IV plus carboplatin area under the curve (AUC) 5 IV q21 days.

Other neoplasms (e.g., endometrial stromal tumors) occasionally develop in the uterine connective tissues as well. Most often, advanced or recurrent connective tissue tumors are of higher grade or are unresectable and thus must be treated systemically. Depending on hormonal receptor status and the type of histology, dramatic responses to hormonal ablation with high-dose progesterone such as megestrol acetate (Megace) 240 to 360 mg PO daily can occur. Others sometimes respond to chemotherapy including etoposide, dactinomycin, doxorubicin combinations, ifosfamide alone or with cisplatin, or cisplatin. Unfortunately, most high-grade sarcomas that are not cured surgically do not have prolonged responses to systemic treatment.

c.   Preserving fertility. Infrequently, a young woman desirous of fertility will develop a well-differentiated endometrioid adenocarcinoma of the endometrium. Barring evidence of advanced disease or magnetic resonance imaging suggesting myometrial invasion, well-informed patients can consider, as primary management, intensive hormonal therapy using high-dose progesterone (e.g., megestrol acetate 240 mg PO daily × 3 months) instead of hysterectomy. A thorough dilation and curettage with or without hysteroscopy follows the limited trial of hormones. If the cancer is resolved, reproductive assistance with ovulation stimulation can be done in hope of completing fertility desires before a need for hysterectomy develops. Generally, however, the odds for achieving a successful pregnancy under these circumstances are considered poor, although successful full-term deliveries have occurred.

III.   Fallopian tube cancer. Despite its direct physical and anatomic relation with the uterus, the rare tubal cancer is biologically and behaviorally more analogous to serous epithelial ovarian cancer. As a practical matter, fallopian tube cancer is staged and managed in a fashion similar to ovarian and not uterine malignancy. The diagnosis of a tubal cancer is usually fortuitous, or comes about retrospectively, after surgery is performed to address some other process. Preoperative symptoms are sometimes present, the classic being a profuse, intermittent watery vaginal discharge. Pelvic pain and an abnormal Pap smear suggesting adenocarcinoma that are not otherwise explained by routine testing such as colposcopy, endocervical curettage, and dilation and curettage can also lead to the diagnosis of fallopian tube cancer. Treatment is primarily surgery followed by postoperative chemotherapy for advanced disease, as in ovarian cancer.

IV.   Ovarian cancer. Ovarian cancer is the leading killer among female pelvic malignancies in the United States. In 2002, there were an estimated 23,300 new cases and 13,900 deaths. Contrary to the common perception, ovarian cancer is a heterologous group of biologically diverse neoplasms, often having only their anatomic site, the ovary, in common. Thus, broad generalizations about ovarian cancer are difficult but are best made by subcategorizing it into three groups based on embryologic origin.

  A.   Histologic types

   1.   Germ cell ovarian cancers. These malignancies typically occur in young women and are curable. They often present as an asymptomatic pelvic mass and, in the past, were usually lethal (e.g., immature teratomas, endodermal sinus tumors, dysgerminomas), even though they were confined to the ovary. Today's therapeutic breakthrough is curative chemotherapy, which, as an added benefit, does not typically compromise future fertility. After surgery, which is done to remove the involved ovary, establish the diagnosis, and stage the disease, the same agents effective against male germ cell tumors (e.g., bleomycin, etoposide, and cisplatin [BEP]) also work well against their less common female counterparts (see Chapter 12).

   2.   Stromal tumors. Stromal tumors of the ovary are rare anachronistic neoplasms occurring at any age but are stereotyped by their occasional sex hormone production. The uncommon, but often discussed, childhood granulosa cell tumor causing precocious puberty is a classic example. After surgical resection, the typical patient with a stromal tumor is observed without further intervention. This management strategy is chosen in part because most stromal tumors are benign or low grade (or of inscrutable malignant potential) and hence are resolved by simple removal. Recurrences can occur, sometimes many years later. If so, or with advanced or unresectable disease, chemotherapy (e.g., bleomycin, etoposide, and cisplatin; see Chapter 12) can be beneficial, even if not curative.

   3.   Epithelial ovarian cancer. Seventy percent of ovarian malignancies belong to the epithelial subgroup (e.g., serous, mucinous, endometrioid, clear cell). In contrast to germ cell tumors, epithelial ovarian cancer (EOC) generally occurs after menopause, is advanced at the time of diagnosis, and is rarely curable. The remainder of this section deals with the diagnosis and management of this common variety of ovarian cancer.

B. Diagnosis and screening of epithelial ovarian cancer

1. Early diagnosis. Diagnosing EOC at an early stage is a difficult, almost fortuitous occurrence because patients usually lack specific symptoms and findings. Little actual merit has come from attempts to screen healthy asymptomatic women for EOCs by using tumor markers with or without ultrasound. CA 125, alone or together with other tumor markers, lacks sufficient sensitivity and specificity for general screening. By its nature, the normal ovary has a dynamic cyclic cyst-forming physiology. By comparison, the chance of developing an EOC—an estimated lifetime risk of 1 in 70 (1.4%) U.S. women—is rare. Although today's ultrasound technology can detect even the tiniest ovarian cysts, uncertainty in the true pathology and need for intervention persist in all but the small "simple" cysts. Consequently, the National Cancer Institute (NCI) and others have concluded that routine screening programs for EOC are inappropriate as a current standard of care.

In contrast, however, two classes of serum tumor markers, monoclonal antibodies (e.g., CA 125 with EOCs) and peptide markers (e.g., α-fetoprotein with endodermal sinus tumors, müllerian-inhibiting factor, and inhibin with granulosa cell tumors) have proved useful in monitoring the treatment of, not the screening for, ovarian cancer. Additionally, preoperative evaluation of tumor markers and pelvic ultrasound may be useful in estimating risk of malignancy and aid in appropriate preoperative patient triage.

2. Risk stratification for screening. As mentioned, screening is not recommended for the general population. However, women deemed at high risk of developing EOC are still being advised to undergo extra surveillance and, at the extreme, prophylactic oophorectomy.

Risk stratification for EOC relies largely on the family history. Fortunately, lacking multiple first-degree relatives with EOC or repetitive generations (maternal or paternal) affected by the cancer, there is little (e.g., 5% to 7% lifetime risk) increase in risk. As part of a comprehensive cancer risk assessment program, some women with a personal or family history of breast, ovarian, or other cancers may elect to undergo genetic testing. During the last several years, multiple genes have been identified that, when mutant, increase the risk of developing ovarian cancer. The breast and ovarian cancer syndrome associated with germline *BRCA1* and *BRCA2* mutations is inherited in an autosomal dominant fashion. *BRCA1* and *BRCA2* function as tumor suppressor genes, based on loss of heterozygosity at this locus in tumors from families with familial ovarian cancer. The precise increase in risk associated with a mutation of *BRCA1* ranges from about 16% to 44%, and this is likely indicative of the specific mutation and penetrance. The risk of ovarian cancer in women harboring a mutation in the *BRCA2* gene is less, with a cumulative risk estimated to be less than 10% by 70 years of age. About 5% to 10% of ovarian cancer cases are likely attributable to such mutations. Women at high risk who harbor a *BRCA1* or *BRCA2* germline mutation and are older than 35 and beyond childbearing may consider prophylactic oophorectomy. Even after oophorectomy, however, serous carcinoma of the peritoneum, a disease similar to EOC, may still occur. Women who retain their ovaries should consider surveillance with gynecologic exam and transvaginal ultrasound with color flow Doppler twice yearly. Increased surveillance in the form of CA 125 levels can also be valuable, especially in the postmenopausal setting. We recommend patients that have a perceived or actual high risk be evaluated in a cancer risk assessment and prevention clinic where a multidisciplinary group of cancer specialists can help to determine actual risk and appropriate surveillance and prevention options. An increased risk of ovarian cancer is also associated with hereditary nonpolyposis colon cancer, with mutations documented in the mismatch repair genes *MSH2, MLH1, PMS1,* and *PMS2.* After risk has been defined by genetic counseling and, if desired, genetic testing, both nonsurgical and surgical options may be considered.

Epidemiologically, low parity with a history of infertility correlates with an increased risk of EOC. In contrast, high parity, tubal ligation, and oral contraceptive use negatively correlate with the risk of EOC, with oral contraceptive use reducing the relative risk up to 50%. Ironically, in this era that clamors for cancer prevention, the use of safe, low-dose birth control pills stands out as a real but often ignored option that may be immediately advantageous.

C. Management

1. The role of surgery. After an initial work-up and assessment of tumor markers, the key first step in the evaluation of a pelvic or abdominal mass with or without ascites is surgery. Indeed, with surgery comes the primary intervention, almost without regard for patient age, clinically presumed diagnosis, or stage of disease. Preoperative diagnostic tests such as needle biopsies and paracenteses are generally meddlesome, risk disseminating disease, and do not alter the ultimate need for surgery. The surgery allows for accurate diagnosis, thorough staging of disease, and, in abdominal disease, valuable tumor debulking.

a. Early disease and surgical staging. At laparotomy, the ovarian mass is resected intact if possible (i.e., without rupture), and diagnosis is established based on frozen-section evaluation (see Table 11.3). During surgery, 20% of EOCs appear visually or grossly confined to the ovary (i.e., stage I), but 30% to 50% of patients have extraovarian microscopic disease; thus the stage of disease is more advanced. Surgical staging then permits postoperative treatment to be realistically directed at the true EOC distribution.

b. Advanced disease. 80% of women have advanced disease (stage III or IV) at diagnosis. Most of the women have disease disseminating throughout the abdominal cavity with ascites. The finding of advanced EOC often portrays a

Table 11.3. FIGO staging system for ovarian cancer

Stage	Definition
I	Growth limited to the ovaries
IA	Growth limited to one ovary; no ascites; no tumor on the external surfaces; capsule intact
IB	Growth limited to both ovaries; no ascites; no tumor on the external surfaces; capsule intact
IC	Tumor either stage IA or IB but with tumor on the surface of one or both ovaries; or with capsule ruptured; or with ascites present containing malignant cells or with positive peritoneal washings
II	Growth involving one or both ovaries with pelvic extension
IIA	Extension and/or metastases to the uterus and/or tubes
IIB	Extension to other pelvic tissues
IIC	Tumor either stage IIA or IIB but with tumor on the surface of one or both ovaries; or with capsule ruptured; or with ascites present containing malignant cells or with positive peritoneal washings
III	Tumor involving one or both ovaries with peritoneal implants outside the pelvis and/or positive retroperitoneal or inguinal nodes; surface liver metastasis equals stage III; tumor is limited to the true pelvis but with histologically verified malignant extension to small bowel, large bowel, or omentum
IIIA	Tumor grossly limited to the true pelvis with negative nodes but with histologically confirmed microscopic seeding of abdominal peritoneal surfaces
IIIB	Tumor of one or both ovaries; histologically confirmed implants of abdominal peritoneal surfaces, none exceeding 2 cm in diameter; nodes negative
IIIC	Abdominal implants greater than 2 cm in diameter and/or positive retroperitoneal or inguinal nodes
IV	Growth involving one or both ovaries with distant metastases; if pleural effusion is present, there must be positive cytologic test results to allot a case to stage IV; parenchymal liver metastases equals stage IV

seemingly insurmountable picture of unresectable peritoneal and bulky pelvic and abdominal tumor. Fortunately, with the proper surgical approach, maximal tumor resection is possible in 80% of patients. Although the surgical risks of debulking are real and substantial, they seem justified by the improved survival experienced by patients whose tumor was optimally debulked relative to those in whom cytoreduction was suboptimal or not carried out. Therefore, if technically feasible, as is usual in experienced hands, optimal debulking remains the recommended surgical intervention for advanced EOC. The value of a focused expertise in managing EOC has been indirectly recognized by the NCI in their recommendation that where the potential for such cases exists, they be managed by fellowship-trained gynecologic oncologists.

2.   Chemotherapy. The need for postsurgery chemotherapy is determined in the context of histology, grade, stage, amount of residual tumor, and other prognostic factors such as DNA ploidy and proliferative index. With the exception of ovarian tumors of low malignant potential (or borderline ovarian tumors) generally treated with bilateral salpingo-oophorectomy alone or the occasional patient with stage I low-grade EOC, most patients benefit from postoperative therapy.

    a.   In early-stage, high-grade EOC, adjuvant chemotherapy has proved to prolong disease-free survival and possibly survival itself. Clear cell histology has also been identified as carrying a worse prognosis. For these patients, judicious adjuvant platinum-based therapy for three to six cycles is a current recommendation. In the past, IP ^{32}P has been used, but this has fallen out of favor, given the high incidence of bowel complications and equivalent survival rates when compared with platinum-based adjuvant chemotherapy. The GOG is formally addressing the issue of treatment duration in early-stage disease. Given the limited data on chemotherapy in early EOC, treatment regimens have been extrapolated from those used in advanced disease. Dosing and timing of treatment are identical to advanced disease, as outlined next.

    b.   Patients with more advanced disease are currently treated with a platinum and paclitaxel regimen after debulking surgery. Appropriate regimens include the following:

1. Carboplatin IV calculated with AUC of 5 to 7.5 (using the Jeliffe formula to calculate the estimated creatinine clearance and the Calvert formula for determining the AUC), *plus* paclitaxel 175 mg/m^2 IV over 3 h
2. Cisplatin 75 mg/m^2 IV, *plus* paclitaxel 135 mg/m^2 IV over 24 h (high neurotoxicity otherwise)
3. Carboplatin IV calculated with an AUC of 5 to 7.5 *plus* cyclophosphamide 500 to 600 mg/m^2 IV
4. Carboplatin IV calculated with an AUC of 5 to 7.5 *plus* docetaxel IV 60 to 80 mg/m^2

    Although paclitaxel and a platinum is the favored regimen, with improvement in response rate and in disease-free and overall survival rates when compared with cyclophosphamide and a platinum, the latter regimen may be favored in certain circumstances such as the diabetic patient who has significant peripheral neuropathy. A newer, and possibly more effective, alternative in this scenario is the taxane docetaxel (Taxotere) and carboplatin. The regimen is typically administered every 3 weeks for six cycles. Recent data suggest that docetaxel, substituting for paclitaxel in combination with carboplatin, may indeed have similar overall efficacy with the up-front treatment of

EOC. Thus, this regimen is an alternative for patients with neuropathy or inability to receive paclitaxel for other reasons.

Overall, the response rate to paclitaxel and carboplatin as first-line treatment of EOC (complete response plus partial response) is 70% to 80%, of which 50% are complete clinical responses and 30% complete pathologic responses. Patients are carefully monitored to determine treatment efficacy. Before receiving each cycle, they undergo physical examination, CA 125 determination, and less frequently other studies. If any parameter suggests treatment failure (i.e., progression of disease), the regimen is immediately curtailed, and strategic options that remain are presented to the patient. Patients opting for second-line treatment, on or off protocol, do so realistically and with a great concern for maintaining the best possible quality of life under difficult circumstances.

3.   Second-look laparotomy. Once a part of standard ovarian cancer treatment, second-look laparotomy is now offered only to selected patients at the end of primary treatment. Patients with a complete clinical response, a normal CA 125 level, and a normal-appearing CT scan may elect to undergo this additional surgery. Most typically, this is appropriate only in a protocol setting, in which the information gained from surgery is used to determine further protocol treatment. Despite a preoperative impression of no evidence of disease, about one-third of second-look laparotomies reveal gross disease. Although controversial, under such circumstances, if optimal secondary debulking is technically feasible without undue morbidity, the effort seems prudent. Of the remaining second-look laparotomies, one-third reveal microscopic residual disease and one-third are negative (i.e., all of the restaging biopsy and cytology studies are normal). Of patients with a pathologic complete response at second-look laparotomy, half are destined to recur.

4.   Intraperitoneal chemotherapy. While the role of IP chemotherapy is unclear in the management of bulky EOC, this therapy deserves mention for the optimally debulked patient. Although most studies fail to show an advantage to IP versus IV therapy, a recently completed GOG study showed improved recurrence-free survival in the IP arm, though there was no effect on ultimate survival. IP chemotherapy probably has the most value after a second-look laparotomy, when at most only microscopic disease was found. In the setting of exceedingly minimal drug-sensitive disease, the limited but very-high-dose drug intensity IP chemotherapy delivers to the peritoneal surfaces at risk of EOC is theoretically advantageous compared with IV administration. An appropriate regimen includes the following:

Cisplatin 100 mg/m^2 IP every 3 weeks × 6, *or* cisplatin 100 mg/m^2 IP, *plus* etoposide (VP-16) 350 mg/m^2 in 2 L of normal saline every 3 weeks × 6

Thiosulfate should be used during high-dose IP cisplatin to protect against nephrotoxicity.

Thiosulfate 4 g/m^2 IV bolus over 30 min at the start of IP therapy and then 2 g/m^2/h continuous IV infusion for a total of 6 h, has been employed.

D.   Follow-up. Even the patients with negative findings at second-look laparotomy may eventually develop recurrent disease. Recurrences are usually identified using CA 125 levels, sometimes months before diagnosed disease. As with initial disease, recurrences are most common within the abdomen. Current treatment has greatly improved survival and quality of life, but patients are not, in the strictest sense, cured. Time to recurrence can range greatly, from a few months to more than 15 years. Nevertheless, if patients are followed long enough, recurrences typically develop. It may be that a recurrence many years later is actually a new or second malignant process (e.g., *de novo* peritoneal disease) and not a treatment failure.

E.   Recurrent and persistent disease. Patients who demonstrate marker-only relapse (elevated CA 125) without symptoms and with no evidence of recurrence by exam or CT scan may be good candidates for observation or enrollment in a clinical trial. Once the decision to utilize chemotherapy is made, the choice of agent is based on balancing anticipated toxicities with scheduling, as various second-line chemotherapy regimens have yielded similar responses. If a patient is not platinum refractory, as defined by recurrence within 6 months of completing primary treatment, it is our bias to re-treat with platinum. Generally, single-agent therapy is used, unless the patient is on protocol or has had a long disease-free interval, where paclitaxel and carboplatin may be retried. Taxanes (paclitaxel and docetaxel) can be given if not used up front or if the patient has received a taxane up front but is not considered taxane resistant. Various schedules of taxanes and other agents with reported activity include the following (used as single agents, not in combinations):

- Paclitaxel 135 to 175 mg/m^2 IV over 3 h q21 days
- Paclitaxel 50 to 80 mg/m^2 IV over 1 h on days 1, 8, and 15 every 28 days
- Docetaxel 60 to 80 mg/m^2 IV every 21 days
- Docetaxel 25 to 35 mg/m^2 IV days 1, 8, and 15 every 28 days
- Liposomal doxorubicin (Doxil) 40 to 50 mg/m^2 IV every 3 weeks
- Topotecan 1.0 to 1.5 mg/m^2 IV on days 1 to 5 every 3 weeks
- Oral etoposide 50 mg/m^2 (30 mg/m^2 for prior radiotherapy) on days 1 to 21 every 28 days
- Gemcitabine 800 to 1,000 mg/m^2 IV on days 1, 8, and 15 every 28 days
- Vinorelbine 30 mg/m^2 IV on days 1, 8, and 15 every 28 days
- Tamoxifen 20 mg PO b.i.d.
- Oral altretamine (hexamethylmelamine, Hexalen) 260 mg/m^2

Responses with second-line treatment range from 20% to 40%. Most are short, but responses can occasionally exceed 1 to 2 years, justifying the concept of second-line chemotherapy for the informed patient who still wishes to try. High-dose therapy including peripheral blood stem cell transplant has not been found to improve survival in EOC. In the relapsed setting, patients should be encouraged to participate in clinical trials.

V.   Gestational trophoblastic neoplasm. Gestational trophoblastic disease encompasses a spectrum of neoplasms arising from fetal chorionic tissue. These tumors range from benign hydatidiform mole, to invasive or metastatic molar tissue, to malignant choriocarcinoma. All histologic classifications of this disease exhibit proliferation of cytotrophoblasts and syncytiotrophoblasts secreting human chorionic gonadotropin (β-hCG), which is a highly sensitive and specific tumor marker for gestational trophoblastic neoplasm (GTN). Historically, metastatic gestational choriocarcinoma was the first solid tumor to be cured with systemic chemotherapy. Today, most GTNs can be cured with systemic chemotherapy, even in the presence of widespread metastases.

A.   Hydatidiform mole. By far the most common form of GTN is the hydatidiform mole. Cytogenetic techniques have established two distinct molar syndromes: complete moles and partial moles. The complete moles arise from a paternal diploid genotype (90% 46XX, 6% 46XY) and constitute 95% of GTNs overall. In contrast, partial moles are associated with triploidy incorporating an extra haploid paternal chromosome (69XXY or 69XYY). All hydatidiform moles have the potential for developing malignant sequelae. Malignant transformation occurs in 20% of complete moles, but only 5% overall develop metastasis. Partial moles are less likely to develop malignant sequelae, usually in the form of nonmetastatic postmolar GTN.

1.   Initial management. The evaluation and primary management of both complete and partial hydatidiform moles consist of surgical evacuation of the uterus and close monitoring of postevacuation β-hCG levels until proof of cure or malignant sequelae occur. Often, the diagnosis of hydatidiform mole is established only retrospectively, following what was presumed to be an otherwise unremarkable spontaneous or elective abortion. If, however, the actual diagnosis is made before evacuating the uterus (typically by antenatal ultrasound), a physical examination, complete blood cell count, chest x-ray film, and baseline β-hCG measurement should be done preoperatively. Liver and thyroid function tests should be considered. Hydatidiform moles can present with a variety of severe medical syndromes; classic among them is early-gestational-age pre-eclampsia. Occasionally, ultrasound identifies a concomitant viable fetus or large ovarian theca lutein cysts. Uncommonly, metastatic disease is found, requiring a more extensive work-up and staging (to be discussed). Considering the complex array of problems associated with hydatidiform moles, if the diagnosis is known preoperatively, clinical management is best rendered by physicians with extensive knowledge of and experience in treating GTN.

2.   Monitoring. After evacuation of a molar pregnancy, serum β-hCG levels are monitored weekly until three consecutive measurements are normal, and then titers are followed monthly for 6 months. Normalization of the β-hCG typically occurs in 12 weeks. Throughout the entire observation period, patients are recommended to practice effective birth control to prevent pregnancy and its attendant β-hCG elevation, which confuses the situation.

3. Malignant transformation. Malignant transformation of a hydatidiform mole expresses itself as a prolonged plateau or rise in the β-hCG titer during the follow-up period. Under these circumstances, prompt referral to an oncologist is recommended to expedite further evaluation and treatment. Staging and management of these patients are described in the next section. The risk of specific hydatidiform mole undergoing malignant transformation may be predicted by a number of factors (e.g., signs of marked trophoblastic growth, including uterine size greater than dates, highly elevated β-hCG titer, prominent ovarian theca lutein cysts, toxemia, hyperthyroidism, age). At some centers, patients deemed at high risk of developing malignant sequelae are recommended to receive single-agent prophylactic chemotherapy to reduce the transformation risk. However, because the accuracy of prognostic factors is less than absolute and the transformation rate of hydatidiform mole overall is only 15%, most experts do not recommend or use prophylactic chemotherapy, even in high-risk patients. Instead, all patients are observed, and treatment is reserved until actual malignant transformation is documented.

B. Malignant gestational trophoblastic neoplasm. The FIGO staging system for GTN and that of the American College of Obstetricians and Gynecologists (ACOG) are shown in Tables 11.4 and 11.5. The ACOG staging has greater clinical utility because it facilitates treatment selection as well as classification. The ACOG staging utilizes the prognostic variables used in the World Health Organization classification system, including age, β-hCG titer, number and sites of metastases, antecedent pregnancy, interval between antecedent pregnancy and start of chemotherapy, and prior chemotherapy. There is a proposal by FIGO to revise its staging system, which will incorporate the risk factor scoring system of the World Health Organization with the anatomic staging system.

Unlike patients with hydatidiform moles, everyone with malignant GTN is ultimately treated with chemotherapy. Before treatment is initiated, patients undergo a more extensive

Table 11.4. FIGO staging for gestational trophoblastic neoplasia

Stage	Definition
I	Strictly confined to uterine corpus
II	Extends outside uterus but limited to genital structures
III	Extends to lungs with or without genital tract involvement
IV	All other metastatic sites

Modified from Pettersson F, et al. *Annual report on the results of treatment of gynecologic cancer. Vol. 19.* Stockholm: International Federation of Gynecology and Obstetrics, 1985.

**Table 11.5.   Modified American
College of Obstetricians and Gynecologists
classification of gestational trophoblastic neoplasm**

I. Nonmalignant GTN
  A. Hydatidiform mole
    1. Complete
    2. Incomplete
II. Malignant GTN
  A. Nonmetastatic GTN: no evidence of disease outside of uterus,
     not assigned to prognostic category
  B. Metastatic GTN: any metastases
    1. Good-prognosis metastatic GTN
       Short duration (<4 mo)
       Low β-hCG level (<40,000 mIU/mL serum β-hCG)
       No metastases to brain or liver
       No antecedent term pregnancy
       No prior chemotherapy
    2. Poor-prognosis metastatic GTN: any high-risk factor
       Long duration (>4 mo since last pregnancy)
       High pretreatment β-hCG level (>40,000 mIU/mL serum
       β-hCG)
       Brain or liver metastases
       Antecedent term pregnancy
       Prior chemotherapy

GTN, gestational trophoblastic neoplasm.

metastatic survey. For example, chest x-ray studies and CT of the chest, abdomen, brain, and pelvis are usually done. In the setting of a normal chest radiograph and a normal pelvic examination, however, metastases are rarely identified by any of the other more sophisticated tests. As such, clinicians experienced in GTN management often exercise cost-effective selectivity in the actual pretreatment evaluation of patients with malignant GTN.

The key treatment monitor for malignant GTN, as with all GTNs, is the serum β-hCG level. For surveillance, the complete blood cell count along with renal and liver function tests are also followed starting from their pretreatment baseline. As a further safeguard, a pretreatment ultrasound to exclude the possibility of an intrauterine pregnancy should be considered. Once the patient's malignant GTN data base is collected, permitting ACOG classification, malignant GTN is divided into two subsets according to the presence or absence of metastatic disease.

1.   Treatment of malignant nonmetastatic gestational trophoblastic neoplasm. Nonmetastatic GTN patients have nearly 100% cure rates using single-agent treatment chemotherapy with either methotrexate or dactinomycin. Methotrexate 0.4 mg/kg IM for 5 days with cycles repeated every 14 days has been standard, but methotrexate 40 mg/m^2

IM weekly has emerged as the preferred alternative because of its simplicity and relative lack of toxicity. An alternative schedule, giving methotrexate 100 mg IV bolus followed by 200 mg/m² over 12 h, has also been found to be effective with minimal toxicity. This regimen is repeated every 2 weeks if there is not a fall in the β-hCG titers. Whichever primary treatment regimen is selected for nonmetastatic GTN, additional controversy exists regarding the number of cycles of therapy required for disease resolution. In the United States, nonmetastatic GTN has been treated using repeated doses, given at short intervals, until one or two negative β-hCG titers are achieved. This tack is in recognition of the subpopulation of trophoblastic cells that can theoretically persist even when the β-hCG titer is zero.

Fortunately, few patients with malignant nonmetastatic GTN fail primary therapy. Most patients who fail methotrexate, however, can still be salvaged using single-agent dactinomycin. Dactinomycin is given in IV doses of 9 to 13 μg/kg/day for 5 days, recycled at 14-day intervals, or as a single IV bolus of 40 μg/kg (1.5 mg/m²) administered every 2 weeks. As mentioned, dactinomycin can also be used as an alternative to methotrexate as initial therapy of nonmetastatic disease. Patients prefer the latter, however, particularly because it does not cause alopecia.

For patients who do not desire continued fertility, hysterectomy is an alternative approach to the use of extended chemotherapy alone. The advantage of hysterectomy is that it reduces the total number of chemotherapy cycles needed to produce remission. However, given the high effectiveness of chemotherapy in treating GTN and the uncertainty of most young patients regarding their future fertility, the hysterectomy option is rarely taken.

2. Treatment of malignant metastatic gestational trophoblastic neoplasm. As defined by the ACOG criteria, patients with malignant metastatic GTN are further separated into low- and high-risk groups. This distinction is of major clinical relevance.

   a. Low-risk (good-prognosis) metastatic gestational trophoblastic neoplasm. This group is treated identically to nonmetastatic GTN discussed already. About two-thirds of low-risk patients have complete remission after single-agent therapy. Similar to their nonmetastatic peers, nearly all low-risk patients with metastases who develop disease resistant to initial therapy are subsequently cured with either an alternative single-agent or combination chemotherapy.

   b. High-risk (poor-prognosis) metastatic gestational trophoblastic neoplasm. Not all patients with metastatic high-risk GTN survive. High-risk metastatic GTNs are treated using multiagent chemotherapy. The overall success rate in high-risk disease ranges between 63% and 80% for multiagent chemotherapy using methotrexate-based and dactinomycin-based combinations. The two most commonly used combination regimens are outlined in Table 11.6. MAC (methotrexate, artino) chemotherapy (see Table 11.6) has

**Table 11.6.   Multiagent chemotherapy for
high-risk metastatic gestational trophoblastic disease**

MAC
    Days 1–5: Methotrexate 0.3 mg/kg IM (11.1 mg/m^2 IV)
                  Dactinomycin 8–10 μg/kg IV (0.30–0.37 mg/m^2)
                  Cyclophosphamide 250 mg IV
    Cycles repeated every 14–21 d
EMA-CO
  Course A
    Day 1:   Dactinomycin 0.5-mg IV bolus
                  Etoposide 100-mg/m^2 IV infusion over 30 min
                  Methotrexate 100-mg/m^2 IV bolus followed by
                      200-mg/m^2 IV infusion over 12 h
    Day 2:   Dactinomycin 0.5-mg IV bolus
                  Etoposide 100-mg/m^2 IV infusion over 30 min
                  Folinic acid (leucovorin), 15 mg IM/PO every 6 h for
                      four doses; begin 12 h after methotrexate infusion
                      is completed
    In patients with CNS metastases, increase methotrexate to
    1 g/m^2 as 24-h IV infusion. Increase folinic acid to 15 mg IM/PO
    every 8 h for nine doses, beginning 12 h after methotrexate
    infusion is completed.
  Course B
    Day 8:   Vincristine 1-mg/m^2 IV bolus
                  Cyclophosphamide 600-mg/m^2 IV infusion
    Day 15:   Recycle course A
                  Patients with CNS metastases or with high-risk
                  World Health Organization prognostic index sources
                  receive 12.5 mg of methotrexate by intrathecal injec-
                  tion on d 8.

Modified from Newlands ES, et al. Developments in chemotherapy for medium-
and high-risk patients with gestation trophoblastic tumors (1979–1984). *Br J
Obstet Gynaecol* 1986;93:63.

been the combination regimen most often reported in U.S.
centers. MAC frequently produces significant toxic side effects, particularly when cycled at intervals of less than 21
days. Because of MAC's severe toxicity, this regimen has
fallen out of favor in deference to less-toxic therapy. The alternative, increasingly preferred regimen is EMA-CO (see
Table 11.6), given on an outpatient basis. This combination
is attractive because its primary complete response rate
appears to be slightly better than that of MAC.

3.   Special situations. In general, high-risk metastatic
and special-situation GTN should be managed by centers experienced with the disease.

    a.   Central nervous system metastases. Patients with
    metastases to the central nervous system (CNS) have a
    greater risk of failing primary therapy than do patients
    with disease limited to the lungs or vagina. Radiation ther-

apy is often administered to patients with CNS metastasis in conjunction with their primary multiagent chemotherapy. Delivered in 10 equal fractions, 3,000 cGy has been safely administered with concurrent chemotherapy. Survival rates approximate 70% to 89% for patients treated with primary brain metastasis; however, the survival rate falls to 30% for those who receive salvage treatment for brain metastasis. Patients with CNS metastasis are at risk of neurologic decompensation caused by cerebral edema and acute hemorrhage. Therefore, dexamethasone is frequently used throughout their course of whole-brain radiation to minimize cerebral edema. Surgical extirpation is generally reserved for patients who demonstrate neurologic decompensation or those who require salvage therapy for recurrent CNS disease.

b.   Metastases to the liver. Liver metastases occur in 2% to 8% of patients presenting for primary therapy of metastatic GTN. Survival rates of 30% to 50% are reported for patients with primary involvement of the liver. Because these metastases tend to be highly vascular and death is frequently caused by intra-abdominal hemorrhage, whole-liver radiation to 2,000 cGy in conjunction with combination chemotherapy is frequently utilized to reduce the risk of hepatic hemorrhage.

c.   Drug-resistant disease. Patients with high-risk metastatic GTN who have not responded to primary chemotherapy have a very poor prognosis. Surgical excision of drug-resistant foci of disease should be considered in patients with limited systemic metastases and has been curative when all else has failed. β-hCG imaging techniques are available to identify small sites of drug-resistant disease. Regimens including cisplatin or etoposide (VP-16) and cisplatin plus ifosfamide plus etoposide in patients who did not respond to EMA-CO can be effective. Other experimental drugs can be considered as a last resort. Total parenteral nutrition and other systemic supports can be essential. In short, no therapeutic approach or support should be ignored on behalf of these compelling patients because they are young and salvage for cure is occasionally still possible.

4.   Posttreatment follow-up. Most women with malignant gestational trophoblastic disease can be cured using chemotherapy alone, thus preserving the potential for future childbearing. During the first year after completion of therapy, pregnancy is deferred so that β-hCG surveillance is not disrupted by an intercurrent pregnancy. Several series of women treated with simple chemotherapy for nonmetastatic or low-risk metastatic GTN have shown normal reproductive capacity after treatment.

VI.   Vulvar cancer. Vulvar cancer is relatively uncommon, accounting for only 4% to 5% of gynecologic malignancies. Squamous histology constitutes 85% of vulvar malignancies, but cancer of other cell types, including melanoma, Bartholin's gland adenocarcinoma, Paget's disease, and sarcoma, can occur as well. Because vulvar squamous cancers anatomically involve external skin and are slow growing, early diagnosis is possible and generally leads to high cure rates. Cancers of the other cell types can be more insidious and have variable prognoses.

A.   Pathology. Squamous cancers of the vulva typically occur in older, often elderly women and may be preceded by or associated with vulvar intraepithelial neoplasia. The risk factors correlating with disease include lower socioeconomic status, smoking, history of lower genital tract malignancies (particularly squamous neoplasia of the cervix), and immune-compromised states. Biologically, squamous cancers tend to be indolent, spread initially by direct extension to adjacent organs (e.g., to the vulva, vagina, urethra, anus), and at some point send tumor emboli to regional lymph nodes (inguinal and femoral nodes) and then to distant nodes. Hematogenous spread to the lungs and distant organs is usually a late finding.

B.   Diagnosis and work-up. Diagnosing vulvar cancer, based simply on gross appearance, is generally not possible. To the contrary, clinical impression is notoriously incorrect, both overestimating and underestimating the degree of neoplasia present. Therefore, a biopsy of abnormal vulvar lesions is needed for definitive diagnosis. After malignancy is diagnosed, establishing the lesion size and location as well as the regional lymph node status by clinical examination is important. Further work-up includes a thorough examination (e.g., colposcopy) of the cervix and vagina looking for concomitant neoplasia, CT of the pelvis and abdomen to evaluate disease and nodes, and a chest radiograph.

C.   Treatment

1.   Surgery. Because of the biologic behavior and anatomic site, vulvar cancer is often ideal for surgical cure. The surgery itself comprises both a radical vulvar excision as well as an inguinal lymphadenectomy. Radiation therapy is a poorly tolerated alternative in that anatomic area, leading to high morbidity with skin breakdown, infection, and pain. Currently, the extent of surgical resection (i.e., the radicalness of the vulvectomy) required to achieve cure is in the midst of reconsideration, but a trend toward less extensive, but still radical, vulvar surgery appears to be emerging. Similarly, with respect to the inguinal dissection, the radicalness of the procedure is being reconsidered, with consideration of performing just superficial rather than superficial and deep node dissection as well as whether ipsilateral or bilateral dissection is needed. These modifications are based on lesion size, location, depth of invasion, and clinical status of the groin nodes. The use of lymphatic mapping and sentinel lymph node biopsy is still investigational but holds promise.

Primary radiation therapy is rarely the best alternative, except in the case of posterior lesions where adequate resection would compromise fecal continence. In this situation, the combination of primary vulvar radiation and concurrent chemotherapy with cisplatin and fluorouracil has been shown to result in significantly smaller lesions amenable to surgical resection. Morbidity, in the form of a mucocutaneous reaction in the vulvoperineal region is frequent, however.

2. Staging, risk stratification, and management principles. Staging of vulvar cancer has been changed from clinical to surgical (Table 11.7). Based on surgicopathologic findings (e.g., depth of invasion, nodal status) coupled with clinical prognostic factors (e.g., lesion size, location), risk stratification is possible and helps with further treatment planning. Depth of invasion greater than 1 mm is the best prognostic factor for inguinal metastasis. Most commonly after surgery, the lesion is found to be completely resected and the lymph nodes are negative. The good-prognosis patients are generally observed and do well. In contrast, if groin nodes are positive, the prognosis is significantly worse, with the numbers of positive nodes being the best predictor of survival. In this circumstance, adjuvant radiation to the inguinal region as well as to the whole pelvis is usually recommended. In this poor-prognosis situation, the use of radiation therapy has increased survival relative to that of the former strategy (ultraradical surgery), including pelvic lymph node dissection.

3. Candidates for chemotherapy. Patients with distant metastasis and those with locally advanced disease who would otherwise require exenterative-type, ultraradical surgery for complete resection are candidates for chemotherapy. The latter group can receive, as an alternative, neoadjuvant chemotherapy with or without preoperative radiation therapy, followed by a less radical resection, as previously mentioned.

Experience with cytotoxic drugs in managing vulvar malignancy is largely restricted to treating squamous cell tumors. As would be expected, most agents effective against squamous neoplasms occurring at other sites also have an effect on the vulva. Cisplatin, bleomycin, fluorouracil, methotrexate, mitomycin, and doxorubicin have some reported activity, albeit brief. Various combinations of these agents have been used, particularly as neoadjuvant treatment or in conjunction with radiation therapy. One commonly used regimen is as follows:

- Cisplatin 50 mg/m^2/day IV on day 1, *plus*
- Fluorouracil 1,000 mg/m^2 on days 1 to 4, continuous IV infusion every 3 weeks
- Cycles may be repeated in 3 or 4 weeks, depending on recovery of the blood cell counts and whether subsequent surgery is planned.

At this time, surgery remains the mainstay of treatment for vulvar cancer. There is a trend toward more limited, less disfiguring procedures, and investigation of the role of lymphatic mapping and sentinel lymph node biopsy is ongoing. Chemotherapy and radiation may be employed singly or in combination in both the neoadjuvant and the adjuvant settings as creative solutions to this disease continue to emerge.

Table 11.7.   1995 FIGO staging for carcinoma of the vulva

Stage	Definition
Stage 0	Carcinoma *in situ;* intraepithelial carcinoma (Tis)
Stage I	Tumor confined to the vulva and/or perineum, ≤2 cm in greatest dimension; nodes are negative (T1, N0, M0)
Stage IA	Lesions ≤2 cm in size confined to the vulva or perineum with stromal invasion no greater than 1 mm No nodal metastases. The depth of invasion is defined as the measurement of the tumor from the epithelial–stromal junction of the adjacent most superficial derma papilla to the deepest point of invasion
Stage IB	Lesions ≤2 cm in size confined to the vulva or perineum with stromal invasion >1 mm; no nodal metastases
Stage II	Tumor confined to the vulva and/or perineum, >2 cm in greatest dimension; nodes are negative (T2, N0, M0)
Stage III	Tumor of any size with (a) adjacent spread to the lower urethra and/or the vagina or to the anus; and/or (b) unilateral regional lymph node metastasis (T3, N0, M0; T3, N1, M0; T1, N1, M0; T2, N1, M0)
Stage IVA	Tumor invades any of the following: upper urethra, bladder mucosa, rectal mucosa, pelvic bone; and/or bilateral regional node metastasis (T1, N2, M0; T2, N2, M0; T3, N2, M0; T4, any N, M0)
Stage IVB	Any distant metastasis, including pelvic lymph nodes (any T, any N, M1)

TNM classification
  Primary tumor

Tis	Preinvasive carcinoma (carcinoma *in situ*)
T1	Tumor confined to the vulva and/or perineum <2 cm in greatest dimension
T2	Tumor confined to the vulva and/or perineum >2 cm in greatest dimension
T3	Tumor of any size with adjacent spread to the urethra and/or vagina and/or to the anus
T4	Tumor of any size infiltrating the bladder mucosa and/or the rectal mucosa, including the upper part of the urethral mucosa and/or fixed to the bone

Regional lymph nodes

N0	No lymph node metastasis
N1	Unilateral regional lymph node metastasis
N2	Bilateral regional lymph node metastasis

Distant metastasis

M0	No clinical metastasis
M1	Distant metastasis (including pelvic lymph node metastasis)

SELECTED READINGS

General

Brierley JD, Catton PA, O'Sullivan B, et al. Accuracy of recorded tumor, node, and metastasis stage in a comprehensive cancer center. *J Clin Oncol* 2002;20:413–419.

Carney ME, Lancaster JM, Ford C, et al. A population-based study of patterns of care for ovarian cancer: who is seen by a gynecologic oncologist and who is not? *Gynecol Oncol* 2002;84:36–42.

McCahill LE, Krouse R, Chu D, et al. Indications and use of palliative surgery—results of Society of Surgical Oncology survey. *Ann Surg Oncol* 2002;9:104–112.

Miaskowski C, Dodd MJ, West C, et al. Lack of adherence with the analgesic regimen: a significant barrier to effective cancer pain management. *J Clin Oncol* 2001;19:4275–4279.

Granai CO, ed. *Surgical Oncology Clinics of North America. Cancers unique to women, vol. 7.* Philadelphia: WB Saunders, 1998.

Muss HB. Older age—not a barrier to cancer treatment [Editorial]. *N Engl J Med* 2001;345:1128–1129.

Rousseau P. The art of oncology: when the tumor is not the target. Spirituality and the dying patient. *J Clin Oncol* 2000;18:2000–2002.

Von Roenn JH. Are we the barrier? [Editorial]. *J Clin Oncol* 2001;19: 4273–4274.

Carcinoma of the Cervix

Ambros RA, Kurman RJ. Current concepts in the relationship of human papilloma virus infection to the pathogenesis and classification of precancerous lesions of the uterine cervix. *Semin Diagn Pathol* 1990;7:158.

American Cancer Society. *Cancer facts and figures—2002.* Atlanta American Cancer Society, 2002.

Benedetti-Panici P, Greggi S, Colombo A, et al. Neoadjuvant chemotherapy and radical surgery versus exclusive radiotherapy in locally advanced squamous cell cervical cancer: results from the Italian Multicenter Randomized Study. *J Clin Oncol* 2002;20:179–188.

Keys HM, Bundy BN, Stehman FB, et al. Cisplatin, radiation, and adjuvant hysterectomy compared with radiation and adjuvant hysterectomy for bulky stage Ib cervical carcinoma. *N Engl J Med* 1999l;340:1154–1161.

Killackey MA, Boardman L, Carroll DS. Adjuvant chemotherapy and radiation in patients with poor prognostic stage Ib/IIa cervical cancer. *Gynecol Oncol* 1993;49:377.

Morris M, Eifel PJ, Lu J, et al. Pelvic radiation with concurrent chemotherapy compared with pelvic and para-aortic radiation for high-risk cervical cancer. *N Engl J Med* 1999;340:1137–1143.

Peters WA III, Liu PY, Barrett RJ II, et al. Concurrent chemotherapy and pelvic radiation therapy compared with pelvic radiation therapy alone as adjuvant therapy after radical surgery in high-risk early-stage cancer of the cervix. *J Clin Oncol* 2000;18:1606–1613.

Reich O, Lahousen M, Pickel H, et al. Cervical intraepithelial neoplasia III: long-term follow-up after cold-knife conization with involved margins. *Obstet Gynecol* 2002;99:193–196.

Rose PG, Bundy BN, Watkins EB, et al. Concurrent cisplatin-based radiotherapy and chemotherapy for locally advanced cervical cancer. *N Engl J Med* 1999;340:1144–1153.

van Nagell JR, et al. Surgical therapy for cervical cancer. In: Gershenson DM, DeCherney AH, Curry SL, eds. *Operative gynecology.* Philadelphia: Saunders, 1993:271.

Whitney CW, Sause W, Bundy BN, et al. Randomized comparison of fluorouracil plus cisplatin versus hydroxyurea as an adjunct to radiation therapy in stage IIb–IVa carcinoma of the cervix with negative para-aortic lymph nodes: a Gynecologic Oncology Group and Southwest Oncology Group Study. *J Clin Oncol* 1999;17: 1339–1348.

Endometrial Carcinoma

American Cancer Society. *Cancer facts and figures—2002.* Atlanta American Cancer Society, 2002.

Aoki Y, Kase H, Watanabe M, et al. Stage III endometrial cancer: analysis of prognostic factors and failure patterns after adjuvant chemotherapy. *Gynecol Oncol* 2001;83:1–5.

Ball HG, et al. A phase II trial of paclitaxel in advanced and recurrent adenocarcinoma of the endometrium: a Gynecologic Oncology Group study. *Gynecol Oncol* 1995;56:120.

Burk TW, Morris M. Surgery for malignant tumors of the uterine corpus. In: Gershenson DM, DeCherney AH, Curry SL, eds. *Operative gynecology.* Philadelphia: Saunders, 1993:371–393.

Creasman WT, et al. Surgical pathologic spread patterns of endometrial cancer: a Gynecologic Oncology Group Study. *Cancer* 1987; 60:2035.

Gurney H, Murphy D, Crowther D. The management of primary fallopian tube carcinoma. *Br J Obstet Gynaecol* 1990;97:822.

Levenback C, Burke TW, Silva E, et al. Uterine papillary serous carcinoma (UPSC) treated with cisplatin, doxorubicin, and cyclophosphamide (PAC). *Gynecol Oncol* 1992;46:317–321.

Morris PJ, Malt RA, eds. *Oxford textbook of surgery, vol. 12.* Oxford: Oxford Medical, 1994:1438–1443.

Morrow CP, et al. Relationship between surgical–pathological risk factors and outcome in clinical stage I and II carcinoma of the endometrium: a GOG study. *Gynecol Oncol* 1991;40:55.

Muntz HG, et al. Primary adenocarcinoma of the fallopian tube. *Eur J Gynaecol Oncol* 1989;10:239.

Silverberg SG, et al. Carcinosarcoma (malignant mixed mesodermal tumor) of the uterus: a Gynecologic Oncology Group pathologic study of 203 cases. *Int J Gynecol Pathol* 1990;9:1.

Society of Gynecologic Oncologists clinical practice guidelines. Practice guidelines: uterine corpus—sarcomas. *Oncology (Huntingt)* 1998; 12:284–286.

Thigpen JT, et al. A randomized comparison of doxorubicin alone versus doxorubicin plus cyclophosphamide in the management of advanced or recurrent endometrial carcinoma: a Gynecologic Oncology Group study. *J Clin Oncol* 1994;12:1408.

Zanotti KM, Belinson JL, Kennedy AW, et al. The use of paclitaxel and platinum-based chemotherapy in uterine papillary serous carcinoma. *Gynecol Oncol* 1999;74:272–277.

Fallopian Tube Cancer

Society of Gynecologic Oncologists clinical practice guidelines. Practice guidelines: fallopian tube cancer. *Oncology (Huntingt)* 1998;12: 287–288.

Carcinoma of the Ovary

Alberts DS, Liu PY, Hannigan EV, et al. Intraperitoneal cisplatin plus intravenous cyclophosphamide versus intravenous cisplatin plus intravenous cyclophosphamide for stage III ovarian cancer. *N Engl J Med* 1996;335:1950–1955.

Arbuck SG. Paclitaxel: what schedule? what dose? *J Clin Oncol* 1994;12:233.

Baker TR, Piver MS, Hempling RE. Long term survival by cytoreductive surgery to less than 1 cm, induction weekly cisplatin and monthly cisplatin, doxorubicin, and cyclophosphamide therapy in advanced ovarian adenocarcinoma. *Cancer* 1994;74:656.

Berek JS, Bertelsen K, DuBois A, et al. Advanced epithelial ovarian cancer: 1998 consensus statements. *Ann Oncol* 1999;10(suppl 1): S87–S92.

Braun S, Schindlbeck C, Hepp F, et al. Occult tumor cells in bone marrow of patients with locoregionally restricted ovarian cancer predict early distant metastatic relapse. *J Clin Oncol* 2001;19:368–375.

Burke W, Daly M, Garber J, et al. Recommendations for follow-up care of individuals with an inherited predisposition to cancer. *JAMA* 1997;277:997–1003.

Cannistra S. Cancer of the ovary. *N Engl J Med* 1993;329:1550–1559.

Friedman JB, Weiss NS. Second thoughts about second look laparotomy in advanced ovarian cancer. *N Engl J Med* 1990;322:1079.

Gallion HH, et al. Molecular genetic changes in human epithelial ovarian malignancies. *Gynecol Oncol* 1992;47:137.

Gershenson DM. Chemotherapy of ovarian germ cell tumors and sex cord stromal tumors. *Semin Surg Oncol* 1994;10:290–298.

Granai CO, Gajewski WH, Arena B. Ovarian cancer: issues and management. *Cancer* 1994;7:1.

Kaye SB, Cassidy PJ, Lewis CR, et al. Mature results of a randomized trial of two doses of cisplatin for the treatment of ovarian cancer. *J Clin Oncol* 1996;14:2113–2119.

Jaeger W, Ackermann S, Kessler H, et al. The effect of bowel resection on survival in advanced epithelial ovarian cancer. *Gynecol Oncol* 2001;83:286–291.

Johannsson OT, Ranstam J, Borg A, et al. Survival of BRCA1 breast and ovarian cancer patients: a population-based study from southern Sweden. *J Clin Oncol* 1998;16:397–404.

Kirmani S, et al. Intraperitoneal cisplatin/etoposide (IP/CDDP/VP-16) for consolidation of pathologic complete response (PCR) in ovarian carcinoma. *Proc Am Soc Clin Oncol* 1990;9:167.

Markman M. Intraperitoneal chemotherapy in the treatment of ovarian cancer. *Ann Med* 1996;28:293–296.

McGuire WP, Hoskins WJ, Brady MF, et al. Assessment of dose-intensive therapy in suboptimally debulked ovarian cancer: a Gynecologic Oncology Group study. *J Clin Oncol* 1995;13:1589–1599.

McGuire WP, Hoskins WJ, Brady MF, et al. Cyclophosphamide and cisplatin compared with paclitaxel and cisplatin in patients with stage III and stage IV ovarian cancer. *N Engl J Med* 1996;334:1–6.

Miki Y, Swenson J, Shattuck-Eidens D, et al. A strong candidate for the breast and ovarian cancer susceptibility gene BRCA1. *Science* 1994;266:66–71.

Muggia FM, Hainsworth JD, Jeffers S, et al. Phase II study of liposomal doxorubicin in refractory ovarian cancer: antitumor activity and toxicity modification by liposomal encapsulation, *J Clin Oncol* 1997;3:987–993.

Narod SA, Risch H, Moslehi R, et al., for the Hereditary Ovarian Cancer Clinical Study Group. Oral contraceptives and the risk of hereditary ovarian cancer. *N Engl J Med* 1998;339:424–428.

NIH Consensus Conference. Ovarian cancer screening, treatment and follow-up. *JAMA* 1995;273:491.

Ozols RF, Schwartz PE, Eifel PJ. Ovarian cancer, fallopian tube carcinoma, and peritoneal carcinoma. *Cancer* 1997;X:1502–1534.

Ozols RF, et al. Update of the NCCN ovarian cancer practice guidelines. *Oncology* 1997;11:95–105.

Piver MS, Jishi MF, Tsukada Y, et al. Primary peritoneal carcinoma after prophylactic oophorectomy in women with a family history of ovarian cancer. *Cancer* 1993;71:2651–2655.

Rose PG, Blessing JA, Mayer AR, et al. Prolonged oral etoposide as second-line therapy for platinum-resistant and platinum-sensitive ovarian carcinoma: a Gynecologic Oncology Group study. *J Clin Oncol* 1998;16:405–410.

Rubin SC, Benjamin I, Behbakht K, et al. Clinical and pathological features of ovarian cancer in women with germ-line mutations of BRCA1. *N Engl J Med* 1996;335:1413–1416.

Sabbatini P, Spriggs D. Salvage therapy for ovarian cancer. *Oncology (Huntingt)* 1998;12:833–846, 848, 851.

Schrag D, Kuntz KM, Garber JE, et al. Decision analysis—effects of prophylactic mastectomy and oophorectomy on life expectancy among women with BRCA1 or BRCA2 mutations. *N Engl J Med* 1997;336:1465–1471.

Stiff PJ, et al. High-dose chemotherapy with autologous transplantation for persistent/relapsed ovarian cancer: a multivariate analysis of survival for 100 consecutively treated patients. *J Clin Oncol* 1997;15:1309–1317.

Thigpen T, Vance RB, McGuire WP, et al. The role of paclitaxel in the management of coelomic epithelial carcinoma of the ovary: a review with emphasis on the Gynecologic Group experience. *Semin Oncol* 1995;22(suppl 14):23–31.

Vasey PA, Atkinson R, Coleman R, et al., on behalf of the Scottish Gynaecological Cancer Trials Group. Docetaxel–carboplatin as first line chemotherapy for epithelial ovarian cancer. *Br J Cancer* 2001;84:170–178.

Wooster R, Bignell G, Lancaster J, et al. Identification of the breast cancer susceptibility gene BRCA2. *Nature* 1995;378:789–792.

Young RC, et al. Adjuvant therapy in stage I and stage II epithelial ovarian cancer: results of two prospective randomized trials. *N Engl J Med* 1990;322:1021.

Gestational Trophoblastic Neoplasm

Ayhan A, Tuncer ZS, Halilzade H, et al. Predictors of persistent disease in women with complete hydatidiform mole. *J Reprod Med* 1996;41:591–594.

Ayhan A, Tuncer S, Tanir M, et al. Central nervous system involvement in gestational trophoblastic neoplasia. *Acta Obstet Gynecol Scand* 1996;75:548–550.

Berkowitz RS, Goldstein DP. Comprehensive review of the treatment of gestational trophoblastic diseases. *N Engl J Med* 1996;335:1740–1748.

Berkowitz RS, Goldstein DP. Recent advances in gestational trophoblastic disease. *Curr Opin Obstet Gynecol* 1998;10:61–64.

Bolis G, et al. EMA/CO regimen in high-risk gestational trophoblas-tic tumor (GTT). *Gynecol Oncol* 1988;31:439.

Cohn DE, Herzog TJ. Gestational trophoblastic diseases: new stan-dards for therapy. *Curr Opin Oncol* 2000;12:492–496.

Crawford RAF, Newlands E, Rustin GJS, et al. Gestational tro-phoblastic disease with liver metastases: the Charing Cross expe-rience. *Br J Obstet Gynaecol* 1997;104:105–109.

Feldman S, et al. Low risk metastatic gestational trophoblastic tumors. *Semin Oncol* 1995;22:166–171.

Holmseley HD, et al. Weekly intramuscular methotrexate for non-metastatic gestational trophoblastic disease. *Obstet Gynecol* 1988; 72:413.

Jones HW. Adjuvant hysterectomy in low-risk gestational trophoblas-tic disease. *Obstet Gynecol Surv* 2001;56:413–414.

Kohorn EI. The new FIGO 2000 staging and risk factor scoring sys-tem for gestational trophoblastic disease: description and critical assessment. *Int J Gynecol Cancer* 2001;11:73–77.

Lurain JR. High-risk metastatic gestational trophoblastic tumors: current management. *J Reprod Med* 1994;39:217–222.

Mangili G, Garavaglia E, Frigerio L, et al. Management of low-risk gestational trophoblastic tumors with etoposide (VP16) in patients resistant to methotrexate. *Gynecol Oncol* 1996;61:218–220.

Mutch DG, et al. Recurrent gestational trophoblastic disease: experi-ence of the Southeastern Regional Trophoblastic Disease Center. *Cancer* 1990;66:978.

Roberts JP, Lurain JR. Treatment of low-risk metastatic gestational trophoblastic tumors with single-agent chemotherapy. *Am J Obstet Gynecol* 1996;174:1917–1922.

Society of Gynecologic Oncologists clinical practice guidelines. Practice guidelines: gestational trophoblastic disease. *Oncology (Huntingt)* 1998;12:455–458, 461.

Theodore C, et al. Treatment of high-risk gestational trophoblastic disease with chemotherapy combinations containing cisplatin and etoposide. *Cancer* 1989;64:1824.

Wong LC, Ngan H, Cheng D, et al. Methotrexate infusion in low-risk gestational trophoblastic disease. *Am J Obstet Gynecol* 2000;183: 1579–1582.

Yordan EL, et al. Radiation therapy in the management of gestational choriocarcinoma metastatic to the central nervous system. *Obstet Gynecol* 1987;69:627–630.

Carcinoma of the Vulva

Burke TW, Levenback C, Coleman RL, et al. Surgical therapy of t1 and t2 vulvar carcinoma: further experience with radical wide ex-cision and selective inguinal lymphadenectomy. *Gynecol Oncol* 1995;57:215–220.

Figge DC, Tamimi HK, Greer BE. Lymphatic spread in carcinoma of the vulva. *Am J Obstet Gynecol* 1985;152:387.

Han SC, Kim DH, Higgins SA, et al. Chemoradiation as primary or adjuvant treatment for locally advanced carcinoma of the vulva. *Int J Radiat Oncol Biol Phys* 2000;47:1235–1244.

Homesley HD, Bundy BN, Sedlis A, et al. Radiation therapy versus pelvic node resection for carcinoma of the vulva with positive groin nodes. *Obstet Gynecol* 1986;68:733–740.

Homesley HD, et al. Assessment of current International Federation of Gynecology and Obstetrics staging of vulvar carcinoma relative to prognostic factors for survival (a Gynecologic Oncology Group study). *Am J Obstet Gynecol* 1991;164:997.

Montana G, Thomas GM, Moore DH, et al. Preoperative chemo-radiation for carcinoma of the vulva with N2/N3 nodes: a Gynecologic Oncology Group study. *Int J Radiat Oncol Biol Phys* 2000; 48:1007–1013.

Society of Gynecologic Oncologists clinical practice guidelines. Practice guidelines: vulvar cancer. *Oncology (Huntingt)* 1998;12:275–282.

Thomas G, et al. Concurrent radiation and chemotherapy in vulvar carcinoma. *Gynecol Oncol* 1989;34:263.

Urologic and Male Genital Malignancies

Scott B. Saxman and Craig R. Nichols

Malignancies that arise from the urinary and male genital tracts are highly diverse in their biologic behavior. They span a spectrum that includes one of the most chemotherapeutically curable of cancers (testicular germ cell tumor [GCT]) and one of the most resistant (renal cell carcinoma [RCC]). The therapeutic approaches to these tumors are also diverse and should be multidisciplinary because chemotherapy, surgery, and radiation therapy all have important roles.

I. Carcinoma of the kidney

A. Background. RCC, which is an adenocarcinoma that arises from the parenchyma of the kidney, accounts for 85% of primary renal neoplasms. Transitional cell carcinomas (TCCs) arise from the cells lining the collecting system. Their behavior and response to therapy are similar to those arising in the bladder (see Section II). Other rare malignancies of the kidney include oncocytomas (well-differentiated adenocarcinomas), undifferentiated carcinomas, and sarcomas. Wilms' tumor (nephroblastoma) is a cancer that is seen predominantly in childhood and is not covered here. The term "hypernephroma" is a misnomer and should no longer be used.

B. Staging. Staging for RCC should include a computed tomography (CT) scan of the chest and abdomen, bone scan, and usually arteriography or venography if nephrectomy is being considered. The TNM staging system is as follows:

Stage I: Tumor 7 cm or smaller confined to the kidney (T1, N0, M0)

Stage II: Tumor larger than 7 cm confined to the kidney (T2, N0, M0)

Stage III: Tumor extending into major veins, adrenal gland, or perinephric tissues but not beyond Gerota's fascia or metastasis to single node (T3, N0, M0; or T1 to 3, N1, M0)

Stage IV: Tumor invading beyond Gerota's fascia or multiple lymph node metastases or distant metastatic disease (T4, any N, M0; any T, N2, M0; or any T, any N, M1)

C. General therapeutic approach. The treatment of choice for RCC is radical nephrectomy, including removal of the perinephric fat and regional lymph nodes. Partial nephrectomy is an option in patients with bilateral RCC or a solitary kidney to prevent the need for dialysis or kidney transplantation. Rarely, patients with solitary metastatic lesions can be cured by surgical removal of the metastasis at the time of nephrectomy. RCC is relatively radioresistant; thus, adjuvant radiation therapy does not improve survival. Radiation therapy can be useful for palliation of painful metastasis. Although it is reasonable to consider patients with inoperable metastatic disease for treatment with biologic agents or chemotherapy, in most patients, these systemic therapies are of minimal benefit. In the context of new biological therapies, nephrectomy is being considered as an adjunct to systemic treatment.

D. Treatment regimens

  1. Biologic response modifiers

   a.   Interleukin-2 (IL-2) mediates its antitumor effects through activation of the patient's immune system. IL-2 alone or in combination with lymphokine-activated killer cells or interferon results in tumor regression in 15% of patients. Although some of these responses have been complete and long-lasting, it is not yet known whether this represents a therapeutic advance because patients in the reported studies were carefully selected. There is a wide dosage range in various protocols. Some generally accepted treatment regimens and schedules are shown in Table 12.1. Although the greatest experience has been with the high-dose bolus regimen, this regimen is difficult to recommend for most patients because of its greater toxicity. Outpatient bolus therapy may be equally efficacious and has less morbidity.

Table 12.1.   Interleukin-2–based regimens for renal cell carcinoma

Regimen	Treatment plan[a]
High-dose bolus IL-2 (inpatient therapy; requires intensive care unit support)	IL-2: 600,000 or 720,000 IU/kg IV over 15 min every 8 h on d 1–5 and 15–19. Repeat cycle in 6–12 wk if stable or responding disease.
Low-dose bolus IL-2 (inpatient therapy, fewer complications, reduced use of vasopressor support, and fewer admissions to intensive care unit)	IL-2: 72,000 IU/kg IV bolus over 15 min every 8 h on d 1–5 and 15–19. Repeat cycle in 5–6 wk if stable or responding disease.
Outpatient subcutaneous IL-2	IL-2: $9–18 \times 10^6$ IU/m^2/d SC for 5 d/wk. Repeat weekly for 4–6 wk; then give a 2- to 3-wk rest period. For stable or responding disease, repeat for two or three cycles.

[a] **Daily premedication and additional symptomatic medication are required on all regimens.** Examples of medication for symptom control include ondansetron 30 mg IV on each day of the IL-2; acetaminophen 650 mg PO before treatment and q4 h p.r.n.; cimetidine 800 mg PO daily; diphenoxylate with atropine (Lomotil) 1 tablet up to six times daily for diarrhea; hydroxyzine 25–50 mg q4–6 h for itching. In any of the schedules, therapy may be stopped prematurely for constitutional symptoms or for cardiovascular, renal, hepatic, neurologic, pulmonary, or hematologic toxicity.

b. Interferon results in regression in 15% of treated patients. The optimal treatment regimen or duration of treatment is not known; it is most commonly used in an intermediate-dose regimen of 5 to 10×10^6 IU/m^2 SC three to five times per week. The average response duration is 6 to 10 months. Response correlates with prior nephrectomy, good performance status, long disease-free interval, and lung-predominant disease.

c. Combination therapy. Combinations of interferon and IL-2 have been tested but have not been shown to be superior to IL-2 or interferon alone.

2. Cytotoxic chemotherapy. The most commonly used regimen is vinblastine 5 to 6 mg/m^2 IV weekly, which produces responses in 10% of patients. The major dose-limiting toxicity is hematologic, and therapy should be delayed when the white blood cell count is less than 3,000/μL or the platelet count is less than 100,000/μL. Chemotherapy does not prolong survival in these patients; therefore, the minimal potential palliative benefit should be carefully weighed against the added toxicity.

3. Hormonal therapy. Hormonal therapy (medroxyprogesterone acetate or tamoxifen) has historically been the mainstay of treatment, initially used because of preclinical data suggesting activity. More recent studies do not support any beneficial effect of these agents. At best, these agents produce responses in fewer than 5% of patients and therefore cannot be recommended.

E. Complications of therapy. Complications of IL-2, particularly with higher doses, include fever, agitation, and a capillary leak syndrome that results in increased interstitial water in the lungs and respiratory insufficiency. This situation usually requires management in an intensive care unit. Interferon can cause nausea, anorexia, fatigue, myalgia, headache, and fever. Complications of cytotoxic therapy include nausea, mucositis, myalgia, and myelosuppression. Hormonal therapy is usually free of side effects other than fluid retention.

F. Recommendations. Most patients with metastatic RCC should be managed expectantly with the aggressive use of narcotics and radiation therapy for pain control or be placed in clinical trials. Well-informed patients with excellent performance status and cardiac and pulmonary function can be considered for treatment with one of the IL-2 or interferon regimens.

II. Bladder cancer

A. General considerations and staging. Cancer arising in the bladder is usually TCC, although occasionally squamous cell carcinoma, neuroendocrine carcinoma, and adenocarcinoma are seen. TCC falls into two major groups: superficial and invasive. The biology and natural history of these two groups differ markedly. When planning treatment for bladder cancer, one must take into account the stage of the tumor (0 to IV), histologic grade (1 to 3), and location of the tumor within the bladder (related to surgical considerations of partial versus total cystectomy).

The standard evaluation of a patient with invasive bladder cancer should include a CT scan of the abdomen and pelvis, chest radiograph, complete blood cell count, and serum chemistry profile. The TNM staging system can be summarized as follows:

TX: Primary tumor cannot be assessed
T0: No evidence of primary tumor
Ta: Noninvasive papillary carcinoma
Tis: Carcinoma *in situ*
T1: Tumor invades subepithelial connective tissue
T2: Tumor invades muscle
T2a: Superficial (inner half)
T2b: Deep (outer half)
T3: Tumor invades perivesical fat
T3a: Microscopically
T3b: Macroscopically (extravesical mass)
T4: Tumor invades any of the following: prostate, uterus, vagina, pelvic wall, or abdominal wall
T4a: Tumor invades the prostate, uterus, or vagina
T4b: Tumor invades the pelvic wall or abdominal wall

Stage groupings are as follows:

Stage 0: Ta or Tis, N0, M0
Stage I: T1, N0, M0
Stage II: T2, N0, M0
Stage III: T3 or T4a, N0, M0
Stage IV: T4b, N0, M0; any T, N1 to 3, M0 to 1

B.   General approach to therapy
   1.   Superficial-stage, low-grade tumors. Patients with stage 0 or I tumors are usually treated with transurethral resection (TUR) and fulguration, with a local control rate higher than 80%. However, TUR does not reduce the risk of recurrence at other sites in the bladder. This risk may be reduced by administration of intravesical therapy. Diffuse carcinoma *in situ* may also be treated with intravesical therapy.
   2.   Deep-stage, high-grade tumors. Patients with larger stage II lesions or with stage III disease are usually managed with partial or radical cystectomy (depending on the size and location of the tumor). Several trials have investigated the roles of preoperative radiation therapy and chemotherapy, with inconclusive results. The role of neoadjuvant therapy remains controversial, and it should not be considered standard care.
   3.   Advanced and metastatic tumors. Patients with locally advanced disease or local recurrences can be considered for radiation therapy. Patients with metastatic disease are candidates for systemic chemotherapy. There is evidence that chemotherapy can prolong survival and that combinations are superior to single agents.
C.   Treatment regimens and evaluation of response
   1.   Intravesical chemotherapy
      a.   Method of administration and follow-up. Intravesical therapy is usually administered in a volume of 40 to 60 mL through a Foley catheter. The catheter is then clamped and the agent retained for 2 h. This procedure delivers a high local concentration to the tumor area while

usually avoiding systemic effects. Patients with superficial bladder cancers require lifelong surveillance with periodic cystoscopy (initially every 3 months, then every 6 months, then annually) because even with intravesical therapy, an increased risk of new primary tumors persists. Patients being treated for diffuse carcinoma *in situ* should have biopsy confirmation of the return of normal mucosa after the installation therapy has been completed. These patients also require lifelong cystoscopic surveillance.

b. Selection of patients for intravesical therapy. Only patients with superficial or small, minimally invasive tumors (T1) should be treated. The grade of the tumor is also a significant predictor of progression. Patients with grade 3 lesions should be considered for more aggressive treatment than intravesical therapy. Possible objectives for intravesical therapy are as follows:

(1) Prevention of relapse in patients with Ta grades 2 and 3 and stage I lesions treated with TUR.

(2) Prevention of occurrence of new bladder tumors. Patients with two or more previously resected bladder tumors should be treated in an effort to prevent development of *de novo* malignancies.

(3) Carcinoma *in situ* may involve the bladder diffusely and thus not be amenable to TUR. A course of installation therapy is usually given, followed by repeat biopsies. Persistence of carcinoma *in situ* is an indication for more aggressive local management such as cystectomy.

c. Specific intravesical therapeutic regimens

Bacillus Calmette–Guérin (BCG) 120 mg weekly for 6 to 8 weeks, *or*

Thiotepa 30 to 60 mg weekly for 4 to 6 weeks, *or*

Mitomycin 20 to 40 mg weekly for 6 to 8 weeks, *or*

Doxorubicin 50 to 60 mg weekly for 6 to 8 weeks

d. Selection of therapy. Although few controlled studies have been done, it appears that thiotepa, mitomycin, and doxorubicin are equally effective. Two separate studies have shown BCG to be superior to thiotepa and doxorubicin in preventing recurrence. Thus, BCG should be considered the agent of choice for intravesical therapy.

e. Response to therapy. About 40% to 70% of patients with existing or residual tumor after TUR respond to therapy. Whether adjuvant intravesical therapy prevents progression to invasive or metastatic bladder cancer or improves survival requires further study.

f. Complications of therapy. All of the agents mentioned can cause symptoms of bladder irritation (pain, urgency, hematuria) and allergic reactions. Thiotepa is systemically absorbed and can occasionally cause myelosuppression. This is rare with mitomycin and doxorubicin. Patients receiving thiotepa should have their blood cell counts monitored closely. Mitomycin can cause dermatitis in the perineal area and hands. BCG is occasionally associated with systemic symptoms including fever, chills, malaise, arthralgias, and skin rash.

2. Adjuvant chemotherapy. Chemotherapy has been studied both preoperatively and postoperatively in patients with deeply invasive tumors or positive lymph nodes. To date, no randomized trial has demonstrated a clear-cut benefit, although the recent Southwestern Oncology Group trial suggested some benefit for neoadjuvant MVAC (methotrexate, vinblastine, doxorubicin, and cisplatin). This question is still under study. Neoadjuvant or adjuvant chemotherapy can be considered one standard of care in this patient population, although data for local therapies without pre- or postoperative chemotherapy are more compelling.

3. Systemic chemotherapy for advanced disease

a. Drugs active against bladder cancer. Drugs active against bladder cancer include cisplatin, doxorubicin, vinblastine, fluorouracil, cyclophosphamide, carboplatin, mitoxantrone, and methotrexate. Of these, cisplatin is probably the most active as a single agent. The combination of methotrexate, vinblastine, doxorubicin, and cisplatin (MVAC) is the most commonly used. A randomized trial showed MVAC to have a survival advantage over single-agent cisplatin.

b. Specific regimens. Combination chemotherapy should be considered standard first-line therapy (Table 12.2). Single agents can be used for patients with congestive heart failure, renal dysfunction, or poor bone marrow reserve who are unable to tolerate more aggressive treatment.

c. Response to therapy. MVAC may be expected to produce a complete response in 15% of patients and a partial response in 35%, for an overall response rate of about 50%.

Table 12.2. Combination chemotherapy and active single agents for cancer of the bladder

Regimen or single agent	Doses and schedules
MVAC	Methotrexate 30 mg/m^2 IV on d 1 Vinblastine 3 mg/m^2 IV on d 2 Doxorubicin 30 mg/m^2 IV on d 2 Cisplatin 70 mg/m^2 IV on d 2 (with vigorous diuresis) Repeat methotrexate and vinblastine on d 15 and 22 if white blood cell count >2,000/µL and platelet count >50,000/µL. Cycles should be repeated every 28 days.
CP	Paclitaxel 200 mg/m^2 over 3 h, followed by: Carboplatin AUC 5 Repeat cycle every 21 d.
Cisplatin	40–60 mg/m^2 IV every 3 wk
Doxorubicin	60 mg/m^2 IV every 3 wk
Cyclophosphamide	1 g/m^2 IV every 3 wk
Fluorouracil	500 mg/m^2 IV weekly

The median survival time is about 13 months. The toxicity of this regimen is substantial and must be weighed against the expected benefit when selecting therapy. Drug delivery can be enhanced by the co-administration of granulocyte colony-stimulating factor. However, there is no evidence that this improves survival. Response to any chemotherapy is monitored by periodic measurement of tumor masses with the expectation that most patients who will respond will do so within the first one to two cycles of treatment. Patients who relapse after or progress during MVAC occasionally respond to a second-line regimen. This should be undertaken for palliative reasons only because any survival benefit is minimal. Such patients should be considered for clinical trials. The couplet of cisplatin and gemcitabine has been compared with MVAC in metastatic TCC. The preliminary report suggests equivalence of these two regimens, although there was some criticism of the power of the study to prove equivalence. Despite this statistical argument, cisplatin plus gemcitabine and carboplatin plus paclitaxel have entered common usage in this patient population.

Management of the non-TCC histologies arising from the bladder is difficult. Local therapies should be identical to TCC, but the role of chemotherapy is limited. Non-TCC histologies respond poorly to chemotherapy. Neuroendocrine tumors of the bladder are usually treated similarly to small cell lung cancer with cisplatin/etoposide-based regimens and local radiation for those with bladder-confined disease.

d.   Complications of systemic therapy. The major dose-limiting toxicity of MVAC is myelosuppression, which often precludes the administration of chemotherapy on days 15 and 22. Cisplatin can cause renal damage, but this can usually be prevented by vigorous hydration and saline diuresis. Mucositis, nausea and vomiting, and malaise are also commonly seen.

e.   Follow-up. Patients can be followed every few months for symptomatic progression. Serial x-ray studies or bone scans are costly and are of minimal value.

III.   Prostate cancer

A.   Background. Carcinoma of the prostate is the most common cancer in the United States, with the exception of nonmelanoma skin cancers. Largely because of aggressive "screening" using prostatic-specific antigen (PSA), the incidence of new cases increased 50% between 1980 and 1990, so that in 1998, about 185,000 new cases were diagnosed. Whether the earlier diagnosis and aggressive surgical or radiotherapeutic management of these patients will change the natural history of prostate cancer and decrease the mortality of this disease of older men remains unknown.

B.   Staging. Staging is usually done using a combination of clinical and pathologic indicators. Pathologic staging is necessary for completely accurate staging of low-stage disease but often is not needed once the disease has become metastatic to the bones or visceral organs. Accurate determination of extension beyond the prostate capsule and into lymph nodes requires pathologic evaluation in most circumstances. The modified Whitmore–Jewett, or American Urologic Association, staging system is the most commonly used in the United States; the TNM system provides more detail about tumor extent and spread:

TX: Primary tumor cannot be assessed

T0: No evidence of primary tumor

T1: Clinically inapparent tumor not palpable or visible by imaging

T1a: Tumor incidental histologic finding in 5% or less of tissue resected

T1b: Tumor incidental histologic finding in more than 5% of tissue resected

T1c: Tumor identified by needle biopsy (e.g., because of elevated PSA)

T2: Tumor confined within prostate

T3: Tumor extends through the prostatic capsule

T4: Tumor is fixed or invades adjacent structures other than seminal vesicles

Stage groupings are as follows:

Stage I: T1a, N0, M0, G1

Stage II: T1a, N0, M0, G2 to 4

   T1b, c, N0, M0, any G

   T2, N0, M0, any G

Stage III: T3, N0, M0, any G

Stage IV: T4, N0, M0, any G

   Any T, N1 to 3, M0, any G

   Any T, any N, M1, any G

In the American Urologic Association system, stages A, B, C, and D correspond closely to stages I, II, III, and IV in the TNM system. Additional prognostic information can be obtained by evaluating the differentiation of the tumor using the Gleason Grading System and the degree of elevation of the PSA.

Staging of prostate cancer should include abdominal and pelvic CT scans, chest radiographs, bone scans, liver function tests, and serum PSA and acid phosphatase measurements.

C.   General considerations and goals of therapy. Selection of therapy for prostate cancer is complex and based on the extent of the disease as well as the age and general medical condition of the patient. Although many biases exist, there are no good randomized studies comparing treatment modalities in patients with organ-confined disease.

With the possible exception of young patients (less than 60 years of age), T1a (A1) prostate cancer should be followed without further therapy because survival is equal to that in age-matched controls. For other patients with organ-confined disease (T1b, c, T2), radical prostatectomy and high-dose radiation therapy are treatment options that probably have equal effectiveness. Observation alone may also be reasonable for patients with low-grade, organ-confined tumors. The choice between these three options must take into account the patient's performance status and the toxicities of each modality, which include anesthesia, blood loss, and incontinence for surgery versus tenesmus, rectal bleeding, and diarrhea for radiation. Stage III (C) tumors are usually treated with radiation therapy, although it is unclear whether this therapy prolongs survival. Very elderly patients or patients who have poor general health can be observed without therapy because the natural history is usually slow, with progression over years rather than months. Patients with metastatic disease are usually treated initially with hormonal therapy with or without radiation therapy to severely affected vertebral bodies or long bones. Patients with asymptomatic metastatic disease can have treatment delayed until symptoms develop, with no decrease in likelihood of benefit from therapy.

D. Treatment of symptomatic metastatic disease

1. Hormonal therapy. Hormonal therapy results in a subjective response in nearly 75% of patients treated, lasting an average of 18 months. Most of these patients also have objective evidence of response, measured either radiographically or by a decreasing PSA level. In general, there is little evidence to suggest that one hormonal manipulation is superior to any other, so the choice can be based on patient preference, existing medical conditions, and cost. No good predictive markers for response currently exist in clinical practice.

a. Orchiectomy is often the treatment of choice because it is relatively inexpensive and obviates the need for injections or daily medications. This procedure can be done on an outpatient basis in all but the sickest of patients with minimal morbidity.

b. Estrogens are effective but less frequently used because of concern about potential cardiotoxicity and thrombophlebitis. Historically, 3 to 5 mg/day of diethylstilbestrol has been given; however, 1 mg/day produces fewer side effects without shortening survival. Painful gynecomastia can be prevented by superficial radiation (5 Gy) to the breast tissue before the start of therapy.

c. Luteinizing hormone–releasing hormone (LHRH) analogs are synthetic peptides administered by parenteral injection that occupy the receptors for LHRH in the pituitary gland. Initially, the release of LH is increased, causing a rise in the serum testosterone level. The continuous administration of therapeutic (superphysiologic) doses of the LHRH analog blocks the physiologic pulsatile LH release from the pituitary, causing a fall in the serum testosterone to castrate levels. These agents can be administered either by SC injection daily or monthly in a depot form. Currently used agents include the following:

Leuprolide 7.5 mg IM depot monthly or 22.5 mg IM depot every 3 months or 30 mg IM depot every 4 months.

Goserelin 3.6 mg SC depot monthly or 10.8 mg SC every 3 months

Advantages of these agents are that they avoid the trauma of orchiectomy as well as the side effects of diethylstilbestrol. Disadvantages include the potential for rapid worsening during the initial few weeks owing to a paradoxical transient increase in testosterone production. This flare can usually be avoided by the concurrent use of antiandrogens. Other disadvantages include the potential for poor patient compliance and the extremely high cost— more than $500 per month.

d.   LHRH analogs and antiandrogens (total androgen blockade) have been used in combination. Synthetic antiandrogens (e.g., flutamide) act by competing with testosterone at the level of the cellular receptor. A recent randomized trial showed no improvement in survival when flutamide was given after orchiectomy. Because of the lack of consistent evidence of benefit as well as added cost and toxicity, total androgen blockade should no longer be considered an absolute standard in treatment of patients with metastatic disease.

e.   Second-line hormonal therapies that have been tried include orchiectomy (if not used as initial therapy), adrenalectomy, hypophysectomy, antiandrogens, progestins, and adrenal suppressants. The response rates to these therapies are low (less than 15%) and of brief duration. Patients who were initially treated with combined-modality therapy occasionally respond to withdrawal of the anti-androgen. This should be considered before proceeding to more toxic therapies.

2.   Cytotoxic chemotherapy. Patients who relapse from or fail to respond to hormonal therapies can be considered for cytotoxic chemotherapy. In general, however, chemotherapy trials have been disappointing, with most agents having response rates lower than 10%. A recent randomized trial demonstrated that patients treated with

Mitoxantrone 12 mg/m^2 every 3 weeks, *and*
Prednisone 5 mg b.i.d.

had improved pain control and reduced need for analgesic medications when compared with patients treated with prednisone alone. This is a reasonable option for patients with symptomatic hormone-refractory disease.

Except for the combination of estramustine and vinblastine, they are most commonly used as single agents. There is no evidence that chemotherapy improves survival in these patients. Other most commonly used alternative drug regimens are shown below:

Doxorubicin 60 mg/m^2 IV every 3 weeks
Docetaxel 80 to 100 mg/m^2 IV every 3 weeks
Cyclophosphamide 1 g/m^2 every 3 weeks
Fluorouracil 500 mg/m^2 IV weekly
Methotrexate 40 mg/m^2 IV weekly
Cisplatin 40 mg/m^2 IV every 3 weeks
Estramustine 600 mg/m^2 PO on days 1 to 42, *and* **vinblastine** 4 mg/m^2 IV weekly for 6 weeks. Courses of estramustine and vinblastine are repeated every 8 weeks.

Patients who have received extensive radiation therapy should have their initial chemotherapy dose reduced by 20%.

Patients who progress with hormonal therapy can still have severe symptomatic worsening if testosterone levels rise. Therefore, patients who have not undergone orchiectomy should continue with estrogen or LHRH therapy.

3. Evaluation of response. Evaluating the response is often difficult because many patients do not have measurable disease. However, the serum PSA or alkaline phosphatase level is often elevated and can be serially measured as a marker for response. Bone scans are difficult to interpret because "hot spots" can reflect either the presence of disease or healing of bone in response to tumor regression.

4. Complications of therapy. All effective hormonal therapies will cause sexual dysfunction, including impotence and decreased libido. Orchiectomy can rarely be complicated by local infection or hematoma. LHRH analogs can cause an initial flare of the disease and are frequently associated with hot flashes. Antiandrogens can cause diarrhea and hepatic dysfunction. Estrogens are associated with thromboembolic disease, fluid retention, and cardiac disease. Chemotherapy side effects include nausea and vomiting, mucositis, marrow suppression, and alopecia.

E. Follow-up. Patients treated with radical prostatectomy can be followed with PSA measurements every 4 months. Patients with a rising PSA level, evidence of local recurrence, and no evidence of metastatic disease can be considered for radiation to the prostatic bed. Otherwise, there is no role for serial PSA measurements (except as a marker for response to hormonal therapy, noted in Section III.D.3) or bone scans because patients are treated only for symptomatic progression. Some patients can be considered for bisphosphonate therapy as well.

IV. Testicular cancer (germ cell tumors)

A. Overview. Although primary neoplasms of the testis can arise from Leydig's or Sertoli's cells, more than 95% of testicular cancers are of spermatogenic or germ cell origin. GCTs are rare, accounting for 1% of all malignancies in men. However, they are important malignancies because they represent the most common solid tumor in young men and because of their high degree of curability. With the advent of cisplatin-based chemotherapy, accurate tumor markers, and aggressive surgical approaches, overall cure rates for patients with disseminated disease approach 80%, and patients with early-stage disease are nearly always cured. GCT is also one of the few solid tumors for which salvage chemotherapy can be curative.

B. Histology. GCTs are categorized as either seminomatous or nonseminomatous (which includes a variety of other histologies such as embryonal cell carcinoma, choriocarcinoma, and yolk sac tumors). Pure seminoma accounts for 40% of patients with GCTs. Although mild elevations of the β-subunit of hCG may be seen, pure seminoma is never associated with an elevation of α-fetoprotein. Nonseminomatous GCT can cause elevations of hCG, α-fetoprotein (AFP), or both.

C. Staging. Pretreatment staging should include serum tumor markers (α-fetoprotein, hCG) and CT of the abdomen and chest. Other radiographic procedures should be undertaken only if symptoms or physical examination dictate.

Stage I: Tumor confined to the testis with or without involvement of the spermatic cord or epididymis
Stage II: Tumor with metastasis limited to retroperitoneal lymph nodes
Stage III: Tumor spread beyond retroperitoneal lymph nodes

D. Treatment strategies and management of specific situations. The therapeutic approach to the patient with testicular cancer depends on the histology of the tumor and the clinical or pathologic stage of the disease.

 1. Seminoma. Most patients with seminoma present with early-stage disease and are nearly always cured with radiation therapy. Patients with stage I disease are treated with 2,500 cGy given to abdominal nodes in daily fractions over 3 to 4 weeks. Patients with lymph node involvement on lymphangiogram or CT scans receive a slightly higher dose of 3,000 to 3,500 cGy. The contralateral testis should be shielded to maintain fertility. Radiation to the mediastinum is contraindicated and can compromise subsequent chemotherapy. Surveillance for clinical stage I seminoma is a competitive option for motivated patients and physicians. Residual radiographic abnormalities are most often scar tissue or necrosis and do not need to be surgically resected. Patients with bulky retroperitoneal disease larger than 5 cm or stage III disease should be treated with chemotherapy (see Section IV.D.2).

 2. Nonseminoma

  a. Stage I disease. Historically, these patients have been pathologically staged and treated with a retroperitoneal lymph node dissection (RPLND). Patients with pathologically confirmed stage I disease do not need any further therapy because less than 10% show relapse. In about 25% of patients, clinical stage I disease is found to be stage II pathologically at RPLND, and treatment for these patients is discussed in the following section. The major complication of RPLND has been retrograde ejaculation with subsequent infertility, although this is rare with the currently used nerve-sparing procedure. The other option for selected patients is surveillance without RPLND. These patients should be chosen carefully and must be committed to careful lengthy follow-up. Because 30% of these patients eventually experience relapse, they must be followed closely with monthly measurements of serum markers and chest radiographs for the first year and every other month the year after that. Abdominal CT scans should also be performed every 2 months the first year and every 4 months thereafter. If patients are selected and followed appropriately, overall survival is the same as for patients undergoing RPLND.

  b. Stage II disease. Patients with lymph nodes larger than 2 to 3 cm should be treated primarily with chemotherapy. If the lymph nodes measure less than 2 cm, an RPLND can be considered. Patients with pathologically confirmed and completely resected stage II disease have a relapse rate of about 30%. Patients with fully resected pathologic stage II disease either can be treated with two cycles of adjuvant chemotherapy after RPLND or can be followed closely and treated with standard chemotherapy if they show relapse. Patients who choose observation should receive monthly chest radiograph and serum marker evaluations and should be treated immediately if the disease recurs. Patients with stage II disease who have elevated markers after RPLND or whose disease is not completely resected should be treated the same as patients with stage III disease.

c.   Stage III disease. About 30% of patients present with stage III disease. The most common site of involvement is the lungs, but liver, bone, and brain can also be involved with metastatic disease. These patients are further categorized as good, intermediate, or poor risk based on the primary site, level of marker elevation, and involvement of brain liver or bone. An international germ cell prognostic classification has been developed based on a retrospective analysis of more than 5,000 patients with metastatic GCTs. Poor-risk patients according to the International Germ Cell Cancer Consensus Classification System include those with the following:

- Mediastinal primary site;
- degree (high) of elevation of AFP, hCG, and LDH; presence of non-pulmonary viceral metastasis (e.g., liver, bone, and brain).

Other adverse factors include:

Advanced chest disease (mediastinal mass more than 50% of the intrathoracic diameter, or more than 10 pulmonary metastases per lung, or multiple pulmonary metastases larger than 3 cm), or
Palpable abdominal mass plus pulmonary metastases.

d.   Recommended therapy. All patients with stage II or III disease who require chemotherapy should receive cisplatin-based chemotherapy, as follows:

BEP Cisplatin 20 mg/m^2 IV over 30 min on days 1 to 5, *and*
Etoposide 100 mg/m^2 IV on days 1 to 5, *and*
Bleomycin 30 U IV push weekly on days 1, 8, and 15

Repeat cycle every 21 days regardless of blood cell counts for two (adjuvant therapy), three (good-risk patients), or four (immediate or poor risk) cycles. For good-risk patients, particularly those with seminoma requiring chemotherapy, four cycles of etoposide and cisplatin without bleomycin may be considered (same doses as BEP).

If the patient has fever associated with granulocytopenia, we would give the next cycle at the same doses, followed by daily SC injections of granulocyte colony-stimulating factor. Other chemotherapy regimens such as VIP (etoposide, ifosfamide, cisplatin) have not improved outcome and are more toxic.

e.   Surgery for residual disease. Patients who have a complete response with chemotherapy should be followed and do not require any further treatment. Patients whose marker levels normalize but who have not achieved a radiographic complete response should undergo complete surgical resection of residual disease. If the resected material reveals only teratoma, necrosis, or fibrosis, then no further therapy is necessary, and the patient should be followed. If there is carcinoma in the resected specimen, the patient should receive two more cycles of BEP chemotherapy.

f.   Follow-up. Most patients who experience relapse do so within the first 2 years, although late relapses do occur. In general, patients should be followed with monthly physical examination, chest x-ray studies, and serum marker measurements during the first year and every 2 months during the second year. Patients should then be followed about every 4 months for the third year, twice the fourth year, and yearly thereafter. Because tumors can arise in the contralateral testis, patients should be taught to do testicular self-examination.

E.   Salvage chemotherapy

1.   Standard-dose therapy. Patients who respond to first-line chemotherapy and then relapse are still curable with salvage regimens such as VIP:

- Vinblastine 0.11 mg/kg (4.1 mg/m^2) IV push on days 1 and 2, *and*
- Ifosfamide 1.2 g/m^2 IV over 30 min on days 1 to 5, *and*
- Cisplatin 20 mg/m^2 IV over 30 min on days 1 to 5

Repeat every 21 days for four cycles. Any radiographic abnormalities that persist after salvage chemotherapy should be surgically resected.

2.   High-dose chemotherapy with autologous bone marrow transplantation. High-dose chemotherapy with carboplatin and etoposide with or without cyclophosphamide followed by autologous bone marrow transplantation (ABMT) should be considered for patients who show relapse after salvage chemotherapy. Overall, about 15% of these patients are long-term survivors. The role of ABMT as first-line salvage therapy is being evaluated and should be considered experimental.

F.   Prognosis. With these strategies, the overall cure rate for patients with stage I disease is more than 98%, stage II disease more than 95%, and stage III disease more than 80%.

G.   Complications of therapy. Because patients are cured, the short- and long-term toxicities are of considerable importance. The short-term toxicities of the described chemotherapy regimens include nausea and vomiting, myelosuppression, renal toxicity, and hemorrhagic cystitis. The major long-term morbidities include infertility, pulmonary fibrosis, and a small but definite risk of secondary leukemia.

H.   Mediastinal and other midline germ cell tumors. GCTs can arise in several midline structures including the retroperitoneum, mediastinum, and pineal gland. All patients with GCTs at these sites should have a testicular ultrasound examination to exclude an occult primary tumor. Mediastinal nonseminomatous GCTs are associated with Klinefelter's syndrome and with rare hematologic malignancies (particularly acute megakaryocytic leukemia). Small mediastinal seminomas can be treated with radiation therapy alone. Widespread tumors or nonseminomatous tumors should be treated with four cycles of BEP chemotherapy. Salvage chemotherapy (including ABMT) in patients with nonseminomatous mediastinal GCT is ineffective.

V.   Cancer of the penis

A.   General considerations. Penile cancer is rare in North America but is a significant health problem in many developing countries. These tumors are nearly always squamous cell in origin and are associated with the presence of a foreskin and poor hygiene. Typically, these tumors present as a nonhealing ulcer or mass on the foreskin or glans. The most common treatment is wide surgical excision or penectomy, depending on the size and location of the lesion. Prophylactic inguinal lymph node dissection is indicated in certain subgroups of patients. Radiation therapy can also provide local control, although 15% to 20% of patients require surgical salvage.

B.   Chemotherapy for systemic disease. Active single agents include bleomycin, cisplatin, and methotrexate, with response rates of 20% to 50%. Combination chemotherapy results in high response rates, but whether survival is improved over that with single agents is unknown. A reasonable regimen is cisplatin 100 mg/m^2 on day 1, with fluorouracil 1,000 mg/m^2/day given by continuous infusion on days 1 to 4. Cycles can be repeated every 21 days.

SELECTED READINGS

Kidney

Atkins MB, Sparano J, Fisher RI, et al. Randomized phase II trial of high-dose interleukin-2 either alone or in combination with interferon alfa-2b in advanced renal cell carcinoma. *J Clin Oncol* 1993; 11:661–670.

Bukowski RM. Natural history and therapy of metastatic renal cell carcinoma: the role of interleukin-2. *Cancer* 1997;80:1198–1220.

Fyfe G, Fisher RI, Rosenberg SA, et al. Results of treatment of 255 patients with metastatic renal cell carcinoma who received high-dose recombinant interleukin-2 therapy. *J Clin Oncol* 1995;13:688–696.

Thrasher JB, Robertson JE, Paulson DF. Expanding indications for conservative renal surgery in renal cell carcinoma. *Urology* 1994; 43:160–168.

Yang JC, Topalian SL, Parkinson D, et al. Randomized comparison of high-dose and low-dose intravenous interleukin-2 for the therapy of metastatic renal cell carcinoma: an interim report. *J Clin Oncol* 1994;12:1572–1576.

Bladder

Herr HW, Schwalb DM, Zhang ZF, et al. Intravesical bacillus Calmette–Guérin therapy prevents tumor progression and death from superficial bladder cancer: ten-year follow-up of a prospective randomized trial. *J Clin Oncol* 1995;13:1404–1408.

Igawa M, Urakami S, Shiina H, et al. Long-term results with M-VAC for advanced urothelial cancer: high relapse rate and low survival in patients with a complete response. *Br J Urol* 1995;76:321–324.

Lacombe L, Dalbagni G, Zhang ZF, et al. Overexpression of p53 protein in a high-risk population of patients with superficial bladder cancer before and after bacillus Calmette–Guérin therapy: correlation to clinical outcome. *J Clin Oncol* 1996;14:2646–2652.

Lamm DL, Blumenstein BA, Crawford ED, et al. A randomized trial of intravesical doxorubicin and immunotherapy with bacille Calmette–Guérin for transitional-cell carcinoma of the bladder. *N Engl J Med* 1991;325:1205–1209.

Loehrer P, Elson P, Dreicer R, et al. Escalated dosages of methotrexate, vinblastine, doxorubicin, and cisplatin plus recombinant human granulocyte colony-stimulating factor in advanced urothelial carcinoma: an Eastern Cooperative Oncology Group trial. *J Clin Oncol* 1994;12:483–488.

Saxman SB, Propert K, Einhorn LH, et al. Long-term follow-up of a phase III intergroup study of cisplatin alone or in combination with methotrexate, vinblastine, and doxorubicin in patients with metastatic urothelial carcinoma: a cooperative group study. *J Clin Oncol* 1997;15:2564–2569.

Tester W, Caplan R, Heaney J, et al. Neoadjuvant combined modality program with selective organ preservation for invasive bladder cancer: results of Radiation Therapy Oncology Group phase II trial 8802. *J Clin Oncol* 1996;14:119–126.

Prostate

Chodak GW, Thisted RA, Gerber GS. Results of conservative management of clinically localized prostate cancer. *N Engl J Med* 1994;330:242.

Eisenberger M, Crawford ED, McLeod D, et al. A comparison of bilateral orchiectomy with or without flutamide in stage D2 prostate cancer. *Proc Am Soc Clin Oncol* 1997;16:2a(abst 3).

Fowler FJ, Barry MJ, Lu-Yao G, et al. Outcomes of external-beam radiation therapy for prostate cancer: a study of Medicare beneficiaries in three surveillance, epidemiology, and end results areas. *J Clin Oncol* 1996;14:2258–2265.

Pienta KJ, Esper PS. Risk factors for prostate cancer. *Ann Intern Med* 1993;118:793.

Pilepich MV, Caplan R, Byhardt RW, et al. Phase III trial of androgen suppression using goserelin in unfavorable-prognosis carcinoma of the prostate treated with definitive radiotherapy: report of Radiation Therapy Oncology Group protocol 85-31. *J Clin Oncol* 1997;15:1013–1021.

Prostate Cancer Trialists Collaborative Group. Maximum androgen blockade in advanced prostate cancer: an overview of 22 randomised trials with 3283 deaths in 5710 patients. *Lancet* 1995;346:265–269.

Small EJ, Vogelzang NJ. Second-line hormonal therapy for advanced prostate cancer: a shifting paradigm. *J Clin Oncol* 1997;15:382–388.

Tannock IF, Osoba D, Stockler MR, et al. Chemotherapy with mitoxantrone plus prednisone or prednisone alone for symptomatic hormone-resistant prostate cancer: a Canadian randomized trial with palliative end points. *J Clin Oncol* 1996;14:1756–1764.

Testis

Baniel J, Foster RS, Gonin R, et al. Late relapse of testicular cancer. *J Clin Oncol* 1995;13:1170–1176.

Beyer J, Kramar A, Mandanas R, et al. High-dose chemotherapy as salvage treatment in germ cell tumors: a multivariate analysis of prognostic variables. *J Clin Oncol* 1996;14:2638–2645.

Einhorn LH. Treatment of testicular cancer: a new and improved model. *J Clin Oncol* 1990;8:1777.

Foster RS, McNulty A, Rubin LR, et al. The fertility of patients with clinical stage I testis cancer managed by nerve sparing retroperitoneal lymph node dissection. *J Urol* 1994;152:1139–1143.

International Germ Cell Cancer Collaborative Group. International Germ Cell Consensus Classification: a prognostic factor-based staging system for metastatic germ cell cancers. *J Clin Oncol* 1997;15:594–603.

Loehrer PJ, Johnson D, Elson P, et al. Importance of bleomycin in favorable-prognosis disseminated germ cell tumors: an Eastern Cooperative Oncology Group trial. *J Clin Oncol* 1995;13:470–476.

Nichols CR, Williams SD, Loehrer PJ, et al. Randomized study of cisplatin dose intensity in poor-risk germ cell tumors: a Southeastern Cancer Study group and Southwest Oncology Group protocol. *J Clin Oncol* 1991;9:1163–1172.

Read G, Stenning SP, Cullen MH, et al. Medical Research Council prospective study of surveillance for stage I testicular teratoma. *J Clin Oncol* 1992;10:1762–1768.

Saxman S. Salvage therapy in recurrent testicular cancer. *Semin Oncol* 1992;19:143.

Saxman SB, Finch D, Gonin R, et al. Long-term follow-up of a phase III study of 3 versus 4 cycles of bleomycin, etoposide and cisplatin in favorable-prognosis germ cell tumors: the Indiana University experience. *J Clin Oncol* 1998;16:702–706.

Williams SD, Stablein DM, Einhorn LH, et al. Immediate adjuvant chemotherapy versus observation with treatment at relapse in pathological stage II testicular cancer. *N Engl J Med* 1987;317:1433–1438.

Penis

Abi-Aad AS, deKemion JB. Controversies in ilioinguinal lymphadenectomy for cancer of the penis. *Urol Clin North Am* 1992;19:319.

Burgers JK, Badalament RA, Drago JR. Penile cancer: clinical presentation, diagnosis, and staging. *Urol Clin North Am* 1992;19:247.

Thyroid and Adrenal Carcinomas

Samir N. Khleif and Haitham S. Abu-Lebdeh

Endocrine cancers account for 1.5% of all cancers diagnosed and for 0.4% of cancer deaths. Thyroid cancer is the most common endocrine malignancy, accounting for 90% of endocrine cancers and for 60% to 70% of the deaths from this group of diseases. Although the role of cytotoxic chemotherapy is limited in endocrine cancer, it is beneficial in selected patients. Pancreatic islet cell carcinomas and other pancreatic malignancies are discussed in Chapter 9. Here, thyroid and adrenal carcinomas are discussed. The pathology, presentation, and biologic behavior of thyroid and adrenal carcinomas are important determinants of therapy, and they are briefly considered.

I. Thyroid carcinoma
A. Background
1. **Incidence.** About 17,000 new cases of thyroid carcinoma are diagnosed each year, which result in about 1,200 deaths due to this cancer. The incidence of thyroid carcinoma is 5.9 per 100,000 women and 2.2 per 100,000 men, and the peak incidence is at age 40 for women and age 60 for men. The prevalence at autopsy is 5 to 15 per 100,000 subjects. Thyroid carcinoma usually affects people between the ages of 25 and 65 years.

2. **Etiology and prevention.** In most instances, the cause of thyroid carcinoma is unknown, although experimentally prolonged stimulation by thyroid-stimulating hormone (TSH) may lead to the development of thyroid carcinoma. Some cases appear to be related to a dose-dependent phenomenon involving radiation to the neck during childhood. Thyroid malignancy has been observed 20 to 25 years after radiation exposure in atomic bomb survivors and in children treated with radiation therapy for benign conditions of the head and neck. The frequency increases exponentially with doses up to 12 Gy and then decreases, so that with doses over 20 Gy, the risk of developing malignancy becomes relatively low because such high doses lead to the destruction of cells rather than nonlethal damage of the deoxyribonucleic acid (DNA). Some cases of thyroid carcinoma (usually medullary carcinoma) are familial, as seen in the multiple endocrine neoplasia (MEN) syndrome, associated with germline mutation of the *RET* proto-oncogene. Although ionizing radiation for benign conditions of the head and neck is no longer being used, thyroid carcinomas related to prior exposure to radiation are still being seen. In cases of accidental nuclear exposure, it is thought that the use of potassium iodide to block the thyroid uptake of radioactive iodine (RAI) in children is helpful in reducing the incidence of subsequent thyroid cancer. This measure was used in Eastern Europe after the Chernobyl accident.

3.   Histologic types. The most common histologic types of thyroid carcinoma are as follows:

   a.   Differentiated thyroid cancer. Differentiated thyroid cancer (DTC) includes papillary carcinoma (75% to 80%) and follicular carcinoma (11%). DTCs are derived from thyroglobulin-producing follicular cells.

   b.   Anaplastic or undifferentiated carcinoma (2%)

   c.   Medullary carcinoma (4%). Medullary carcinomas are derived from thyroid parafollicular or C cells. These cells produce both immunoreactive calcitonin and carcinoembryonic antigen (CEA).

   d.   Hürthle cell carcinoma (3%). Hürthle cell carcinoma used to be considered a variant of follicular carcinoma. It is now considered as a separate pathologic entity.

   e.   Thyroid lymphoma (5%)

4.   Prognosis

   a.   Cell types. Papillary and mixed papillary and follicular histologies are considered to have similar biologic and prognostic behaviors. Patients with these cancers have an excellent prognosis, with less than 15% mortality at 20 years. Patients with pure follicular carcinoma do not do as well as those with papillary elements, at least in part because there is a tendency for the follicular carcinoma to spread through the bloodstream, whereas the papillary carcinoma spreads more by lymphatic channels. The 10-year relative survival rates are 85% and 93%, respectively. Recent studies have shown that patients having follicular carcinoma with vascular invasion have a relatively bad prognosis, whereas patients with follicular carcinoma without vascular invasion do almost as well as those with papillary carcinoma. About 25% of medullary carcinomas are familial, as part of three clinical syndromes (MEN-IIa, MEN-IIb, and familial non-MEN medullary thyroid carcinoma). Regional lymph node and distant metastases are common in patients with medullary carcinomas and occur in early stages of the disease. The 10-year survival rate after surgical resection is 40% to 60%. Patients with anaplastic thyroid carcinoma have an abysmal prognosis, with a median survival time of 4 months, although occasional patients may be cured with combined radiotherapy and chemotherapy.

   b.   Other factors. In addition to the cell type, the prognosis of thyroid carcinoma is shown to be worse if the following factors are present:

- A large tumor size, especially more than 4 cm.
- Patient age more than 40 years.
- Distant metastases. DTC tends to metastasize to the lung or bone. Patients with bone metastases have survival rates at 5, 10, and 15 years of 53%, 38%, and 30%, respectively.
- Abnormal DNA content in tumor cells in the papillary type; the more pronounced the aneuploidy, the more aggressively the cancer behaves.
- Male sex, which may be related to the fact that men tend to be older at the time of diagnosis and are more likely to have a worse histologic type.

In contrast to most other cancers, limited regional lymph node metastasis of DTC does not influence survival substantially, and radiation-induced thyroid carcinoma is not associated with a worse prognosis.

B. Diagnosis and staging. Any solitary thyroid nodule should be considered a possible malignant tumor until proved otherwise, especially in patients younger than 25 years and men older than 60 years. Although toxic nodular goiters are less likely to contain carcinoma, a nodule in the setting of hyperthyroidism does not automatically confer benignity. The overall incidence of cancer in a "cold" nodule is 5% to 10%. Because most thyroid tumors spread primarily by local extension and regional nodal metastasis, assessment of the extent of disease is concentrated on the neck. Presurgical studies include careful physical examination, thyroid function tests, and cytology by fine-needle aspiration (FNA). Unlike core-needle biopsy, FNA biopsy yields an aspirate of cells and not tissue fragment. FNA does not require local anesthesia and is considered safer and easier to perform.

Other studies such as indirect laryngoscopy, radionuclide scanning, esophagogram, and computed tomography (CT) scan of the neck could be performed on a case-by-case basis. In a few instances, a core-needle biopsy might be considered. If there is a strong clinical suspicion of thyroid lymphoma and FNA is not diagnostic, then a core-needle biopsy might be considered as an alternative to a surgical biopsy that requires general anesthesia. The accuracy of needle aspiration biopsy ranges between 50% and 97%, depending on the experience of the pathologist and the institution. Chest radiography should be performed before surgery to rule out pulmonary metastasis. If there is any clinical or laboratory suggestion of bone metastases, skeletal x-rays, CT scan, or a radionuclide bone scan should be performed. Patients with thyroid carcinoma are typically euthyroid. Thyroid carcinoma rarely destroys thyroid function to the point of frank hypothyroidism. However, elevated TSH levels with increased thyroid peroxidase antibodies may be seen with Hashimoto's thyroiditis, which may co-exist in 20% of patients with thyroid lymphoma.

The most widely accepted staging system is the pathologic TNM classification, which assesses tumor size and extent (T1, less than 2 cm; T2, 2 to 4 cm; T3, greater than 4 cm), lymph node metastasis, and distant metastasis (Table 13.1). With use of pTNM staging, any anaplastic thyroid cancer is considered stage IV, and there are no stage III or IV patients with differentiated thyroid cancer who are younger than 45 years. This staging system does not provide all the information needed. Other staging or risk-group assignment systems are used to providing prognostic information.

C. Treatment. The therapeutic approach to patients with thyroid carcinoma depends considerably on the histologic type.

  1. Differentiated thyroid carcinoma

    a. Surgery is the only definitive therapy. Although the surgical approach may differ among surgeons and institutions, many surgeons prefer a bilateral near-total thyroidectomy, taking into consideration that with DTC, the incidence of disease in the contralateral lobe is 20% to 87%. Limited lymph node involvement does not substantially in-

Table 13.1.   pTNM staging system for thyroid cancer

Stage	Papillary or follicular, age <45	Papillary or follicular, age >45 medullary any age	Anaplastic any age
I	M0	T1N0M0	—
II	M1	T2N0M0	—
III	—	T3N0M0	—
		T1-3N1aM0	
IV	—	T4AnyNM0	Any
		T1-3N1bM0	
		AnyTAnyNM1	

fluence the survival rate, but it is associated with an increase in local recurrence. Total thyroidectomy with modified neck dissection is often preferred for those who have lateral cervical lymph node involvement. Mortality after thyroidectomy in DTC approaches 0%. Complications include permanent recurrent laryngeal nerve damage in 2% of patients and permanent hypoparathyroidism in 1% to 2%.

b.   Thyroid-stimulating hormone suppression is an essential component in the treatment of DTC because there is good evidence that cells are usually responsive to TSH. TSH suppresses the growth of malignant as well as normal thyroid tissue, and therefore the recurrence rate is reduced; in a few patients, metastatic lesions are diminished markedly. This hormonal suppression can be achieved by the administration of exogenous thyroid hormone. Usually 125 to 200 μg of levothyroxine (T_4) daily is used to obliterate the pituitary response to thyrotropin-releasing hormone (TRH) and thus keep the TSH level in the range of 0.1 to 0.4 mIU/L. Complete TSH suppression (0.01 to 0.1 mIU/L) should be reserved for high-risk patients to avoid long-term adverse effects on bone and heart. Side effects and dose-limiting factors include symptoms of thyrotoxicosis, angina, and cardiac arrhythmia.

c.   Radiotherapy. Destruction of residual normal thyroid tissue after thyroidectomy with radioactive iodine (RAI) is termed radioactive remnant ablation (RRA). RRA is widely used in practice in the United States. When ablation is carried out postoperatively, it is usually done 4 to 6 weeks after thyroidectomy. RRA allows for better subsequent imaging with RAI when looking for metastasis. It also improves the sensitivity for thyroglobulin measurements (since remnant thyroid tissue is destroyed) and may destroy microscopic cancer cells within the remnant. A dose of 30 mCi (1,110 MBq) to 150 mCi (5,550 MBq) is usually used. Most centers use the lower dose of 30 mCi, which is estimated to expose the whole body to about 6 rems. RRA is different from RAI therapy where larger doses of RAI are used to destroy persistent cancer or distant metastasis. For patients who are at low risk (tumor size less than 1 cm), ablation is controversial. Many physicians still ablate to allow for an easier follow-up. RRA is strongly recommended for patients who are at high risk of recurrence or metastasis (patients older than 45 years or with large lesions).

Treatment with RAI (^{131}I) is usually recommended for patients with DTC and known postoperative residual disease, patients with distant metastases, and patients with locally invasive lesions. For patients with nodal metastases that are not large enough to excise, a dose of 100 to 175 mCi of RAI treatment is given (3,700 to 6,475 MBq). Locally invasive cancer that is not completely resected is treated with 150 to 200 mCi (5,550 to 7,400 MBq). Patients with distant metastasis are treated with 200 mCi (7,400 MBq). The exception is lung metastasis; a dose of up to 80 mCi (2,960 MBq) is generally thought to avoid radiation-induced fibrosis. Another approach is to use quantitative dosimetry methods to calculate RAI dose based on tumor uptake or dosimetry based on blood levels.

Although the effect of RAI on survival is not well determined, it is well accepted that the use of RAI and T_4 suppressive therapy markedly decreases the recurrence rate. Effective use of RAI treatment requires the following:

1. Tumor cells that are capable of receiving and concentrating iodide (i.e., DTC), *and*
2. Appropriate patient preparation by withholding thyroid hormone administration for 2 to 4 weeks to provide the iodine-concentrating cells with the highest endogenous TSH stimulation.

T_3 is cleared from the body much more rapidly than T_4. The shorter period of withdrawal minimizes the period of hypothyroidism. Accordingly, patients are switched from suppression therapy with T_4 to a corresponding dose of T_3 for 2 to 4 weeks to allow metabolic disposal of the T_4. This is followed by 2 weeks of T_3 withdrawal. Ideally, TSH of at least 25 to 30 μm/mL is required for successful ablation or radiotherapy. Potential side effects expected after radioiodine therapy include temporary bone marrow depression, nausea, sialoadenitis with possible permanent cessation of salivary flow (radiation mumps), skin reaction over the tissue concentrating the radioiodine, and pulmonary fibrosis. The use of high doses (cumulative effect) may be associated with acute myelogenous leukemia, bladder and breast cancer, and transient bone marrow depression. Once ablation is successful, patients are placed on suppressive therapy. Patients with lung metastases treated with RAI have a 20-year survival rate of 54%. Scintigraphy should be performed 4 to 10 days after therapy to detect any residual carcinoma. Most DTCs grow very slowly. The rate of recurrence is 0.5% to 1.6%/year. Therefore, lifelong annual serum thyroglobulin assays are recommended. Scintigraphy is suggested if the thyroglobulin is found to be elevated. Some centers also advocate the use of neck ultrasounds for follow-up. The role of external radiation therapy in DTC is limited. It is considered for tumors that concentrate little or no iodine. It is also used for localized bony metastasis.

2. Medullary thyroid carcinoma. With familial medullary carcinoma, the disease is almost always bilateral. Regional lymph node involvement is common in early stages. Therefore, total thyroidectomy, central lymph node dissection, and lateral ipsilateral modified radical neck dissection are required. The overall 10-year survival rate after surgical resection is 40% to 60%. Serum calcitonin levels should be measured 8 to 12 weeks postoperatively to assess disease burden and residual cancer. Search for germline and not somatic *RET* proto-oncogene mutations identifies most familial cases. For other family members with a positive *RET* proto-oncogene, surgery is recommended as early as an age of 2 years. Postoperative annual evaluation is recommended by measuring levels of calcitonin and CEA, both of which are secreted by the medullary thyroid carcinoma cells, as a follow-up for residual disease or recurrence. Suppressive therapy is of no benefit because medullary cells do not have TSH receptors. RAI and cytotoxic chemotherapy are of little utility. Cisplatin, streptozocin, carmustine, methotrexate, and fluorouracil have shown little, if any, benefit. However, some studies have shown doxorubicin chemotherapy to produce occasional responses of metastatic disease (see Section I.C.4). Local radiation therapy is useful in some patients as palliative therapy.

3.   Anaplastic thyroid carcinoma. Most anaplastic tumors are unresectable at the time of presentation. A more complete thyroid resection is associated with longer survival than biopsy alone. Combination chemotherapy or chemotherapy plus radiation therapy has shown encouraging results for local control, and few partial and complete remissions have been seen.

4.   Chemotherapy

a.   Single-agent chemotherapy. The most widely applied cytotoxic agents are doxorubicin, bleomycin, cisplatin, and etoposide. Each of these medications has demonstrated some activity against anaplastic and medullary thyroid carcinomas. Improved survival may be achieved in patients who respond to sequential exposure to these agents. Doxorubicin has proved to be the best single chemotherapeutic agent with the highest response rate. Doxorubicin in a dosage of 60 to 75 mg/m^2 IV every 3 weeks has resulted in objective responses in 20% to 45% (median 34%) of patients with advanced refractory metastatic thyroid carcinoma. The response rate is probably highest for the medullary type and lowest for undifferentiated thyroid carcinoma. A high single dose of doxorubicin, which should be increased in patients with no response, appears to be essential for a therapeutic effect. Because of its apparently lower cardiotoxicity, epirubicin, although almost as effective as doxorubicin, may be given at higher doses and over longer periods and is therefore preferred by some investigators. Paclitaxel infusion over 96 h may be a potential chemotherapeutic agent for treatment of undifferentiated forms of thyroid cancer.

b.   Combination chemotherapy. Combination chemotherapy usually includes doxorubicin. Cisplatin 40 mg/m^2 IV plus doxorubicin 60 mg/m^2 IV given every 3 weeks have yielded a higher rate and quality of response than doxorubicin alone. These results included complete remission in

12% of patients, several of whom survived more than 2 years. Toxicity was no worse with the combination therapy. Other combination-chemotherapy regimens are doxorubicin, bleomycin, vincristine, and melphalan, with a response rate of 36%, and doxorubicin, bleomycin, and vincristine, with an improved 64% response rate. Doxorubicin 10 mg/m^2 IV has been used in combination with external radiotherapy 90 min before the first radiation treatment and weekly thereafter. In this combination, the radiotherapy was given at a dose of 1.6 Gy/treatment twice a day for 3 consecutive days weekly for 6 weeks. Patients with undifferentiated thyroid carcinoma treated in this fashion showed an improvement in the median survival compared with historical control subjects. In general, the highest response is observed in patients with pulmonary metastasis. If anaplastic thyroid carcinoma responds to chemotherapy, a prolongation of the median survival time from 3 to 5 months to 15 to 20 months can be achieved.

5. Non-Hodgkin's lymphoma. Non-Hodgkin's lymphoma is more thoroughly addressed in Chapter 22. The discussion here briefly highlights its significance concerning thyroid malignancies. By definition, lymphoma of the thyroid is, at the time of diagnosis, confined to the gland or to the gland and regional lymph nodes. The major histologic type is non-Hodgkin's lymphoma. Autoimmune thyroiditis is a predisposing factor. Lymphoma of the thyroid usually presents with rapid enlargement of the gland within a few weeks and is bilateral in 25% of patients. If the tumor is confined to the thyroid, surgical excision alone yields a 5-year survival rate of 70% to 90%. Once the lymphoma extends beyond the thyroid gland, however, surgical therapy does not improve survival, and radiation therapy and chemotherapy are indicated.

II. Adrenal carcinoma
A. Adrenocortical carcinoma
1. Incidence and etiology. Adrenocortical carcinoma is a rare tumor, with fewer than 200 new cases occurring yearly in the United States. It accounts for 0.05% to 0.20% of all cancers and for 0.2% of cancer deaths. It has a prevalence of 2 per 1 million population worldwide. The peak incidence of adrenocortical carcinoma occurs during the fourth and fifth decades of life. The incidence in women in most reports is about 2.5 times higher than that in men, who tend to be older at diagnosis. Women have a tendency to develop a functional (hormone-secreting) carcinoma, whereas men usually develop a nonfunctional malignancy. There is no family predilection, and no etiologic factors have been established. Most cancers are monoclonal, suggesting that a genetic alteration in a progenitor cell contributes to tumorigenesis. Sometimes, it occurs in the context of tumor-predisposing syndromes such as Li–Fraumeni or Beckwith–Wiedemann syndrome.

2. Clinical picture. Adrenal carcinoma may present in several modes.

   a. An abdominal mass maybe detected incidentally by abdominal imaging for some other purpose.

   b. A functioning tumor with endocrine signs and symptoms of Cushing's syndrome, virilization, or feminization maybe detected. Forty percent to 60% of patients present with functioning tumor. Such manifestations are due to an increase in the production of a wide variety of steroid hormones. Ten percent of adrenocortical carcinomas are associated with virilization and 12% with feminization. Adrenal carcinoma is the cause of 10% of all cases of Cushing's syndrome.

   c.   Other frequent presenting symptoms include upper abdominal pain, weight loss, palpable abdominal mass, anorexia, and malaise. Usually, these symptoms are associated with advanced disease.

3.   Pathology and diagnosis. Most malignant adrenal masses represent carcinomatous metastatic lesions, primarily from the lung and breast. Whether the coincidental finding of an adrenal mass requires complete screening of the patient for a hidden primary adrenal tumor depends on the clinical situation. There may be some difficulty distinguishing adenoma from carcinoma (Table 13.2). CT scan and magnetic resonance imaging (MRI) are helpful in diagnosing adrenocortical carcinoma. A CT finding of a large unilateral adrenal mass with irregular borders and a heterogeneous and hypervascular interior is almost always an indication of adrenal cancer. On MRI, adrenal cancer has intermediate to high signal intensity on T2-weighted images in contrast to benign lesions, which have low signal intensity. In addition, MRI is a helpful tool in delineating adrenocortical carcinoma before surgery. Iodocholesterol scanning is rarely indicated. It shows poor uptake in carcinomas compared with adenomas. Adrenocortical carci-

Table 13.2.   Diagnosis of malignancy in adrenocortical neoplasms

Reliability	Clinical criteria	Pathologic criteria
Diagnostic of malignancy	Weight loss, feminization, nodal or distant metastases	Tumor weight >100 g, tumor necrosis, fibrous bands, vascular invasion, mitoses
Consistent with malignancy	Virilism, Cushing's syndrome and virilism, no hormone production	Nuclear pleomorphism
Suggestive of malignancy	Elevated urinary 17-ketosteroid levels	Capsular invasion
Unreliable	Hypercortisolism, hyperaldosteronism	Tumor giant cells, cytoplasmic size variations, ratio between compact and clear cells

Adapted from Page DL, DeLellis RA, Hough AJ. Tumors of the adrenal. *In:* Hartmann WH, Sobin LH, eds. *Atlas of tumor pathology.* Washington, D.C.: Armed Forces Institute of Pathology, 1986.

noma can be further divided into two categories according to the pathologic patterns of cellular arrangement and the cellular pleomorphism:

> **a.   Well-differentiated adrenocortical carcinoma,** which occurs more commonly in women and usually presents with a functioning tumor, *and*
>
> **b.   Anaplastic carcinoma,** which is more common in men and is often associated with a lack of hormone production.

4.   Staging and prognosis. Most patients (70%) present with stage III or IV disease. Adrenocortical carcinoma is a highly malignant cancer with an overall 5-year mortality rate of 75% to 90%, depending on the stage and morphology of the disease. The most commonly used staging system (derived from the TNM classification system) for adrenocortical carcinoma is presented in Table 13.3.

Metastases of adrenocortical carcinoma most commonly occur in the lung (60%), lymph nodes (43%), liver (53%), and bone (10%). The median survival time of patients with well-differentiated carcinoma is 40 months, whereas patients with anaplastic carcinoma have a more dismal median survival time of 5 months. The median survival time of patients with stage I, II, or III disease is 24 to 28 months and for stage IV disease 12 months. Intratumoral hemorrhage, number of mitotic figures per high-power field, and tumor size correlate with survival rates.

5.   Treatment. Because of the extremely low incidence of this disease, few medical centers have sufficient experience treating it, and an effort should be made to refer these patients to centers that have clinical trials pertaining to this disease. This caveat notwithstanding, several guidelines regarding its treatment can be given.

> **a.   Surgery.** In up to half of patients, adrenocortical carcinomas can be resected, although incompletely in some patients; however, the remainder of patients have either local invasion that is too extensive or metastases to the abdomen, liver, lung, or other locations. Of the patients whose tumors are resected for cure, 40% remain disease-free. The remainder die, usually with extensive metastatic disease, within an average of less than 1 year. Patients who undergo complete resection should initially be followed on a monthly basis (with measurements of steroid levels if they have a functioning tumor) to detect recurrence. Serial MRI may also be used to evaluate for recurrence.
>
> **b.   Radiotherapy.** Radiation therapy provides symptomatic relief from pain due to local or metastatic disease, es-

Table 13.3.   TNM staging system for adrenocortical cancer

Stage	Size (cm)	Nodes or local invasion	Metastasis
I	≤5	−	−
II	>5	−	−
III	Any	+	−
IV	Any	Both present or absent	+

pecially bony metastases. It has also been used to prevent local recurrence after surgical resection (40 to 55 Gy over 4 weeks), but the benefit is uncertain, and there is no proof that it improves survival.

c.   **Chemotherapy.** Indications for chemotherapy include recurrent, metastatic, and nonresectable adrenocortical carcinoma. Agents used are the following:

(1)   **Adrenocortical suppressants**

(a)   **Mitotane (*o,p*'-DDD, Lysodren).** An unconventional chemotherapy and a close chemical relative of the insecticide 1,1-bis(*p*-chlorophenyl)-2,2,2-trichloroethane (DDT), mitotane has been used to treat adrenocortical carcinoma since 1960. It inhibits steroid biosynthesis and with prolonged use destroys adrenal cells. The cytotoxic effect of mitotane has been considered transient and inconsistent. Included in its effects is the destruction of the adrenocortical cells. The part that is most affected by this action is the zona reticularis and the least affected is the zona glomerulosa. Forty percent of the medication is absorbed from the gastrointestinal tract. The drug is highly lipid soluble and is subsequently concentrated in both normal and malignant adrenocortical cells. Reports of its plasma half-life range from 18 to 159 days.

(i)   **Dosage and administration.** Treatment with mitotane is started at 2 to 6 g/day PO in three divided doses, then gradually increased monthly by 1 g/day until 9 to 10 g/day is reached or until the maximum tolerated dose is achieved with no side effects. Blood levels of *o,p*'-DDD should be maintained at more than 14 μg/mL to demonstrate a therapeutic response. Mitotane serum level was shown in a retrospective study to be the only significant prognostic factor for tumor response. Levels of more than 20 μg/mL have a higher incidence of toxicity.

(ii)   **Response and follow-up.** Objective tumor regression usually occurs within 6 weeks after the initiation of therapy and is seen in 70% of patients as a decrease in excessive hormone production. However, the reduction in hormone production is not regularly accompanied by an objective tumor response. In about 30% to 40% of patients, the tumor size is reduced significantly, but complete remission is unlikely. The median duration of response is 10.5 months. If no clinical benefit is demonstrated at the maximum tolerated dose after 3 months, the case may be considered a clinical failure. Postoperative adjuvant therapy with mitotane has resulted in no improvement in survival. The combination of mitotane and radiation therapy has not conferred any additional benefit over mitotane alone.

(iii)   **Side effects.** Nausea and vomiting occur in 80% of patients. Severe neurotoxicity, which may occur during long-term treatment, presents as somnolence, depression, ataxia, and weakness in 40% of patients. Reversible diffuse electroencephalographic changes may also occur. Adrenal insufficiency occurs in 50% of patients (without replacement), and dermatitis develops in 20% of patients. Because the maximal dosage is often limited by the severity of, and the patient's tolerance to, the side effects, the total dose may range widely from patient to patient.

(iv)   Glucocorticoid replacement. During mitotane treatment, it is necessary to prevent hypoadrenalism. Replacement can be achieved by administering cortisone acetate 25 mg PO in the morning and 12.5 mg PO in the evening or equivalent glucocorticoid plus fludrocortisone acetate 0.1 mg PO in the morning. Plasma cortisol should be used to monitor adrenal function during mitotane use. If severe trauma or shock develops, mitotane should be discontinued immediately and larger doses of corticosteroids (e.g., hydrocortisone 100 mg t.i.d.) should be administered.

(v)   Nonresponders to mitotane. These patients can be treated with other adrenocortical suppressants including metyrapone (750 mg PO every 4 h), which reduces cortisol production by inhibiting 11β-hydroxylase. However, this results in accumulation of deoxycorticosterone and can induce hypertension and hypokalemic alkalosis.

Another agent is aminoglutethimide (250 mg PO every 6 h initially, with a stepwise increase in dosage to a total of 2 g/day or until limiting side effects that resemble those of mitotane appear). The latter drug inhibits conversion of cholesterol to pregnenolone. Metyrapone can induce hypertension and hypokalemic alkalosis. Neither of these medications has antitumor effects, but they are effective in relieving the signs and symptoms of excessive hormonal secretion. Combining both in smaller doses might reduce the side effects seen in taking higher doses of either agent alone. Another medication that can be used is ketoconazole 600 mg/day. It is a potent adrenal inhibitor that produces clinical alleviation of the signs and symptoms within 4 to 6 weeks. In addition, it may cause regression of pulmonary and hepatic metastases, although the mechanism is not clear. Other drugs that might be of benefit in controlling symptoms include those that block the action of steroids in their target tissues, including antimineralocorticoid and antiandrogenic agents and, more recently, antiglucocorticoid agents such as mifepristone (RU 486). None of these medications has an effect on tumor regression.

(2)   Cytotoxic chemotherapy. Cytotoxic drugs are usually used in patients who show no response to mitotane. Because of the small number of patients who require such therapy, the experience with this treatment is limited despite many clinical trials. No cytotoxic drug has shown definite effectiveness in the treatment of adrenocortical carcinoma, although doxorubicin, cisplatin, and suramin have been reported to produce partial responses in patients with metastatic disease. Few combination-chemotherapy regimens have been effective. Cyclophosphamide 600 mg/m^2 IV plus doxorubicin 40 mg/m^2 IV plus cisplatin 50 mg/m^2 IV given in cycles every 3 weeks led to partial remission in 2 of 11 patients with adrenocortical carcinoma. The only combination that has induced complete remission is cisplatin 40 mg/m^{2}IV plus etoposide 100 mg/m^2 IV plus bleomycin 30 U IV given every 4 weeks. Three of four patients responded, one with complete remission. Severe side effects occurred in patients in both of these studies.

Chemotherapy can also be given in combination with mitotane. Cisplatin 75 to 100 mg/m^2 was combined with mitotane 4 g PO daily. This resulted in a 30% objective response that lasted for 7.9 months. The survival duration in this study was 11.8 months. Other combinations of natural-product chemotherapy with mitotane are being tested; this may be pharmacologically advantageous because mitotane has been shown to be a multidrug resistance–blocking agent.

   d. Arterial embolization. Another modality used for palliation of adrenocortical carcinoma is arterial embolization. It is used to decrease the bulk of the tumor, suppress tumor function, and relieve pain. Embolic agents used include polyvinyl alcohol foam and surgical gelatin.

B. Pheochromocytoma

   1. Description and diagnosis. Pheochromocytoma is a tumor that arises from chromaffin cells mainly in the adrenal medulla (90% of cases), paraganglia, as well as other sites (e.g., urinary bladder, heart, and organ of Zuckerkandl). It is an uncommon tumor, with an estimated 800 cases diagnosed in the United States every year. It is found in up to 0.3% of autopsy subjects and is responsible for less than 0.1% to 0.5% of all cases of hypertension. Pheochromocytoma can be hereditary, as part of the MEN syndrome (MEN-IIa, MEN-IIb), or familial with no other manifestation of the MEN syndrome; when part of the MEN syndrome, it is almost always benign. Also, it may be found as part of von Hippel–Lindau disease and Carney's syndrome. The risk of developing a contralateral tumor in hereditary pheochromocytoma is more than 50%. The incidence of malignant pheochromocytoma ranges between 5% and 45%. The only definite proof of malignancy is the presence of tumor in secondary sites where chromaffin tissue is not normally present. The diagnosis of pheochromocytoma depends on a thorough history and physical examination, increased catecholamine levels in the plasma and the urine (including epinephrine, norepinephrine, dopamine, and total metanephrines), cross-sectional imaging such as CT or MRI, or [131I]meta-iodobenzylguanidine ([131I]MIBG) scintigraphy. The overall 5-year survival rate for patients with malignant pheochromocytoma is 36% to 44%. Although pheochromocytoma is a rare tumor, early detection and treatment are crucial, owing to its high morbidity and potential mortality (stroke and myocardial infarction). Patients with pheochromocytoma can present with sustained or episodic hypertension. Hypertension does not usually correlate with the amount of catecholamine production, and its severity varies widely among patients.

2. Treatment

a. Surgery. Surgery is the only definitive therapy for pheochromocytoma. It is done for localized and regional unilateral or bilateral disease. Surgery requires careful preoperative preparation to achieve control of the blood pressure, blood volume, and heart rate. Phenoxybenzamine, an α-adrenergic receptor blocker, is started 1 to 2 weeks before surgery in a dose of 10 to 20 mg PO three or four times daily. Some patients require the addition of β-blockers (e.g., propranolol 80 to 120 mg/day), which are indicated for persistent supraventricular tachycardia or the presence of angina. To prevent hypertensive crisis secondary to unopposed vasoconstriction, the β-blocker should never be given before the α-antagonist. Other α-adrenergic blockers are used for the same purpose, including prazocin, which is a selective α_1-antagonist that has also been used successfully for preoperative preparation of pheochromocytoma. Intraoperatively, blood pressure can be controlled by titration with nitroprusside.

Catecholamine and metanephrine levels should be measured 1 week after surgery to confirm total removal of the tumor. Surgical mortality is estimated around 2% and usually correlates with the severity of hypertension. Patients whose localized disease is fully resected should have normal life expectancy. Close postoperative follow-up is mandatory because of the possibility of postoperative residual tumor and because 10% of patients have metastasis and another 10% have multiple primary tumors at the time of diagnosis.

The follow-up should include a history, physical examination, and catecholamine and metanephrine measurements at 3 months, followed by a similar evaluation yearly for life. Redevelopment of any sign or symptom suggesting pheochromocytoma or a rising trend in catecholamine levels requires imaging, including [131I]MIBG scintigraphy. A few centers recommend that [131I]MIBG scintigraphy be done yearly regardless of the catecholamine levels or the clinical picture; this is not frequently practiced in the U.S.A. The recurrence rate of pheochromocytoma postoperatively is 5%/year. Contralateral adrenalectomy of a normal gland is generally not recommended in patients with a high incidence of bilateral disease (e.g., MEN-II), despite the high risk of subsequent involvement. In patients with metastatic disease, there is no evidence to support improved survival after local debulking.

b. Chemotherapy and radiation therapy. These are reserved for locally invasive, metastatic, and inoperable lesions. Response to both of these treatments is evaluated by regression of tumor size and a decrease in the catecholamine levels. Owing to the small number of patients with pheochromocytoma, limited data are available regarding the effect of chemotherapy. Because of the functional and biologic similarities between pheochromocytoma and neuroblastoma, the combination of cyclophosphamide and dacarbazine, which induces an 80% response in neuroblastoma, was used in two series to treat pheochromocytoma. The chemotherapy regimen consisted of cyclophosphamide 750 mg/m^2 IV plus vincristine 1.4 mg/m^2 IV on day 1 and dacarbazine 600 mg/m^2 IV on days 1 and 2; it was repeated in 21- to 28-day cycles. Analysis of 23 patients showed objective tumor size regression in 61% of patients, and the urinary catecholamine levels decreased in 74% of patients. The median response time averaged 28 months. Improvement of blood pressure control and performance status occurred with minimal toxicity. Because streptozocin has yielded favorable results in the treatment of neuroendocrine tumor in the gastrointestinal tract, it was used as a single agent in a patient with malignant pheochromocytoma. Streptozocin showed promising results, with a 73% reduction in urinary vanillylmandelic acid level and significant tumor size regression.

c.   Radiation therapy. [131I]MIBG is actively taken up and concentrated by pheochromocytoma cells with high sensitivity and specificity. Consequently, a high dose of [131I]MIBG is used to treat pheochromocytoma. This treatment has shown some evidence of response in terms of tumor size regression and decreased catecholamine levels. The uptake of [131I] MIBG by pheochromocytoma requires the presence of an active neuronal pump mechanism, which limits the use of this agent to patients with pheochromocytoma who have the ability to concentrate [131I]MIBG in the cells. Therefore, initial screening of the ability of the pheochromocytoma to concentrate small doses of [131I]MIBG is necessary to determine the probable efficacy of the treatment. In addition, combination [131I]MIBG and chemotherapy produced additive effects in reducing tumor burden. External radiation to doses of 4,000 to 5,000 cGy in 4 to 5 weeks may provide local control to an inoperable tumor and may be used to control local bone metastasis.

d.   Supportive pharmacologic therapy. α-Blockers should be used to prevent severe hypertension-related morbidity and mortality, especially in untreated patients and those receiving chemotherapy. Another pharmacologic agent that can be used is α-methyl-L-tyrosine (metyrosine), which inhibits tyrosine hydroxylase, a rate-limiting step in catecholamine biosynthesis. Metyrosine allows the use of lower doses of α-blockers and has been shown to be effective in catecholamine-induced cardiomyopathy. Other medications include β-blockers, which are used to control arrhythmia, angiotensin-converting enzyme inhibitors, and calcium-channel blockers, which are also used for hypertension control.

SELECTED READINGS

Thyroid Carcinoma

Bucsky P, Parlowsky T. Epidemiology and therapy of thyroid cancer in childhood and adolescence. *Exp Clin Endocrinol Diabetes* 1997; 105(suppl 4):70–73.

Farid NR. Molecular pathogenesis of thyroid cancer: the significance of oncogenes, tumor suppressor genes, and genomic instability. *Exp Clin Endocrinol Diabetes* 1996;104(suppl 4):1–12.

Galloway RJ, Smallridge RC. Imaging in thyroid cancer. *Endocrinol Metab Clin North Am* 1996;25:93–113.

Giuffrida D, Gharib, H. Anaplastic thyroid carcinoma: current diagnosis and treatment. *Ann Oncol* 2000;11:1083–1089.

Harmer CL. Radiotherapy in the management of thyroid cancer. *Ann Acad Med Singapore* 1996;25:413–419.

Modigliani E, Franc B, Niccoli-Sire P. Diagnosis and treatment of medullary thyroid cancer. Best practice and research. *Clin Endocrinol Metab* 2000;14:631–649.

Moley JF. Medullary thyroid cancer. *Surg Clin North Am* 1995;75: 405–420.

Noguchi M, Katev N, Miwa K. Therapeutic strategies and long-term results in differentiated thyroid cancer. *J Surg Oncol* 1998;67: 52–59.

Robbins J. Prognostic factors in the management of thyroid cancer. *J Endocrinol Invest* 1995;18:159–160.

Soh EY, Clark OH. Surgical considerations and approach to thyroid cancer. *Endocrinol Metab Clin North Am* 1996;25:115–139.

Tezelman S, Clark OH. Current management of thyroid cancer. *Adv Surg* 1995;28:191–221.

Thyroid Carcinoma Task Force. AACE/AAES medical/surgical guidelines for clinical practice: management of thyroid carcinoma. *Endocr Pract* 2001;7:203–220.

Yeh SD, La Quaglia W. [131]I therapy for pediatric thyroid cancer. *Semin Pediatr Surg* 1997;6:128–133.

Adrenocortical Carcinoma

Bornstein SR. Stratakis CA. Chrousos GP. Adrenocortical tumors: recent advances in basic concepts and clinical management. *Ann Intern Med* 1999;130:759–771.

Boscaro M, Fallo F, Barzon L, et al. Adrenocortical carcinoma: epidemiology and natural history. *Minerva Endocrinol* 1995;20:89–94.

Cook DM. Adrenal mass. *Endocrinol Metab Clin North Am* 1997;26: 829–852.

Dogliotti L, Berruti A, Pia A, et al. Cytotoxic chemotherapy for adrenocortical carcinoma. *Minerva Endocrinol* 1995;20:105–109.

Dunnick RN. Adrenal carcinoma. *Radiol Clin North Am* 1994;31:99.

Gicquel C, Baudin E, Lebouc Y, Schlumberger M. Adrenocortical carcinoma. *Ann Oncol* 1997;8:423–427.

Haak HR, Hermans J, Van deVelde CJ, et al. Optimal treatment of adrenocortical carcinoma with mitotane: results in a consecutive series of 96 patients. *Br J Cancer* 1994;69:947.

Kasperlik-Zaluska AA, Migdalska BM, Makowska AM. Impact of adjuvant mitotane on the clinical course of patients with adrenocortical cancer: two years later [Letter]. *Cancer* 1996;78:1520–1521.

Kendrick ML, Lloyd R, Erickson L, et al. Adrenocortical carcinoma: surgical progress or status quo? *Arch Surg* 2001;136:543–549.

Khan TS, Imam H, Juhlin C, et al. Streptozocin and *o,p'*-DDD in the treatment of adrenocortical cancer patients: long-term survival in its adjuvant use. *Ann Oncol* 2000;11:1281–1287.

Khorram-Manesh A, Ahlman H, Jansson S, et al. Adrenocortical carcinoma: surgery and mitotane for treatment and steroid profiles for follow-up. *World J Surg* 1998;22:605–611.

Kopf D, Goretzki PE, Lehnert H. Clinical management of malignant adrenal tumors. *J Cancer Res Clin Oncol* 2001;127:143–155.

Luton JP, Cerdas S, Billaud L, et al. Clinical features of adrenocortical carcinoma, prognostic factors, and the effect of mitotane therapy. *N Engl J Med* 1990;322:1195–1201.

McGrath PC, Sloan DA, Schwartz RW, et al. Current advances in the diagnosis and therapy of adrenal tumors. *Curr Opin Oncol* 1998;10:52–57.

Miller JA, Norton JA. Multiple endocrine neoplasia. *Cancer Treat Res* 1997;90:213–225.

Wooten MD, King DK. Adrenal cortical carcinoma: epidemiology and treatment with mitotane and review of the literature. *Cancer* 1993;72:3145–3155.

Pheochromocytoma

Averbuch SD, Steakley CS, Young RC, et al. Malignant pheochromocytoma: effective treatment with a combination of cyclophosphamide, vincristine, and dacarbazine. *Ann Intern Med* 1988;109:267–273.

Bravo EL. Pheochromocytoma. *Curr Ther Endocrinol Metab* 1997;6:195–197.

Francis IR, Korobkin M. Pheochromocytoma. *Radiol Clin North Am* 1996;34:1101–1112.

Kebebew E, Duh QY. Benign and malignant pheochromocytoma: diagnosis, treatment, and follow-up. *Surg Oncol Clin North Am* 1998;7:765–789.

Kenady DE, McGrath PC, Sloan DA, et al. Diagnosis and management of pheochromocytoma. *Curr Opin Oncol* 1997;9:61–67.

Loh KC, Fitzgerald PA, Matthay KK, et al. The treatment of malignant pheochromocytoma with iodine-131 metaiodobenzylguanidine (^{131}I-MIBG): a comprehensive review of 116 reported patients. *J Endocrinol Invest* 1997;20:648–658.

Neumann HP, Bender BU, Januszewicz A, et al. Inherited pheochromocytoma. *Adv Nephrol Necker Hosp* 1997;27:361–376.

O'Riordan JA. Pheochromocytomas and anesthesia. *Int Anesthesiol Clin* 1997;35:99–127.

Pacak K, Linehan WM, Eisenhofer G, et al. Recent advances in genetics, diagnosis, localization, and treatment of pheochromocytoma. *Ann Intern Med* 2001;134:315–329.

Page DL, DeLellis RA, Hough AJ. Tumors of the adrenal. In: Hartmann WH, Sobin LH, eds. *Atlas of tumor pathology.* Washington, D.C.: Armed Forces Institute of Pathology, 1986.

Plouin PF, Duclos JM, Soppelsa F, et al. Factors associated with perioperative morbidity and mortality in patients with pheochromocytoma: analysis of 165 operations at a single center. *J Clin Endocrinol Metab* 2001;86:1480–1486.

Sisson JC, Shapiro B, Shulkin BL, et al. Treatment of malignant pheochromocytomas with 131-I metaiodobenzylguanidine and chemotherapy. *Am J Clin Oncol* 1999;22:364–370.

Werbel SS, Ober KP. Pheochromocytoma: update on diagnosis, localization, and management. *Med Clin North Am* 1995;79:131–153.

Young WF Jr. Pheochromocytoma: issues in diagnosis and treatment. *Compr Ther* 1997;23:319–326.

Melanoma and Other Skin Malignancies

Walter D. Y. Quan, Jr.

More than 1 million Americans were diagnosed with skin cancer in 2002. About 95% of these cases were either basal or squamous carcinoma of the skin. Melanoma accounted for approximately 54,000 cases in 2002 and is responsible for approximately 7,400 deaths annually, far surpassing the sum total of deaths due to all other skin malignancies combined. Melanoma is increasing in incidence at a higher rate than any other cancer (except for non–small cell lung cancer in females) in the United States. Less common tumors of the skin include Merkel's cell cancer, Kaposi's sarcoma (see Chapter 25), and mycosis fungoides (MF).

I. Melanoma
A. Natural history
1. **Etiology and epidemiology.** Melanoma arises from pigment-producing melanocytes that migrate to the skin and eye during embryologic development. Approximately 5% of melanoma occurs in extradermal sites such as the eye and mucous membranes of the oropharynx, vagina, and anus. In about 5% of cases, patients present with either regional lymph node involvement or metastatic organ involvement without any obvious primary being identified. Melanoma occurs more commonly in men than women and has a peak age at incidence of approximately 50 years. Owing to the young age of many melanoma patients, this disease takes a striking toll in terms of the average number of years of life lost per patient in this country. The incidence of the disease has increased rapidly in the United States to the point where melanoma is now the sixth most common cancer. The substantial increase in incidence is presumably due to increased exposure to sunlight (primarily ultraviolet radiation), with the greatest risk of melanoma felt to be in those who have intermittent intense sun exposure, particularly in fair-skinned, light-haired individuals. The cultural emphasis on sun-tanned skin as an indicator of physical health and beauty has played a major role in this increase. Depletion of the ozone layer may contribute as well. Sunny parts of the United States have the highest incidence of the disease, especially Southern California, Florida, and Texas. One particular melanoma subtype, lentigo malignant melanoma, may be more closely associated with long-term occupational sun exposure as is seen in farmers and fishers, for instance. Patient education in prevention, including use of sun-protective clothing, performing outdoor activities at times other than the brightest sunlit hours of the day, use of topical sunscreens, refraining from use of sun-tan parlors, use of skin self-examination, and avoiding sun-tanning

("tanned skin = damaged skin"), should be emphasized. Individuals with xeroderma pigmentosa, an autosomal recessive disorder, typically incur multiple basal and squamous skin cancers and melanoma because their skin lacks the ability to repair damage induced by ultraviolet radiation.

2. Precursor lesions, genetics, and familial melanoma. Melanoma may arise not only from dysplastic nevi but also from congenital and acquired nevi. Dysplastic nevi may be sporadic or familial. Individuals who have more than 100 benign nevi may also be at risk for melanoma. Ten percent of patients with melanoma have a family history of this cancer. Careful follow-up should be carried out in patients with these risk factors. Suspicious-appearing lesions or lesions that appear to have changed should be excised. The familial atypical multiple mole melanoma (FAMMM) syndrome is characterized by earlier mean age at diagnosis (34 years) and multiple lesions. The most common germline mutation seen in familial melanoma occurs in the tumor suppressor gene *CDKN2A*. Both *CDKN2A* and *PTEN* mutations have been seen in nonfamilial melanoma. Multiple chromosomal abnormalities have been identified and associated with melanoma, including chromosomal regions 10q, 9p, 6q, 7, 1p, and 11.

3. Types and appearance of primary lesions. Clinical features ("ABCD") suspicious for melanoma are as follows:

*   **A**symmetry of a lesion
*   **B**orders that are irregular
*   **C**olor that is multihued
*   **D**iameter greater than 6 mm (i.e., "larger than the diameter of a pencil eraser")

Other characteristics of concern could include history of recent growth, change in pigmentation, ulceration, itching, or bleeding. Skin lesions that behave like melanoma should be examined with the immunochemical stains S-100 and HMB-45 as 1% to 2% of melanoma lesions are amelanotic.

There are four clinical types of primary cutaneous melanoma. **Superficial spreading melanoma** is the most common type, accounting for 70% of melanomas. It is commonly found on the trunks of males and lower extremities of females. **Nodular melanoma** comprises 10% to 15% of melanomas and has an early vertical growth phase. It is commonly found on the trunks of men. **Lentigo malignant melanoma** accounts for approximately 10% of cases. It is characterized by flat, large (1- to 5-cm) lesions located on the arms, hands, and face of the elderly (median age 70 years) in particular and is known for a relatively longer radial phase. **Acral lentiginous melanoma** is seen in approximately 3% to 5% of cases and occurs primarily on the palmar surfaces of the hands, plantar surfaces of the feet, and under nails on the digits. This melanoma subtype is most commonly seen in individuals with darker-pigmented skin.

In general, melanoma is felt to show two distinct growth phases: an initial radial phase during which the melanoma enlarges in a horizontal/superficial pattern above the basal lamina of the skin, followed eventually by a vertical growth phase characterized by the cancer "diving deep" toward subcutaneous fat. It is during the vertical growth phase that metastases are felt to be at highest risk.

4. Patterns of metastases. While much attention is rightly attached to assessing lymph node status (see below), melanoma has a proclivity for hematogenous spread as well. Common sites of metastases include lung, liver, bone, subcutaneous areas, and, primarily in late stages, brain. However, melanoma can spread to virtually any site hematogenously. Following diagnosis, approximately 25% of patients will develop visceral (non–lymph node) metastases. As many as an additional 15% may develop disease limited to lymph nodes alone. Patients who present with lymph node or metastatic involvement without any obvious primary site may have undergone spontaneous remission of the primary, a phenomenon that may be attributable to some degree of immune system involvement. Patients with "cancer of unknown primary" should have their biopsy material stained with the immunohistochemical stains S-100 and HMB-45 in consideration of the possibility of melanoma.

5. Ocular melanoma. Ocular melanoma is the most common malignancy of the eye in adults. It may occur in any eye structure that contains melanocytes, although uveal tract sites predominate, with choroid, ciliary body, and iris in decreasing frequency. Standard therapy may consist of either enucleation (often utilizing a "no touch" technique) or brachytherapy with radioisotopes such as [125]I. This tumor metastasizes most frequently to the liver and appears to be less sensitive to both biologic agents and chemotherapy than is cutaneous melanoma.

B. Staging. Melanoma is staged according to the recently updated American Joint Committee on Cancer staging system (see Tables 14.1 to 14.3). All patients should have a careful history and physical examination with special attention to the skin including scalp, mucous membranes, and regional lymph nodes. Laboratory studies should include complete blood count, blood urea nitrogen (BUN), serum creatinine, liver panel, alkaline phosphatase, and serum lactate dehydrogenase. A chest x-ray or computed tomography (CT) scan is done to evaluate for pulmonary lesions. Elevation of liver function tests warrants CT scan of the liver. Elevation of alkaline phosphatase level or unexplainable bone pain suggests the need for bone scanning. Primary lesions equal to or thicker than 1.0 mm are at higher risk of regional lymph node involvement; therefore, the use of sentinel node surgery is recommended (see Section I.C).

C. Surgical treatment. The standard surgery for suspected melanoma lesions is excisional biopsy rather than incision or "shave" biopsies. Importantly, a subsequent wide excision is required to provide adequate tumor-free margins as melanoma is notorious for local recurrences. While there is some variation in recommendations, most would advocate a 1-cm tumor-free margin for melanomas less than 1 mm in thickness and 1- to 2-cm margins for deeper primary lesions if technically possible. Additionally, for primary lesions ≥ 1 mm, sentinel node mapping is recommended. Based on work by Morton and others

Table 14.1.   Revised TMN classification for melanoma

T status Classification	Thickness (mm)	Ulceration
T1	≤1.0	a = no ulceration *and* Clark's level III or less
		b = with ulceration *or* Clark's level IV or V
T2	1.01–2.0	a = no ulceration
		b = with ulceration
T3	2.01–4.0	a = no ulceration
		b = with ulceration
T4	>4.0	a = no ulceration
		b = with ulceration

N status Classification	Number of lymph nodes	Involvement
N1	1	a = microscopic
		b = macroscopic
N2	2–3	a = microscopic
		b = macroscopic
		c = "in-transit met" or "satellite" present but no lymph nodes involved
N3	≥4	Note: This classification applies also if "in-transit met" or "satellite" lesions present *with* metastatic nodes.

M status Classification	Metastatic site	Serum LDH
M1a	Distant subcutaneous, skin, or node	Not elevated
M1b	Lung	Not elevated
M1c	All other visceral sites	Not elevated
M1c	Any	Elevated

LDH, lactate dehydrogenase.

Table 14.2.   Clark's levels of invasion

Level	Description
I	Limited to the epidermis
II	Invades papillary dermis
III	Extends to papillary–reticular dermal junction
IV	Invades reticular dermis
V	Invades subcutaneous fat

Table 14.3. **Approximate survival based on stage grouping**

Stage	TNM (pathologic)	5-yr survival (%)
IA	T1a	95
IB	T1b	90
	T2a	89
IIA	T2b	77
	T3a	
IIB	T3b	65
	T4a	
IIC	T4b	45
IIIA	N1a	53
	N2a	49
IIIB	N1b	51
	N2b	46
IIIC	N3	27
IV	M1a	19
All other	M	<10

From Balch CM, Buzaid AC, Soong SJ, et al. Final version of the American Joint Committee on Cancer staging system for cutaneous melanoma. *J Clin Oncol* 2001;19:3635–3648.

(1992), it is known that lymph node "drainage areas" are accessed via a specific lymph node (sentinel node) into which lymph-borne metastases generally first occur. The absence of tumor involvement in this lymph node precludes the need for elective lymph node dissection. While blue dye was originally used in this procedure, current refinements of this technique include the use of technetium-based radionuclides.

D. Adjuvant therapy. Eastern Cooperative Oncology Group (ECOG) 1684 was a large randomized adjuvant trial of interferon-α_{2b} (IFN-α_{2b}) in patients with deep primary lesions (> 4 mm thick) or regional lymph node involvement that showed statistically significant improvement in overall survival compared to observation. The IFN dose used in this trial was 20×10^6 IU/m^2 IV 5 days/week for 4 weeks followed by 10×10^6 IU/m^2 SC 3 days/week for 48 weeks. Toxicity (flu-like symptoms, hepatic dysfunction, and neurologic symptoms) was significant, but quality-of-life analysis demonstrated overall benefit. The follow-up study, ECOG 1690, also showed a significant disease-free survival advantage over the observation arm but not a benefit in overall survival. The difference between these two studies may be that patients on the observation arm in the subsequent trial (1690) may have been treated with biotherapy (including IFN) at the time of relapse. A recent European randomized study comparing 18 months of low-dose interferon-alfa (3 MU SC t.i.w.) versus observation showed a statistically significant improvement in disease-free survival (but not overall survival) in the IFN-treated group. Given that it is clear that patients with deep cutaneous primaries and/or lymph node involvement are at high risk for metastatic recurrence and that the majority of patients who suffer metastatic relapse will die of their disease, it is reasonable to treat such high-risk patients with either IFN or entrance into a clinical trial. An adjuvant trial looking to modify the high-dose protocol above would seem reasonable. A current cooperative group trial is comparing high-dose IFN with biochemotherapy (described below.) A particularly fertile area of exploration is the administration of therapeutic vaccines (see vaccine discussion below). A recent study by McClay et al. (2000) has examined the combination of cisplatin and tamoxifen as adjuvant therapy with some suggestion of benefit; however, no randomized comparison with either an observation arm or adjuvant IFN at the doses above is available. Regional perfusion chemotherapy in patients with high-risk extremity melanoma has been reported by the European Organisation for Research and Treatment of Cancer (EORTC)/World Health Organization (WHO), which found no substantial benefit.

E. Therapy of metastases
  1. General considerations about systemic therapy
  a. Patient selection. While, in general, melanoma is considered relatively resistant to systemic therapy, certain favorable prognostic factors do lend themselves to a higher chance of response. These include ECOG performance status 0 or 1; subcutaneous, lymph node, or pulmonary metastasis; no prior chemotherapy; normal marrow, renal, and hepatic function; and absence of central nervous system (CNS) metastases. Some investigators have noted that females are more likely than males to respond to chemotherapy. The biologic basis for this finding has not been fully elucidated. Typical response rates for commercially available single agents are listed in Table 14.4. These response rates are highly dependent upon site of metastasis. When reviewing potential therapy for patients, patient characteristics as well as the natural history of the disease must be considered, including that the median survival of patients in Phase II studies that have 0% response rates can reach 7 months.
  2. Biologic agents. This class of agents, along with experimental therapy/clinical trials, represents the most signifi-

Table 14.4. Systemic therapy for melanoma: single agents in metastatic melanoma

Agent	Response rate (%)
Dacarbazine	20
Nitrosoureas (carmustine/lomustine/semustine)	18
Interleukin-2	16
Cisplatin	16
Interferon-alfa	15
Carboplatin	15
Temozolomide	15
Paclitaxel	14
Docetaxel	14
Vinca alkaloids (vinblastine/vincristine)	12

cant hope for the future in the treatment of this disease. The currently available agents in this class are as follows:

a. Interferon-α$_{2a}$ (Roferon) and **interferon-α**$_{2b}$ (Intron-A) have been examined at a wide range of doses, schedules, and routes from 3 to 50×10^6 IU/m^2 given SC, IM, or IV, administered three to five times per week. These agents have been found to have response rates of approximately 15% in a variety of studies. Additionally, some patients may have stable disease lasting many months or longer. In regards to dosing, some investigators believe that higher doses of IFN (20 MIU/m^2 IV, such as those given in adjuvant therapy) act more by inhibiting tumor cell proliferation, while lower doses of IFN (less than 5 MIU/m^2 SC) may be more immunostimulatory. A possible starting dose for subcutaneous IFN would be 3 MU SC three times per week.

b. Interleukin-2 (IL-2; Proleukin, aldesleukin) appears to be the most active single agent for patients with visceral metastases. It is most commonly used in a "high-dose" regimen of 600,000 IU/kg given in 15-min IV infusions every 8 h for a total of 14 doses. This schedule produces responses in 15% to 20% of patients, many of long duration. A recent review of National Cancer Institute data showed a response rate of 50% in patients with disease limited to cutaneous/subcutaneous sites. Because this drug is associated with a capillary leak syndrome that can include hypotension, fluid retention, renal and hepatic hypoperfusion, and pulmonary edema, the dose and schedule above require inpatient care. It should be used only by those experienced in its administration. Inpatient continuous-infusion schedules (18 MIU/m^2 given over 24 h for up to 5 consecutive days) may also be administered. Patients receiving this dose must also be closely monitored. Moderate-dose IL-2 (22 MIU/m^2 given by 15-min infusions for 5 consecutive days for 2 consecutive weeks) when given with low-dose cyclophosphamide (see Section I.D.5 below) can be administered on an outpatient basis and is relatively well tolerated but requires significant premedication and daily physician examination. The role of low-dose SC administration of IL-2 is unclear; some investigators feel that such low-dose regimens are less likely to yield durable responses. It should be noted that the older literature may express IL-2 dosing in other than International Units. Therefore, when comparing various studies, a "rule of thumb" for conversions is 1 mg $= 3 \times 10^6$ Cetus Units $= 6 \times 10^6$ Roche Units $= 18 \times 10^6$ IU.

c. Thalidomide, an inhibitor of angiogenesis, is currently being explored.

d. Combinations of biologic agents. The role of combinations of biologic agents is an area of ongoing study. IL-2 and IFN-α have been utilized together, but most studies have found no advantage in response rates or response durations to this combination compared with either agent alone. The use of IFN following therapeutic vaccine therapy resulted in higher response rates than what is usually seen with IFN alone. Current studies are examining IFN and thalidomide in combination.

3. Chemotherapy

a.   Single-agent chemotherapy. While many of the cytotoxic agents commonly used in other tumor types are inactive in this disease, several agents do possess some degree of activity in melanoma (Table 14.4). Responses are obtained primarily in lung and nonvisceral sites and occur in ambulatory patients with few or no symptoms of their disease.

(1)   Dacarbazine (DTIC) has historically been the most widely utilized single agent for the treatment of metastatic melanoma. The most commonly used doses are 200 mg/m^2 IV on days 1 to 5 every 3 weeks or 750 to 800 mg/m^2 IV on day 1 every 4 to 6 weeks. Most responses to this agent occur in subcutaneous or lymph node sites.

(2)   Nitrosoureas have been used in melanoma and probably have about equal efficacy. Carmustine (BCNU) 150 mg/m^2 IV is given as a single dose every 4 to 6 weeks, *or* lomustine (CCNU) is given in a dosage of 100 to 130 mg/m^2 PO once every 4 to 6 weeks.

(3)   Platinum-containing drugs. Cisplatin 100 mg/m^2 IV every 3 weeks *or* carboplatin 400 mg/m^2 IV every 3 weeks appears to have similar efficacy.

(4)   Taxanes. Paclitaxel (Taxol) 135 to 215 mg/m^2 is given in 3-h IV infusions every 3 weeks, *or* docetaxel (Taxotere) 60 to 100 mg/m^2 is given in 1-h IV infusions every 3 weeks.

(5)   Temozolomide (an oral imidazole) is a new oral DTIC derivative with significant CNS penetrance and therefore the potential for clinical responses in the difficult subpopulation of patients with CNS metastases. Typical doses are 150 to 200 mg/m^2 PO daily for 5 days every 28 days.

(6)   Vinca alkaloids have been used primarily in combinations. Vincristine 2 mg IV given every 4 weeks and vinblastine are representative of this class of agents.

b.   Multiagent chemotherapy. Despite decades of trials, no combination chemotherapy has emerged as a standard therapy. While multiple regimens have shown high response rates in single-arm Phase II or nonrandomized trials, there are no convincing randomized trial data to show both statistically significant improvements in response rate and median survival compared with single-agent therapy (usually dacarbazine alone). Two of the most commonly used regimens are shown in Table 14.5.

4.   Hormones. Although hormone receptors have been identified on some melanoma cell lines, these, unlike the ones seen in breast cancer, do not appear to be functional. Tamoxifen and megestrol acetate have no significant antitumor activity when used alone in patients with metastatic disease. There has been some *in vitro* evidence and some indirect clinical evidence that these drugs may potentiate the activity of some cytotoxic agents.

5.   Biochemotherapy. In one carefully implemented large study employing initial use of chemotherapy followed by biotherapy with both IFN and IL-2 (Table 14.5), 17% of patients

Table 14.5.   Multiagent systemic therapy for melanoma

Regimen	Drug dosages
BCDT ("Dartmouth regimen")	BCNU (carmustine) 150 mg/m^2/d on day 1 every 6 wk Cisplatin 25 mg/m^2/d on days 1–3 every 3 wk DTIC (dacarbazine) 220 mg/m^2/d on days 1–3 every 3 wk Tamoxifen 20 mg PO daily
CVD	DDP (cisplatin) 20 mg/m^2/d on days 1–4 for 3 wk VLB (vinblastine) 1.6 mg/m^2/d on days 1–4 for 3 wk DTIC (dacarbazine) 800 mg/m^2 on day 1 only for 3 wk
Biochemotherapy[a]	CVD as above, *together with:* Interleukin-2 9 MIU/m^2/q.d. by continuous IV infusion days 1–4 (96 h)[b] Interferon-α_{2b} 5 MU/m^2 SC on days 1–5, 7, 9, 11, 13 G-CSF 5 µg/kg SC q.d. on days 7–16 Repeat cycle every 21 days for maximum of four cycles.
Cyclophosphamide and moderate-dose interleukin-2	Cyclophosphamide 350 mg/m^2 IVPB on day 1 Interleukin-2 22 MIU/m^2 IVPB on days 4–8, 11–15 Repeat cycle every 21 days for three cycles. Thereafter give every 28–42 d.

G-CSF, granulocyte colony-stimulating factor.
[a] See Legha SS. Durable complete responses in melanoma treated with interleukin 2 in combination with interferon alfa and chemotherapy. *Semin Oncol* 1997;24:S4–S39.
[b] On day 1, begin interleukin-2 2–3 h after chemotherapy.

achieved measurable complete responses that were durable (greater than 18 months). Moreover, 9% of patients experienced complete responses lasting longer than 3 years, leading to the conclusion that the regimen has curative potential. Substantial toxicity is encountered in such studies, and experience and strong medical support are required for their implementation. Moreover, a meta-analysis of small studies (some randomized) has reported 29% versus 41% objective response rates and 8.6- versus 9.8-month median survival durations for polychemotherapy regimens versus biochemotherapy, respectively—a modest gain, indeed, for a toxic and complex regimen. A current cooperative group study is comparing polychemotherapy with the same regimen plus biotherapy.

6. Other biochemotherapy regimens. An alternative approach involving biochemotherapy utilizes IL-2 with doses of chemotherapeutic agents that are chosen to theoretically augment an immune response. Cyclophosphamide, for instance, may increase lymphokine-activated killer (LAK) cell activity, decrease the dampening effect of suppressor T cells on the immune response, or allow for space in the bone marrow for repopulation by LAK cells. Mitchell et al. (1989) have shown activity of an outpatient combination of low-dose cyclophosphamide and IL-2 with an overall response rate (5% complete response [CR], 21% partial response [PR]) similar to those seen with high-dose inpatient IL-2 regimens.

F. **Regional therapy**

1. **Local perfusion.** For patients with subcutaneous metastases limited to a single extremity, arteriovenous cannulation and perfusion of that limb with agents such as melphalan, cisplatin, or tumor necrosis factor-α often with hyperthermia yield higher tissue concentrations of the drugs than what are achievable by IV administration. Phase II studies often show impressive response rates. Whether there is any survival advantage to this therapy compared with systemic treatment remains controversial. Because of issues involving factors such as cost, the equipment required, and the physician training needed to implement this approach, its practicality is unclear. Hepatic arterial infusion therapy is theoretically appealing for ocular melanoma metastatic only to the liver. This therapy looks to be more active than systemic chemotherapy in ocular melanoma, although it is unclear that such an approach improves median survival.

2. **Intralesional therapy with bacillus Calmette-Guérin** (BCG), IFN-α, granulocyte–macrophage colony-stimulating factor, and other agents has also been used with varying degrees of success.

3. **Treatment of central nervous system metastases.** Dexamethasone 10 mg IV followed by 6 mg every 6 h IV or PO is given to reduce cerebral edema. As soon as possible, radiation should be started by either stereotactic, gamma knife, or three-dimensional conformal techniques. For solitary lesions, surgical resection followed by radiotherapy may yield a significant group of survivors over 1 year who experience good quality of life. The role of temozolomide needs to be further explored in this group of patients.

4. **Radiotherapy** is of variable efficacy in the treatment of the regional or bony metastases but sometimes may yield gratifying symptomatic benefit.

5. **Surgery,** when utilized judiciously, can result in long-term disease-free survivals of up to 20% in individuals with isolated metastatic sites. Special considerations for surgical resection of metastases include gastrointestinal metastases that threaten significant morbidity such as impending bowel obstruction and single brain metastasis prior to the start of biologic therapy (as long-term steroid use, which is frequently needed in the setting of brain metastasis, is antagonistic with biologic agents). The role of adjuvant therapy in patients who have undergone metastatectomies needs to be

elucidated. A reasonable approach is to treat such patients with IFN as described above.

G.   Experimental and future therapies are of great importance in this disease. Only a few salient approaches will be discussed here. A variety of references are available for further reading below.

   1.   Therapeutic vaccines are an area of intense interest, and much potential is expected in the coming years. In general, toxicity from vaccine therapy tends to be quite low, usually limited to local reactions to the vaccine or the immunologic adjuvant that may be combined with the antigenic stimulus. Most vaccine studies have dealt primarily with patients who have been rendered surgically free of all macroscopic disease. Fewer studies have been done in patients with metastatic disease. Two examples of the latter include a polyvalent melanoma cell vaccine and Melacine (approved for use in metastatic disease in Canada), which have achieved objective responses in patients with metastatic tumor. A purified ganglioside, GM-2KLH/QS-21, which demonstrated prolongation of survival of patients in whom the vaccine is optimally immunogenic, was tested in an adjuvant setting (ECOG E1694) but found to be inferior to IFN. Other approaches that have been or are currently being investigated include vaccines based on recently discovered melanoma antigens such as MART-1, anti-idiotype vaccine, partially purified polyvalent vaccine, and vaccinia-infected melanoma cell lysates. Potential advantages to vaccine-based therapy include relatively little toxicity, the possibility of long-term disease stabilization, and an immunologic effect that may continue long after dose administration.

   2.   Cellular therapy. The administration of *ex vivo* activated cells such as cytotoxic T cells theoretically specific for melanoma continues to be of interest. Currently, there is no evidence that the addition of bulk cultured T cells to IL-2 therapy, for instance, is superior to IL-2 alone. The use of gene-modified T cells that might be more potent is an area of investigation. Alternatively, cytotoxic T cells immunized to specific tumor epitopes offer theoretical potential. The addition of LAK cells to IL-2 has not been clearly shown to be better than IL-2 alone, although Rosenberg and colleagues (1993) identified a survival trend ($p = 0.064$) in favor of the LAK/IL-2 arm. Recent studies have examined the infusion of dendritic cells that have been pulsed with melanoma antigen.

   3.   Antiangiogenic factors are a logical approach in this disease, given its vascularity. Several epidermal growth factor–like antibodies are undergoing clinical trials.

II.   Nonmelanoma skin cancer

A.   Etiology and epidemiology. It is estimated that more than 1 million cases of either basal cell cancer (BCC) or squamous cell carcinoma (SCC) will occured in the United States in 2002. BCC exceeds SCC by a four-to-one ratio. Both are seen predominantly in the elderly, and sun exposure is felt to be the highest risk factor, particularly in individuals with fair complexions and light-colored eyes and hair. It is common (30% to 50%, by some estimations) to see multiple BCCs or

SCCs in the same individual. Other etiologic factors include prior irradiation to the skin for benign disorders, chronic inflammation, scarring or burns, and arsenic exposure. Patients who are chronically immunosuppressed such as in chronic lymphocytic leukemia and renal transplantation are also at increased risk, as are individuals with genetic disorders including xeroderma pigmentosum. There is evidence that human immunodeficiency virus infection may predispose to a clinically more aggressive SCC or BCC.

B. Diagnosis and clinical features

  1. Diagnosis of both SCC and BCC is made by biopsy, incisional, excisional, or sometimes "shave," depending on the clinical situation. Staging systems are not typically utilized for these tumors as both have generally low potential for metastases. BCC often presents as a nodular, ulcerative lesion ("rodent ulcer"), that is, as a nodule with pearly or translucent edges and a central ulceration. Perhaps 0.1% of BCCs metastasize, usually occurring only in the setting where a long-standing lesion has been neglected. Lymph node metastases are the most common site (60%), with lung and bone less frequently.

  SCCs often arise from crusty-appearing sun-damaged skin areas with a higher rate of metastases (2%) than BCCs. Patients whose SCC arises from causes other than actinic damage (immunosuppression, e.g.) may display a more rapid course with higher rates of metastases (20% to 50%). Neglected lesions, large ulcerated lesions, and poorly differentiated histology are risk factors for metastases. The great majority of metastases initially occur in lymph nodes (90%), with perhaps 50% of patients developing metastases to other sites such as lung and bone.

  2. Local treatment. Surgical excision, electrodesiccation, curettage, Moh's chemosurgery, radiation therapy, and cryotherapy are of similar efficacy (about 95% cure rate) and may be chosen based on individualized factors including the area involved, treatment facilities available, and physician skill. In general, surgical excision is recommended for SCC because adequate margins can be ensured. This is of importance as SCC has more metastatic potential than BCC. BCC, because of its rare metastases, can be treated with any of the measures above, including cryotherapy. For both SCC and BCC, radiation may be a treatment of choice for areas in which poor cosmetic result would occur after excision, such as near eyelids, ear lobes, or tip of the nose. Moh's chemosurgery is an involved procedure in which thin layers are meticulously removed, chemically fixed, and reviewed microscopically immediately to ultimately be assured of clear margins. Some reports suggest that this therapy may have a slight advantage in terms of local control, although it is highly operator dependent.

  3. Treatment of metastatic disease

  Both BCC and SCC may be treated with cisplatin-containing regimens. Response rates as high as 70% have been reported.

One of the more active regimens appears to be cisplatin 75 mg/m^2 IVPB (IV Piggy Back) (with appropriate hydration) and doxorubicin 50 mg/m^2 IV, both every 3 weeks.

C. Merkel's cell carcinoma

1. Etiology and epidemiology. Merkel's cell cancer is a rare cutaneous neuroendocrine tumor that arises in the basal layer of the epidermis. Its microscopic appearance is that of small blue cells with scant cytoplasm and hyperchromatic nuclei ("small cell cancer of the skin"). Merkel's cell cancer is 20 times more likely to occur in Caucasians than non-Caucasians, occurs more frequently in males than females, and affects persons at a median age of 65 to 70 years. Sun exposure is felt to be the major risk factor.

2. Clinical features. Initially, it may be seen as a blue or bluish red, nontender, firm skin lesion, starting as a nodule but increasing in size rapidly over weeks to months. The most commonly involved sites are the face and neck (50%) and the extremities (40%). There is no universally accepted staging system for this uncommon tumor. In general, Merkel's cell cancer has a tendency toward an aggressive, recurrent course similar in some ways to small cell lung cancer or melanoma. Most patients experience recurrence within 12 months of initial treatment. These recurrences may be local or involve regional lymph nodes with metastatic involvement later. The most frequent distant metastatic sites are liver, lung, and bones.

3. Treatment. The rarity of this tumor precludes any prospective randomized treatment data. Nevertheless, standard therapy for this disease includes surgical resection with 2-cm margins, if possible, followed by lymph node dissection. Sentinel node surgery would seem to have a role in this situation, as a negative result could preclude the morbidity of the more extensive surgery. Because of the risk of local recurrence, radiation therapy to the primary site and to the site of pathologically involved lymph nodes can be considered. For metastatic disease, the two most common regimens used have been cyclophosphamide, doxorubicin, and vincristine (CAV) or cisplatin and etoposide (EP) at doses utilized for small cell lung cancer. Response rates for these regimens are about 60%. There has been no established role for adjuvant chemotherapy.

D. Mycosis fungoides

1. Etiology and epidemiology. MF is a T cell–derived lymphoma arising from lymphocytes that classically mark positive for the T-helper phenotype (CD4). It is an uncommon lymphoma, with just over 500 new cases diagnosed in the United States per year. It is seen predominantly in males with a median age of approximately 60 years. The lymphocytic infiltrate seen in this disease is present in the upper aspect of the dermis, obscures the junction between the dermis and epidermis, and characteristically infiltrates the epidermis in clusters of cells that are called Pautrier's microabscesses. Biopsies early in the course of the disease (the "premycotic phase") may show nonspecific, nondiagnostic skin changes.

2. Clinical features. Patients with this disorder tend to display a skin rash that is erythematous, somewhat scaling, and pruritic. Over time, patches, plaques, and even ulcers can be seen. Patients may exhibit erythroderma and lymphadenopathy. Sézary's syndrome occurs with the presence of a leukemic phase. The course of MF may be variable, from a minority of patients who have "skin-only" involvement to more extensive disease with visceral metastases that can include liver, lungs, spleen, and gastrointestinal tract. Staging is according to the TMN(B) system (Tables 14.6 and 14.7). Patients with stage IA to IIA have an excellent prognosis with median survival greater than 11 years. Individuals with stage IIB to III disease have median survival of 3 to 4 years. Among patients with T4 (erythroderma), a subgroup who are younger (less than 65 years), lower in stage (III), and without any evidence of blood involvement has been shown to have a favorable prognosis with median survival of approximately 10 years. Stage IVA/IVB has poor prognosis with median survival less than 1.5 years. A subgroup of cases of MF may undergo transformation to a large cell lymphoma, CD30+, which also heralds a poor prognosis.

3. Treatment. For individuals whose disease is confined only to the skin, electron beam radiation, PUVA (the combination of a photosensitizing substance such as psoralen and ultraviolet radiation), extracorporeal photopheresis, or topical application of nitrogen mustard can lead to complete response of disease and potentially cure. Thick plaque disease may be better treated with electron therapy as PUVA and topical nitrogen mustard may be less able to penetrate the depth of the lesions. Patients who fail on one of the local/topical therapies can be treated with a different type of local therapy. For visceral disease or Sézary's syndrome, systemic

Table 14.6.   TMNB classes for mycosis fungoides

T1	Limited patch/plaque lesions <10% of total skin surface
T2	Generalized patch/plaque lesion ≥10% of total skin surface
T3	Tumors
T4	Erythroderma, generalized skin involvement
N0	No clinically palpable lymph nodes
N1	Enlarged lymph nodes but microscopically negative
N2	Nonpalpable lymph nodes but microscopically involved
N3	Clinically palpable lymph nodes that are microscopically involved
M0	No visceral involvement
M1	Visceral involvement
B0	Absence of peripheral blood involvement
B1	Peripheral blood involvement

Table 14.7.   Clinical stages for mycosis fungoides

Stage	T	N	M
IA	T1	N0	M0
IB	T2	N0	M0
IIA	T1–2	N1	M0
IIB	T3	N0–1	M0
IIIA	T4	N0	M0
IIIB	T4	N1	M0
IVA	T1–4	N2–3	M0
IVB	Any	Any	M1

Note: B symptoms have no specific bearing on this staging system.

therapy such as interferon-alfa 3 MU SC t.i.w. given continuously or gradually escalated to a cumulative weekly dose of
18 MU can yield response rates of over 60%. "Traditional" anti-
lymphoma chemotherapy agents such as cyclophosphamide,
doxorubicin, vincristine, and prednisone (CHOP) appear
less active in this lymphoma than in other non-Hodgkin's
lymphoma. Fludarabine and pentostatin have some activity.
IL-2–diptheria toxin fusion protein has recently been approved
for refractory disease.

Acknowledgment: It is my privilege to acknowledge Dr. Larry Nathanson,
who authored the previous five editions of this chapter. Dr. Nathanson has had
a distinguished career as a melanoma investigator and is responsible for many
of the insights that are incorporated into current care of the patient with
melanoma.

SELECTED READINGS

Melanoma

Atkins MB, Kunkel L, Sznol M, et al. High-dose recombinant inter-
leukin-2 therapy in patients with metastatic melanoma: long-term
survival update. *Cancer J Sci Am* 2000;6(suppl 1):S11–S14.

Balch CM, Buzaid AC, Soong SJ, et al. Final version of the American
Joint Committee on Cancer staging system for cutaneous melanoma.
J Clin Oncol 2001;19:3635–3648.

Balch CM, Houghton AN, Milton GW, et al., eds. *Cutaneous melanoma.*
3rd ed. Philadelphia: Lippincott–Raven, 1998:1.

Balch CM, Soong SJ, Gershenwald JE, et al. Prognostic factor analysis of 17,600 melanoma patients: validation of the American Joint
Committee on Cancer melanoma staging system. *J Clin Oncol*
2001;19:3622–3634.

Balch CM, Urist MM, Karakousis CP, et al. Efficacy of 2 cm surgical
margins for intermediate thickness cutaneous melanoma (1–4 mm):
results of a multi-institutional randomized surgical trial. *Ann Surg*
1993;218:262.

Bedikian AY, Legha SS, Mavligit G, et al. Treatment of uveal
melanoma metastatic to the liver. *Cancer* 1995;76:1665.

Bedikian AY, Weiss GR, Legha SS, et al. Phase II trial of docetaxel in patients with advanced melanoma previously untreated with chemotherapy. *J Clin Oncol* 1995;13:2895.

Buzaid AC, Anderson CM. The changing prognosis of melanoma. *Curr Oncol Rep* 2000;2:322–328.

Buzaid AC, Tinoco L, Ross MI, et al. Role of computed tomography in the staging of patients with local–regional metastases of melanoma. *J Clin Oncol* 1995;13:2104.

Chang E, Rosenberg SA. Patients with melanoma metastases at cutaneous and subcutaneous sites are highly susceptible to interleukin-2-based therapy. *J Immunother* 2001;24:88–90.

Dalgleish A. The case for therapeutic vaccines. *Melanoma Res* 1996;6:5.

Hwu P. The gene therapy of cancer. *PPO Updates* 1995;9:1–13.

Garrison M, Nathanson L. Prognosis and staging in melanoma. *Semin Oncol* 1996;23:725.

Haluska FG, Hodi FS. Molecular genetics of familial melanoma. *J Clin Oncol* 1998;16:670.

Jemal A, Thomas A, Murray T, et al. Cancer statistics, 2002. *Ca Cancer J Clin* 2002;52:23–47.

Kirkwood JM, Ibrahim JG, Sondak VK, et al. High- and low-dose interferon alfa-2b in high risk melanoma: first analysis of Intergroup Trial E1690/S9111/C9190. *J Clin Oncol* 2000;18:2444–2458.

Kirkwood JM, Ibrahim JG, Sosman JA, et al. High-dose interferon alfa-2b significantly prolongs relapse-free and overall survival compared with the GM2-KLH/QS-21 vaccine in patients with resected stage IIb–III melanoma: results of Intergroup Trial E1694/S9512/C509801. *J Clin Oncol* 2001;19:2370–2380.

Kirkwood JM, Strawderman MH, Ernstoff MS, et al. Interferon alfa 2b adjuvant therapy of high-risk resected cutaneous melanoma: the Eastern Cooperative Oncology Group trial EST 1684. *J Clin Oncol* 1996;14:7.

Lau R, Wang F, Jeffery G, et al. Phase I trial of intravenous peptide-pulsed dendritic cells in patients with metastatic melanoma. *J Immunother* 2001;24:66–78.

Legha SS. Durable complete responses in melanoma treated with interleukin 2 in combination with interferon alfa and chemotherapy. *Semin Oncol* 1997;24:S4–S39.

Legha SS, Ring S, Eton O, et al. Development of a biochemotherapy regimen with concurrent administration of cisplatin, vinblastine, darcarbazine, interferon alfa, and interleukin-2 for patients with metastatic melanoma. *J Clin Oncol* 1998;16:1752–1759.

Margolin K, Liu P-Y, Flaherty L, et al. Phase II study of BCNU, DTIC, cisplatin (DDP) and tamoxifen (Tam) in advanced melanoma: a Southwest Oncology Group study. *J Clin Oncol* 1998;16:664–669.

McClay EF, McClay MET, Monroe L, et al. The effect of tamoxifen and cisplatin on the disease-free and overall survival of patients with high risk malignant melanoma. *Br J Cancer* 2000;83:16–21.

Mitchell MS, Darrah D, Yeung D, et al. Phase I trial of adoptive immunotherapy with cytolytic T lymphocytes immunized against a tyrosinase epitope. *J Clin Oncol* 2002;20:1075–1086.

Mitchell MS, Jakowatz J, Harel W, et al. Increased effectiveness of interferon alfa-2b following active specific immunotherapy for melanoma. *J Clin Oncol* 1994;12:402.

Mitchell MS, Kempf RA, Harel W, et al. Low-dose cyclophosphamide and low-dose interleukin-2 for malignant melanoma. *Bull NY Acad Med* 1989;65:128–144.

Morton DL, Foshag LJ, Hoon DSB, et al. Prolongation of survival in metastatic melanoma after active specific immunotherapy with a new polyvalent melanoma vaccine. *Ann Surg* 1992;216:463.

Morton DL, Wen DR, Wong JH, et al. Technical details of intra-operative lymphatic mapping for early stage melanoma. *Arch Surg* 1992;127:392.

Nathanson L, ed. *Current research and clinical management of melanoma.* Boston: Kluwer Academic, 1993.

Nathanson L. Interferon adjuvant therapy of melanoma. *Cancer* 1996;78:944.

Nathanson L. Melanoma and other skin malignancies. In: Skeel RT, ed. *Handbook of cancer chemotherapy.* 5th ed. Philadelphia: Lippincott Williams & Wilkins, 1999*a*:362.

Nathanson L. Malignant melanoma. In: Foley JF, Vose JM, Armitage JO, eds. *Current therapy in cancer.* 2nd ed. Philadelphia: Saunders, 1999*b*:245–254.

Phan GQ, Attia P, Steinberg SM, et al. Factors associated with response to high-dose interleukin-2 in patients with metastatic melanoma. *J Clin Oncol* 2001;19:3477–3482.

Pollock PM, Trent JM. The genetics of cutaneous melanoma. *Clin Lab Med* 2000;20:667–690.

Quan WDY Jr. Immunotherapy for cancer: harnessing the host immune defenses—biologic mechanisms and results in melanoma and renal cell carcinoma. *Disease a Month* 1997;43:755–782.

Quan WDY Jr, Bindus C, Casal R, et al. Administration of moderate dose bolus iv interleukin-2 in the office/outpatient setting. *Proc Am Soc Clin Oncol* 1997;16:444a.

Rosenberg SA. Cancer vaccines based on the identification of genes encoding cancer regression antigens. *Immunol Today* 1997;18:175.

Rosenberg SA, Lotze MT, Yang JC, et al. Prospective randomized trial of high-dose interleukin-2 alone or in conjunction with lymphokine-activated killer cells for the treatment of patients with advanced cancer. *JNCI* 1993;85:622–632.

Schuchter L. Review of the 2001 AJCC staging system for cutaneous malignant melanoma. *Curr Oncol Rep* 2001;3:332–337.

Schwartzentruber D. Guidelines for the safe administration of high-dose interleukin-2. *J Immunother* 2001;24:287–292.

Wang F, Bade E, Kuniyoshi C, et al. Phase I trial of a MART-1 peptide vaccine with incomplete Freund's adjuvant for resected high-risk melanoma. *Clin Cancer Res* 1999;5:2756–2765.

Nonmelanoma Skin Cancer

Fleming ID, Amonette R, Monaghan T, et al. Principles of management of basal and squamous carcinoma of the skin. *Cancer* 1995; 75:699.

Goessling W, McKee PH, Mayer RJ. Merkel cell carcinoma. *J Clin Oncol* 2002;20:588–598.

Guthrie T Jr. Squamous cell and basal cell carcinoma of the skin. In Foley JF, Vose JM, Armitage JO, eds. *Current therapy in cancer.* 2nd ed. Philadelphia: Saunders, 1999:255–257.

Guthrie TH Jr, Porubsky ES, Luxenberg MN, et al. Cisplatin-based chemotherapy in advanced basal and squamous cell carcinomas of the skin: results in 28 patients including 13 patients receiving multi-modality therapy. *J Clin Oncol* 1990;8:342–346.

Jumbou O, N'Guyen JM, Tessier MH, et al. Long-term follow-up in 51 patients with mycosis fungoides and Sezary syndrome treated by interferon-alfa. *Br J Dermatol* 1999;140:427–431.

Kim YH, Hoppe RT. Mycosis fungoides and the Sezary syndrome. *Semin Oncol* 1999;26:276–289.

Preston DS, Stern RS. Non-melanoma cancers of the skin. *N Engl J Med* 1992;327:1649.

Rupoli S, Barulli B, Guiducci B, et al. Low-dose interferon-alpha 2b combined with PUVA is an effective treatment of early stage mycosis fungoides: results of a multicenter study. Cutaneous-T Cell Lymphoma Multicenter Study Group. *Haematologica* 1999;84:809–813.

Safai B. Management of skin cancer. In: DeVita VT, Hellman S, Rosenberg SA, eds. *Cancer: principles and practice of oncology.* 5th ed. Philadelphia: Lippincott–Raven, 1997:1879.

Siegel RS, Pandolfino T, Guitart J, et al. Primary cutaneous T-cell lymphoma: review and current concepts. *J Clin Oncol* 2000;18:2908–2925.

15

Primary and Metastatic Brain Tumors

Benjamin E. Lawler and Tracy T. Batchelor

I. Primary brain tumors
A. Incidence

According to population-based estimates from the Central Brain Tumor Registry of the United States, there were 35,519 primary brain tumors (PBTs) diagnosed in 2001. The overall incidence of these tumors in the United States is 11.3 cases per 100,000 person-years, with 4.2 per 100,000 person-years for benign tumors and 6.8 per 100,000 person-years for malignant tumors. This represented 1% to 2% of all cancers diagnosed in 2000 and accounted for over 13,000 deaths in the same year. The age-adjusted 5-year relative survival for all PBTs from 1989 to 1996 was 30.8%. Survival rates for PBT by age are as follows: 0 to 19 years: 61.1%; 20 to 44 years: 49%; 45 to 64 years: 13.3%; and 65 years or older: 4.7%. The only established risk factor for PBT is ionizing radiation at high doses, which has been associated with an increased incidence of nerve sheath tumors, meningiomas, and gliomas.

B. Gliomas

Gliomas account for two-thirds of PBTs and include astrocytic, oligodendroglial, and ependymal tumors. The astrocytomas are the most frequent type, and these tumors have a wide spectrum of clinical behavior. The more malignant types—anaplastic astrocytoma and glioblastoma multiforme (GBM)—are not generally curable, though each may respond to radiation and chemotherapy. These are graded based on the presence or absence of the following histologic features: nuclear atypia, mitoses, endothelial proliferation, and necrosis.

1. **Grades I and II Astrocytoma.** Pilocytic astrocytomas are World Health Organization (WHO) grade I tumors that most commonly arise in the posterior fossa. These tumors are most common in the pediatric population and can be cured if a total surgical resection is possible. WHO grade II astrocytomas (low-grade astrocytomas) are most commonly seen in the third and fourth decades. This tumor typically appears as a nonenhancing diffuse hypointense mass on T1-weighted magnetic resonance imaging (MRI). The median survival for persons with these tumors is 7.5 years with a 5-year survival of 60%.

If feasible, a gross total resection should be performed and then the patient should be followed regularly with serial MRI studies and clinical examinations. Randomized clinical trials have shown that there is no overall survival benefit when radiation is given at the time of the original diagnosis. There is controversy regarding the management of WHO grade II astrocytoma in "high-risk" patients; for example, an elderly patient's tumor is more likely to progress more rapidly than in a much younger patient. One option in this setting is to administer involved field radiation (IFR) up to 60 Gy.

In the event of tumor progression on computed tomography (CT) or MRI, further surgery, if possible, may be performed and/or IFR is recommended. If, at the time of the recurrence, the histopathology demonstrates a higher-grade astrocytoma, chemotherapy can be initiated, which will be discussed in Section I.B.2 on malignant astrocytomas.

2. Grades II and III Astrocytoma. Malignant astrocytomas occur in 3 to 4 per 100,000 people in the United States. Anaplastic astrocytoma (WHO grade III) occurs most commonly in the fourth and fifth decades, while GBM (WHO grade IV) occurs most commonly in the fifth and sixth decades. Median survival times are 24 to 36 and 9 to 12 months, respectively. These two types of tumors are indistinguishable by MRI, as both appear as diffuse hypointense lesions on T1-weighted images and both readily enhance after contrast agent administration. These tumors can have cystic areas associated with them, areas of hemorrhage, and are most commonly seen in the cerebral hemispheres.

Diagnosis is made histologically, after either a stereotactic biopsy or gross resection. Surgical debulking is the preferred initial treatment to minimize neurologic morbidity; gross total resection is associated with longer survival. Following surgery, IFR up to 60 Gy is given. Positive prognostic factors in these tumors include high Karnofsky performance score, gross total resection, and younger age.

a. Chemotherapy. Chemotherapy for malignant astrocytomas is controversial. The Medical Research Council (MRC) Brain Tumor Working Party reported a Phase III comparative trial of IFR with adjuvant (procarbazine, lomustine [CCNU], and vincristine) versus no adjuvant chemotherapy in patients with newly diagnosed malignant glioma and found no significant difference in survival. Prior studies have shown questionable benefit from adjuvant chemotherapy in anaplastic astrocytoma, though no benefit in GBM. It is unclear if there is any benefit in routinely giving chemotherapy to older patients with malignant gliomas. Since older patients with GBM are not likely to respond to conventional chemotherapy, if appropriate, they may be entered into therapeutic trials.

b. Chemotherapy regimens. The chloroethylnitrosoureas are the best-studied chemotherapeutic agents for malignant gliomas and include carmustine (BCNU) and lomustine (CCNU), the latter typically given in combination with procarbazine and vincristine (PCV). BCNU and CCNU act by alkylating deoxyribonucleic acid (DNA) and ribonucleic acid (RNA) and may also inhibit several key enzymatic processes by carbamoylation of amino acids in proteins. Alkylating chemotherapeutic agents are inhibited by the DNA repair enzyme O^6-methylguanine-DNA methyltransferase (MGMT). However, when the MGMT promoter is methylated, studies have shown alkylating agents to be more effective. This finding is currently being studied for potential treatment benefit. The following are regimens that have been used both in the adjuvant setting and for patients who have recurrence after surgery, radiotherapy, or both.

(1)   BCNU may be administered as adjuvant monotherapy and is given in either one dose or in two to three divided consecutive daily doses for a total of 150 to 200 mg/m^2 IV every 6 weeks.

(2)   PCV is a combination of three antineoplastic agents given in a 6-week cycle:

Lomustine 110 mg/m^2 PO on day 1
Vincristine 1.4 mg/m^2 (maximum 2.2 mg) IV on days 8 and 29
Procarbazine 60 mg/m^2 PO days 8 through 21 of the 42-day cycle

PCV is typically administered for 6 to 12 months or until tumor progression.

(3)   Gliadel wafers are a depot source of BCNU that can be surgically implanted at the time of resection. The U.S. Food and Drug Administration (FDA) approved the 3.85% BCNU wafer after a Phase III, double-blind, placebo-controlled clinical study involving 222 patients undergoing surgery for recurrent malignant glioma showed that gliadel wafers increased median survival from 20 to 28 weeks.

(4)   Temozolomide is approved for the treatment of recurrent anaplastic astrocytoma. It is an imidotetrazine analog of dacarbazine (DTIC) and acts by alkylating DNA. Temozolomide is given orally in 28-day cycles. **The first cycle is dosed at 150 mg/m^2 PO daily for 5 consecutive days in a 28-day treatment cycle. If this is tolerated, then the remaining cycles are given at 200 mg/m^2 PO daily for 5 consecutive days.** In one study involving recurrent anaplastic astrocytomas, temozolomide had a 35% response rate and a 26% stable disease rate. Since these results are comparable with those of PCV and the chloroethylnitrosoureas and temozolomide has more a favorable side effect profile, it is used both as first-line adjuvant chemotherapy for anaplastic astrocytomas and for recurrent anaplastic astrocytomas. Temozolomide does not have significant activity against GBM.

Recurrent malignant astrocytoma may be treated by surgical debulking, radiosurgery, or chemotherapy. In general, recurrent malignant gliomas are resistant to most types of therapy, and consideration of treatment within the context of a clinical trial is appropriate.

3.   Oligodendroglioma (World Health Organization grades II and III)

a.   Characteristics. Well-differentiated (WHO grade II) and anaplastic (WHO grade III) oligodendrogliomas are glial tumors that are found almost exclusively in the cerebral hemispheres and represent between 4% and 15% of all gliomas. The peak incidence occurs in the fourth through sixth decades of life. Oligodendrogliomas have increased cellularity with homogeneous, hyperchromatic nuclei surrounded by clear cytoplasm: the "fried-egg appearance."

Allelic loss of the short arm of chromosome 1p and the long arm of chromosome 19q is common. Microcalcifications and increased vascularity are also seen. These tumors are hypo-intense on T1-weighted MRI scans and hyperintense on T2-weighted images and are located in the deep white matter. Low-grade oligodendroglioma has a more circumscribed appearance than its anaplastic counterpart and is commonly confused with low-grade astrocytomas, vascular malformations, or craniopharyngiomas. Calcifications are more commonly seen in oligodendrogliomas than in mixed gliomas (oligoastrocytomas). The median survivals for WHO grade II oligodendrogliomas and WHO grade III oligodendrogliomas have been reported as 9.8 to 16.7 and 3.9 years, respectively.

b.   Treatment. Although the optimal treatment for these tumors remains controversial, the general approach is similar to that for astrocytomas. In all cases, if a tumor is suspected, a stereotactic biopsy should be performed or confirmed tumors should be resected, if feasible. Residual or unresectable low-grade oligodendrogliomas can be followed with serial MRI studies and clinical examinations. Following the initial resection of an anaplastic oligodendroglioma, radiation has been a standard recommendation. However, since grade III tumors have shown 60% to 100% response rates to PCV, this form of chemotherapy is administered either prior to IFR or in the postradiation period. Although there are high initial response rates to PCV, in general, adjuvant chemotherapy has not been demonstrated to improve survival in this type of tumor. Temozolomide has shown a 26% response rate when used for recurrence of oligodendroglial tumors and is an option in this setting.

4.   Ependymoma (World Health Organization grades II and III)

a.   Characteristics. Ependymomas are slow-growing neuroepithelial tumors found along the ventricular system and in the spinal canal. They represent 3% to 9% of all neuroepithelial tumors, with a bimodal peak incidence at 6 and at 30 to 40 years. Infratentorial ependymomas are more common in the pediatric population, while in adults, the tumors occur with equal incidence in the posterior fossa and spinal cord. Ependymomas represent 50% to 60% of spinal neuroepithelial neoplasms. Indicators of poor outcome include age below 3 years, anaplastic histopathology, an incomplete resection, and no postoperative radiation. In one adult series, survival at 5 years was 57%. Spinal ependymomas have better outcomes than cerebral lesions, and supratentorial lesions have better outcomes than infratentorial ependymomas. These tumors can disseminate along cerebrospinal fluid (CSF) pathways, and staging should include MRI of the brain and entire spine and CSF cytopathology if a lumbar puncture can be safely performed.

b.   Treatment. Surgical removal is the treatment of choice for both ependymomas (WHO grade II) and anaplastic ependymomas (WHO grade III), and patients who have undergone gross total resection achieve longer survival than those who have had only biopsy or subtotal removal. The role of radiation and chemotherapy in the treatment of this tumor is controversial. If an ependymoma (WHO grade II) is totally resected, then postoperative observation is a reasonable option. If residual tumor remains after resection or there is recurrence of tumor, IFR is typically recommended. However, in a child under 3 years of age, chemotherapy is given, with the possibility of using radiation after the age of 3. Radiation in children younger than 3 has been shown to cause significant morbidity. In an anaplastic ependymoma (WHO grade III), regardless of the type of resection performed, treatment involves radiation and, occasionally, chemotherapy.

The most commonly used chemotherapy regimen is derived from the Pediatric Oncology Group protocol, which uses two 28-day cycles of cyclophosphamide plus vincristine followed by one 28-day cycle of cisplatin plus etoposide.

Chemotherapy is started 2 to 4 weeks after surgery and is given in alternating 28-day cycles. Regimen 1 using vincristine and cyclophosphamide is given twice sequentially. Twenty-eight days later, regimen 2 using cisplatin and etoposide is given once. The entire sequence (1, 1, 2, 1, 1, 2) is then repeated for 1 to 2 years.

  (1) **Vincristine** 1.6 mg/m^2 (0.065 mg/kg), maximal dose 1.5 mg, IV push on days 1 and 8, and **cyclophosphamide** 1,600 mg/m^2 (65 mg/kg), infused over a 30-min period on day 1. Repeat this cycle on day 29. After completion of the second cycle, give:
  (2) **Cisplatin** 100 mg/m^2 (4 mg/kg) as a 6-h infusion on day 1 and a 1-h IV infusion of **etoposide** 160 mg/m^2 (6.5 mg/kg) on days 3 and 4. This cycle is not repeated until two more cycles of vincristine and cyclophosphamide have been given again.

This treatment was repeated in one study until disease progression or until the patients reached 3 years of age, at which time they received radiation.

C. Medulloblastoma (World Health Organization grade IV)

  1. Characteristics. Medulloblastomas are malignant embryonal tumors of the posterior fossa. Eighty percent are found in children under the age of 15, and this neoplasm accounts for 20% of all pediatric brain tumors. Medulloblastomas represent 1% of tumors in patients older than 20 years. The tumors are invasive and tend to metastasize through the CSF to the rest of the CNS. The staging evaluation for these patients should include gadolinium-enhanced MRI of the entire neuraxis (brain and spinal cord) and lumbar puncture for CSF cytopathology if the latter can be safely performed. If disseminated disease is found at the time of the diagnosis (poor-risk category), radical tumor resection confers little to no survival benefit. Histologically, the tumor has poorly differentiated, densely packed, hyperchromatic, nucleated, small, round, blue cells.

  2. Treatment. Treatment for local disease involves surgical resection, followed by craniospinal radiation (CSR) in adults at a dose of 36 Gy with a boost to the tumor bed to 54 Gy. In the average-risk patient, this treatment approach is associated with a 60% 5-year progression-free survival. In an attempt to minimize the long-term side effects of radiation in children, one study showed acceptable results with 23.4 Gy of CSR given, with a boost to the tumor bed to 55.8 Gy, followed by chemotherapy. This approach resulted in progression-free survival results of 79% at 5 years.

There are multiple chemotherapy regimens for medulloblastomas, all of which were developed in the pediatric population. A common approach involves the protocol used for ependymomas (etoposide, cisplatin, cyclophosphamide, and vincristine). In patients with recurrent medulloblastoma, high-dose chemotherapy with autologous stem cell rescue may be beneficial.

D. Primary central nervous system lymphoma
Primary CNS lymphoma (PCNSL) is a diffuse large B-cell lymphoma arising within the CNS. This tumor accounts for 1.5% to 6% of all PBTs, and it has a peak incidence in the sixth and seventh decades of life. Ocular involvement is seen in 5% to 20% of cases and leptomeningeal spread in up to 40% of cases. Sixty percent of tumors are supratentorial and commonly involve the periventricular regions and corpus callosum. Twenty-five percent to 50% of cases have multifocal disease at the time of diagnosis. The lesions are hypointense to isointense on T1-weighted MRI and enhance homogeneously on postgadolinium images. The tumors are responsive to corticosteroids, and as a result, these drugs should be avoided until a diagnosis has been established. The only role for surgery in PCNSL is to establish the diagnosis by biopsy. These tumors should not be resected except in the rare circumstance of brain herniation from mass effect.

Staging examinations for patients with PCNSL should include gadolinium-enhanced MRI of the brain and spine, ophthalmologic evaluation with slit lamp examination, and a lumbar puncture for CSF cytopathology analysis. Bone marrow biopsy and CT imaging of the body are not necessary unless systemic disease is clinically suspected.

Whole-brain radiation therapy (WBRT) results in a 90% response rate, but the median survival with WBRT alone is less than 12 months. PCNSL is sensitive to many types of chemotherapy, with all successful regimens involving the use of high-dose methotrexate at either 3.5 or 8 g/m^2. Either alone or in combination with other chemotherapeutic drugs, methotrexate-based treatment is associated with radiographic response rates of 50% to 100% and survival durations of 40 to 90 months without the use of WBRT.

II. Cerebral metastases
A. Incidence. The overall incidence of cerebral metastases to the brain is significantly higher than that of PBT in adults. The incidence is approximately 2.8 to 11.1 per 100,000 cases per year in the United States. It is suspected that 20% to 25% of patients dying of cancer each year have brain metastases. Most commonly, cerebral metastases arise from cancer of the lung, breast, skin (melanoma), kidney, and colon.

B. **Treatment**
  1. **Surgery.** Because metastatic cancers often do not extensively infiltrate the surrounding normal brain parenchyma, these tumors can usually be resected. However, this approach should be attempted only when the tumors are accessible and few in number, as revealed by CT or MRI, and when the patient's cancer is under good control systemically. In these circumstances, surgery followed by WBRT results in longer survival than WBRT alone (40 versus 15 weeks for cerebral metastases from lung cancer).
  2. **Radiation therapy.** WBRT is employed for metastatic cancers. Small tumors (generally less than 4 cm in diameter) that are solitary or persistent after whole-brain irradiation may be treated with stereotactic radiosurgery (linear accelerator, cobalt source/gamma knife, proton radiosurgery). This technique uses a stereotactic frame and specialized external-beam focusing. It permits a high dose of radiation to be delivered to a small region in a single fraction. However, cerebral radiation necrosis is a common complication and may necessitate either surgery or prolonged use of corticosteroids. The decision to proceed with either radiosurgery or resection should be individually tailored and based on status of the primary tumor, performance status, location of the tumor, and number of tumors.
  3. **Chemotherapy.** Chemotherapy has a limited role in the treatment of cerebral metastases. However, there are exceptions as metastases from breast cancer occasionally respond well to the usual regimens for breast tumors. Lymphomatous brain masses may also respond to methotrexate-based chemotherapy.
  4. **Evaluation for a primary tumor.** Occasionally, a patient presents with brain metastases as the first manifestation of cancer. In most cases, there is little benefit to be gained by an extensive search for the primary tumor if the history, physical examination, chest radiograph, blood cell count, and chemistry profile are unrevealing because the prognosis for patients with brain metastases is generally poor. An exception to this rule is a young male in whom metastatic testicular cancer (and occasionally other germ cell tumors) can be cured despite brain metastases. In these patients, measuring α-fetoprotein and β-human chorionic gonadotropin levels is warranted. In addition, small cell lung cancer sometimes responds well to chemotherapy and radiation therapy. Therefore, it is reasonable to perform a chest CT scan and biopsy of any lung tumor if the patient has a good performance status.
III. **Leptomeningeal metastases.** The treatment of leptomeningeal metastases includes radiation therapy to symptomatic areas of the CNS (e.g., to the base of the brain for cranial nerve dysfunction) and intrathecal (IT) chemotherapy with methotrexate, cytosine arabinoside (ara-C), or thiotepa.
  A. **Chemotherapy regimens**
    1. Methotrexate 12 mg/m^2 (maximum 15 mg) IT per dose is the most commonly used IT chemotherapeutic agent. It is administered once or twice a week until the cytologic examination shows clearance of malignant cells from the CSF, then once a month as maintenance.

2.   Cytarabine (ara-C) 50 mg is available in a sustained-delivery form (Depocyt, Depotec, depofoam) for IT administration that allows treatment every 2 weeks. This is an advantage over conventional IT drugs, which must be delivered two to three times each week. Concurrent administration of oral corticosteroids (dexamethasone 4 mg b.i.d. on days 1 to 5) is required with the sustained-release form of cytarabine as the main side effect from this medication is arachnoiditis.

3.   Thiotepa 12 mg is a third IT chemotherapeutic agent that may be used if there is no response to methotrexate or cytarabine. However, the short CSF half-life of this agent may compromise its efficacy.

B.   Administration. All chemotherapeutic agents for IT administration should be freshly prepared in preservative-free diluent. Since drugs that are administered into the lumbar subarachnoid space result in lower concentrations of the drugs in the upper spine and brain, it is advisable to administer these drugs through an Ommaya reservoir, a device that is implanted under the scalp and connected by a catheter, through a burr hole, to the frontal horn of the lateral ventricle. This method allows more reliable delivery of drug to the CSF and better distribution of drug along CSF pathways and avoids the necessity of repeated lumbar punctures for the patient.

C.   Complications. Complications of IT chemotherapy include arachnoiditis and leukoencephalopathy. The latter is more likely to occur if the perforated tubing of the Ommaya catheter becomes lodged in brain tissue rather than the lateral ventricle. Myelosuppression is not usually significant unless the patient undergoes spinal irradiation or systemic chemotherapy as well. Oral leucovorin is generally given after IT methotrexate (10 mg leucovorin PO every 6 h for six to eight doses, starting 24 h after the methotrexate) to prevent bone marrow toxicity.

IV.   Treatment of cerebral edema

A.   Corticosteroids. These drugs are usually started soon after the diagnosis of a brain tumor is established. However, if PCNSL is suspected on the basis of the CT or MRI, then corticosteroids should be withheld until after a biopsy has been done. In the rare patient with PCNSL who requires emergent antiedema measures, mannitol may be administered (see below). **Dexamethasone 10 mg IV followed by 4 mg every 6 h PO or IV** reduces or eliminates the lethargy, headaches, visual blurring, and nausea caused by cerebral edema and also often reduces some of the focal neurologic signs and symptoms such as hemiparesis. The corticosteroid dose should be tapered and discontinued after a complete surgical resection has been performed or after radiation therapy has been completed and resumed if symptoms recur. The dose should be held at the lowest dose that maximizes therapeutic benefit and minimizes side effects (e.g., gastric irritation, insomnia, mood swings, cushingoid body features, increased appetite, and proximal myopathy).

B.   Treatment of refractory cerebral edema

1.   Increase dexamethasone. When moderate doses of dexamethasone do not effectively control cerebral edema, the dose may be increased transiently to 10 to 24 mg IV every 4 to 6 h. This dose should usually not be maintained for longer than 48 to 72 h.

2. An osmotic diuretic in an urgent situation may act more rapidly than a corticosteroid. Mannitol 75 to 100 g IV (as a 15% to 25% solution) is given by rapid infusion over 20 to 30 min and repeated at 6- to 8-h intervals as needed. Careful monitoring of electrolytes, serum osmolarity, fluid intake and output, and body weight is essential to avoid dehydration. The osmotic diuresis may be discontinued when there is improvement in the signs and symptoms from cerebral edema and when the corticosteroids or other measures to reduce cerebral edema have taken effect.

V. Treatment of seizures

A. Seizures are a common presenting feature in patients with brain tumors, with an incidence of approximately 20%. Prophylactic treatment for patients with brain tumors who have not had a seizure is not beneficial. However, it is common practice to administer a prophylactic anticonvulsant for a period of time after a biopsy or a craniotomy. If the patient has not had a seizure and has undergone only an uncomplicated biopsy or resection, the anticonvulsant may be discontinued after 4 to 8 weeks. If a patient does have a seizure and is to be placed on an anticonvulsant, phenytoin (Dilantin) at 300 mg/day is often recommended. Alternative monotherapies include carbamazepine, phenobarbital, and valproic acid. If the patient has further seizures despite having sufficient serum levels of an anticonvulsant, then a second agent may be added. For those on long-term anticonvulsant therapy, it is important to check drug levels at intervals, especially after dosages of other medications have been changed or new medications have been added.

B. Common side effects of anticonvulsant treatment include sedation, nausea, rashes, diplopia, dysmetria, ataxia, and hepatic dysfunction. A rare but serious toxicity is Stevens–Johnson syndrome, which is an immune complex–mediated hypersensitivity disorder. There may be an increased risk of this complication in patients undergoing simultaneous cranial irradiation and corticosteroid taper. This may present as a rash beginning as macules that may develop into papules, vesicles, bullae, urticarial plaques, or confluent erythema. A fever is present in 85% of cases.

C. Cytochrome P-450 induction. Several commonly used anticonvulsants (phenytoin, phenobarbital, carbamazepine) may induce the hepatic cytochrome P-450 enzyme system with potentially important clinical implications. This may result in increased metabolism and reduced plasma levels of chemotherapeutic drugs that undergo hepatic metabolism. This has been demonstrated in a trial of the topoisomerase I inhibitor irinotecan (CPT-11) in patients with recurrent malignant gliomas. It was found that the maximum tolerated dose of CPT-11 was approximately fourfold higher in patients taking cytochrome P-450–inducing anticonvulsants than in patients not on these drugs. This emphasizes the importance of using anticonvulsants only when clearly indicated.

SELECTED READINGS

Brem H, Piantadosi S, Burger PC, et al. Placebo-controlled trial of safety and efficacy of intraoperative controlled delivery by biodegradable polymers of chemotherapy for recurrent gliomas. The Polymer–Brain Tumor Treatment Group. *Lancet* 1995;345:1008–1012.

Burger PC, Vogel FS, Green SB, et al. Glioblastoma multiforme and anaplastic astrocytoma. Pathologic criteria and prognostic implications. *Cancer* 1985;56:1106–1111.

Cairncross G, Macdonald D, Ludwin S, et al. Chemotherapy for anaplastic oligodendroglioma. National Cancer Institute of Canada Clinical Trials Group. *J Clin Oncol* 1994;12:2013–2021.

DeAngelis LM. Brain tumors. *N Engl J Med* 2001;344:114–123.

Duffner PK, Horowitz ME, Krischer JP, et al. Postoperative chemotherapy and delayed radiation in children less than three years of age with malignant brain tumors. *N Engl J Med* 1993;328:1725–1731.

Esteller M, Garcia-Foncillas J, Andion E, et al. Inactivation of the DNA-repair gene MGMT and the clinical response of gliomas to alkylating agents. *N Engl J Med* 2000;343:1350–1354.

Glantz MJ, Cole BF, Forsyth PA, et al. Practice parameter: anticonvulsant prophylaxis in patients with newly diagnosed brain tumors—report of the Quality Standards Subcommittee of the American Academy of Neurology. *Neurology* 2000;54:1886–1893.

Hubbard JL, Scheithauer BW, Kispert DB, et al. Adult cerebellar medulloblastomas: the pathological, radiographic, and clinical disease spectrum. *J Neurosurg* 1989;70:536–544.

Jeyapalan SA. Batchelor TT. Diagnostic evaluation of neurologic metastases. *Cancer Invest* 2000;18:381–394.

Kaye AH, Laws Jr ER. *Brain tumors. An encyclopedic approach.* 2nd ed. New York: Churchill Livingstone, 2001.

Kleihues P, Cavenee WK. *WHO classification of tumors, pathology and genetics, tumours of the nervous system.* Lyon: IARC Press, 2000.

Levin VA, Silver P, Hannigan J, et al. Superiority of post-radiotherapy adjuvant chemotherapy with CCNU, procarbazine, and vincristine (PCV) over BCNU for anaplastic gliomas: NCOG 6G61 final report. *Int J Radiat Oncol Biol Phys* 1990;18:321–324.

Medical Research Council Brain Tumor Working Party. Randomized trial of procarbazine, lomustine, and vincristine in the adjuvant treatment of high-grade astrocytoma: a Medical Research Council trial. *J Clin Oncol* 2001;19:509–518.

Mellet LB. Physicochemical consideration and pharmacokinetic behavior in delivery of drugs to the central nervous system. *Cancer Treat Rep* 1977;61:527.

Packer RJ, Sutton LN, Elterman R, et al. Outcome for children with medulloblastoma treated with radiation and cisplatin, CCNU, and vincristine chemotherapy. *J Neurosurg* 1994;81:690–698.

Patchell RA, Tibbs PA, Walsh JW, et al. A randomized trial of surgery in the treatment of single metastases to the brain. *N Engl J Med* 1990;322:494–500.

Plotkin SR. Batchelor TT. Primary nervous-system lymphoma. *Lancet Oncol* 2001;2:354–365.

Prados MD. Future directions in the treatment of malignant gliomas with temozolomide. *Semin Oncol* 2000;27(suppl 6):41–46.

Reddy AT, Packer RJ. Chemotherapy for low-grade gliomas. *Childs Nerv Syst* 1999;15:506–513.

Shapiro WR, Green SB, Burger PC, et al. Randomized trial of three chemotherapy regimens and two radiotherapy regimens in post-operative treatment of malignant glioma. Brain Tumor Cooperative Group Trial 8001. *J Neurosurg* 1989;71:1–9.

Trojanowski T, Peszynski J, Turowski K, et al. Quality of survival of patients with brain gliomas treated with postoperative CCNU and radiation therapy. *J Neurosurg* 1989;70:18–23.

Walker MD, Green SB, Byar DP, et al. Randomized comparisons of radiotherapy and nitrosoureas for the treatment of malignant glioma after surgery. *N Engl J Med* 1980;303:1323–1329.

Wasserstrom WR, Glass JP, Posner JB. Diagnosis and treatment of leptomeningeal metastasis from solid tumors: experience with 90 patients. *Cancer* 1982;49:759.

Soft Tissue Sarcomas

Robert S. Benjamin

I. Classification and approach to treatment

A. Types of soft tissue sarcomas. The soft tissue sarcomas are a group of diseases characterized by neoplastic proliferation of tissue of mesenchymal origin. Thus, they differ from the more common carcinomas, which arise from epithelial tissue. Sarcomas can arise in any area of the body and from any origin; however, they most commonly arise in the soft tissue of the extremities, trunk, retroperitoneum, or head and neck area. There are more than 20 different types of sarcomas, classified according to lines of differentiation toward normal tissue. For example, rhabdomyosarcoma shows evidence of skeletal muscle fibers with cross-striations, liposarcoma shows fat production, and angiosarcoma shows vessel formation. Precise characterization of the types of sarcoma is often impossible, and these tumors are called *unclassified sarcomas*. All of the primary bone sarcomas may arise in soft tissue, leading to such diagnoses as extraskeletal osteosarcoma, extraskeletal Ewing's sarcoma, and extraskeletal chondrosarcoma. A common diagnosis at present is malignant fibrous histiocytoma (MFH). This tumor is characterized by a mixture of spindle (or fibrous) cells and round (or histiocytic) cells arranged in a storiform pattern with frequent areas of pleomorphic appearance and frequent giant cells. There is no evidence of differentiation toward any particular tissue type. Many tumors previously called pleomorphic fibrosarcoma, pleomorphic rhabdomyosarcoma, and so forth are now classified as MFH. As immunohistochemistry and molecular diagnostic techniques improve, it is likely that some of the tumors currently classified as MFH will be reclassified as pleomorphic something else. Furthermore, there are strong opponents of the term MFH, and tumors previously classified as such will probably be reclassified as unclassified pleomorphic sarcomas.

B. Metastases. Metastatic spread of all sarcomas tends to be through the blood rather than through the lymphatic system. The lungs are by far the most frequent site of metastatic disease. Local sites of metastasis by direct invasion are the second most common area of involvement, followed by bone and liver. (Liver metastases are common with intra-abdominal sarcomas, especially gastrointestinal stromal tumors [GISTs]; however, and metastases to soft tissue are common with myxoid liposarcomas.) Central nervous system (CNS) metastases are extraordinarily rare except in alveolar soft-part sarcoma.

C. Staging. Staging of sarcomas is complex and demands an expert sarcoma pathologist. Tumors have been staged according to two systems: the American Joint Committee on Cancer (AJCC) staging system and the Musculoskeletal Tumor Society staging system. The new International Union Against Cancer (UICC)/AJC staging system with international acceptance takes portions from each of the older systems and more appropriately identifies patients at increased risk of metastatic disease. Further revisions to this system are still underway, and a final, widely accepted system is still not universally accepted. Since current and older publications still refer to the older systems, however, all will be included.

1. The old American Joint Committee on Cancer staging system
  a.   Tumor grade. The primary determinant of stage is tumor grade.

  Grade 1 tumors are stage I.
  Grade 2 tumors are stage II.
  Grade 3 tumors are stage III.
  Any tumor with lymph node metastases is automatically stage III.
  Any tumor with gross invasion of bone, major vessel, or major nerve is stage IV.

  b.   Stage. Further divisions of stages I to III into A and B are based on tumor size.

  A = tumor smaller than 5 cm
  B = tumor size 5 cm or larger

  In stage III, lymph node metastases are classified as IIIC. In stage IV, local invasion is called IVA, and IVB represents distant metastases.

2. The Musculoskeletal Tumor Society staging system. The Musculoskeletal Tumor Society stages sarcomas according to grade and compartmental localization. The Roman numeral reflects the tumor grade.

Stage I: low grade
Stage II: high grade
Stage III: any-grade tumor with distant metastasis

  The letter reflects compartmental localization. Compartments are defined by fascial planes.

Stage A: intracompartmental (i.e., confined to the same soft tissue compartment as the initial tumor)
Stage B: extracompartmental (i.e., extending outside of the initial soft tissue compartment into the adjacent soft tissue compartment or bone)

  A stage IA tumor is a low-grade tumor confined to its initial compartment, a stage IB tumor is a low-grade tumor extending outside the initial compartment, and so forth.

3. The new American Joint Committee on Cancer staging system. The stage is determined by tumor grade, tumor size, and tumor location relative to the muscular fascia. There are now four tumor grades.

Grade 1: well differentiated
Grade 2: moderately differentiated
Grade 3: poorly differentiated
Grade 4: undifferentiated

  Tumor size is now divided at less than or equal to 5 cm or more than 5 cm (in the old AJCC system, it was less than 5 cm or more than or equal to 5 cm).

T1 = ≤5 cm
T2 = >5 cm

Tumor status is subdivided by location relative to the muscular fascia.

Ta = superficial to the muscular fascia
Tb = deep to the muscular fascia

The AJCC stage grouping is as follows:

Stage I	T1a, 1b, 2a, 2b	N0	M0	G1 to 2
Stage II	T1a, 1b, 2a	N0	M0	G3 to 4
Stage III	T2b	N0	M0	G3 to 4
Stage IV	Any T	N1	M0	Any G
	Any T	N0	M1	Any G

The new staging system divides patients according to necessary therapy.

Stage I patients are adequately treated by surgery alone.
Stage II patients require adjuvant radiation therapy.
Stage III patients require adjuvant chemotherapy.
Stage IV patients are managed primarily with chemotherapy, with or without other modalities.

D. Evaluation. Patients are evaluated and followed according to the plan in Table 16.1.
E. Primary treatment
  1. Surgery and radiotherapy. Treatment of the primary tumor involves surgery with or without radiation therapy. If radiation therapy is not used, surgery must be radical. Although this may often involve amputation or complete excision of the involved muscle group from origin to insertion, more and more frequently, wide local resection is performed, with or without adjuvant radiation, depending on stage and extent of negative margins.
  2. Adjuvant chemotherapy. The role of adjuvant chemotherapy remains controversial, with both positive and negative results reported. A recent meta-analysis indicated a highly significant decrease in the risk of disease recurrence (either local or distant) and death in patients treated with adjuvant chemotherapy; thus, *some investigators believe that adjuvant therapy is clearly indicated for patients whose histologic type, grade, or location is known to convey a poor prognosis.* A meta-analysis of individual patient data confirms a survival benefit for patients with primary sarcomas of the extremities as well as increased local or distant disease-free interval for all patients treated with doxorubicin (Adriamycin)–based adjuvant chemotherapy. A recent Italian cooperative group study using epirubicin and ifosfamide for patients with current stage III disease also demonstrated survival and disease-free survival advantage for patients treated with chemotherapy.
F. Prognosis. Prognosis is related to stage, with a 5-year survival rate of 99% for new AJCC/UICC stage I, 82% for stage II, and 52% for stage III. Corresponding rates of disease-free survival at 5 years are 78% for stage I, 64% for stage II, and 36% for stage III. Long-term results are still worse. The survival rate for

Table 16.1.   Soft tissue sarcoma evaluation

Tests[a]	Initial	During treatment	Follow-up (if no evidence of disease)
History and physical examination	X	Before each treatment	Yr 1: q2 mo; yr 2, 3: q3 mo; yr 4: q4 mo; yr 5: q6 mo; then yearly
CBC, differential, and platelet counts[b]	X	Twice weekly	Yearly
Electrolytes[b]	X	Before each treatment	—
Chemistry profile[b]	X	Before each treatment	q4 mo
Urinalysis	If giving ifosfamide	As indicated by symptoms	—
PT, APTT, fibrinogen	X	—	—
Chest radiograph	X	Before each treatment	Same as for history and physical examination
CT scan chest	If chest radiograph appears normal	To confirm chest radiograph findings (if initially abnormal) or for surgical planning	If chest radiograph becomes equivocal
MRI primary (if not intra-abdominal), *or*	X	Preoperatively	—
Ultrasound primary	—	—	Yr 1: q4 mo; yr 2, 3: q6 mo

CT of abdomen and pelvis	If myxoid liposarcoma or retroperitoneal or pelvic primary tumor	If baseline, every third cycle	If baseline, yr 1: q4 mo; yr 2, 3: q6 mo
ECG	If cardiac history	—	—
Cardiac nuclear scan (for ejection fraction)	If cardiac history	If doxorubicin dose is to exceed standard limits for schedule	Yearly for 2 yr, then as clinically indicated
Central venous catheter	X	—	—
Bone marrow or screening MRI of spine and pelvis	If small cell tumor	—	—
Bone scan	If indicated by history	—	—
Plain film	If indicated by history	—	—

CBC, complete blood cell count; PT, prothrombin time; APTT, activated partial thromboplastin time; CT, computed tomography; MRI, magnetic resonance imaging; ECG, electrocardiography.

[a] Tests may be ordered more frequently based on clinical indications.

[b] Required more frequently if patient is on a medical treatment program.

stage IV disease is less than 10%; however, a definite fraction of patients in this category can be cured. Most patients with stage IV disease, if left untreated, die within 6 to 12 months; however, there is great variation in actual survival, and patients may go on with slowly progressive disease for many years.

G.   Treatment response. Response to treatment is measured in the standard fashion for solid tumors with the addition of tumor necrosis, both radiologically and pathologically.

1.   Complete remission. This implies complete disappearance of all signs and symptoms of disease.

2.   Partial remission. Standard Response Evaluation Criteria in Solid Tumors (RECIST) criteria (Chapter 2, Section IV.B.1) are generally employed. This requires a 30% or greater decrease in measurable disease, calculated by comparing the sum of the longest diameters of all lesions before and after therapy. When disease can be followed objectively by magnetic resonance imaging (MRI) or computed tomography (CT), marked tumor necrosis attributable to chemotherapy demonstrated by imaging or pathology is at least the equivalent of a partial response by RECIST criteria.

3.   Stable disease or improvement. Lesser degrees of tumor shrinkage are categorized by some physicians as stable disease and by others as improvement or minor response. Stable disease implies a smaller than 20% increase in disease for at least 8 weeks. For all response categories, no new disease must appear during response.

4.   Progression. New disease in any area or a 20% or more increase in measurable disease constitutes progressive disease.

5.   Survival. All patients whose disease responds objectively to chemotherapy survive longer than do patients with progressive disease, and the degree of prolongation of survival is directly proportional to the degree of antitumor response that can be measured.

II.   Chemotherapy

A.   General considerations and aims of therapy. Although there are numerous types of soft tissue sarcomas, there are few differences among them regarding responsiveness to a standard soft tissue sarcoma regimen. GISTs and alveolar soft-part sarcomas and, to a lesser extent, clear cell sarcomas and epithelioid sarcomas respond less frequently to standard regimens than do the other soft tissue sarcomas. GISTs, in particular, should not be treated with doxorubicin- and ifosfamide-based chemotherapy. GISTs are usually characterized by mutated *c-Kit* and have a high response rate with prolonged remissions after treatment with imatinib mesylate (Gleevec, STI-571). Angiosarcomas can respond to paclitaxel, while other sarcomas do not. Two tumors—Ewing's sarcoma and rhabdomyosarcoma—particularly in children, are responsive to dactinomycin, vincristine, or etoposide. The other tumors are not. The goal of therapy for patients with advanced disease is primarily palliative, although a small fraction (about 20%) of patients who achieve complete remission are, in fact, cured. The first aim, therefore, is to achieve complete remission. Several investigators, including the author, have shown that the prognosis is the same whether complete remission is obtained by chemotherapy alone or by chemotherapy with adjuvant surgery, that is, surgical removal of all residual disease. Short of complete remission, partial remission causes some palliation, with relief of symptoms and prolongation of survival by about 1 year. Any degree of improvement or stabilization of previously advancing disease likewise increases survival.

B.   Effective drugs. The most important chemotherapeutic agent is doxorubicin, which forms the backbone of all combination-chemotherapy regimens. Ifosfamide, an analog of cyclophosphamide that has documented activity even in patients who are refractory to combinations containing cyclophosphamide, is usually included in front-line chemotherapy combinations. It is always given together with the uroprotective agent mesna to prevent hemorrhagic cystitis. Dacarbazine (DTIC), a marginal agent by itself, adds significantly to doxorubicin in prolonging remission duration and survival as well as increasing the response rate. Cyclophosphamide adds marginally, if at all, but is included in some effective regimens.

The key to effective sarcoma chemotherapy is the steep dose–response curve for doxorubicin. At a dose of 45 mg/m^2, the response rate is lower than 20% compared with a 37% response rate at a dose of 75 mg/m^2. A similar dose–response relationship exists for ifosfamide and for combination chemotherapy, and the regimens with the best reported results are those using the highest doses.

C.   Primary chemotherapy regimen (adjuvant or advanced). The most effective primary chemotherapy regimens include doxorubicin and ifosfamide (high-dose AI) or doxorubicin and dacarbazine (ADIC), with or without the addition of cyclophosphamide (CyADIC) or ifosfamide and mesna (MAID). The CyADIC regimen is a modification of the standard CyVADIC regimen, which includes vincristine. Because analysis has shown that vincristine makes no significant contribution and produces neurotoxicity, its addition at a dose of 2 mg maximum or 1.4 mg/m^2 weekly for 6 weeks and then once every 3 to 4 weeks is recommended only for treatment of rhabdomyosarcoma and Ewing's sarcoma.

By giving doxorubicin and dacarbazine by continuous 72- or 96-h infusion, with the two drugs mixed in the same infusion pump, nausea and vomiting are markedly reduced, and the chemotherapy can be continued until a cumulative doxorubicin dose of 800 mg/m^2 is reached, with less cardiac toxicity than with standard doxorubicin administration and a cumulative dose of 450 mg/m^2.

1.   The high-dose AI regimen is as follows:

Doxorubicin by continuous 72-h infusion at 75 mg/m^2 IV (25 mg/m^2/day for 3 days), *and*

Ifosfamide 2.5 g/m^2 IV over 2 to 3 h daily for 4 days.

Mesna 500 mg/m^2 is mixed with the first ifosfamide dose, and 1,500 mg/m^2 is given as a continuous infusion over 24 h for 4 days in 2 L of alkaline fluid.

Filgrastim (granulocyte colony-stimulating factor) 5 µg/kg SC is given on days 5 to 15 or until granulocyte recovery to 1,500/µL.

Repeat cycle every 3 weeks.

2. The continuous-infusion CyADIC regimen is as follows:

Cyclophosphamide 600 mg/m^2 IV on day 1, *and*

Doxorubicin, by continuous 96-h infusion at 60 mg/m^2 IV (15 mg/m^2/day for 4 days), *and*

Dacarbazine by continuous 96-h infusion at 1,000 mg/m^2 IV (250 mg/m^2/day for 4 days) mixed in the same bag or pump as the doxorubicin. Doses should be divided into four consecutive 24-h infusions.

Repeat cycle every 3 to 4 weeks.

3. The continuous-infusion ADIC regimen is as follows:

Doxorubicin by continuous 96-h infusion at 90 mg/m^2 IV (22.5 mg/m^2/day for 4 days), *and*

Dacarbazine by continuous 96-h infusion at 900 mg/m^2 IV (225 mg/m^2/day for 4 days) mixed in the same bag or pump as the doxorubicin. Doses should be divided into four consecutive 24-h infusions.

Repeat cycle every 3 to 4 weeks.

4. The MAID regimen is as follows:

Mesna by continuous 96-h infusion at 8,000 mg/m^2 IV (2,000 mg/m^2/day for 4 days).

Doxorubicin by continuous 72-h infusion at 60 mg/m^2 IV (20 mg/m^2/day for 3 days).

Ifosfamide by continuous 72-h infusion at 6,000 mg/m^2 IV (2,000 mg/m^2/day for 3 days). Doses should be divided into three consecutive 24-h infusions. (Some investigators prefer to infuse ifosfamide over 2 h rather than 24 h because of higher single-agent activity with the shorter infusions.)

Dacarbazine by continuous 72-h infusion at 900 mg/m^2 IV (300 mg/m^2/day for 3 days) mixed in the same bag or pump as the doxorubicin. Doses should be divided into three consecutive 24-h infusions.

Repeat cycle every 3 to 4 weeks.

5. Dose modification. Doses of doxorubicin, cyclophosphamide, ifosfamide, and mesna should be increased by 25% and may be decreased by 20% for each course of therapy to achieve a lowest absolute granulocyte count of about 500/µL if growth factors are not used. *The maximum doxorubicin dose is limited to 600 to 800 mg/m^2*, depending on the duration (48 to 96 h) of infusion, at which point therapy should be discontinued unless cardiac biopsy specimens indicate that it is safe to continue. With Ewing's sarcoma and rhabdomyosarcoma, therapy may be continued, and dactinomycin 2 mg/m^2 in a single dose or 0.5 mg/m^2 daily for 5 days may be substituted for the doxorubicin, with continuation of the regimen for a total of 18 months.

6. An alternative regimen for children with rhabdomyosarcoma is an alternating regimen, using ifosfamide and etoposide alternating with the so-called VAdriaC regimen.

Vincristine 1.5 mg/m^2 is given weekly × 3 for the first two cycles of VAdriaC and then on day 1 only.

Doxorubicin is given at a dose of 60 to 75 mg/m^2 as a 48-h continuous infusion, *and*

Cyclophosphamide 600 mg/m^2 is given daily for 2 days (with mesna).

After 3 weeks,

Ifosfamide is given at a dose of 1,800 mg/m^2 daily for 5 days (with mesna), *and*

Etoposide is given at a dose of 100 mg/m^2 daily for 5 days.

Chemotherapy cycles are alternated every 3 weeks for 39 weeks.

7. A less-intensive, older, but still effective regimen for children with good-prognosis rhabdomyosarcoma is the so-called pulse VAC regimen. Dactinomycin is given at a total dose of 2 to 2.5 mg/m^2 by divided daily injection over 5 to 7 days (e.g., 0.5 mg/m^2 daily for 5 days) repeated every 3 months for a total of five courses. Cyclophosphamide pulses of 275 to 330 mg/m^2 daily for 7 days are begun at the same time but are given every 6 weeks with vincristine 2 mg/m^2 on days 1 and 8 of each cyclophosphamide cycle. Cyclophosphamide cycles are terminated prematurely if the white blood cell counts fall below 1,500/μL. Chemotherapy continues for 2 years. (The necessity of the 2-year duration of the chemotherapy program is not certain.)

D.   Secondary chemotherapy. Secondary chemotherapy for patients with sarcoma is relatively unrewarding, with response rates lower than 10% for almost all conventional drugs or regimens tested. The best commercially available drug is ifosfamide, which, if not used in primary treatment, produces a response in about 20% of patients. High-dose ifosfamide (12 g/m^2 or higher) may produce responses in patients resistant to lower doses in combination. Gemcitabine in our hands has a response rate of 18% and has become our standard drug for salvage therapy. Methotrexate, with a response rate of about 15% regardless of schedule, is the only other active agent. Patients who do not respond to doxorubicin, ifosfamide, or gemcitabine should be entered in a Phase II study of a new agent to see if some activity can be established because other reasonably good alternatives do not exist.

E.   Complications of chemotherapy. Side effects of sarcoma chemotherapy can be classified into three categories: life threatening, potentially dangerous, and unpleasant.

1.   Life-threatening complications of chemotherapy are infection or bleeding. Thrombocytopenia lower than 20,000/μL occurs with this type of chemotherapy when growth factors are used to maintain dose intensity, but bleeding is rare and can be minimized by transfusing platelets at 10,000/μL. About 20% to 40% of patients have documented or suspected infection related to drug-induced neutropenia at some time during their treatment course. These infections are rarely fatal if treated promptly with broad-spectrum, bactericidal antibiotics at the onset of the febrile neutropenia episode.

2.   Potentially dangerous side effects of chemotherapy include the following:

a.   Mucositis, which occurs in fewer than 25% of patients, may interfere with oral intake or may act as a source of infection.

b.   Granulocytopenia predisposes the patient to infection but, because of its brevity, rarely causes infection.

c.   Cardiac damage from doxorubicin rarely causes clinical problems at the doses recommended, with usually reversible congestive heart failure occurring in fewer than 5% of patients.

d.   Renal insufficiency is a rare complication of ifosfamide. Fanconi's syndrome, particularly manifested by a significant loss of bicarbonate, is a dose-related complication of ifosfamide, occurring in 10% to 30% of patients at standard ifosfamide doses and in close to 100% with high-dose regimens.

e.   Central nervous system toxicity of ifosfamide is rarely a serious complication. Patients frequently demonstrate minor confusion, disorientation, or difficulty with fine movements. Somnolence and coma are rarely seen in patients without hypoalbuminemia and/or acidosis.

f.   Hemorrhagic cystitis, a rare complication of cyclophosphamide therapy, used to be the dose-limiting toxicity of ifosfamide. It can be prevented in most cases by administration of another agent, mesna, before and after each ifosfamide dose, allowing higher doses of ifosfamide to be used.

3.   Unpleasant but rarely serious problems include nausea and vomiting (primarily from dacarbazine and ifosfamide) and alopecia (from doxorubicin, cyclophosphamide, and ifosfamide).

F.   Special precautions

1.   Ifosfamide. Patients must be kept well hydrated with an alkaline pH to prevent CNS toxicity and minimize nephrotoxicity. Sodium bicarbonate or sodium acetate should be added to IV fluids at an initial concentration of 100 to 150 mEq/L, and fluid administration should be adjusted to produce a urine output of at least 2 L/day and to maintain the serum bicarbonate concentration at 25 mEq/L or higher.

2.   Doxorubicin. Avoid extravasation. Continuous infusions must (and short infusions should) be administered through a central venous catheter. Attention to cumulative dose administered (varying according to the schedule of administration) is critical to minimize the risk of cardiac toxicity.

SELECTED READINGS

Adjuvant chemotherapy for localised resectable soft-tissue sarcoma of adults: meta-analysis of individual data. *Lancet* 1997;350:1647–1654.

Antman KH, Crowley J, Balcerzak SP, et al. An intergroup phase III randomized study of doxorubicin and dacarbazine with or without ifosfamide and mesna in advanced soft tissue and bone sarcomas. *J Clin Oncol* 1993;11:1276.

Antman KH, Montella D, Rosenbaum C, et al. Phase II trial of ifosfamide with mesna in previously treated metastatic sarcoma. *Cancer Treat Rep* 1985;69:499.

Benjamin RS, Legha SS, Patel RS, et al. Single agent ifosfamide studies in sarcomas of soft tissue and bone: the M.D. Anderson experience. *Cancer Chemother Pharmacol* 1993;31:S174–S179.

Elias A, Ryan L, Sulkes A, et al. Response to mesna, doxorubicin, ifosfamide, and dacarbazine in 108 patients with metastatic or unresectable sarcoma and no prior chemotherapy. *J Clin Oncol* 1989;7:1208.

Fata F, O'Rielly E, Ilson D, et al. Paclitaxel in the treatment of patients with angiosarcoma of the scalp or face. *Cancer* 1999;86:2034–2037.

Frustaci S, Gherlinzoni F, De Paoli A, et al. Adjuvant chemotherapy for adult soft tissue sarcomas of the extremities and girdles: results of the Italian Randomized Cooperative Trial. *J Clin Oncol* 2001;19:1238–1247.

Greene FL, Page DL, Fleming ID, et al. for the American Joint Committee on Cancer. *AJCC cancer staging manual.* 6th ed. New York: Springer, 2002.

Harrison L, Franzese F, Gaynor J, et al. Long-term results of a prospective randomized trial of adjuvant brachytherapy in the management of completely resected soft tissue sarcomas of the extremity and superficial trunk. *Int J Radiat Oncol Biol Phys* 1993; 27:259–265.

Joensuu H, Roberts PJ, Sarlomo-Rikala M, et al. Effect of the tyrosine kinase inhibitor STI571 in a patient with a metastatic gastrointestinal stromal tumor. *N Engl J Med* 2001;344:1052–2056.

Lindberg RD, Martin RG, Romsdahl MM, et al. Conservative surgery and radiation therapy for soft tissue sarcomas. In: Martin RG, Ayala AG, eds. *Management of primary bone and soft tissue tumors.* Chicago: Year Book, 1977:289–298.

Patel SR, Benjamin RS, eds. Sarcomas: part I and II. *Hematol Oncol Clin North Am* 1995;9:513–942.

Patel SR, Gandhi V, Jenkins J, et al. Phase II clinical investigation of gemcitabine in advanced soft tissue sarcomas and window evaluation of dose-rate on gemcitabine triphosphate accumulation. *J Clin Oncol* 2001;19:3483–3489.

Patel SR, Vadhan-Raj S, Burgess MA, et al. Results of two consecutive trials of dose-intensive chemotherapy with doxorubicin and ifosfamide is highly active in patients with soft-tissue sarcomas. *Am J Clin Oncol* 1998;21:317–321.

Patel SR, Vadhan-Raj S, Papadopoulos N, et al. High-dose ifosfamide in bone and soft-tissue sarcomas: results of phase II and pilot studies. Dose response and schedule dependence. *J Clin Oncol* 1997;15:2378–2384.

Pisters P, Leung D, Woodruff J, et al. Analysis of prognostic factors in 1,041 patients with localized soft tissue sarcomas of the extremities. *J Clin Oncol* 1996;14:16799–1689.

Therasse P, Arbuck SG, Eisenhauer EA, et al. New guidelines to evaluate the response to treatment in solid tumors. *JNCI* 2000;92:205–216.

van Oosterom AT, Judson I, Verweij J, et al. Safety and efficacy of imatinib (STI571) in metastatic gastrointestinal stromal tumours: a phase I study. *Lancet* 2001;358:1421–1423.

Wunder J, Healey J, Davis A, et al. A comparison of staging systems for localized extremity soft tissue sarcoma. *Cancer* 2000;88:2721–2730.

Zalupski MM, Ryan J, Hussein M, et al. Defining the role of adjuvant chemotherapy for patients with soft tissue sarcoma of the extremities. In: Salmon SE, ed. *Adjuvant therapy of cancer VII.* Philadelphia: Lippincott, 1993:385–392.

17

Bone Sarcomas

Robert S. Benjamin

There are four major sarcomas of bone, each differing somewhat in clinical behavior, chemotherapy responsiveness, and prognosis. All present as painful bony lesions, and all metastasize preferentially to lung and then to other bones. The prognosis of untreated sarcomas of the bone is inversely proportional to their chemotherapy responsiveness. The sarcomas are considered in order of greatest to least chemotherapeutic responsiveness: Ewing's sarcoma, osteosarcoma, malignant fibrous histiocytoma of bone, and chondrosarcoma.

Response to treatment is evaluated according to the usual criteria used for solid tumors and identical to that reported in Chapter 16 for soft tissue sarcomas. Angiography is particularly helpful in defining the response of primary bone tumors to chemotherapy, and the angiographic response correlates well with pathologic tumor destruction. Complete resection and examination of the total specimen often are required to determine response to therapy in a primary or even a metastatic lesion and to confirm complete remission.

I.   Staging. Bone tumors are staged exclusively according to the criteria of the Musculoskeletal Tumor Society.
   A.   The Roman numeral reflects the **tumor grade.**

Stage I: low grade
Stage II: high grade
Stage III: any-grade tumor with distant metastasis

   B.   The companion letter reflects **tumor compartmentalization.**

Stage A: confined to bone
Stage B: extending into adjacent soft tissue

   C.   Thus, a stage IA tumor is a low-grade tumor confined to bone, and a stage IB tumor is a low-grade tumor extending into soft tissue, and so forth. Patients are evaluated and followed according to the plan in Table 17.1.
II.   Ewing's sarcoma
   A.   General considerations and aims of therapy
      1.   Tumor characteristics. Ewing's sarcoma is a highly malignant, small, round-cell tumor of bone. It occurs most commonly in the second decade of life, and 90% of patients are younger than 30 years. There is a slight male predominance. The most common locations are the pelvis or the diaphysis of long tubular bones of the extremities. Often, systemic symptoms of fever and leukocytosis suggest infection. Radiographically, the predominant feature is osteolysis, although sclerosis does occur. Frequently, the periosteal reaction has the so-called onion skin pattern with layering of subperiosteal new bone, frequently with spicules radiating out from the cortex. Prognosis,

Table 17.1. Primary bone sarcoma evaluation

Tests[a]	Before therapy	On initial treatment	Preoperative	On subsequent treatment	Follow-up
History and physical examination	X	Before each treatment	X	Before each treatment	Yr 1: q2 mo; yr 2, 3: q3–4 mo; yr 4: q4 mo; yr 5: q6 mo; then yearly
CBC, differential, and platelet counts[b]	X	Twice weekly	X	Twice weekly	Yearly
Chemistry profile[b]	X	Before each treatment	X	Before each treatment	Yr 1: q4–6 mo; then yearly
Calculated creatinine clearance	X	For methotrexate	—	For methotrexate	—
Electrolytes, Mg[b]	X	Before each treatment	X	Before each treatment	—
Urinalysis	If ifosfamide is given	As indicated by symptoms	X	Before each treatment	—
PT, APTT, fibrinogen	X	Before each intra-arterial (IA) treatment and q.d. while on IA treatment	X	—	—

continued

Table 17.1.   *Continued*

Tests[a]	Before therapy	On initial treatment	Preoperative	On subsequent treatment	Follow-up
Plain films of primary tumor	X	q2 cycles	X	q3 mo	Yr 1: q4–6 mo; then yearly
CT of primary tumor	X	After two to four cycles	X	—	At end of treatment for head and neck or pelvic primaries
MRI of primary tumor	—	For surgical planning only	—	—	—
Bone scan	X				
Sestamibi scan[c]	X	After two to four cycles	If needed to assess response	—	—
Chest radiograph	X	Before each treatment	X	Before each treatment	Yr 1: q2 mo; yr 2, 3: q3–4 mo; yr 4: q4 mo; yr 5: q6 mo; then yearly
Chest CT	If chest radiograph appears normal	If chest radiograph is equivocal or for surgical planning	—	If chest radiograph is equivocal or for surgical planning	If chest radiograph is equivocal or for surgical planning

	Before each preoperative treatment				
Angiogram	—	—	—	—	—
Bone marrow	Only for small cell tumors with metastases	—	—	—	—
ECG	If cardiac history	—	If cardiac history	—	—
Cardiac scan	If cardiac history	—	If doxorubicin dose exceeds standard limits for schedule	—	—
Central venous catheter	X	—	—	—	—
Bone tumor conference	X	—	—	—	If further multidisciplinary decisions are required

CBC, complete blood cell count; PT, prothrombin time; APTT, activated partial thromboplastin time; CT, computed tomography; MRI, magnetic resonance imaging; ECG, electrocardiogram.

[a]Tests may be ordered more frequently based on clinical indications.

[b]Required more frequently if patient is on a medical treatment program.

[c]Name of the thallium–technetium isotope used for scanning. Tradename is Cardiolyte. Procedure is suggested but optional.

until the era of modern chemotherapy, was extremely poor, with a 5-year survival rate lower than 10% and almost half of patients dying within 1 year of diagnosis. Because Ewing's sarcoma is a high-grade tumor and, by definition, is almost always accompanied by a soft tissue mass, it usually is staged as IIB or IIIB depending on the demonstration of metastatic disease in lung, bone, or both.

2.   Primary treatment. Because of the poor prognosis and because of the mutilative surgery involved in resection of the primary lesion, radiotherapy has been the primary modality for local tumor control. As techniques for limb salvage surgery have become more widely practiced, attempts to use surgery rather than radiation therapy are again increasing. There are indications that the use of surgery not only increases the rate of local control but also may improve overall prognosis. While this may, in fact, be the case, the conclusions need to be tempered by the fact that patients with the worst prognosis are not offered surgical resection.

B.   Chemotherapy

1.   CyVADIC regimen. A good chemotherapeutic regimen for Ewing's sarcoma, particularly in adult patients, is the continuous-infusion CyVADIC regimen, which is mentioned in Chapter 16 (see Section II.C).

Cyclophosphamide 600 mg/m^2 IV on day 1.

Vincristine, 1.4 mg/m^2 (2 mg maximum) IV weekly for 6 weeks, then on day 1 of each cycle.

Doxorubicin (Adriamycin) 60 mg/m^2 IV by 96-h continuous infusion through a central venous catheter (15 mg/m^2/day for 4 days).

Dacarbazine (DTIC) 1,000 mg/m^2 IV by 96-h continuous infusion (250 mg/m^2/day for 4 days) mixed in the same bag or pump as the doxorubicin. Doses should be divided into four consecutive 24-h infusions.

Repeat cycle every 3 to 4 weeks.

2.   Dose modifications. Courses are repeated with a 25% increase or decrease in the doses of cyclophosphamide and doxorubicin, depending on morbidity. Courses are repeated in 3 to 4 weeks as soon as recovery to 1,500 granulocytes/µL and 100,000 platelets/µL occurs. Complications are as described in Chapter 16 (see Section II.E), with the addition of peripheral neuropathy from vincristine. When the cumulative dose of doxorubicin has reached 800 mg/m^2, therapy is discontinued.

3.   Alternative regimens. Alternative regimens omit dacarbazine; vary doses of cyclophosphamide up to 4,200 mg/m^2; give dactinomycin with, or in place of, doxorubicin; and in some patients, add other drugs. The most common pediatric regimen at present alternates two regimens every 3 weeks: ifosfamide plus etoposide; and vincristine, doxorubicin plus cyclophosphamide, with dactinomycin substituted for doxorubicin after a cumulative (bolus) dose of 375 mg/m^2 (VAdCA). In a recent intergroup study, this regimen was superior to VAdCA alone. The schedule of drug administration is as follows:

a. Initial combination

Ifosfamide 1,800 mg/m^2 IV daily $\times$ 5 (with mesna), *and*
Etoposide 100 mg/m^2 IV daily $\times$ 5.

b. Three weeks later, start

Vincristine 1.5 mg/m^2 IV on day 1, *and*
Doxorubicin 75 mg/m^2 IV on day 1, *and*
Cyclophosphamide 1,200 mg/m^2 IV on day 1.

c. Three weeks later, return to the first regimen, and so forth. At a cumulative doxorubicin dose of 375 mg/m^2, substitute dactinomycin 1.25 mg/m^2. Chemotherapy continues for a total of 1 year.

d. Another version of the alternating regimen starts with an intensive VAC regimen with the doxorubicin and vincristine given by 72-h continuous infusion and the cyclophosphamide dose increased to 4,200 mg/m^2 divided into two equal doses on days 1 and 2.

4. Responses. Most patients with metastatic disease obtain complete remission; however, almost all patients, especially those with bone metastases, experience relapse and ultimately die of disease. When chemotherapy is used in the therapy of primary disease with surgery or radiation therapy, prognosis depends on the size and location of the primary tumor. Patients with large flat-bone lesions have a lower than 30% cure rate compared with a 60% to 70% cure rate for those patients with long-bone lesions, which are generally smaller. An alarming complication of the chemotherapy and radiation therapy combination is a high frequency of second malignancies in cured patients, with 4 of 10 patients in one series developing secondary sarcomas within the radiated fields. This complication is another reason for considering surgical intervention rather than radiation because chemotherapy is required for cure whether or not the primary lesion can be controlled with radiation.

5. Secondary chemotherapy. Occasional responses have been seen with etoposide (VP-16), other alkylating agents (especially ifosfamide), the nitrosoureas, and cisplatin. A combination of etoposide and ifosfamide is now frequently used in patients for whom those drugs were not used in initial therapy. High-dose ifosfamide (14 g/m^2 divided over 3 to 7 days, either as a 2-h infusion with each dose or as a continuous infusion) with mesna or high-dose doxorubicin (90 mg/m^2) plus dacarbazine (900 mg/m^2) as a 96-h continuous infusion is occasionally effective in producing brief remissions in patients for whom these agents were not used or were used at substantially lower doses during initial therapy. Nonetheless, secondary responses are extremely poor, and the survival of a relapsed patient with Ewing's sarcoma is measured in weeks.

6. High-dose chemotherapy. The standard chemotherapy used for Ewing's sarcoma is accompanied by severe but transient myelosuppression. The availability of hematopoietic growth factors to reduce infectious complications provides an added measure of safety but is not routinely required. Our policy has been to use growth factors only in patients who have had febrile–neutropenic episodes during a previous course of chemotherapy rather than to reduce the doses of the myelosuppressive drugs.

Bone marrow transplantation or peripheral stem cell rescue programs are still being investigated in patients presenting with poor prognostic features (large pelvic primary tumors, metastatic disease) but have not yet been demonstrated to improve prognosis. Such regimens have been tried with negative results in patients relapsing after standard chemotherapy and have been demonstrated to have no significant benefit. Clearly, this approach should not be used in patients with relapse.

III. Osteosarcoma

A.   General considerations. Osteosarcoma is a tumor with a poor prognosis in the absence of effective chemotherapy. It is the most common primary bone sarcoma. Frequently, it affects patients 10 to 25 years old and tends to be located around the knee in about two-thirds of patients, with two-thirds of those tumors involving the distal aspect of the femur. As with other sarcomas of bone, pulmonary metastases are most common, followed by bone metastases. Because conventional osteosarcoma is a high-grade tumor by definition and is accompanied by a soft tissue mass in 90% or more of patients, it is usually staged as IIB or IIIB, depending on the demonstration of metastatic disease in lung or bone.

B.   Role of chemotherapy. Chemotherapy is usually employed in the neoadjuvant or adjuvant situation, and its value preoperatively has been conclusively demonstrated. Patients who show a complete response to preoperative chemotherapy with tumor destruction of at least 90% have significantly improved survival. Response rates in evaluable tumors range from 30% to 80%. Cure of primary disease with adjuvant chemotherapy is 50% to 80%.

C.   Effective agents. The four major standard single agents in the treatment of osteosarcoma are cisplatin, doxorubicin, ifosfamide, and high-dose methotrexate. In addition, the combination of bleomycin, cyclophosphamide, and dactinomycin (BCD) has been effective.

D.   Recommended regimen. A variety of regimens may be recommended based on preliminary or more extensive evaluation.

1.   Doxorubicin and cisplatin

Doxorubicin 90 mg/m^2 IV by 96-h continuous infusion through a central venous catheter, *and*
Cisplatin 120 mg/m^2 intra-arterially (for primary tumor) or IV on day 6.
Repeat every 4 weeks.

Three to four courses of therapy should be administered preoperatively. Postoperative therapy depends on the response of the primary tumor. Patients with tumor necrosis of 90% or more should continue on the same regimen for three to six postoperative courses or until a cumulative doxorubicin dose of 800 mg/m^2 is reached. If cisplatin must be discontinued earlier, decrease the doxorubicin dose to 75 mg/m^2 IV by 72-h continuous infusion and substitute ifosfamide 2,500 mg/m^2 IV over

3 h daily for 4 days (the dose-intensive AI regimen for soft tissue sarcoma; see Chapter 16, Section II.C.1).

2.   After primary chemotherapy, if there is less than 90% tumor necrosis at surgery, **switch to the alternative regimen** as follows:

a.   High-dose methotrexate 12 g/m^2 IV every 2 weeks for 8 weeks with leucovorin rescue (see Section III.E.2).

b.   Three weeks later, administer ifosfamide 2 g/m^2 IV over 2 h for 5 consecutive days, with mesna 1,200 mg/m^2 IV in three divided doses each day (i.e., 400 mg/m^2 IV every 4 h × 3) or by continuous infusion after a loading dose of 400 mg/m^2 mixed with the first ifosfamide dose. Three weeks later, repeat the course.

c.   Three weeks later, administer a 96-h continuous infusion of doxorubicin 75 mg/m^2 plus dacarbazine 750 mg/m^2 (ADIC). Three to 4 weeks later, repeat the course.

d.   Three to 4 weeks later, repeat the entire cycle of four courses of methotrexate, two courses of ifosfamide, and two courses of ADIC. End with four more courses of high-dose methotrexate.

3.   There are many alternative approaches to chemotherapy, adding high-dose methotrexate and/or ifosfamide to the induction regimen and continuing with the same three to four drugs postoperatively. The combination of bleomycin, cyclophosphamide, and dactinomycin (BCD) is rarely, if ever, used anymore.

E.   Special precautions in administration

1.   Cisplatin. Prehydration is necessary, with overnight infusion of IV fluids at 150 mL/h or 1 L of fluid over 2 h (for adults), followed by at least 6 L of fluid containing potassium chloride (KCl; at least 20 mEq/L) and magnesium sulfate (MgSO$_4$; at least 4 mEq/L) for the first 1 or 2 days or after cisplatin administration. The addition of mannitol (66 mL of a 15% solution) before cisplatin, followed by 266 mL of a 15% solution mixed with normal saline in a total volume of 1 L to run simultaneously with the cisplatin over 2 to 3 h, is preferred by many investigators. Particular care in electrolyte balance, including frequent determinations of magnesium levels, is necessary. In the presence of severe hypomagnesemia, magnesium sulfate up to 1 to 2 mEq/kg may be infused over 4 h.

2.   High-dose methotrexate. The pretreatment-calculated creatinine clearance rate should be at least 70 mL/min.

a.   Methotrexate administration and alkalization of urine. Before administration of high-dose methotrexate, 0.5 mEq/kg of sodium bicarbonate is infused IV over 15 to 30 min in an attempt to create an alkaline urine. Allopurinol 300 mg/day for 3 days is given starting 1 day before the methotrexate infusion. Methotrexate is dissolved in no more than 1,000 mL of 5% dextrose in water, with a final concentration of about 1 g/100 mL. The total dose ranges from 8 g/m^2 for patients over 40 years old to 12 g/m^2 for children and young adults. The dose should be increased on subsequent courses if an immediate postinfusion methotrexate level is less than 10^{-3} M. Sodium bicarbonate 50 mEq is added per liter of methotrexate solution, which is infused over 4 h. After completion of the methotrexate infusion, 10 mL/kg of an IV infusion of 5% dextrose in water with 50 mEq/L of bicarbonate is given over 2 h if the patient is unable to drink or if the 24-h methotrexate levels of the previous high-dose methotrexate treatment have been higher than 1.5×10^{-5} M. The IV infusion is then discontinued, and the patient is encouraged to drink sufficient fluid to produce about 1,600 mL/m² of alkaline urine for the first 24 h and 1,900 mL/m² daily for the next 3 days. Sodium bicarbonate 14 to 28 mEq PO every 6 h is administered to ensure alkaline urine. The pH of the urine is measured, and if it is less than 7, an extra dose of bicarbonate is administered.

b.   Leucovorin rescue. Twenty-four hours after the start of the methotrexate infusion, leucovorin 15 to 25 mg is administered PO every 6 h for at least 10 doses or IM if the oral medication is not tolerated.

c.   Serum methotrexate levels. These levels should be followed and should fall about 1 log/day. When methotrexate concentration falls below 10^{-7} M, leucovorin may be safely discontinued. IV hydration is required whenever oral intake is inadequate to produce sufficient urine output as previously defined, for abnormal serum methotrexate concentration, for persistent vomiting, or for early toxicity.

3.   Ifosfamide. Patients must be kept well hydrated with an alkaline pH to prevent central nervous system (CNS) toxicity and minimize nephrotoxicity. Sodium bicarbonate or sodium acetate should be added to IV fluids at an initial concentration of 100 to 150 mEq/L and fluid administration adjusted to produce a urine output of at least 2 L/day and maintain the serum bicarbonate concentration at 25 mEq/L or higher.

F.   Complications. Complications of chemotherapy depend on the drugs. For doxorubicin, the major complication is infection owing to neutropenia. Other complications include stomatitis, nausea and vomiting, and delayed cardiac toxicity, as discussed in the management of soft tissue sarcomas (see Chapter 16, Section II.E). Ifosfamide produces myelosuppression, nausea and vomiting, and alopecia, similar to doxorubicin. Hemorrhagic cystitis, once the dose-limiting toxicity, is rarely seen because the use of mesna has become routine. The most serious toxicities of ifosfamide are nephrotoxicity and CNS toxicity. Nephrotoxicity in the form of Fanconi's syndrome is a frequent problem, the morbidity of which can be minimized by the routine use of alkaline infusions and correction of electrolyte levels with oral replacement therapy. Only rarely does the nephrotoxicity progress to renal failure. Correction of acid–base balance and hypoalbuminemia can essentially prevent the CNS toxicity (see Chapter 16, Section II.E). Dactinomycin causes similar side effects to those of doxorubicin, but not cardiac toxicity. Methotrexate predominantly causes stomatitis, but it may cause myelosuppression and renal, hepatic, and CNS abnormalities. Cisplatin and dacarbazine cause severe nausea and vomiting. In addition, cisplatin nephrotoxicity is primarily a tubular defect, with hypomagnesemia as the most prominent manifestation, but hypocalcemia, hypokalemia, and hyponatremia also occur. Delayed cumulative nephrotoxicity can cause impaired glomerular function as well.

Ototoxicity may occur but is less common. Delayed neurotoxicity also occurs. Both cisplatin and methotrexate can, by causing renal toxicity, exacerbate their other side effects.

G. Recurrence and treatment of refractory disease. Patients with osteosarcoma who are refractory to a combination of doxorubicin and cisplatin may respond to high-dose methotrexate; patients refractory to high-dose methotrexate may respond to doxorubicin plus cisplatin; and patients refractory to both may respond to ifosfamide or, rarely, to BCD. However, treatment of refractory disease is usually disappointing, and participation in studies of new agents is indicated for patients whose disease cannot be resected. Surgical resection of pulmonary metastases remains the only viable secondary therapy for most patients. For this reason, careful follow-up for detection of metastases while they are still at the stage of resectability is indicated.

H. High-dose chemotherapy. The standard chemotherapy used for osteosarcoma is accompanied by severe but transient myelosuppression. The availability of hematopoietic growth factors to reduce infectious complications provides an added measure of safety but is not routinely required. Our policy has been to use growth factors only in patients who have had febrile–neutropenic episodes during a previous course of chemotherapy rather than to reduce the doses of the myelosuppressive drugs.

Bone marrow transplantation or peripheral stem cell rescue programs are being investigated in patients presenting with poor prognostic features (e.g., poor-prognosis histologic subtypes, pelvic primary tumors, metastatic disease) but are not yet demonstrated to improve prognosis.

IV. Malignant fibrous histiocytoma of bone. This entity, characterized by a purely lytic lesion in bone, has an exceptionally poor prognosis when treated with surgery alone, although the number of reported patients is small. It may be extremely difficult to distinguish from fibroblastic osteosarcoma and may be best considered as a fibroblastic osteosarcoma with minimal (i.e., no detectable) osteoid production. The tumor responds well to the CyADIC regimen for soft tissue sarcomas, with more than half of patients obtaining at least partial remission. In addition, cisplatin at a dose of 120 mg/m^2 every 4 weeks has caused remissions, even in patients who did not respond to primary therapy. A particularly attractive approach for patients with large, unresectable primary tumors is the administration of cisplatin by the intra-arterial route. Complete tumor destruction in one patient and a good partial remission in a second patient are the reported results among three patients so treated. Systemic doxorubicin may be added, as for osteosarcomas (see Section III.D.1). Alternatively, responses have been seen after high-dose methotrexate-based regimens for osteosarcomas (see Section III.D.2). After local tumor destruction, surgery may be employed to remove residual disease. Because of the poor prognosis, adjuvant chemotherapy with the continuous-infusion CyADIC regimen is recommended until an 800-mg/m^2 cumulative doxorubicin dose has been reached.

V. Chondrosarcoma. The chemotherapy for chondrosarcoma is totally inadequate, and no regimen can be recommended except for the rare patients with mesenchymal chondrosarcoma, a subtype that may respond to CyADIC chemotherapy or cisplatin, or with dedifferentiated chondrosarcoma, which should be treated the same way as osteosarcoma. Most patients have conventional chondrosarcoma and are candidates only for surgical management. Metastatic disease should be treated with Phase II protocols in an attempt to determine some effective type of chemotherapy that may be recommended in the future.

SELECTED READINGS

Bacci G, Briccoli A, Ferrari S, et al. Neoadjuvant chemotherapy for osteosarcoma of the extremity: long-term results of the Rizzoli's 4th protocol. *Eur J Cancer* 2001;37:2030–2039.

Bacci G, Ferrari S, Bertoni F, et al. Prognostic factors in nonmetastatic Ewing's sarcoma of bone treated with adjuvant chemotherapy: analysis of 359 patients at the Istituto Ortopedico Rizzoli. *J Clin Oncol* 2000a;18:4–11.

Bacci G, Ferrari S, Bertoni F, et al. Neoadjuvant chemotherapy for peripheral malignant neuroectodermal tumor of bone: recent experience at the Istituto Rizzoli. *J Clin Oncol* 2000b;18:885–892.

Bacci G, Ferrari S, Longhi A, et al. Neoadjuvant chemotherapy for high grade osteosarcoma of the extremities: long-term results for patients treated according to the Rizzoli IOR/OS-3b protocol. *J Chemother* 2001;13:93–99.

Benjamin RS, Murray JA, Carrasco CH, et al. Preoperative chemotherapy for osteosarcoma: a treatment approach facilitating limb salvage with major prognostic implications. In: Jones SE, Salmon SE, eds. *Adjuvant therapy of cancer, vol IV*. New York: Grune & Stratton, 1984:601–610.

Chawla SP, Benjamin RS, Abdul-Karim FW, et al. Adjuvant chemotherapy of primary malignant fibrous histiocytoma of bone: prolongation of disease free and overall survival. In: Jones SE, Salmon SE, eds. *Adjuvant therapy of cancer, vol IV*. New York: Grune & Stratton, 1984:621–629.

Gehan EA, Sutow WW, Uribe-Botero G, et al. Osteosarcoma: the M. D. Anderson experience, 1950–1974. In: Terry WD, Windhorst D, eds. *Immunotherapy of cancer: present status of trials in man*. New York: Raven Press, 1978.

Grier H, Krailo M, Link M, et al. Improved outcome in non-metastatic Ewing's sarcoma (EWS) and PNET of bone with the addition of ifosfamide (D) and etoposide (E) to vincristine (W), Adriamycin (Ad), cyclophosphamide (C), and actinomycin (A): a Children's Cancer Group (CCG) and Pediatric Oncology Group (POG) report. *Proc Am Soc Clin Oncol* 1994;13:A1443.

Kushner BH, Meyers PA, Gerald WL, et al. Very-high-dose short-term chemotherapy for poor-risk peripheral primitive neuroectodermal tumors, including Ewing's sarcoma in children and young adults. *J Clin Oncol* 1995;13:2796–2804.

Rosen G, et al. The successful management of metastatic osteogenic sarcoma: a model for the treatment of primary osteogenic sarcoma. In: van Oosterom AT, Muggia FM, Cleton FJ, eds. *Therapeutic progress in ovarian cancer, testicular cancer and the sarcomas*. Hingham: Leiden University Press, 1990:244–265.

18

Acute Leukemias

Andrew M. Evens and Martin S. Tallman

The acute leukemias are a heterogeneous group of disorders characterized by neoplastic transformation and abnormal differentiation of hematopoietic progenitor cells. These immature cells proliferate and accumulate primarily in the bone marrow and peripheral blood, ultimately resulting in inhibition of normal hematopoiesis. These diseases are rapidly fatal if untreated. Prior to the 1960s, the treatment of acute leukemia was primarily palliative, but over the last 40 years, great therapeutic advances have been made and many patients can now be cured of their disease. The general treatment approach for most patients with acute leukemia includes eradication of the leukemic clone with intensive systemic chemotherapy. Despite this strategy, many patients under ages 55 to 60 and the majority of older adults die from their disease. Many questions still need to be answered with regard to the optimum treatment for these diseases. Therefore, all patients with acute leukemia should be considered candidates for well-designed, early-phase and/or prospective, randomized clinical trials and should be treated in centers where appropriate comprehensive, intensive care can be provided.

   I.   Diagnosis and classification. Acute leukemia is a clonal disorder that arises in an early hematopoietic stem cell, which proliferates and accumulates, leading to a hypofunctional bone marrow. This results in varying degrees of neutropenia, anemia, and thrombocytopenia with corresponding clinical consequences such as infection, fatigue, dyspnea, and bleeding. The acute leukemias are divided into acute myeloid leukemia (AML) and acute lymphoblastic leukemia (ALL) forms based on the stem cell of origin. Although the peripheral blood smear may be highly suggestive of acute leukemia, examination of the bone marrow aspirate and biopsy is essential. Classification into AML and ALL categories is usually based on the morphologic, immunohistochemical, and immunophenotypic characteristics of the blast cells. Chromosome analysis and genetic study techniques may also aid in establishing an accurate diagnosis and have proven important in determining prognosis. The principles used to diagnose and classify acute leukemia are briefly presented below.
   A.   Acute myeloid leukemia. The French–American–British (FAB) classification was initially described in 1976 and was based solely on morphologic and cytochemical features of the leukemic cell clone. Despite important advances in cytogenetics and immunophenotyping, the FAB classification remains the foundation on which the diagnosis of AML is established. Normally, myeloblasts and promyelocytes constitute fewer than 5% of the nucleated cells in the marrow. The category of refractory anemia with excess blasts in transformation, previously classified within the myelodysplastic syndromes, has been eliminated according to the updated World Health Organization

(WHO) classification, and the lower limit of bone marrow blasts sufficient to establish a diagnosis of AML is now 20%. The diagnosis of AML is established by demonstrating that leukemic cells (myeloblasts, promyelocytes, monoblasts, promonocytes, megakaryoblasts) constitute now more than 20% of the nucleated marrow cells (or more than 20% of the nonerythroid nucleated cells in the case of erythroleukemia). Classically, histochemical stains have been used to demonstrate that cells are of nonlymphoid origin. Common histochemical stains that are positive in nonlymphoid cells are Sudan black B and peroxidase (myeloblasts, promyelocytes), nonspecific esterases that are inhibited by sodium fluoride (monoblasts), and the periodic acid–Schiff stain (pronormoblasts in erythroleukemia). Antigens commonly demonstrated by flow cytometry techniques include CD13 and CD33 on myeloblasts and monoblasts, CD14 on monoblasts, and von Willebrand factor, GPIIb (CD41), and GPIIIa (CD61) on megakaryoblasts. Electron microscopy is useful for demonstrating the presence of myeloperoxidase and platelet peroxidase in the FAB M0 and M7 variants, respectively. Recent advances in our understanding of the pathogenesis of AML as well as insights into karyotype abnormalities and molecular genetics have led to a new classification generated by the WHO that correlates morphology, cytochemistry, immunophenotype, molecular genetics, and clinical features. A simplified version of the WHO classification of AMLs is as follows:

AMLs with recurrent cytogenetic translocations
    AML with t(8;21)
    Acute promyelocytic leukemia (APL; AML with t[15;17] *PML/RAR*-α)
    AML with abnormal bone marrow eosinophils (inv[16] or t[16;16])
    AML with 11q23 (MLL) abnormalities
AML with multilineage dysplasia
    With prior myelodysplastic syndrome (MDS)
    Without prior MDS
AML and MDSs, therapy related
    Alkylating agent related
    Epipodophyllotoxin related
    Other types
AML not otherwise categorized (correlated with FAB subtype)
    AML minimally differentiated (FAB M0)
    AML without maturation (FAB M1)
    AML with maturation (FAB M2)
    Acute myelomonocytic leukemia (FAB M4)
    Acute monocytic leukemia (FAB M5)
    Acute erythroid leukemia (FAB M6)
    Acute megakaryocytic leukemia (AmegL; FAB M7)
    Acute basophilic leukemia
    Acute panmyelosis with myelofibrosis
Acute biphenotypic leukemias

Cytogenetics at presentation has emerged as the most important prognostic factor for patients with AML. Three prognostic groups have been defined by cytogenetic abnormalities detected at presentation that are based on response to induction therapy, risk of relapse, and overall survival (OS) (Table 18.1).

B. Acute lymphoblastic leukemia. Whereas mature lymphocytes may account for up to 25% of the nucleated cells in the adult bone marrow, recognizable lymphoblasts are not a component of normal marrow. Diagnosis and classification of ALL are based on characteristic cell morphology, immunohistochemistry, and immunophenotypic and cytogenetic features. In general, the diagnosis of ALL is established by demonstrating that leukemic lymphoblasts constitute more than 25% of the nucleated marrow cells. Because of its lack of reproducibility, the morphologic subclassification of ALL by the FAB system has been abandoned. In general, ALL is subclassified according to B-cell or T-cell lineage based on antigen expression immunophenotype. Approximately 70% to 75% of adult ALL cases are of precursor B-cell origin, 20% to 25% are of T-cell origin, and 5% are mature B cell (or Burkitt-type leukemia, FAB L3). Immunologic markers classically suggesting B-cell lineage are the common ALL antigen (CALLA, CD10; common or pre-pre–B-cell ALL), intracytoplasmic heavy chains (pre–B-cell ALL), and surface membrane immunoglobulin (Ig; B-cell ALL). Ia, CD19, and CD22 are common generic markers for cells of B lineage, whereas CD20 is seen in more mature B-lineage cells. T-Cell ALL arises from stage I (prothymocyte) and stage II thymocytes. Immunologic markers classically suggesting T-cell lineage are CD2 (sheep red blood cell [RBC] receptor), CD3, CD7, CD38 (panthymocyte), and CD71 (transferrin receptor). The enzyme terminal deoxynucleotidyl transferase (TdT) can

Table 18.1.   AML prognostic groups based on cytogenetics at presentation[a]

SWOG/ECOG cytogenetic classification

Favorable
  t(15;17)—with any other abnormality
  inv(16) or t(16;16)[b] or del(16q)—with any other abnormality
  t(8;21)[b]—without del(9q) or complex karyotype
Intermediate
  +8, −Y, +6, del(12p) or normal karyotype
Unfavorable
  −5 or del(5q), −7 or del(7q), inv(3q), abnormalities of 11q23, 20q, 21q, del(9q), t(6;9), t(8;21) with del(9q) or with complex karyotype, t(9;22), abnormalities of 17p, complex karyotypes (3 or more abnormalities)
Unknown
  All other clonal chromosomal aberrations with less than 3 abnormalities

[a] Determined by conventional cytogenetic techniques, fluorescent *in situ* hybridization, or polymerase chain reaction.
[b] Karyotypes in these two groups are part of "core-binding factor-type" acute leukemia.

be demonstrated in cells of early B-cell (before pre–B-cell) and T-cell (through thymocyte) lineage. If prominent lymphadenopathy is noted at presentation, the diagnosis of high-grade lymphoma such as Burkitt's (or Burkitt's-like) and lymphoblastic lymphoma should be considered. The differentiation between high-grade lymphoma and ALL is based on the amount of bone marrow involvement, with a diagnosis of ALL favored if malignant lymphoid cells constitute more than 25% of the bone marrow. The WHO has also integrated genetic abnormalities into the classification of ALL, secondary to their prognostic importance. A simplified version of the WHO classification of ALL is as follows:

Precursor B-cell acute lymphoblastic leukemia

Cytogenetic subgroups	Prognosis
t(9;22) (*BCR/ABL*)	Unfavorable
t(4;11)	Unfavorable
t(1;19)	Unfavorable
t(12;21)	Favorable

Precursor T-cell acute lymphoblastic leukemia
Burkitt's cell leukemia

C.   Acute mixed-lineage and stem cell leukemias. With the expansion of immunophenotyping panels and the increased use of electron microscopy and gene rearrangement studies for the characterization of acute leukemia, increasing degrees of infidelity of myeloid and lymphoid markers can be demonstrated. Minimal deviation from the expected markers is not uncommon and may produce well-defined syndromes that do not alter the basic cellular lineage (e.g., CD13/CD33 ALL, CD7 AML, TdT AML). There are no consensus guidelines for the diagnosis of true acute mixed-lineage leukemia, which is probably a rare disorder. In stem cell leukemia, the cells express only rudimentary hematopoietic markers (e.g., Ia antigen, TdT, CD34). The identification of entities such as CD13/CD33 ALL and stem cell leukemia may be of prognostic importance and have therapeutic implications.

II.   Initial support. Once the diagnosis of acute leukemia has been established, the next 24 to 48 h are spent preparing the patient for the initiation of cytotoxic chemotherapy. The following issues need to be addressed in almost all individuals facing induction chemotherapy.

A.   Hydration and correction of electrolyte imbalance. Dehydration needs to be corrected and adequate urine output maintained to prevent renal failure due to the deposition of cellular breakdown products resulting from the tumor lysis syndrome. In the absence of cardiac disease, normal saline with or without 5% dextrose is infused to maintain the urine output at more than 100 mL/h. The concomitant use of loop diuretics may be necessary in patients with congestive heart failure. Although a variety of electrolyte problems may occur in patients with acute leukemia, hypokalemia is the most troublesome, particularly in patients with AML. Serum potassium levels should be monitored closely because a normal serum potassium level often does not reflect the diminished potassium stores of most patients.

B.   Prevention of uric acid nephropathy. Hyperuricemia is common at presentation and may also occur with the tumor lysis caused by chemotherapy. Allopurinol is the mainstay of prevention of uric acid nephropathy. The usual initial adult dose is 300 mg (150 mg/m^2) b.i.d. for 2 to 3 days, which is then decreased to 300 mg once a day. Allopurinol should be stopped after 10 to 14 days to lessen the risk of rash and hepatic dysfunction. If chemotherapy needs to be initiated urgently, allopurinol at a dose of 600 mg b.i.d. is well tolerated for 1 to 2 days. With the advent of allopurinol, the role of urine alkalinization has become less clear. Although urine alkalinization increases uric acid solubility, it decreases the solubility of urinary phosphates and may promote phosphate deposition in patients susceptible to the tumor lysis syndrome (e.g., B-cell ALL and T-cell lymphoblastic leukemia). A commonly employed method of urine alkalinization is to hydrate the patient with D5W to which two syringes of sodium bicarbonate (44 mEq of NaHCO$_3$ per syringe) have been added per liter.

C. Coagulopathy. Coagulation abnormalities are not uncommon in patients with newly diagnosed acute leukemia. In addition to thrombocytopenia, patients may also present with consumption coagulopathy (disseminated intravascular coagulation [DIC]). This is particularly common in patients with APL in which there is evidence of both consumptive coagulopathy as well as primary fibrinolysis that may be associated with life-threatening bleeding. Consumption coagulopathy is also more common in patients with leukemia cells that show monocytic differentiation, such as patients with M4 or M5 morphology. Frequent monitoring of coagulation tests is important with replacement products such as cryoprecipitate or fresh frozen plasma in appropriate patients. Sepsis may also contribute to coagulopathy in newly diagnosed patients.

D. Blood product support. Most patients with acute leukemia present with bone marrow failure, so symptomatic anemia and thrombocytopenia must be corrected (see Chapter 28). It is recommended that human leukocyte antigen (HLA) typing be obtained before initiating therapy, because patients who are severely myelosuppressed during chemotherapy do not have enough lymphocytes for HLA typing. However, occasionally an inadequate number of circulating lymphocytes and the presence of blast cells preclude the ability to carry out HLA typing prior to initial therapy. HLA-matched platelet transfusions may need to be administered to patients who develop alloimmunization and become refractory to pooled or single-donor platelets.

E. Fever or infection. Patients frequently have a fever or an infection at initial diagnosis. The approach to fever and infection is discussed in Chapter 27. The cardinal rule is that all patients with acute leukemia and fever are presumed to have an infection until proved otherwise. Given the additional myelosuppressive and immunosuppressive effects of chemotherapy, severe infections should be treated aggressively before initiating chemotherapy. However, the antibiotic treatment frequently needs to be administered concurrently with induction chemotherapy. Patients with acute leukemia need a careful physical examination daily. There should be close attention toward potential sites of infection, including the fundi, sinuses, oral cavity, intertriginous areas, perineum (attempts are made to avoid internal rectal examination during neutropenia), and catheter sites. A dental consultation at the time of diagnosis is often useful.

F.   Vascular access. Because of the need for several sites of venous access for at least 1 month, a multiple-lumen implantable catheter (e.g., Hickman catheter or peripherally inserted central catheter [PICC] line) must be placed as soon as possible. An implantable port is not recommended for leukemic patients because there is higher risk of infection and hematoma at the access site. Because of the coagulopathy in patients with APL, the placement of a long indwelling catheter is avoided until the coagulopathy has been corrected. A risk of life-threatening bleeding is present even if most or all of the routine coagulation studies are normal.

G.   Suppression of menses. A serum human chorionic gonadotropin (β-hCG) assay (pregnancy test) should be done in all premenopausal women before initiating chemotherapy. Because menorrhagia may occur owing to the severe thrombocytopenia that is seen during induction chemotherapy, preventing menses becomes desirable. Medroxyprogesterone (Provera) may be used for hormonal support of the progestational endometrium. Medroxyprogesterone 10 mg PO b.i.d. should be started 5 to 7 days before the presumed starting time of the next menstrual period. It may be increased to 10 mg t.i.d. or higher if breakthrough bleeding occurs. Depo-Provera is contraindicated in the thrombocytopenic and neutropenic patient.

H.   Birth control and fertility. Given the potential teratogenic effects of cytotoxic chemotherapy, appropriate measures for preventing conception must be addressed with women who are undergoing chemotherapy and who may still be in their reproductive years. Although there are no clear data linking chemotherapy in the male partner to teratogenic effects in the fetus, it is prudent to suggest that appropriate birth control measures be undertaken in this situation as well. Late effects of chemotherapy, such as infertility, need to be considered in younger patients. Sperm cryopreservation should be offered to men of reproductive age prior to initiation of chemotherapy. Gonadal function in women seems to be less affected by cytotoxic chemotherapy. Furthermore, current egg cryopreservation procedures are not yet refined. Treatment with a gonadotropin-releasing hormone (GnRH) agonist analog to induce a temporary prepubertal milieu should be considered in women of reproductive age.

I.   Psychosocial support. Patients with acute leukemia are usually previously healthy individuals who have suddenly had to accept the possibility of their own imminent mortality. Intensive psychological and spiritual support by the health care team, family, and religious leaders is critical for maintaining the patient's sense of well-being (see Chapter 32).

J.   Optimization of co-morbid disease treatment. Patients with good performance status are best able to tolerate chemotherapy. Co-morbid disease such as heart failure, diabetes, and chronic lung disease should be aggressively treated before initiating induction chemotherapy.

III. Therapeutic principles of and approach to therapy for acute leukemia

   A. Therapeutic aim. The goals of chemotherapy are to eradicate the leukemic clone and re-establish normal hematopoiesis in the bone marrow. Long-term survival is seen only in patients in whom a complete remission (CR) is attained. Although leukemia therapy is toxic and infection is the major cause of death during therapy, the median survival time of untreated (or unresponsive) acute leukemia is 2 to 3 months, and most untreated patients die of bone marrow failure and its complications. The doses of chemotherapy are never reduced because of cytopenia, since lowered doses still produce the unwanted side effects (further marrow suppression) without having as great a potential for eradicating the leukemic clone and ultimately improving marrow function.

   B. Forms of chemotherapy

   1. Induction chemotherapy is initial intensive chemotherapy given in an attempt to eradicate the leukemic clone and to induce a CR. The term CR depicts patients who achieve recovery of normal peripheral blood counts with recovery of bone marrow cellularity, including the presence of less than 5% blast cells, in the absence of extramedullary disease. The aim of induction chemotherapy is to reduce the leukemia cell population by several logs from the clinically detectable leukemia tumor burden of 10^{12} cells that is commonly seen at diagnosis to below the cytologic detectable level of 10^9 cells. It is important to note that because achievement of initial CR represents only a 3- to 6-log leukemia cell reduction, a substantial leukemia cell burden persists, and patients usually relapse within months if further therapy is not administered.

   2. Postremission chemotherapy is additional chemotherapy given after a CR has been obtained in a further attempt to eradicate the residual, but often undetectable, leukemic cells. In many younger patients, given the generally high induction rate for acute leukemia, future advances are likely to be made through improved postremission chemotherapy. In the older patient population, all patients should be candidates for experimental protocols evaluating options for both induction and postremission therapy.

   a. Consolidation. This involves repeated courses of the same drugs at the same or higher doses as those used to induce the remission, which are given soon after the remission has been achieved. Consolidation often requires further hospitalization.

   b. Maintenance. This pertains mainly to ALL, which includes low doses of drugs designed for outpatient use given for months to years. In AML, this applies generally only to APL.

   C. Definition of response. The criteria are based on the peripheral blood counts and the status of the bone marrow at the time of marrow recovery, not at the time of marrow aplasia.

   1. Complete response (complete remission, CR) is the return of the complete blood count to a "normal" absolute neutrophil count (ANC) of more than 1,500/μL and to a platelet count of more than 100,000/μL in conjunction with a normal bone marrow (i.e., normal cellularity, less than 5% blasts or promyelocytes and promonocytes, an absence of obvious leukemic cells [e.g., containing Auer rods]) and absence of extramedullary disease.

2. Partial response is the persistence of morphologically identifiable residual leukemia (5% to 15% leukemic cells in the bone marrow).

IV. Therapy for adult acute myeloid leukemia

A. General plan of therapy. The day that induction chemotherapy is started is arbitrarily called day 1. Bone marrow aspiration and biopsy are repeated on about days 10 to 14. If the bone marrow is severely hypoplastic with fewer than 5% residual blasts or if the bone marrow is aplastic, no further chemotherapy is given, and the patient is supported until bone marrow recovery occurs (usually 1 to 3 weeks). A bone marrow examination is repeated 2 weeks later (about days 26 to 28). Once a CR has been documented, the potential benefit of further consolidation therapy should be determined on an individual basis. The overall approach to induction and consolidation therapy used at Northwestern University is shown in Table 18.2.

Table 18.2. Therapeutic options for AML other than APL (outside of a clinical trial)[a]

Initial cytogenetics	Induction chemotherapy	Postremission therapy	
		HLA-matched donor	No donor
Favorable	Standard 7 + 3[b]	HDAC × 3–4 cycles, or 2–3 cycles followed by autologous HSCT	HDAC × 3–4 cycles, or 2–3 cycles followed by autologous HSCT
Intermediate	Standard 7 + 3	Allogeneic HSCT (as soon as possible), or HDAC × 2–4 cycles	HDAC × 2–4 cycles + autologous HSCT
Unfavorable	Standard 7 + 3	Allogeneic HSCT (as soon as possible)	HDAC × 2–4 cycles ± autologous HSCT

HDAC, high-dose cytarabine (ara-C); HSCT, hematopoietic stem cell transplantation.
[a]All individuals with acute leukemia should be treated in clinical trials.
[b]7 + 3, cytarabine 100 mg/m² continuous infusion days 1–7 and anthracycline (i.e., daunorubicin 45–60 mg/m²) by bolus infusion days 1–3.

B.   Acute myeloid leukemia other than acute promyelocytic leukemia

1.   Induction therapy. Factors that influence the choice of the chemotherapeutic program to be employed include the patient's cardiac function, age, and performance status. The initial drug doses outlined below are based on the presence of normal hepatic function. They are not modified based on peripheral blood counts. Cytarabine is the most active agent against AML and is the agent around which most active regimens are built. Remission rates for AML vary depending on cytogenetics at presentation. Following induction therapy, patients with favorable cytogenetics have CR rates of 80% to 90%, while 50% to 60% of patients with unfavorable cytogenetics enter CR. According to age, 70% to 80% of adults less than age 55 to 60 can be expected to enter CR as opposed to 45% to 55% for older adults. This not only is attributable to better tolerance of intensive therapy but also is a function of a lower proportion of younger adults presenting with unfavorable cytogenetics.

a.   "7 + 3." During the last 30 years, a series of clinical trials has identified an induction regimen that is now considered standard. Approximately 30% to 40% of patients achieve CR with either cytarabine or daunorubicin given as a single agent. However, CR is routinely achieved in more than 60% of patients when these agents are combined. The most widely used induction chemotherapy regimen currently administered is cytarabine 100 mg/m^2 by continuous IV infusion for 7 days and daunorubicin 45 to 60 mg/m^2/day IV for 3 days (known as "7 + 3"). Several randomized trials have compared daunorubicin at 45 mg/m^2 with various other anthracyclines and anthracenediones such as idarubicin (12 mg/m^2) and mitoxantrone (12 mg/m^2). In older adults, a randomized trial showed no benefit to one anthracycline/anthracenedione over the other. Therefore, one of these alternative agents or daunorubicin at a higher dose such as 60 mg/m^2 should be incorporated into induction therapy with cytarabine. Although many investigators have strong personal biases regarding the choice of anthracycline or anthracenedione for induction therapy, we would consider daunorubicin, idarubicin, and mitoxantrone as essentially equivalent choices based on current data. All three should be considered potentially cardiotoxic.

A commonly administered induction regimen is presented below:

Cytarabine 100 mg/m^2/24 h continuous IV infusion on days 1 to 7, *and*
Daunorubicin 45 to 60 mg/m^2 IV bolus on days 1 to 3, *or*
Idarubicin 12 mg/m^2 IV bolus on days 1 to 3, *or*
Mitoxantrone 12 mg/m^2 IV bolus on days 1 to 3.

b.   Other regimens. Many permutations to the standard "7 + 3" regimen have been studied over the years in attempts to improve the CR rate of induction therapy and prolong survival. The addition of other agents such as 6-thioguanine

(DAT) and etoposide (3 + 7 + 3) to the "7 + 3" regimen have improved the CR and response duration in some studies, but these regimens produce increased toxicity without improvement in OS. Furthermore, the risk of secondary acute leukemia from topoisomerase inhibitors needs to be considered in patients who are potentially long-term survivors. Dose intensification through use of intermediate- to high-dose cytarabine (HDAC) of 1,500 to 3,000 mg/m^2, respectively, either alone or following "7 + 3" has produced similar CR rates with longer CR duration in some trials, but the treatment-related toxicities were increased and OS was not clearly improved. HDAC has been examined through a protocol that contained a second induction course on day 16 of TAD (6-thioguanine, cytarabine, and daunorubicin) or HAM (HDAC plus mitoxantrone) for double induction (TAD-TAD versus TAD-HAM). CR and OS rates were similar in these two treatment groups. TAD-HAM was associated with a higher CR (65% versus 49%) and 5-year survival (25% versus 18%) in the defined unfavorable subgroup with lactate dehydrogenase higher than 700 U/L, day 16 bone marrow greater than 40% blasts, or unfavorable cytogenetics.

c.   Residual disease. Patients who have residual disease at day 28 should be considered primary treatment failures and have alternative therapy initiated. If a significant response has been demonstrated at the day 10 to 14 marrow (greater than 50% to 60% reduction in leukemic infiltration) but residual leukemia persists, a second course of similar chemotherapy is given (versus an alternative regimen such as HDAC). Patients with significant involvement of leukemia on day 10 to 14 (less than 40% to 50% leukemic reduction) should be changed to an alternative chemotherapy regimen. There is no dose modification for the second course based on blood cell counts. The doses of drugs may be decreased for the second cycle if hepatic dysfunction develops and is attributable to drug toxicity.

d.   Impaired cardiac function. The use of an anthracycline or an anthracenedione is contraindicated for induction therapy in patients with severe underlying cardiac disease, particularly if the patient has had a recent myocardial infarction or has an ejection fraction of less than 50%. The choice of therapy in this situation is HDAC. Unique complications of HDAC include ulcerative keratitis and neurotoxicity. Because cytarabine is secreted in tears, ulcerative keratitis can be prevented by instilling eye drops (saline, methylcellulose, or steroid) every 4 h while awake and Lacri-Lube ophthalmic ointment (Allergan Pharmaceuticals) at bedtime, starting at the time HDAC is initiated and continuing for 2 to 3 days after the last dose of HDAC. The optimum dose and schedule of HDAC therapy are not known (i.e., number of doses, dosage, infusion rate). Neurotoxicity (e.g., cerebellar dysfunction, somnolence) occurs more frequently in older patients and as the number of doses of HDAC increases. Renal and hepatic dysfunction contributes to the development of neurotoxicity. Because neurotoxicity appears to be decreased with shorter infusion times, 1- to 2-h infusions are generally recommended as opposed to the original infusion rate over 2 to 3 h.

Commonly employed HDAC regimens are as follows:

Cytarabine 2 to 3 g/m^2 IV infusion over 1 to 2 h every 12 h for 12 doses, *or*

Cytarabine 2 to 3 g/m^2 IV infusion over 2 h every 12 h on days 1, 3, and 5.

Reducing the dose of cytarabine in the face of renal dysfunction may decrease the risk of neurotoxicity. The following schema has been suggested to decrease neurotoxicity in the face of renal dysfunction. For a baseline serum creatinine level of 1.5 to 1.9 mg/dL or an increase in serum creatinine of 0.5 to 1.2 mg/dL from baseline, reduce the cytarabine to 1 g/m^2 per dose. For a baseline serum creatinine of more than 2 mg/dL or an increase of serum creatinine of greater than 1.2 mg/dL from baseline, reduce the cytarabine dose to 100 mg/m^2/day.

2. Postremission therapy. The fact that most patients with AML relapse despite attaining a CR suggests that further postremission therapy is indicated to attempt to eradicate the residual but undetected leukemic clone. There are three general treatment options for postremission therapy: consolidation chemotherapy, autologous hematopoietic stem cell transplantation (HSCT), or allogeneic HSCT. Although the optimum postremission strategy remains to be defined, almost all younger adults with AML benefit from further therapy. The type of postremission therapy should be determined based on age and on prognostic factors, in particular, cytogenetics at presentation. Patients with AML in first CR should be considered candidates for experimental protocols examining postremission therapy options. For patients who cannot be enrolled in protocol studies, the approach to post-induction therapy used as a guide at Northwestern University is shown in Table 18.2.

a. Acute myeloid leukemia with favorable cytogenetics. Patients with t(8;21), inv(16), and t(16;16) are encompassed within the core-binding factor (CBF) leukemias. There is increasing evidence that several courses of HDAC represent the best treatment option for this group of patients. The treatment-related mortality of standard allogeneic HSCT makes this option currently prohibitive in this group of patients. Elevated white blood cell (WBC) count (specifically, WBC index: WBC × [% of marrow blasts/100]) has been demonstrated to be an important prognostic factor in multivariate analysis for disease-free survival (DFS) and OS in t(8;21) AML. The French AML Intergroup reported the 3-year DFS and OS for t(8;21) patients with low WBC index (under 2.5) to be 74% and 74%, respectively, compared with the high WBC index (20 or above) group with 33% and 47%, respectively. Further evaluation in clinical trials of prognostic factors such as WBC index may help define subsets of t(8;21) AML that may benefit from more intensive postremission therapy.

Current published data suggest that HDAC offers a distinct advantage over standard-dose cytarabine consolidation in patients less than 60 years of age. More than 40% to 50% of patients will be in a continuous CR 5 years after consolidation with HDAC. The addition of other agents to HDAC consolidation therapy, with agents such as daunorubicin or amasacrine, has been studied, although improvements in long-term outcomes have not been proven. Consolidation should be initiated when the peripheral blood counts have returned to normal (ANC more than 1,500/μL and platelet count more than 100,000/μL), marrow cellularity is normal, infections have resolved, and mucositis has cleared.

HDAC options include the following:

1. Cytarabine 3 g/m² IV infusion over 3 h every 12 h on days 1, 3, and 5 (better tolerated) for two to four monthly courses, *or*
2. Cytarabine 3 g/m² IV infusion over 2 h every 12 h on days 1 to 6 for one to three monthly courses (most patients cannot tolerate more than one or two courses of standard HDAC), *or*
3. *For patients over age 60* **and/or** *patients with renal dysfunction (including creatine less than 2.0 mg/dL):* Cytarabine 1.5 g/m² IV infusion over 3 h every 12 h on days 1, 3, and 5 for two to three monthly courses.

b.   Acute myeloid leukemia with intermediate-risk cytogenetics. Long-term survival for patients presenting with intermediate cytogenetics is 40% to 45%. For patients less than age 60, data support that an allogeneic HSCT may be considered for postremission therapy. The largest collection of prospective cohort data in this subgroup by the Medical Research Council (MRC) documented superior 3-year relapse rates of 18% (versus 55% and 35% for chemotherapy consolidation and autologous HSCT, respectively) and 3-year survival rates of 65% for patients undergoing allogeneic HSCT for postinduction therapy (48% and 56%, respectively). The U.S. Intergroup Study did not demonstrate this similar advantage for allogeneic HSCT, although a much smaller cohort of patients was reported. The optimal timing of allogeneic HSCT is not known, although retrospective data collected from the International Bone Marrow Transplant Registry (IBMTR) demonstrated that there is not additional benefit in receiving consolidation chemotherapy prior to HSCT. In other words, patients in postinduction CR may proceed immediately to allogeneic HSCT.

Patients who do not have an HLA-identical sibling should receive consolidation chemotherapy incorporating HDAC or similar therapy. The optimal number and duration of HDAC are not known, but 2 g/m² to 3 g/m² is preferred for two to four cycles in younger patients. In healthy patients, this may be followed by autologous HSCT.

Autologous HSCT has been studied in this subgroup of patients but has not been shown to represent an advantage over consolidation chemotherapy alone in randomized studies conducted during the last decade.

c. Acute myeloid leukemia with unfavorable cytogenetics. CR rates approach 60%, but this group of patients has been demonstrated to have the poorest long-term outcome with reported 5-year OS of 11% with rates ranging from 3 to 20% depending on the specific cytogenetic abnormality found at diagnosis (i.e., 3% to 5% of patients with monosomy 5 and complex karyotype are alive at 3 years). The U.S. Intergroup Study demonstrated a significant long-term survival advantage for patients with unfavorable cytogenetics who received allogeneic HSCT for consolidation as compared with autologous HSCT or conventional chemotherapy (combined relative rate [RR] of death of 2.00, confidence interval of 0.98 to 4.06, for latter two treatments versus allogeneic HSCT). Although the total number of patients analyzed in this trial and other similar trials has been small, matched-sibling allogeneic HSCT likely represents the therapy with the best current potential to prevent relapse. Moreover, select reports in younger patients have demonstrated long-term survival rates of 35% to 45% in patients undergoing mismatched-sibling allogeneic HSCT and matched unrelated donor (MUR) HSCT. Despite 100-day mortality rates of approximately 35% to 40%, these strategies may represent the best therapeutic choice for select patients due to the dismal long-term outcome with unfavorable cytogenetics. Low-intensity myeloablation or nonmyeloablative HSCT procedures have allowed less fit and older patients to proceed to allogeneic HSCT for consolidation, but these techniques should still be considered experimental. For less fit patients or patients without a suitable matched donor, enrollment in experimental clinical trials testing novel strategies should be aggressively pursued for patients with unfavorable cytogenetics. Alternative-donor transplantation is an area of active investigation.

d. Acute megakaryocytic leukemia. AmegL (FAB M7) is a rare AML subtype (1% to 2%) not encompassed in the "unfavorable" group that has very poor long-term outcome. The Eastern Cooperative Oncology Group (ECOG) described the 20 of 1,649 patients with newly diagnosed AML found to have AmegL. The median age of patients described was 42 years, and 50% of patients entered CR with a median OS of 10.4 months (2 patients remain alive). There have been only anecdotal reports of allogeneic HSCT for patients with AmegL. Novel therapeutic strategies are needed, including agents such as arsenic trioxide (As_2O_3), which has recently been demonstrated to inhibit growth and survival in megakaryocytic leukemia cell lines.

3. Relapsed acute myeloid leukemia.

   a. Background. Despite many advances, many adults with AML who achieve a remission will ultimately relapse. The goals for relapsed AML vary from achievement of second

CR with intensive chemotherapy and/or HSCT to best supportive care. The success of achieving a second CR varies greatly, depending less on cytogenetic characteristics but more on duration of first CR, age, and active co-morbidities of the patient. The median duration of second CR is usually less than 6 months without HSCT, with long-term DFS rates of less than 10 months. Moreover, most standard salvage chemotherapy regimens induce significant toxicity. Survival is improved in patients who proceed to allogeneic HSCT with long-term OS rates that may approach 30% to 40%. Unfortunately, because of the lack of suitable availability of donors and patient morbidities, many patients are not eligible for allogeneic HSCT.

b. Options for reinduction therapy. Options for reinduction therapy include treatment with the immunoconjugate agent gemtuzumab ozogamicin, intensive chemotherapy with conventional chemotherapeutic agents, investigational therapies on a clinical trial, immediate HSCT for the individual with a suitable allogeneic donor or cryopreserved autologous stem cells available, palliative intent chemotherapy, or best supportive care. Individuals who received an allogeneic HSCT during remission may be eligible for donor lymphocyte infusions as an immunologic maneuver to generate a graft-versus-leukemia (GVL) effect. The determination of the optimal therapy depends in part on the duration of the first remission, whether HSCT is planned, if a second CR is achieved, and the manner in which the relapse was detected. Individuals with remission less than 6 to 12 months in duration are best treated with investigational agents on clinical trials or, if feasible, immediate HSCT depending on the marrow blast percentage. Individuals with a remission greater than 18 to 24 months may be treated with more conventional salvage treatment that commonly includes a HDAC-containing regimen.

c. Gemtuzumab ozogamicin. An advance in the treatment of patients with relapsed and refractory AML was the synthesis of gemtuzumab ozogamicin, a recombinant humanized monoclonal antibody against the CD33 antigen conjugated with calicheamicin, a highly potent antitumor antibiotic. The majority of AML blast cells (80% to 90%) express the CD33 surface antigen, while pluripotent hematopoietic stem cells/tissues and nonhematopoietic cells do not express CD33. Three multicenter trials demonstrated an overall response rate of 30% (16% CR with full platelet recovery) characterized by 5% or less blasts in the bone marrow, recovery of neutrophil count to 1,500/μL, and RBC and platelet transfusion independence following two doses of gemtuzumab ozogamicin. Median relapse-free survival was 6.8 months, median survival was 5.9 months, 1-year OS was 31%, and no differences were noted in age or between duration of first remission. (Of note, patients with myelodysplasia or first CR of less than 3 months were not enrolled in these trials.) Gemtuzumab ozogamicin has been generally well tolerated with the most common side effect that patients experienced being a transient infusion-related syndrome (fevers, chills/rigors, nausea, pain, and hypotension). Notwithstanding, a significant minority of patients treated with gemtuzumab ozogamicin have developed hepatic toxicity manifested as weight gain, ascites, jaundice, and abnormalities in the hepatic transaminases. A direct association of gemtuzumab ozogamicin with liver injury may be confounded by prior and/or concomitant antileukemic cytotoxic therapies received by patients, but reports including patients who had received no prior antileukemic cytotoxic therapy (including patients who received single-agent gemtuzumab ozogamicin) have infrequently documented significant liver injury. Results of liver histologic examination in five of seven patients who died with persistent liver dysfunction demonstrated sinusoidal injury with extensive sinusoidal fibrosis, centrilobular congestion, hepatocyte necrosis, and striking deposition of sinusoidal collagen, suggesting that gemtuzumab ozogamicin targets CD33+ cells residing in hepatic sinusoids. This veno-occlusive disease–like syndrome or sinusoidal obstructive syndrome has occurred in a very small percentage of patients.

d.   Standard chemotherapy. The selection of conventional salvage therapy, the optimal dose of cytarabine, and the benefits of the addition of an anthracycline or other agents all remain important unanswered issues. A randomized trial conducted by the Southwestern Oncology Group (SWOG) failed to demonstrate a significant benefit to the addition of mitoxantrone to cytarabine 3 g/m^2 every 12 h for six doses. The German AML Cooperative Group Trial compared cytarabine 3 g/m^2 versus cytarabine 1 g/m^2 administered twice daily on days 1, 2, 8, and 9 in patients less than 60 years of age. All patients received mitoxantrone. There was no substantial difference in CR rate or median OS. Thus, dose-intense cytarabine should probably be viewed as an essential component of a conventional salvage program, but escalation to 3 g/m^2 is probably not justified given the increased toxicity. There appears to be no value to adding standard-dose anthracyclines. However, there are multiple single-arm trials using escalated doses of anthracyclines that may present a reasonable alternative. It is critical to minimize the toxicity and likelihood of persistent complications since many individuals will be offered HSCT if remission is achieved.

e.   Experimental strategies. Patients with relapsed AML should strongly be considered for experimental protocols. Experimental agents incorporating targeted strategies include the following: (1) Antiangiogenic protein tyrosine kinase inhibitors that target the vascular endothelial growth factor receptors (VEGF-Rs) and platelet-derived growth factor (PDGF) receptor families. The antiangiogenic agent thalidomide is being examined. (2) Troxacitabine, a novel dioxolane nucleoside analog that has recognized activity in refractory and advanced leukemia. (3) Alteration of signal transduction pathways via enzyme-specific inhibitors of farnesyl protein transferase (FTI), such as the orally administered agent R115777, developed as a potential inhibitor of

Ras protein signaling. The protein kinase C active agent bryostatin is actively being evaluated before and after HDAC therapy. Internal tandem duplications (ITDs) of the receptor tyrosine kinase *FLT3* gene have been found in 20% to 30% of patients with AML. It has been demonstrated to be an important adverse prognostic factor, independent of conventional karyotypic findings. Tyrosine kinase inhibitors that are active against *FLT3* are being examined. (4) Transcriptional therapy, through histone deacetylase inhibitors and deoxyribonucleic acid (DNA) hypomethylating agents are being studied. (5) Immunotherapeutic approaches are being evaluated, such as interleukin-2, adoptive immunotherapy (low-intensity allogeneic HSCT), and vaccine approaches. (6) Drug resistance modulation has been examined, such as therapy targeting P-glycoprotein (Pgp)-mediated cellular export of anthracyclines. Pgp overexpression has been reported in 30% to 40% of relapsed or secondary AML patients and is associated with *in vitro* resistance to anthracyclines, in part due to reduced cellular accumulation of anthracyclines, ultimately translating to lower CR rates and inferior survival. Pgp-mediated efflux of cytotoxic drugs can be inhibited by the Pgp antagonist cyclosporin and the cyclosporin analog PSC 833. A prospective, randomized trial conducted by the SWOG demonstrated a significant improvement in outcome of poor-risk AML patients with the incorporation of cyclosporin used for multidrug resistance (MDR) modulator properties. LY335979 (Zosquidar) is one of the most potent MDR-modulating agents reported to date. A feature distinguishing this modulator from others is the lack of alteration in pharmacokinetics of other concomitantly administered cytotoxic agents such as daunorubicin or etoposide. Interestingly, overexpression of Pgp may also play a role in predicting MDR with gemtuzumab ozogamicin.

f. Recommendations. Depending on prior therapy, age, and perceived ability to tolerate subsequent systemic treatment, chemotherapeutic options using commercially available drugs would include the following:

(1) **Gemtuzumab ozogamicin.** A dosage of 9 mg/m^2 as a 2-h IV infusion is used on days 1 and 15. No dose adjustments for anemia or thrombocytopenia should be made. Benadryl may be administered prior to infusion. Acetaminophen has the potential to contribute to hepatotoxicity (increased free radicals) and theoretically should be avoided. Cyclo-oxygenase-2 (Cox-2) inhibitors may be administered as premedication.

(2) **"7 + 3."** Up to half of patients who undergo induction with the "7 + 3" regimen respond to a repeat course of "7 + 3." Patients who relapse within 6 to 12 months of the last chemotherapy are unlikely to respond to the same regimen again. Thus, a different regimen should be considered.

(3) **HDAC.** Fifty percent to 70% of patients respond to HDAC. Although HDAC combination regimens may have

a slightly higher response rate, their increased toxicity may not make them significantly better than single-agent HDAC. Patients who relapse within 6 to 12 months of HDAC intensification are unlikely to have a significant response to further HDAC. The doses given for the HDAC are those originally described for each regimen. Options include the following:

HDAC (see Section IV.B.2.a above), *or*

HDAC plus anthracycline *or* HDAC 3 g/m^2 IV infusion over 2 h every 12 h on days 1 to 4, *plus* mitoxantrone 10 mg/m^2/day IV on days 2 to 5 or 2 to 6, *or*

(4) CAT.

Cyclophosphamide 500 mg/m^2 IV every 12 h on days 1 to 3, *and*

Topotecan 1.25 mg/m^2/day by continuous infusion on days 2 to 6, *and*

Cytarabine 2 g/m^2 IV over 4 h daily for 5 days on days 2 to 6.

(5) MEC. This regimen may produce significant gastrointestinal and cardiac toxicity. It is not recommended for patients over 60 years of age or those with borderline cardiac function. A variation of MEC currently used by the ECOG is as follows:

Etoposide 40 mg/m^2/day IV infusion over 1 h on days 1 to 5, *followed immediately by*

Cytarabine 1 g/m^2/day IV infusion over 1 h on days 1 to 5, *and*

Mitoxantrone 4 mg/m^2/day IV sidearm push on days 1 to 5, given after completion of HDAC each day.

(6) Etoposide 100 mg/m^2/day IV on days 1 to 5 **and mitoxantrone** 10 mg/m^2/day IV on days 1 to 5 represents an active and well-tolerated combination that is commonly used for relapsed or refractory leukemia.

(7) High-dose etoposide 70 mg/m^2/h continuous IV infusion for 60 h **and high-dose cyclophosphamide** 50 mg/kg (1,850 mg/m^2)/day IV infusion over 2 h on days 1 to 4 is a highly toxic but active regimen that does not require bone marrow support. It is active against HDAC-resistant AML (30% CR). This regimen may be useful for young patients who are good candidates for allogeneic HSCT while waiting for an unrelated donor search to be completed. This regimen may also be associated with substantial toxicity.

4. Acute myeloid leukemia in older adults.

a. Background. AML in older patients is a common problem as more than half of all newly diagnosed patients with AML are over the age of 64. Refinements in supportive care and chemotherapy programs have likely benefited older patients with AML, but long-term survival rates have improved little over the last 20 to 30 years for patients over age 55 diagnosed with AML. The 5-year OS for this group of patients treated in ECOG protocols in the

1990s was 12% with median survival rates of just over 8 months. Owing to the effects of co-morbid disease and age on normal physiology, older adults are less able to withstand the inherent toxicity of induction chemotherapy than young adults. There are also intrinsic differences in the biology of older adults with AML (e.g., a higher percentage of the leukemic cells express Pgp at diagnosis, elderly patients have an increased background of secondary leukemia and/or myelodysplasia) that predispose to drug resistance. Moreover, AML in older adults is associated with a greater number of high-risk cytogenetic abnormalities (i.e., abnormalities of chromosomes 5 and 7 and complex karyotypes). As reported by the MRC, the favorable cytogenetic risk group (see Table 18.1) was less common in patients over age 55 (7% versus 26% in younger than 55), while complex karyotypes were more common (13% versus 6%). Furthermore, patients over 55 with complex karyotype predicted a poor outcome with OS of 2% at 5 years. The MRC recognized a predictive hierarchical cytogenetic classification for older adults similar to previous analysis for younger patients, although 5-year OS for favorable cytogenetic group patients over 55 was 34% compared with 65% for younger patients (and 13% and 41%, respectively. for intermediate cytogenetic risk). **The decision to forgo therapy in an older patient with AML should not be made a priori based solely on age;** rather, the decision to treat or not to treat should be based on more substantive factors such as the presence of co-morbid disease, performance status before diagnosis, quality of life before diagnosis, and projected long-term survival.

b.   Induction therapy. In general, 55% to 70% of elderly patients without complex karyotype cytogenetics can achieve a CR with induction chemotherapy (20% to 30% for complex karyotypes). Although attenuated doses of "7 + 3" have been recommended in the past, **full-dose therapy is now generally recommended in older adults without significant co-morbidities,** in part owing to improvements in supportive care. The role of growth factors (granulocyte–macrophage colony-stimulating factor [GM-CSF] or granulocyte colony-stimulating factor [G-CSF]) to stimulate earlier marrow recovery in order to allow older patients to tolerate better full doses of induction is unclear. Growth factors have been shown to decrease the neutropenic period by 2 to 5 days and may decrease the number of severe neutropenic infections (compared with placebo), but improvements in CR rate or overall survival have not been consistently demonstrated. Results of cost–benefit analyses for the use of growth factors in the older patient population have been variable. Induction treatment options include the following:

(1)   **Standard "7 + 3"** (see Section IV.B.1.a).

(2)   **"7 + 3" using idarubicin.** A recent French randomized trial has shown a higher CR rate with idarubicin compared with daunorubicin for patients aged 55 to 75 years.

Cytarabine 100 mg/m²/day IV continuous infusion on days 1 to 7, *and*

Idarubicin 8 mg/m²/day IV bolus on days 1 to 5.

(3) **"7 + 3" plus growth factors.** G-CSF 5 µg/m² SC (or GM-CSF 250 µg/m² SC) beginning on day 8 until absolute granulocytes reach more than 500 for 2 or 3 successive days.

(4) **Etoposide** 100 mg/m²/day IV on days 1 to 5 **and mitoxantrone** 10 mg/m²/day IV on days 1 to 5 represent an active combination.

(5) **Modified HDAC** decreases the cytarabine dose to try to diminish the neurotoxicity that is dose limiting in older adults. Modified HDAC is generally believed to be more toxic than the "7 + 3" regimen. We do not routinely recommend the use of HDAC for induction in older patients given the lack of data to support a higher CR rate and the significantly increased morbidity and mortality associated with HDAC during the induction period. In selected older patients with excellent performance status and a decreased ejection fraction, one can consider using modified HDAC. Although the optimum dose and schedule are not known, 1.5 to 2 g/m² IV over 2 h every 12 h for 8 to 12 doses is commonly used.

c. **Postremission therapy.** There are limited data that indicate postremission maintenance chemotherapy with long-term attenuated chemotherapy that prolongs relapse-free survival in older adults, although there is no evidence for prolongation of OS. Older patients may tolerate one to two cycles of lower doses of HDAC or intermediate cytarabine (1.5 g/m² every 12 h days 1, 3, and 5) than is usually given for younger adults, although a beneficial impact of HDAC consolidation chemotherapy on long-term outcome is not proven. The CALGB trial of varying doses of cytarabine (100 mg/m²/day, 400 mg/m²/day, and 3 g/m²) reported similar 5-year DFS and OS within each arm (each less than 15% and 8%, respectively). Other reports have demonstrated that prolonged consolidation courses (over four cycles) will likely not benefit long-term outcomes. Other more novel therapeutic strategies are needed. Current strategies include incorporation of less intensive therapy, such as incorporation of agents such as gemtuzumab ozogamicin, FTIs, and *bcl-2* antisense oligonucleotides into consolidation (and induction) therapy. Autologous HSCT may be considered for fit patients, although, as in younger patients, the exact integration of this therapy is not known. Low-intensity allogeneic HSCTs have allowed allogeneic HSCT in older patients, but this modality should still be considered experimental in this setting. **Current treatment options include the following:**

1. HDAC 1.5 g/m² IV infusion over 3 h every 12 h on days 1, 3, and 5 (better tolerated) for one to two monthly courses (*with careful attention to cerebellar toxicity and to renal function; if either is noted to be apparent, HDAC should be immediately discontinued*).

2. Cytarabine 100 mg/m²/day for 5 days for two to three courses but there are no data to show that these strategies are effective.

d. Relapsed disease. The treatment of older individuals with relapsed AML presents an extremely difficult dilemma. In general, such patients have been excluded from clinical trials. A reasonable approach may be to make treatment decisions according to the duration of the first CR and the health of the individual. Healthy individuals may be managed as younger adults (see Section IV.B.3). If the duration of first CR was not at least 6 months to a year, the likelihood of a response is likely to be too low to justify the routine administration of salvage therapy. For individuals with a remission longer than 18 months, readministration of the same drugs used in induction may be reasonable. Treatment is generally delayed until significant neutropenia or thrombocytopenia is present.

C. Acute promyelocytic leukemia. APL is an uncommon form of AML (approximately 10% to 15%) that presents unique management challenges but now represents the most curable subtype of AML in adults, with cure rates exceeding 70% with contemporary therapeutic strategies.

1. **Coagulopathy**

a. Manifestations. APL predisposes to the development of a potentially devastating coagulopathy that is due to a combination of DIC and primary hyperfibrinolysis. Pooled data through the late 1980s suggested that under the best of circumstances with cytotoxic induction chemotherapy, 5% of these patients would die of central nervous system (CNS) hemorrhage within the first 24 h of hospitalization and another 20% to 25% would die of CNS hemorrhage during induction chemotherapy. With intensive supportive care and the introduction of all-*trans*-retinoic acid (ATRA) therapy, the most recent studies suggest that less than 5% of patients will die of hemorrhage during induction chemotherapy, while overall induction mortality in APL remains approximately 10%. If looked for carefully, essentially all patients with APL have clinical or laboratory features of DIC. Even with severe thrombocytopenia, in most patients, the bleeding usually stops quickly at the site of bone marrow examination. Subtle laboratory signs suggestive of an underlying consumptive coagulopathy in APL include a prolongation of the prothrombin time (more than 0.1 s) or a normal (or low) rather than increased fibrinogen titer (fibrinogen is an acute-phase reactant that may be normally elevated in acute leukemia at presentation). Patients are at risk of bleeding with relatively normal coagulation studies because of fibrinolysis, the markers of which are not easily or routinely measured.

b. Therapy for promyelocytic coagulopathy. The first rule of managing DIC is to treat the underlying cause. Thus, once the patient has been stabilized, the rapid initiation of induction therapy is the cornerstone of the management of APL. Heparin has been used in the past with the goal of therapy to slow the rate of consumption of coagulation factors and platelets and thus prevent the development of microvascular thromboses and an uncontrolled hemorrhagic state. But since the incorporation of ATRA into induction therapy, coagulopathy and bleeding have diminished significantly, and the risks of heparin therapy likely outweigh the benefits in most patients. Patients who have uncontrolled bleeding despite aggressive transfusion therapy and those with disproportionate fibrinolysis may benefit from ε-aminocaproic acid (EACA) given as either 1 g PO every 2 h or as a 3- to 4-g IV bolus *followed by* continuous IV infusion at 1 g/h. Tranexamic acid 6 g/24 h by continuous IV infusion for up to 6 days has also been suggested. These agents should be used with caution in patients with renal insufficiency. These agents are rarely needed with contemporary ATRA-containing regimens.

2. **Chemotherapy.** Therapy for APL has represented the most exciting recent advancement in the treatment of acute leukemia. ATRA is a derivative of vitamin A that is able to induce a high rate of clinical remission by promoting cell maturation without producing marrow hypoplasia. Induction therapy consists of combination ATRA plus anthracycline-based chemotherapy.

a. **Anthracyclines** can induce remission in 60% to 90% of patients with APL when used as single agents. Leukemic cells from patients with APL are particularly sensitive to anthracyclines, perhaps because of significantly lower Pgp expression and other resistance markers in APL cells compared with other AML subtypes. Despite theoretic advantages to idarubicin (longer half-life and good CNS penetration), there is no clear choice of anthracycline in induction for APL. No prospective, randomized trial has compared daunorubicin with idarubicin. It appears, however, that the dose of anthracycline is critical. In a retrospective analysis, SWOG reported excellent survival in APL patients (70% leukemia-free survival at 10 years) when a higher daunorubicin dose at 70 mg/m^2/day (days 1 to 3) was used compared with doses used in most studies of 45 to 50 mg/m^2. Owing to the high remission rates with anthracycline therapy in combination with ATRA, many study groups have demonstrated that cytarabine can be omitted during induction.

b. **ATRA** as a single agent induced a remission in 72% to 81% of patients with APL in large randomized trials, although the remission durations were short. The impact of ATRA on patients with APL may not necessarily be an improvement in initial CR rate but rather on the relapse rate and on the number of patients cured in this disease. The European APL group studied concurrent ATRA and chemotherapy versus a sequential approach of ATRA followed by chemotherapy for postremission therapy. Two-year event-free survival (EFS) was superior in the concurrent approach (84% versus 77%) with the difference attributable to a significant decrease in the risk of relapse. It appears reasonable to initiate treatment with ATRA first for 2 to 3 days in patients with life-threatening bleeding to ameliorate the coagulopathy before initiating anthracycline-based therapy, provided the WBC count is not high (less than 10,000/µL). Otherwise, concurrent ATRA plus anthracycline-based therapy has been routine practice and may have the advantage of decreasing the incidence of **retinoic acid syndrome** (RAS), the major toxicity associated with ATRA. The incidence of RAS in patients treated with ATRA alone is 15% to 25%, while recent studies reports rates near 10%. These decreased rates reflect in part earlier clinical recognition of RAS with quicker initiation of dexamethasone therapy, but concurrent administration of chemotherapy with ATRA may also be a contributing factor. The most important goal of postremission therapy in APL is complete eradication of the leukemic clone by polymerase chain reaction (PCR) analysis, because persistence of minimal residual disease (MRD) predicts relapse.

c. Treatment program

(1) Induction. ATRA 45 mg/m^2/day PO is divided into two doses with food given every day until CR plus an anthracycline, either daunorubicin 50 to 60 mg/m^2/day for 3 days or idarubicin 12 mg/m^2 every other day for 4 days. The role of cytarabine in induction remains unclear.

(2) Consolidation. One to two cycles of: anthracycline-based chemotherapy, daunorubicin 50 to 60 mg/m^2/day IV for 3 days to PCR negativity, or alternatively anthracyclines/anthracenedione: idarubicin 5 mg/m^2/day on days 1 to 4 (first consolidation), mitoxantrone 10 mg/m^2/day on days 1 to 5 (second consolidation), or idarubicin 12 mg/m^2 on day 1 only (third consolidation). HDAC or intermediate-dose cytarabine can be considered for patients who remain PCR positive after such consolidation. An alternative consideration is As_2O_3, discussed below.

(3) Maintenance. ATRA 45 mg/m^2/day PO, divided into two doses with food for 15 days every 3 months plus 6-mercaptopurine 100 mg/m^2/day plus MTX 10 mg/m^2/week all for 2 years. Follow-up of PCR for *PML-RARα* every 3 to 6 months for 2 years and then every 6 months for 2 years has been considered in the past. However, since contemporary strategies now result in a relapse rate of only 5% to 20%, this schedule may not be necessary in all patients but rather can be carried out in high-risk patients.

d. Retinoic acid syndrome. RAS occurs in 10% to 15% of patients, most commonly 7 to 14 days after starting ATRA. It has rarely been observed during recovery from chemotherapy-induced aplasia as well as during ATRA maintenance. RAS is a "capillary leak" syndrome. The cardinal clinical manifestations are fever, respiratory distress, and pulmonary infiltrates, which are seen in 80% to 90% of cases. Weight gain, plural or pericardial effusion, and renal failure may occur. Although a rising WBC count may be a risk factor for RAS, it may occur with a WBC count below 5,000/µL. If the WBC count is greater than 5,000 to 10,000/µL before initiating treatment, ATRA and chemotherapy should be given concurrently. If the

WBC count rises to more than 10,000/µL during ATRA monotherapy, induction chemotherapy should be started. Regardless of the WBC count or the risk of neutropenic sepsis, at the first sign of dyspnea or pulmonary infiltrates with or without fever, dexamethasone (10 mg IV b.i.d.) should be initiated, and there should be consideration for ATRA discontinuation until RAS resolves. The benefit of prophylactic corticosteroids in patients who develop leukocytosis (over 10,000/µL) has been explored and should be studied in a randomized fashion.

3. **Minimal residual disease (MRD).** Primary resistant disease does not occur in APL. Although residual disease in other forms of AML needs further vigorous treatment if long-term survival is to be attained, data suggest that "promyelocytic maturation" and bone marrow recovery may occur in patients with minimal residual disease in APL. Reverse transcriptase (RT)–PCR for *PML-RARα* has been shown to be an effective method to detect MRD in patients with APL in apparent CR. The Gruppo Italiano Malattie Ematologiche Maligne dell'Adulto (GIEMEMA) Associazione Italiana di Ematologia e Oncologia Pediatrica (AIEOP) trial reported a prospective study of 163 patients induced into remission with ATRA plus chemotherapy. Of 21 patients with a positive PCR, 20 relapsed within a median of 3 months, whereas the 3-year estimate of relapse risk for patients who tested negative at least twice after consolidation was less than 10%. Furthermore, it appears that early treatment of APL patients in molecular relapse with chemotherapy significantly improves outcome compared with delaying treatment until morphologic evidence of relapse.

4. **Prognostic factors.** Despite an excellent response rate and a high relapse-free survival rate with the use of the current regimens, patients with a high WBC at presentation are the highest risk of relapse. The Program for the Study and Treatment of Hematological Malignancies, Spanish Society of Hematology (PETHEMA), and GIMEMA groups identified WBC higher than 10,000/µL and a platelet count less than 40,000/µL as prognostic for relapse. Expression of CD56, which reflects the neural crest adhesion molecule believed to be involved in trafficking of leukemia cells, has also been shown to be a significant unfavorable prognostic in APL. Older patients, arbitrarily defined as older than 65 to 70 in various studies, have been recognized to have inferior outcomes compared with younger patients. It appears that a major cause of failure in older adults is death in CR. The death rate among patients in CR in the European APL 93 Trial was 19%. Alternative consolidation strategies are warranted in older adults with APL, such as As_2O_3, liposomal ATRA, or anti-CD33 antibody-based approaches.

5. **Relapsed acute promyelocytic leukemia.** The current treatment of choice for patients with relapsed APL is As_2O_3, particularly in patients exposed to ATRA within the prior 12 months. Preclinical mechanisms of action of As_2O_3 include apoptosis and APL cell differentiation. Chinese investigators demonstrated CR rates of more than 85% and

2-year DFS of more than 40% in relapsed APL patients. A
U.S. multicenter study of As_2O_3 induction and consolidation
therapy for relapsed APL confirmed the high CR rates and
long-term survival, and importantly more than 85% of patients who attained CR converted from positive *PML-RARα*
to negative per RT-PCR testing by the completion of their
consolidation therapy. The incorporation of As_2O_3 into the induction and consolidation phases for APL is actively being
studied. The most important side effects documented with
As_2O_3 include electrocardiogram abnormalities including QT
prolongation and ventricular arrhythmias (which may be
exacerbated by hypokalemia and/or hypomagnesemia) and
an APL differentiation syndrome. Despite the high initial CR
rates in relapsed disease, many patients relapse following
arsenic-based treatment. Results of retrospective studies have
demonstrated that HSCT may be an effective option at this
point or upon achievement of second CR following As_2O_3 therapy, particularly autologous HSCT when molecular negative
cells are harvested and reinfused. Other therapies active in
APL, such as liposomal ATRA and gemtuzumab ozogamicin,
need to continue to be explored through experimental trials.
D.   Secondary acute myeloid leukemia.
   1.   Background. Secondary AML that develops following
   exposure to alkylating agents is often associated with abnormalities of chromosomes 5 and/or 7. AML that develops after
   alkylating agent exposure characteristically has a long latency, often has an antecedent MDS, and often is associated
   with cytogenetic abnormalities that involve chromosomes 5
   and 7. Patients who develop AML following exposure to topoisomerase II inhibitors have a relatively short latency period,
   myelomonocytic or monocytic differentiation, and rearrangement of chromosome 11q23. Patients with therapy-related
   MDS and AML may have a high response rate but very short
   remission duration when treated with intensive (high-dose)
   cytarabine chemotherapy. There is increasingly frequent recognition of apparent therapy-related MDS and AML following
   high-dose chemotherapy with HSCT. In one study, the estimated cumulative probability of developing therapy-related
   MDS or AML was approximately $8.6 \pm 2.1\%$ at 6 years among
   612 patients undergoing high-dose chemotherapy and HSCT
   for Hodgkin's disease and non-Hodgkin's lymphoma. The most
   important risk factor appears to be large cumulative doses of
   alkylating agents. However, patient age and previous radiotherapy, particularly total-body irradiation as part of the conditioning regimen, are additional risk factors.
   2.   Therapy. The advisability of chemotherapy needs to be
   assessed in each individual situation. Recent data suggest
   that secondary AML with favorable cytogenetics (e.g., t[8:21],
   t[15:17], inv [16]) has a response rate similar to that of *de
   novo* AML with the same cytogenetic features. Therapeutic
   options include supportive care, "7 + 3," and HDAC. In addition, younger patients with secondary AML should be considered for allogeneic HSCT in first remission. All patients
   should be treated on a clinical trial if at all possible.

E.   Acute myeloid leukemia during pregnancy. The outcomes of both the mother and the fetus must be considered when discussing the therapeutic options for a pregnant woman who develops AML. Therapeutic abortion must be considered if AML develops during the first trimester. If therapeutic abortion is not an option or if AML develops during the second or third trimester, induction chemotherapy may be undertaken. Except for a modest increase in fetal deaths and an increased risk of premature labor, "7 + 3" appears to be well tolerated by both the patient and the fetus.

F.   Role of hematopoietic stem cell transplantation in acute myeloid leukemia.

   1.   Matched-sibling allogeneic hematopoietic stem cell transplantation has emerged as an important and potentially curative postremission strategy for many patients with AML. Initial studies in patients with relapsed and refractory disease given high-dose chemotherapy (cyclophosphamide and total-body irradiation) and HLA-matched sibling bone marrow–derived stem cells demonstrated that 10% to 15% of such patients, who would otherwise have died of the disease, appeared to be cured. Subsequently, similar studies were conducted in patients in first CR, that is, earlier in the natural history of the disease when, theoretically, the leukemic cells had not developed resistance to chemotherapy and patients were in better condition to tolerate such an intensive approach. The apparent cure rate increased to approximately 50% despite a treatment-related mortality (TRM) rate of approximately 20%. Multiple studies from single institutions and cooperative groups have confirmed these results. The important benefit attributable to the success of this strategy is the phenomenon of GVL effect whereby the donor cells recognize the recipient's cells, including leukemia cells, as foreign, with resulting cytotoxicity. Such an immunologic reaction is also believed to be partly responsible for graft-versus-host disease (GVHD) manifested by skin rash, abnormal liver function, and abdominal pain, diarrhea, and hematochezia. A major focus in current research involves the identification of targets responsible for GVL, such as minor histocompatability antigens, in order to exploit this desired effect while minimizing GVHD.

   2.   Matched unrelated donors. MUD transplant registries have grown, and this, coupled with more sensitive tissue-typing techniques, has become an effective approach for more patients. However, there are limitations to this strategy, including donor availability, length of time to identify the donor, and significant TRM (historically, approximately 30% to 35%), and the exact role of MUD transplantation in patients with AML has not been established. Improved OS has been associated with transplantation earlier in the natural history of the disease (for example, first CR) and in patients with a low tumor burden. The presence of circulating leukemic blasts has been associated with poor outcome. Finally, transplantation of a marrow cell dose above 3.65×10^8/kg has been associated with faster neutrophil and platelet engraftment as well as decreased incidence of severe GVHD. The leukemia-free survival for patients with AML in remission with poor prognostic features undergoing MUD transplantation with greater than 3.65×10^8/kg of recipient body weight is approximately 45%. Patients undergoing MUD transplantation in CR have a significantly lower risk of relapse than patients transplanted in relapse or after primary induction failure.

3.   Haploidentical transplantation. Another alternative donor is a haploidentical family member. Almost every patient will have such a suitable donor available, and there is little reason for delay in proceeding to transplant beyond that present for an HLA-matched sibling donor transplant. A group from the University of Perugia, Italy, has pioneered this approach using a relatively nontoxic conditioning regimen of thiotepa, a single dose of total-body irradiation of 800 cGy, fludarabine, and antithymocyte globulin. The TRM rate is approximately 10%, and among 27 high-risk patients with AML in first CR, the 5-year EFS is approximately 45%. Among the important components of the strategy appear the megadoses of CD34 cells (10×10^6 cells/kg), which are T depleted and may effectively promote chimerism. This treatment is associated with delayed immune reconstitution and opportunistic infections, particularly cytomegalovirus. Nevertheless, this approach is promising and warrants further research.

4.   Umbilical cord transplants. Finally, hematopoietic stem cells procured from umbilical cords from related and unrelated donors can also restore hematopoiesis with acceptable risks of GVHD. Such stem cells have advantages compared with stem cells procured from adults, including the capacity to form more colonies in cultures, a higher cell cycle rate, and autocrine production of growth factors. The immaturity of the lymphocytes from umbilical cords could theoretically reduce the risks of GVHD and allow for more successful HLA-mismatched transplants. This approach has been limited by the size of the recipient since it has often been difficult to collect enough stem cells. *Ex vivo* expansion of stem cells is an area of active research that may expand the application of umbilical cell transplantation.

5.   Autologous transplantation. The lack of a suitable HLA-matched donor and TRM limit the application of allogeneic transplantation. Alternatively, autologous HSCT is potentially available to all patients and has very low TRM rates (currently 3% or less in contemporary series and in a recent ECOG trial where there were no transplant-related deaths among 60 consecutive patients studied). Peripheral blood stem cells can be collected when the patient achieves CR and cryopreserved until autologous HSCT takes place. Following high-dose chemotherapy or chemoradiation therapy, the stem cells are reinfused. Despite the lack of potential GVL effect, this approach has been associated with 3- to 5-year DFS rates of 40% to 70%. The role, if any, of purging the stem cells of clonogenic leukemia cells is not established. To decrease the relapse rate following autologous HSCT, many (mostly small) studies have explored posttransplanted immunologic manipulations with interferon or interleukin-2, but any definitive benefits are not established.

6. Relapse. Relapse after HSCT performed during first remission occurs in about 20% of patients undergoing allogeneic transplantation and 40% of patients undergoing autologous transplantation. Salvage of these patients is difficult, especially if relapse occurs within 3 months of transplantation. Although 35% of patients may achieve a remission with subsequent "7 + 3" reinduction, long-term leukemia-free survival is rare. A second allogeneic HSCT can be considered in highly selected patients who have achieved a second remission after reinduction chemotherapy, whose disease has relapsed at least 6 months after the initial HSCT, and who have no residual organ damage. However, TRM in this setting is high. The use of donor lymphocyte infusions has been reported to be successful in a small number of patients who are not candidates for a second HSCT. The addition of interleukin-2 or interferon to the donor lymphocyte infusion to improve the antileukemic effect requires further investigation. Preliminary data have also suggested that G-CSF (5 μg/kg/day SC) can stimulate the normal hematopoietic clone in posttransplantation chimeras.

7. Prospective studies of hematopoietic stem cell transplantation. Several studies have compared prospectively the benefits of intensive consolidation with HDAC, autologous, and HLA-matched HSCT. Autologous HSCT involves the administration of higher chemotherapy doses but is limited by the lack of GVL effect associated with allogeneic transplantation. Furthermore, there is a theoretic risk of infusion of occult residual leukemic cells. Allogeneic transplantation provides the best antileukemic potential but is consistently associated with a higher risk of TRM. All of these studies assign younger patients with an HLA-matched donor to allogeneic HSCT and randomize other patients to either consolidation chemotherapy or autologous HSCT or between the latter two strategies. The interpretation of these important studies requires caution. First, in all studies, a significant number of patients randomized to autologous transplantation do not receive the assigned treatment. Second, although allogeneic transplantation offers the potential for GVL effect and is associated with the lowest risk of relapse, higher TRM, compared with autologous transplantation and consolidation chemotherapy, diminishes the impact of the greater antileukemic potential and therefore a benefit in OS is not observed. Third, it is likely that the mortality rate associated with both autologous and allogeneic transplantation will likely continue to decrease as the techniques of transplantation improve, such as the introduction of autologous peripheral blood stem cell transplantation and improvements in T-cell depletion techniques for allogeneic transplantation. Furthermore, recent studies suggest that the outcome for allogeneic transplantation in patients older than 40 may not be worse than for younger patients. There are improvements in all three postremission strategies that require frequent reappraisal of the benefits and hazards of each approach.

V.   Therapy for adult acute lymphoblastic leukemia

A.   Overview. ALL is the most common leukemia in childhood, while it comprises approximately 20% to 25% of acute leukemia cases in adults. Over the last 20 to 30 years, significant advances have been made in the prognostication and treatment of childhood and adult ALL. The emphasis in recent years has been on the development of therapeutic regimens that contain more intensive induction and postremission therapies. Moreover, current treatment strategies are based in part on biologic and clinical features leading to more patient-tailored therapy. With the advent of these more aggressive and patient-tailored regimens, long-term DFS has improved. Current treatment protocols for adult ALL result in initial CR rates in 80% to 90% of patients, with approximately 35% to 40% overall long-term DFS. Whether this is due to a true improvement in chemotherapy as opposed to the biases of patient selection and better supportive care is not clear. These regimens have usually been developed as complete programs without testing the contributions of the individual components. These improved regimens (and the components thereof) need to be tested in rigorous, randomized, prospective trials. All patients with ALL should be considered as candidates for chemotherapy in randomized, prospective clinical trials.

B.   Prognostic features. As with AML, specific prognostic factors can be used to determine the intensity of induction and postremission therapy for adult ALL. Moreover, clinical and biologic features predict CR rates, remission duration, and DFS. In multivariate analysis, age over 60 is associated with a particularly poor prognosis, with shorter remission durations and lower survival. Presenting WBC of greater than $30,000/\mu L$ is an adverse prognostic factor predicting shorter remission durations that pertains more to precursor B-lineage ALL (threshold WBC greater than 50,000 to $100,000/\mu L$ may be important for T-cell ALL). Time required to achieve CR (more than 4 weeks) following induction chemotherapy has been demonstrated to be an adverse prognostic factor in several clinical trials. A recent report from the GIMEMA ALL group demonstrated that response (defined as peripheral blast count of at least $1,000/\mu L$ on day 0) to 7 days of initial prednisone treatment prior to induction was prognostic in predicting disease outcome in adult ALL patients. As with AML, karyotypic and molecular abnormalities are one of the most important prognostic factors predicting outcome in ALL. The t(9;22) (Philadelphia chromosome) results in formation of the *BCR/ABL* fusion gene, which is the most common cytogenetic abnormality, occurring in up to 30% of adults with ALL, compared with 5% of children. The BCR/ABL fusion protein in ALL is smaller with a molecular mass of 185 or 190 kDa compared with the 210-kDa BCR/ABL protein seen in almost all chronic myelogenous leukemia (CML) patients (including blast crisis). The presence of t(9;22) in ALL is associated with a very poor outcome with median survival rates of 6 to 14 months and long-term DFS of 0% to 10%, depending in part on intensity of induction and consolidation therapy. Other chromosomal abnormalities associated with poor outcomes include t(4;11), trisomy 8, and monosomy 7. Patients with t(10;14) karyotype (or other abnormality involving 14q11-13), del(12p), or t(12p) (without associated Philadelphia chromosome) all have an excellent prognosis with long-term DFS rates exceeding 70% to 75%. Furthermore, rearrangement of the *TEL* gene in children with precursor B-cell ALL has been demonstrated to be a very favorable genetic marker, with 91% DFS at 5 years in one study. The *TEL/AML1* fusion gene is formed by t(12;21), but none of the *TEL*-rearranged cases (detected by Southern blot analysis) had cytogenetic evidence of t(12;21) in this study. The subset of T-cell ALL and the expression of myeloid antigens on lymphoblasts (30% to 35% of adults with ALL) were both previously associated with a worse outcome. Newer multiagent, intensive induction regimens have appeared to overcome these factors. In fact, the German Multicenter Studies for Adult ALL (GMALL) group has reported superior long-term EFS of 50% to 60% for the group of thymic ALL patients. Earlier studies using immunophenotypic subclassification of leukemic cells had demonstrated mature B-cell ALL (FAB L3) to be associated with shorter remission rates and worse survival. Survival rates have improved significantly in adults with Burkitt's ALL through regimens adapted from childhood protocols using shorter, intensive, multiagent chemotherapy plans, which have resulted in long-term survival rates of more than 50% in this group of patients.

C. General plan. The goal of intensified induction therapy is to eliminate leukemia cells prior to the emergence of drug-resistant clones and to allow for rapid restoration of normal hematopoiesis. The general plan of therapy for adult ALL is somewhat different from that for AML. Four or five chemotherapeutic agents are typically incorporated into induction therapy. Approximately 80% to 90% of patients will enter CR. Similar to AML, risk-adapted strategies should be followed (especially cytogenetics) to aid in the determination of the most appropriate postremission therapy. Patients not proceeding to allogeneic HSCT will receive postremission treatment categorized as intensification and consolidation phases, which is subsequently followed by prolonged maintenance therapy. As discussed above, the contributions of each individual component/phase is not exactly known. Aggressive prophylaxis (or treatment) throughout all phases of therapy for sanctuary sites such as the CNS is important. The overall approach to the treatment of ALL used at Northwestern University is shown in Table 18.3, which incorporates results from the International ALL Clinical Trial conducted by the ECOG and MRC.

D. Allogeneic hematopoietic stem cell transplantation. Recent reports have demonstrated that many adults with ALL in first CR will benefit from an allogeneic HSCT procedure.

1. Philadelphia chromosome positive. As described earlier, adult Ph[1]-positive patients have a very poor long-term outcome with standard chemotherapy regimens. Allogeneic HSCT is the only postremission therapy demonstrated to provide long-term DFS for Ph[1]-positive patients. Moreover, results from the MRC/ECOG International ALL Trial support MUD HSCT over standard chemotherapy postremission therapy for Ph[1]-positive patients in first CR. In this trial,

Table 18.3.   Initial therapeutic options for ALL outside a clinical trial[a]

Immunophenotype	Cytogenetics	Age (yr)	Therapy[b] (→ postremission therapy)
Precursor B-cell lineage	Philadelphia+	<60	MRC/ECOG (Hoelzer/Linker)[c] → allogeneic HSCT (matched sibling or MUD if matched sibling is not available)
		>60	MRC/ECOG (Hoelzer/Linker) → intensification/consolidation/maintenance
	Philadelphia−	<60	MRC/ECOG (Hoelzer/Linker) → allogeneic HSCT[d] (matched sibling), or consolidation/maintenance (if matched sibling not available)
		>60	MRC/ECOG (Hoelzer/Linker) → intensification/consolidation/maintenance
T-cell lineage		<60	MRC/ECOG (Hoelzer/Linker) → allogeneic HSCT[d] (matched sibling), or consolidation/maintenance (if matched sibling not available)
		>60	MRC/ECOG (Hoelzer/Linker) → intensification/consolidation/maintenance
Mature B cell (Burkitt's, FAB L3)		<70	B-NHL 86, or hyper-CVAD (autologous or allogeneic HSCT in first CR should be consider experimental)
		>70	B-NHL 86, or hyper-CVAD

MRC, Medical Research Council; ECOG, Eastern Cooperative Oncology Group; HSCT, hematopoietic stem cell transplantation; MUD, matched unrelated donor.

[a] All individuals with acute leukemia should be treated in clinical trials.

[b] Intensive CNS treatment represents an integral component of all ALL protocols.

[c] CALGB 8811 represents an active regimen for precursor B-cell and T-cell ALL.

[d] Patients with very favorable cytogenetics (e.g., t[12p] without *BCR/ABL*) and patients with "thymic ALL" may be subgroups that do not benefit from allogeneic HSCT.

patients receive Hoelzer/Linker-based induction therapy with high-dose MTX intensification. Every ALL patient under age 50 with a matched sibling proceeds to HSCT in first CR, and Ph[1]-positive patients under age 50 proceed to MUD HSCT if a matched sibling is not available. Patients without an allogeneic match are randomized to either standard consolidation/ maintenance therapy for 2.5 years or autologous HSCT. Despite the initial high rates of death in CR for matched-sibling HSCT and MUD HSCT of 37% and 43%, respectively (of note, matched-sibling HSCT mortality rate in first CR was 53% from 1993 to 1996 compared with 27% for 1997 to 2000), compared with 14% for autologous HSCT and 8% for chemotherapy, relapse risk at 5 years for patients receiving allogeneic HSCT (matched sibling or MUD) was 29% versus 81% for patients receiving autologous HSCT or chemotherapy. The 5-year EFS and OS for the allogeneic HSCT group (matched sibling and MUD combined) are higher at 38% and 43%, respectively, than 17% and 19%, respectively, for the autologous HSCT/chemotherapy group. This and other trials have recognized that patients with other high-risk characteristics such as high WBC counts at presentation and achievement of late CR (more than 4 to 6 weeks) have a poor long-term outcome.

2.   Philadelphia chromosome negative. Prior studies have not demonstrated an advantage to allogeneic HSCT for patients without adverse cytogenetics or other high-risk prognostic factors (i.e., standard-risk ALL). However, many of these trials have lacked sufficient numbers of patients, have used varied patient selection criteria, or did not allow for direct, prospective comparisons. Results from the prospective International MRC/ECOG ALL Trial have demonstrated favorable results for Ph[1]-negative patients treated with matched-sibling allogeneic HSCT compared with a combined cohort of autologous HSCT and consolidation chemotherapy. Data are available on 239 patients with intended allogeneic HSCT, of which 170 were Ph[1] negative, and 291 patients randomized to autologous HSCT or standard chemotherapy, of which 264 were Ph[1] negative. The actuarial 5-year EFS for the allogeneic HSCT is 54% compared with 34% for the randomized group (100-day mortality for Ph[1]-negative allogeneic patients was 21%). This survival advantage for allogeneic HSCT included patients with standard-risk ALL disease (defined as Ph[1] negative, age under 36 years, time to CR less than 4 weeks, and WBC less than 30,000/µL for B-cell lineage and less than 100,000/µL for T-cell lineage) with 5-year EFS rates and 5-year relapse rates of 66% and 17%, respectively, versus 45% and 50%, respectively, for the randomized group ($p = 0.06$ and 0.001, respectively). Particular subgroups of patients with good long-term EFS such as chromosome 12 and 14 changes (and possibly thymic ALL patients) may not benefit from allogeneic HSCT in first CR. Further evaluation is warranted to determine the optimal intensity of postremission therapy. However, allogeneic HSCT confers the most potent antileukemic effect for adult patients with ALL; despite the initial high early toxicity, matched-sibling **allogeneic**

HSCT should be considered for most ALL patients in first CR, including standard-risk patients.

E.   **Precursor B-cell lineage and T-cell acute lymphoblastic leukemia.** Although T-cell ALL previously had a poor prognosis with standard induction and maintenance chemotherapy, with the advent of more intensive chemotherapy regimens, response rates and long-term DFS are comparable with those for precursor B-cell ALL. There was a 100% response rate, with 59% of responders projected to have long-term DFS, with the regimen devised by Linker and colleagues (2002) for T-cell ALL patients. CALGB 8811 produced a 100% CR rate with a 63% relapse-free survival rate at 3 years for a similar group of patients. Precursor B-cell and T-cell ALL are treated with similar regimens in most contemporary protocols.

1.   **Normal cardiac function.** In the presence of normal cardiac function, adults with ALL are usually treated with an anthracycline-containing program. Complete programs are described below.

   a.   **Hoelzer/Linker regimens.** Historically, regimens for the induction of adult ALL have been built around vincristine, prednisone, and daunorubicin (VPD). L-Asparaginase is commonly added. The overall CR rate is 70% to 85%. Although L-asparaginase proved to be of value in the preanthracycline era, its role in anthracycline-based adult programs is unclear. Given the significant toxicity of L-asparaginase, many investigators no longer recommend its use, especially in older patients. The newer pegalated form of L-asparaginase (pegaspargase) offers a more prolonged half-life and has been shown to be effective in children who had a prior hypersensitivity reaction to other forms of L-asparaginase. This agent continues to be evaluated in clinical trials. Attempts to further improve overall CR rates have been evaluated through more intensified induction protocols with the incorporation of agents such as cytarabine, cyclophosphamide, etoposide, mitoxantrone, and MTX. It has been difficult to demonstrate improved CR rates with additional agents added to VPD-based therapy or using multiple phases of induction therapy, but it appears that the incorporation of additional chemotherapeutic drugs may benefit some patients. The MRC/ECOG ALL treatment regimen (Hoelzer/Linker-based therapy) should be considered for patients regardless of age who are thought to be able to withstand the rigors of an intensive program.

   (1)   **Induction in MRC/ECOG regimen (Hoelzer/ Linker-based protocol) (consisting of two phases)**

   Phase I, weeks 1 through 4.
   Vincristine 2 mg IV push on days 1, 8, 15, 22, *and*
   Prednisone 60 mg/m² PO on days 1 to 28 (followed by rapid taper over 7 days), *and*
   Daunorubicin 60 mg/m² IV push on days 1, 8, 15 and 22, *and*
   L-Asparaginase 10,000 U IV (or IM) once daily on days 17 to 28.

The vincristine dose should be modified to 50% for paresthesia proximal to the DIP (distal interphalyngeal) joints and stopped entirely for major muscle weakness, cranial nerve palsy, or severe ileus.

Daunorubicin and vincristine doses should be modified on a weekly basis according to the serum bilirubin.

Direct bilirubin	Dose of vincristine to give	Dose of daunorubicin to give
2 to 3 mg/dL	100% calculated	50% calculated
more than 3 mg/dL	50% calculated	25% calculated

Phase II, weeks 5 through 8, should be postponed until the total WBC exceeds $3 \times 10^3/\mu L$.

Cyclophosphamide 650 mg/m^2 IV days 1, 15 and 29, *and*
Cytarabine 75 mg/m^2 IV days 1 to 4, 8 to 11, 15 to 18, 22 to 25, *and*
6-Mercaptopurine 60 mg/m^2 PO once daily days 1 to 28.

(2) Central nervous system treatment and prophylaxis. If CNS leukemia is present at diagnosis, MTX intrathecally (IT) or via an Omaya reservoir is given weekly until blasts are not present in spinal fluid. Also, 24-Gy cranial irradiation and 12 Gy to the spinal cord are administered concurrently with Phase II induction. If CNS leukemia is not present at diagnosis, MTX 12.5 mg IT day 15 only in Phase I and MTX 12.5 mg IT days 1, 8, 15, and 22 in Phase II are given.

(3) Intensification therapy. This begins 4 weeks from day 28 of induction Phase II and again can be postponed until the WBC exceeds $3 \times 10^3/\mu L$.

MTX 3 g/m^2 IV days 1, 8, and 22 (with leucovorin rescue starting at 24 h, 10 mg/m^2 PO or IV q6 h × 12 or until the serum MTX concentration is less than $5 \times 10^{-8} M$), *and*
L-Asparaginase 10,000 U days 2, 9, and 23.

(4) Consolidation therapy (for patients not proceeding to allogeneic HSCT). Given after intensification when the WBC is higher than 3,000/μL and the platelet count is higher than 100,000/μL.

(a) Cycle I consolidation.

Cytarabine 75 mg/m^2 IV on days 1 to 5, *and*
Vincristine 2 mg IV on days 1, 8, 15, and 22, *and*
Dexamethasone 10 mg/m^2 PO on days 1 to 28, *and*
Etoposide 100 mg/m^2 IV on days 1 to 5.

(b) Cycle II consolidation (begins 4 weeks from day 1 of first cycle or when WBC exceeds 3,000/μL).

Cytarabine 75 mg/m^2 IV on days 1 to 5, *and*
Etoposide 100 mg/m^2 IV on days 1 to 5.

(c) Cycle III consolidation (begins 4 weeks from day 1 of second cycle or when WBC exceeds 3,000/μL).

Daunorubicin 25 mg/m^2 IV on days 1, 8, 15, and 22, *and*
Cyclophosphamide 650 mg/m^2 IV on day 29, *and*
Cytarabine 75 mg/m^2 IV on days 31 to 34, 38 to 41, *and*
6-Thioguanine 60 mg/m^2 PO on days 29 to 42.

(d) Cycle IV consolidation (begins 8 weeks from day 1 of third cycle or when WBC exceeds 3,000/µL).

Cytarabine 75 mg/m^2 IV on days 1 to 5, *and*
Etoposide 100 mg/m^2 IV on days 1 to 5.

(5) Maintenance for adult acute lymphoblastic leukemia usually consists of MTX and 6-mercaptopurine-based therapy. Pulses of vincristine and prednisone are given as "reinforcement" because they have relatively little toxicity. Maintenance therapy should be continued for 2.5 years from start of intensification.

6-Mercaptopurine 75 mg/m^2/day PO, *and*
Vincristine 2 mg IV every 3 months, *and*
Prednisone 60 mg/m^2 PO for 5 days every 3 months with vincristine, *and*
MTX 20 mg/m^2 PO or IV once per week for 2.5 years.

b. CALGB 8811 consists of a five-drug combination devised to achieve more rapid cytoreduction during the induction phase. For B-cell–lineage ALL, it produced an 82% CR rate with 41% DFS at 36 months. Patients in remission receive multiagent consolidation treatment, CNS prophylaxis, late intensification, and maintenance chemotherapy for a total of 24 months. CALGB 8811 should be considered for patients, regardless of age, who are thought to be able to withstand the rigors of an intensive program.

(1) Induction.

Cyclophosphamide 1,200 mg/m^2 IV on day 1, *and*
Daunorubicin 45 mg/m^2 IV on days 1, 2, and 3, *and*
Vincristine 2 mg IV on days 1, 8, 15, and 22, *and*
Prednisone 60 mg/m^2/day PO on days 1 to 21, *and*
L-Asparaginase 6,000 IU/m^2 SC on days 5, 8, 11, 15, 18, and 22.

For patients older than 60 years:

Cyclophosphamide 800 mg/m^2 on day 1, *and*
Daunorubicin 30 mg/m^2 on days 1, 2, and 3, *and*
Prednisone 60 mg/m^2/day on days 1 to 7.

(2) Early intensification (two cycles).

IT MTX 15 mg on day 1, *and*
Cyclophosphamide 1,000 mg/m^2 IV on day 1, *and*
6-Mercaptopurine 60 mg/m^2/day PO on days 1 to 14, *and*
Cytarabine 75 mg/m^2/day SC on days 1 to 4, 8 to 11, *and*
Vincristine 2 mg IV on days 15 and 22, *and*
L-Asparaginase 6,000 U/m^2 SC on days 15, 18, 22, and 25.

(3) Central nervous system prophylaxis and interim maintenance.

Cranial irradiation 2,400 cGy on days 1 to 12, *and*
IT MTX 15 mg on days 1, 8, 15, 22, and 29, *and*
6-Mercaptopurine 60 mg/m²/day PO on days 1 to 70, *and*
MTX 20 mg/m² PO on days 36, 43, 50, 57, and 64.

(4) Late intensification.

Doxorubicin 30 mg/m² IV on days 1, 8, and 15, *and*
Vincristine 2 mg IV on days 1, 8, and 15, *and*
Dexamethasone 10 mg/m²/day PO on days 1 to 14, *and*
Cyclophosphamide 1,000 mg/m² IV on day 29, *and*
6-Thioguanine 60 mg/m²/day PO on days 29 to 42, *and*
Cytarabine 75 mg/m²/day SC on days 29 to 32 and 36 to 39.

(5) Prolonged maintenance (monthly until 24 months from diagnosis).

Vincristine 2 mg IV on day 1, *and*
Prednisone 60 mg/m²/day PO on days 1 to 5, *and*
MTX 20 mg/m² PO on days 1, 8, 15, and 22, *and*
6-Mercaptopurine 60 mg/m²/day PO on days 1 to 28.

c. Other VPD-based regimens. A number of variations on the basic VPD program have been described. VPD should be used for patients who are thought not to be able to tolerate a more intensive chemotherapy program. Some options are shown in parentheses.

(1) Induction.

Vincristine 2 mg IV on days 1, 8, 15, (22), *and*
Prednisone 40 or 60 mg/m² PO on days 1 to 28 or days 1 to 35, followed by rapid taper over 7 days, *and*
Daunorubicin 45 mg/m² IV on days 1 to 3, *and*
L-Asparaginase 500 IU/kg (18,500 IU/m²) IV on days 22 to 32.

(2) Central nervous system prophylaxis is given as six doses of IT MTX and whole-brain irradiation starting on about day 36 (see Section V.J).

(3) Maintenance for adult acute lymphoblastic leukemia. Maintenance is usually started once the marrow suppression and the oral toxicity of the CNS prophylaxis have cleared. Maintenance may be given in a pulse or a continuous manner. Although allopurinol is usually not needed after remission is achieved, the dose of 6-mercaptopurine should be decreased by 75% when given concomitantly with allopurinol.

Pulse maintenance is an 8-week cycle consisting of three courses of MTX and 6-mercaptopurine given every 2 weeks, followed by a 2-week pulse of vincristine and prednisone.

MTX 7.5 mg/m² PO on days 1 to 5, weeks 1, 3, and 5, *and*
6-Mercaptopurine 200 mg/m² PO on days 1 to 5, weeks 1, 3, and 5, *and*
Vincristine 2 mg IV on day 1, weeks 7 and 8, *and*
Prednisone 40 mg/m² PO on days 1 to 7, weeks 7 and 8.

Oral MTX should be taken in a single daily dose because splitting the daily dose significantly increases the mucositis. About three doses of IT MTX are needed once maintenance has started. The schedule should be coordinated so that the IT MTX is given on day 1 of the 5 scheduled days of oral MTX. On those days when IT MTX is given, the oral MTX is not given. Pulse maintenance is given for 3 years.

Dose adjustments for hematologic toxicity from the MTX and 6-mercaptopurine should be made based on blood cell counts obtained before the start of each course.

Dose	ANC (/μL)	Platelets (/μL)
100%	≥2,000	≥100,000
75%	1,500 to 1,999	75,000 to 99,999
50%	1,000 to 1,499	50,000 to 74,999
0%	<1,000	<50,000

(4) Intensification with cytarabine and daunorubicin given as "7 + 3" and "5 + 2" does not improve remission duration or overall survival compared with pulse maintenance in randomized, prospective trials.

2. Acute lymphoblastic leukemia in older adults. Although older patients are often considered a poor risk because of their co-morbid disease and the increased incidence of the Ph[1] chromosome, they cannot tolerate more intensive therapy. Thus, they are usually treated in the manner described above. In general, full doses of VPD-based induction protocols are used in elderly patients with ALL. Some investigators decrease the dose of vincristine by 50%. The MRC/ECOG and CALGB 8811 regimens should be considered for patients who are thought to be able to tolerate more intensive therapy.

3. Impaired cardiac function

a. Induction. Underlying cardiac disease may preclude the use of an anthracycline for induction therapy. Vincristine, prednisone, and asparaginase in the doses described above represents suboptimal therapy. An active program is **MOAD,** which is given in sequential 10-day courses (minimum three, maximum five) until remission is achieved. Once a CR has been attained, two additional courses of MOAD are given.

MTX 100 mg/m[2] IV on day 1 (increase by 50% courses 2 and 3 and by 25% each additional course until mild toxicity is achieved), *and*

Vincristine 2 mg IV on day 2, *and*

L-Asparaginase 500 IU/kg (18,500 IU/m[2]) IV infusion on day 2, *and*

Dexamethasone 6 mg/m[2]/day PO on days 1 to 10.

b. Consolidation therapy is repeated every 10 days for six courses.

MTX (final dose from induction) IV on day 1, *and*

L-Asparaginase 500 IU/kg (18,500 IU/m[2]) IV infusion on day 2.

c. Cytoreduction begins on day 30 of the last consoli-dation cycle of MTX and L-asparaginase. Cytoreduction is given monthly for 12 months.

Vincristine 2 mg IV on day 1, 30 min before MTX, *and*
MTX 100 mg/kg (3.7 g/m²) IV infusion over 6 h on day 1, *and*
Leucovorin 5 mg/kg (185 mg/m²) divided into 12 doses
    starting 2 h after the MTX infusion over days 1 to 3, *and*
Dexamethasone 6 mg/m²/day PO on days 2 to 6.

d. Maintenance begins on day 30 of the last course of cytoreduction. It is repeated monthly until relapse.

Vincristine 2 mg IV on day 1, *and*
Dexamethasone 6 mg/m²/day PO on days 1 to 5, *and*
MTX 15 mg/m² PO weekly, *and*
6-Mercaptopurine 100 mg/m² PO daily.

F.   Detection and monitoring of minimal residual dis-ease in acute lymphoblastic leukemia. Similar to AML, the aim of induction therapy in ALL is to reduce the leukemia cell population from 10^{12} cells to below the cytologic detectable level of 10^9 cells. At this point, a substantial leukemia cell burden persists (i.e., MRD) and patients relapse within months with-out subsequent therapy. As described above, standard ALL pro-tocols require approximately 2 to 3 years of systemic therapy. Patients will subsequently be followed with bone marrow exams approximately every 3 to 6 months for 2 to 3 additional years. Most ALL patients in continuous CR for 7 to 8 years are considered "cured," although late relapses have been reported. Various techniques such as PCR allow detection of approxi-mately 1 to 5 blasts/100,000 nucleated cells. Routine light mi-croscopic examination identifies approximately 5,000 blasts/ 100,000 cells. MRD is established an independent predictor of outcome in childhood ALL. One trial demonstrated the risk of relapse for children with less than 15 compared to more than 15 blasts/100,000 mononuclear cells measured by clonal PCR using Ig and T-cell receptor (TCR) gene rearrangements after induction and consolidation therapy was 4% and 47%, respec-tively ($p < 0.001$). The precise blast "cutoffs" that determine MRD and the optimal timepoint to evaluate MRD need further study. Additional detailed evaluation is warranted with MRD and adult ALL as there are varied methodologies for detecting MRD such as cytogenetics, fluorescence *in situ* hybridization, Southern blotting, immunophenotyping, and PCR techniques for Ig and TCR rearrangements or leukemia-specific chromoso-mal rearrangements, and there are limitations with specific techniques. Furthermore, large randomized studies are needed to incorporate MRD results into the treatment paradigm for adults with ALL.

G.   B-Cell acute lymphoblastic leukemia. B-Cell ALL is a rare ALL subtype constituting only 2% to 4% of cases of adult ALL. The leukemic cells are characterized by L3 morphology, by expression of monoclonal surface Ig (sIg) and by specific non-random chromosomal translocations (t[8;14] [q24;q32], t[2;8] [q12;q24], t[8;22] [q24;q11]). In the past, the results of the treat-ment of B-cell ALL in both children and adults had been poor, with a CR rate of about 35% and leukemia-free survival (LFS) of 0% to 33%. Over the last 20 years, survival rates have improved in children through the use of shorter-duration, dose-intensive systemic chemotherapy protocols and early prophylaxis/treatment of the CNS. The current pediatric studies designed specifically for B-cell ALL by the French and German study group have substantially improved the CR rate to about 90% and the LFS to 50% to 87%. The changes involve the use of higher doses and fractionation of the cyclophosphamide to expose the rapidly dividing B cells to the active alkylating metabolites of cyclophosphamide over a longer period as well as the use of high-dose MTX. These regimens are of brief duration and require no maintenance. With use of these therapeutic strategies in children as a template, clinical trials with young adults have demonstrated that short-duration, multiagent, dose-intensive chemotherapy regimens combined with aggressive CNS therapy result in long-term survival rates in nearly 70% to 80%. The German BFM group reported their experience in adapting these treatments to adults with B-cell ALL. The CR rate increased from 44% to 74%, the probability of LFS increased from 0% to 71%, and the OS rate increased from 0% to 51% when the intensive treatment was compared with a standard ALL regimen. Unfortunately, long-term DFS in older adults with Burkitt's leukemia/lymphoma remains suboptimal at 15% to 25%. Long-term outcomes in human immunodeficiency virus (HIV)–associated Burkitt's leukemia/lymphoma are improved, in part secondary to more effective chemotherapy regimens but also from enhanced HIV care.

    1. **Study B-NHL 86** consists of six alternating courses of regimens A and B.

        a. **Prephase therapy** is given to avoid tumor lysis syndrome and to correct possible metabolic abnormalities.

        Cyclophosphamide 200 mg/m^2 IV infusion over 1 h on days 1 to 5, *and*

        Prednisone 60 mg/m^2/day PO in three divided doses days 1 to 5.

        b. **Regimen A** begins 1 week after the first dose of Cytoxan.

        MTX 15 mg *plus* cytarabine 40 mg *plus* dexamethasone 4 mg IT on day 1, *and*

        Vincristine 2 mg IV on day 1, *and*

        Ifosfamide 800 mg/m^2 IV on days 1 to 5, *and*

        Teniposide 100 mg/m^2 IV on days 4 and 5, *and*

        Cytarabine 150 mg/m^2 IV every 12 h on days 4 and 5, *and*

        Dexamethasone 10 mg/m^2 PO on days 1 to 5, *and*

        MTX 150 mg/m^2 IVPB bolus over 30 min on day 1, *immediately followed by* MTX 1,350 mg/m^2 IV infusion over 23.5 h (total MTX dose is 1,500 mg/m^2 IV in 24 h), *and*

        Leucovorin rescue 30 mg/m^2 IV 36 h after the beginning of high-dose MTX infusion, *followed by* oral leucovorin 30 mg/m^2, 15 mg/m^2, and three doses of 5 mg/m^2 given at 42, 48, 54, 68, and 78 h, respectively, for an appropriate decrease in MTX levels. If the MTX level at 42 h is more

than 0.5 µmol/L (5×10^{-7} M), give leucovorin 50 mg/m²
IV every 6 h through 60 h. If the MTX level at 68 h is
more than or equal to 0.1 µmol/L (10^{-7} M), give leucovorin 30 mg/m² IV every 6 h for four more doses.

c. Regimen B.

MTX 15 mg *plus* cytarabine 40 mg *plus* dexamethasone
4 mg IT on day 1, *and*
Vincristine 2 mg IV on day 1, *and*
MTX 150 mg/m² IVPB bolus over 30 min on day 1, *then*
MTX 1,350 mg/m² IV infusion over 23.5 h (total MTX
1,500 mg/m² IV in 24 h). This is followed by leucovorin
rescue as per cycle A, *and*
Cyclophosphamide 200 mg/m² IVPB over 1 h on days 1 to
5, *and*
Doxorubicin 25 mg/m² IVP over 15 min on days 4 and 5,
and
Dexamethasone 10 mg/m² PO on days 1 to 5.

d. For patients older than 50 years, an intermediate
dose of MTX (see below) is used instead of high-dose MTX
owing to prolonged hematologic toxicity and mucositis.
   On day 1, give MTX 50 mg/m² loading dose by IVPB over
30 min, followed by MTX 450 mg/m² IV infusion over the
next 23.5 h (total MTX dose 500 mg/m²/day). This is followed by leucovorin rescue 12 mg/m² IV starting 32 h after
the beginning of MTX infusion; then repeat the same dose
every 6 h for a total of four doses. Thereafter, oral leucovorin (12 mg/m²) is given until the MTX level is less than
0.01 µM (1×10^{-8} M).
   e. Central nervous system prophylaxis. Patients in
CR after the first two cycles of chemotherapy (A and B) receive prophylactic cranial irradiation of 2,400 cGy in addition to the triple IT therapy as described above.
2. Hyper-CVAD, evaluated by the M. D. Anderson group,
uses alternating courses of chemotherapy for a total of eight
cycles to treat patients with ALL FAB L3. CR was obtained
in 21 of 26 patients (81%), with 12 of 21 patients in continuous remission at a median follow-up of 3.5 years. The 3-year
OS rate was 49% with age, anemia, and peripheral blasts
identified as independent worse prognostic factors. The overall median age of patients in this trial was 58 years with the
median age for patients under age 60 (14 patients, 54%) of 38
years. The 3-year survival rate for patients under age 60 was
77%, while that for patients over age 60 (12 patients, 46%)
was 17% ($p < 0.01$).
   a. Odd cycles (1, 3, 5, and 7).

Cyclophosphamide 300 mg/m² IV every 12 h on days 1 to
3, *and*
Mesna 600 mg/m²/day by continuous infusion, days 1 to 3,
and
Vincristine 2 mg IV on days 4 and 11, *and*
Doxorubicin 50 mg/m² IV on day 4, *and*
Dexamethasone 40 mg/day on days 1 to 4 and days 11 to 14.
IT therapy: MTX 12 mg day 2 each course, *and*

Cytarabine 100 mg day 7 each course (if CNS leukemia is present, increase therapy to twice weekly until the CSF cell count normalizes).

b. Even cycles (2, 4, 6, and 8).

MTX 1 g/m^2 IV over 24 h on day 1, *and*

Leucovorin 50 mg IV to start 12 h after MTX, then 15 mg IV every 6 h until serum MTX less than 1×10^{-8} *M, and*

Cytarabine 3 g/m^2 IV infusion over 1 h every 12 h × four doses on days 2 and 3 (reduce cytarabine dose to 1 g/m^2 for patients over 60 years old), *and*

IT therapy: MTX 12 mg day 2 each cycle, *and*

Cytarabine 100 mg day 7 each cycle (if CNS leukemia is present, increase therapy to twice weekly until the CSF cell count normalizes).

c. Maintenance therapy for 2 years.

6-Mercaptopurine 50 mg PO t.i.d., *and*

MTX 20 mg/m^2/week PO.

Incorporation of rituximab into the Hyper-CVAD treatment program was studied in a single institution study of 19 patients with newly diagnosed mature B-cell ALL or Burkitt's lymphoma (median age 50). The CR rate in 15 evaluable patients was 93%.

H. Relapsed acute lymphoblastic leukemia. Although a second remission can usually be achieved in adults with ALL, it tends to be short-lived. This is particularly true in patients treated with the contemporary intensive regimens described above. If a second remission can be attained, suitable patients with relapsed ALL should be considered as candidates for HSCT. None of the regimens used for relapse is distinctly superior to the others, and any perceived differences are likely attributable to the usual biases of study selection. Chemotherapeutic options using commercially available agents are shown.

1. "7 + 3" (cytarabine and daunorubicin) as used for the induction of AML is active in ALL. Vincristine and prednisone may be added.

2. HDAC as a single agent has modest activity in ALL, with a CR rate of about 34% and a median remission duration of 3.6 months in data from combined studies. The addition of idarubicin or mitoxantrone increases the response rate to 60%, but the median response time remains 3.4 months.

3. Cytarabine and fludarabine comprise an active noncardiotoxic combination. The median response duration is 5.5 months. Neurotoxicity is low. A second course can be given in 3 weeks if needed.

a. Induction.

Cytarabine 1 g/m^2/day IV over 2 h on days 1 to 6, *and*

Fludarabine 30 mg/m^2/day IV over 30 min 4 h before cytarabine on days 2 to 6.

b. Consolidation is given monthly for two or three courses.

Cytarabine 1 g/m^2/day IV over 2 h on days 1 to 4, *and*

Fludarabine 30 mg/m^2/day IV over 30 min 4 h before cytarabine on days 1 to 4.

c. **Maintenance.**

6-Mercaptopurine 50 mg PO t.i.d., *and*
MTX 20 mg/m²/week PO.

4. **Sequential MTX and** L-asparaginase is another option.
Stomatitis was dose limiting. Twenty-three percent of
treated patients had allergic reactions to L-asparaginase.
  a. **Induction.**

MTX 50 to 80 mg/m² IV on day 1, *and*
L-Asparaginase 20,000 IU/m² IV 3 h after MTX on day 1,
  followed by
MTX 120 mg/m² IV on day 8, *and*
L-Asparaginase 20,000 IU/m² IV on day 9.
Repeat day 8 and 9 doses for MTX and L-asparaginase
  every 7 to 14 days until remission is attained.

  b. **Maintenance** is repeated every 2 weeks.

MTX 10 to 40 mg/m² IV on day 1, *and*
L-Asparaginase 10,000 IU/m² IV on day 1.

5. **Etoposide and cytarabine** are given every 3 weeks for
up to three courses until marrow hypoplasia and remission
are achieved. They are then repeated monthly until relapse.

Etoposide 60 mg/m² IV every 12 h on days 1 to 5, *and*
Cytarabine 100 mg/m² IV bolus every 12 h on days 1 to 5.

6. **Hyper-CVAD** (see Section V.G.2).
7. **Imatinib (STI-571, Gleevec)** is a selective and potent
inhibitor of the tyrosine kinase activity of BCR/ABL that has
demonstrated significant antileukemic activity in CML.
Twenty lymphoid blast crisis and refractory adult Ph¹-positive
ALL patients were treated with STI-571 in a dose-escalating
pilot trial (300 to 1,000 mg). The overall response rate was 70%
with 20% complete hematologic remission with a decrease in
bone marrow blasts to 5% or less in 11 (55%) patients. There
was no definite correlation between STI-571 dose and response and no difference in response rates or durability of response between lymphoid blast crisis and Ph¹-positive patients.
However, duration of response was short, with a median duration of remission of 58 days (range 42 to 123 days). Major
cytogenetic response was observed in three patients. The
GMALL studied STI-571 in 59 ALL patients (median age 47,
ages 17 to 76), including 23 refractory patients. There was a
58% CR, and they demonstrated that day 14 bone marrow
predicted response. They also recognized the unusual toxicity of subdural hygroma in a significant minority of patients
in this trial. Mechanisms of STI-571 resistance, such as
amplified *BCR/ABL* gene, increased expression of BCR/ABL
protein, increase in MDR1 protein, and *BCR/ABL* gene mutations, are actively being studied. STI-571 is being evaluated
in several ALL clinical trials incorporated as a component of
front-line treatment as well as maintenance therapy.
I. **Hematopoietic stem cell transplantation in acute
lymphoblastic leukemia**
  1. **Autologous hematopoietic stem cell transplantation**
  for patients in first remission appears to offer no advantage

over chemotherapy in the small prospective trials reported to date, secondary mainly to high rates of relapse. In the large international MRC/ECOG ALL clinical trial (over 1,300 patients registered), patients in first CR without an HLA-matched sibling donor are randomized following an intensification phase with high-dose MTX to either autologous HSCT or standard consolidation/maintenance therapy. The results of this prospective, randomized trial are eagerly awaited.

2. Allogeneic matched-sibling hematopoietic stem cell transplantation (see Section I.D)

3. Matched unrelated donor hematopoietic stem cell transplantation. Less than 30% of patients in the group of patients suitable for allogeneic HSCT have an HLA-matched sibling donor. MUD HSCT is an option available to ALL patients less than 40 to 50 years of age. TRM is still high (40% to 50% at 100 days), but outcomes have been improved, in part through the use of better matching at the HLA loci with molecular methods instead of only serology. The National Marrow Donor Program reported on 127 poor-risk ALL patients (defined as presence of t[9;22], t[4;11], or t[1;19]) who received a MUD HSCT between 1988 and 1999. The cumulative TRM incidence at 2 years was 61% (54% in first CR, 75% in second CR, and 64% in primary induction failure), while the OS at 2 years from transplant was 40%, 17%, and 5%, respectively. The DFS for patients transplanted in CR1 was 32% at 4 years with a 13% cumulative incidence of relapse for this group of patients. For Ph[1]-positive patients in first CR, we advocate MUD HSCT for fit patients if a matched-sibling donor is not available.

4. Alternative-donor hematopoietic stem cell transplantation. Mismatched family member and haploidentical HSCTs have been evaluated and are options, but these procedures should still be considered experimental in ALL.

5. Relapse after hematopoietic stem cell transplantation. Although up to 50% of patients can attain another remission with reinduction chemotherapy (vincristine and prednisone plus daunorubicin and/or L-asparaginase), fewer than 5% to 10% are leukemia-free after 3 years. If a second remission can be attained with chemotherapy, a second allogeneic HSCT may improve survival, especially in those who have relapsed more than 1 year after the initial transplantation. Nonmyeloablative HSCT procedures or use of donor lymphocyte infusions alone have been largely ineffective owing to lack of GVL effect in ALL, although further study incorporating higher ablative chemotherapy dosing is warranted. Results of autologous HSCT for relapsed ALL have been disappointing with high relapse rates.

J. Central nervous system prophylaxis. In the era before prophylaxis of the CNS, more than half of children and adults experienced relapse solely in the CNS. Treatment of the CNS sanctuary after a CR has been attained has dramatically decreased the risk of CNS relapse. The timing of CNS prophylaxis depends on the intensity of postremission therapy and the perceived risk of developing CNS leukemia. Two equivalent options exist:

1. Cranial irradiation and intrathecal methotrexate. Cranial irradiation with IT MTX has been the classic method of CNS prophylaxis. It has usually been initiated within 2 weeks of attaining a CR when classic maintenance is given.

a. Cranial irradiation is usually given to the cranial vault (anteriorly to the posterior pole of the eye and posteriorly to C2) in 0.2-Gy fractions for a total of 18 to 24 Gy. The spine is not irradiated because marrow toxicity significantly limits the ability to give further chemotherapy. Common acute complications of radiation include stomatitis, parotitis, alopecia, marrow suppression, and headaches. Long-term complications include dental caries. Like children, young adults may develop learning disorders, impaired growth, and leukoencephalopathy.

b. Intrathecal methotrexate. MTX is used instead of radiation therapy for prophylaxis of the spinal cord. A commonly used program is 12 mg/m^2 (maximum 15 mg) of preservative-free MTX diluted in preservative-free saline or Elliot's B solution given IT once a week for 6 weeks. Some investigators also give 10 mg of hydrocortisone succinate IT to try to prevent lumbar arachnoiditis because the latter may limit the ability to give all six of the planned doses of intrathecal MTX. After cerebrospinal fluid (CSF) is obtained for appropriate studies, 5 mL of CSF is withdrawn into a syringe containing MTX diluted in 10 mL of vehicle. This produces a final MTX concentration of 1 mg/mL or less (higher concentrations increase the risk of arachnoiditis). The IT MTX is then given in an "in-and-out" manner. One to 2 mL of the MTX solution is injected into the spinal canal. Then, 0.5 to 1 mL of spinal fluid is withdrawn back into the syringe. This in-and-out process is repeated until all of the MTX has been given. This method is used to ensure that the MTX is actually given into the subarachnoid space. Leucovorin 5 to 10 mg may be given orally every 6 h for four to eight doses to ameliorate the mucositis, although this usually is not needed unless the patient is receiving concurrent systemic MTX. Complications of MTX include chemical arachnoiditis and leukoencephalopathy.

2. Chemoprophylaxis. Given the toxicity of whole-brain irradiation in patients younger than 25 years, other strategies of CNS prophylaxis have been developed. The combination of systemic intermediate- to high-dose MTX with IT MTX is considered to be as effective as cranial irradiation with IT MTX. HDAC used for intensification is also an active adjunct to IT MTX. The incorporation of either or both high-dose MTX and HDAC may make cranial irradiation less important.

K. Experimental strategies for acute lymphoblastic leukemia. Blast cells express various antigens including CD20 and CD 22 in precursor and mature B-cell ALL and CD52 in subsets of T-cell ALL. Monoclonal antibodies under study alone or in combination in ALL include rituximab (anti-CD20), anti-B4-bR (anti-CD19), B43-PAP (anti-CD19), anti-CD22, genistein (anti-CD19), anti-CD-7-ricin, and anti-CD52 (Campath-1H). Further studies are underway to evaluate the overall response and durability of response to the tyrosine kinase inhibitor STI-571. Other small-molecule inhibitors including FTIs will continue to be evaluated. The detection and importance of MRD will continue to be examined in adult ALL. Other therapeutic agents including ara-G (506U78) and purine analogs will continue to be studied all in order to continue to improve outcomes of adult ALL.

VI. Management problems. Although patients receiving therapy for acute leukemia often have a "predictable" course, certain clinical manifestations require further individualization of the therapeutic approach.

A. Central nervous system leukemia. Leukemic involvement of the CNS bodes poorly for the adult with acute leukemia, given the morbidity of the associated neurologic dysfunction, the inability to control CNS leukemia on a long-term basis, and the common association with active marrow disease. CNS involvement occurs most frequently with hyperleukocytosis and with the monoblastic, mature B-cell (Burkitt's), and T-cell lymphoblastic leukemias.

1. Diagnosis. The occurrence of CNS involvement in ALL at diagnosis is well recognized. In ALL patients with high peripheral blast counts and no CNS symptoms, it is usually prudent to perform the lumbar puncture after chemotherapy has decreased the blast count and blasts have been eradicated from the peripheral blood. In this way, contamination of the CSF specimen in the event of a traumatic lumbar puncture is prevented. Common clinical features of CNS leukemia (in ALL and AML) include headache, altered sensorium, and cranial nerve palsy (especially cranial nerve VI). Features suggestive of CNS involvement indicate the need for an immediate lumbar puncture because neurologic dysfunction is most amenable to therapy within the first 24 h and infectious meningitis must be excluded in the immunocompromised host. The diagnosis of CNS leukemia is made by finding five or more blast cells on a cytospin preparation of 1 mL of CSF. Essentially all patients with CNS leukemia have an elevated CSF protein level as well; however, in the absence of infection, elevated protein by itself is suggestive, but not diagnostic, of CNS leukemia.

2. Treatment. Although the therapy for CNS leukemia is usually only palliative, it should be initiated as soon as possible. The rapid initiation of therapy may reverse or prevent cranial nerve palsies, which are a morbid complication for both patients and caretakers. Treatment of CNS leukemia is usually concomitant with cranial irradiation and IT chemotherapy. Cranial irradiation is usually given to a total of 30 Gy in 1.5- to 2-Gy fractions. IT chemotherapy is given in the manner described for CNS prophylaxis (see Section V.J). IT chemotherapy is repeated every 3 to 4 days, with appropriate laboratory studies being done with each lumbar puncture. When blast cells are no longer seen on the cytospin preparation, two more doses of IT drug are given, usually followed by a monthly "maintenance" IT injection. IT MTX 12 mg/m^2 (maximum 15 mg) is most commonly used for ALL. Oral leucovorin 5 to

10 mg PO every 6 h for four to eight doses, starting at the time of the lumbar puncture, may be added to decrease systemic toxicity. Cytarabine 50 mg given IT is most commonly used for AML. The addition of 10 mg of IT hydrocortisone succinate may ameliorate chemical arachnoiditis and have some antileukemic effect as well. Some investigators advocate instilling IT cytarabine and MTX at the same time or alternating doses of cytarabine and MTX. Some advocate the routine use of an intraventricular reservoir for treating patients with CNS leukemia. The use of systemic therapy with high-dose cytarabine 1 to 3 g/m^2 IV infusion over 2 h every 12 h is also effective for the treatment of CNS leukemia. A practical approach is to initiate IT chemotherapy until the time that the HDAC is started. Further IT therapy can then be given based on the results of subsequent CSF analysis after the HDAC is completed. A slow-release formulation of cytarabine (DepoCyt) that maintains cytotoxic concentrations for approximately 14 days has been demonstrated to be effective for the treatment of lymphomatous meningitis and solid tumors and is under evaluation in acute leukemia.

B. Hyperleukocytosis (absolute blast counts of more than 100,000/µL) predisposes to rheologic problems.

    1. Leukostasis (vascular plugging) occurs almost exclusively with AML. Cerebral and cardiopulmonary dysfunction due to vascular obstruction, vessel wall necrosis with hemorrhage, or both are the most common clinical manifestations. Hyperleukocytosis is an oncologic emergency. Given the increased risk of early death with hyperleukocytosis, therapy should be rapidly initiated as soon as the diagnosis is made. If the patient is hemodynamically stable, leukapheresis is the most rapid way to lower the blast count. The goal of the leukapheresis session is to lower the blast count to less than 100,000/µL if possible. With very high blast counts (more than 200,000/µL), decreasing the blast count by 50% may have to be the initial goal because mathematic modeling suggests that prolonged leukapheresis after a "3-L exchange" does not significantly decrease the blast count further. Leukapheresis may be repeated daily. Systemic chemotherapy should be initiated immediately after emergent leukapheresis or if leukapheresis cannot be performed. Hydroxyurea 3 to 5 g/m^2/day split into three doses daily is most commonly used. Hydroxyurea is stopped at the time more specific induction chemotherapy is initiated. In patients presenting with hyperleukocytosis, an allopurinol dose of 600 mg b.i.d. is well tolerated for the first 2 days, followed by 300 mg b.i.d. for 2 to 3 days. Emergent cranial radiation for hyperleukocytosis and cranial nerve palsies (or other severe neurologic deficit) is another treatment modality that may be used.

    2. Hyperviscosity. Blood viscosity increases as the blast count rises. Fortunately, concomitant anemia produces a decrease in viscosity. Aggressive packed RBC (PRBC) transfusion in patients with hyperleukocytosis may precipitate symptoms of hyperviscosity. PRBC transfusions should be used judiciously (e.g., 1 U at a time until symptoms of anemia resolve), with a blast count of more than 200,000/μL, especially in patients with AML. Unless the patient has symptoms due to anemia, a packed cell volume (hematocrit) of 20% to 25% is a reasonable goal.

C. Extramedullary leukemia. Infiltration of organs outside the marrow may occur with acute leukemia. Diffuse organ infiltration (e.g., multiple skin nodules/leukemia cutis and gum infiltration with acute monoblastic leukemia) is best treated with systemic chemotherapy. Testicular involvement can occur in less than 5% of adults with acute leukemia and is most commonly seen with Ph[1]-positive ALL. Isolated accumulations of leukemic cells may occur with AML (granulocyte sarcoma, chloroma) and less often with ALL (lymphoblastoma). These foci are best treated with local irradiation at curative doses (30 Gy). Although most commonly associated with active marrow disease, chloromas and lymphoblastomas may occur as a sole site of relapse or as an initial presentation in association with a normal bone marrow. In either case, they universally herald the subsequent development of leukemic infiltration of the bone marrow. An intuitive approach is to treat these patients with "adjuvant" induction chemotherapy.

VII. Growth factors. Several randomized trials have recently been completed evaluating the effect of hematopoietic growth factors (G-CSF, GM-CSF) as adjuncts to the treatment of patients with AML. Most studies have shown a 2- to 6-day reduction in the duration of severe neutropenia. There has been no evidence for a selective advantage for regrowth of the leukemia clone when growth factors are given before marrow hypoplasia is achieved. The CALGB conducted a double-blinded trial in ALL, randomizing 198 patients to placebo or G-CSF (5 μg/kg/day) at day 4 of induction. For patients treated with G-CSF, there was a shorter time to neutrophil recovery with induction (16 versus 22 days; $p = 0.001$) and consolidation treatment, a reduced number of hospital days from 22 to 28 ($p = 0.02$), and a higher CR rate with induction therapy (90% versus 81%; $p = 0.10$), especially in patients over age 60 (81% versus 55%; $p = 0.10$). However, in this trial and others, there was no long-term benefit as measured by improvement in DFS or OS. Similar data have been reported with AML induction and consolidation therapy with reductions in duration of neutropenia and potentially fewer hospital days, but there have been no consistent data for superior long-term outcomes. Furthermore, there appears to be no role at this time for the priming of leukemia cells by growth factors to enhance the effect of chemotherapy. It is clear that growth factors administered after consolidation chemotherapy can shorten the duration of neutropenia, without a significant effect on treatment outcome. The use of growth factor can be cost saving if patients are hospitalized only for chemotherapy administration or for serious complications during the neutropenic period. Consolidation chemotherapy followed by growth factor support can be administered on an outpatient basis, with less than half of patients being readmitted to the hospital for neutropenic fever. A long-acting pegalated growth factor (pegfilgrastim) that utilizes a "self-regulating" function for clearance allowing for one-time dosing has been approved and warrants study in hematologic malignancies.

SELECTED READINGS

Annino L, Vegna ML, et al. Treatment of adult acute lymphoblastic leukemia (ALL): long-term follow- up of the GIMEMA ALL 0288 randomized study. *Blood* 2002;99:863–71.

Appelbaum FR, Rowe JM, Radich J, et al. Acute myeloid leukemia. In: Schecter GP, Broudy VC, Williams ME, eds. *Hematology 2001: the American Society of Hematology education program book.* Washington, D.C.: American Society of Hematology, 2001:62–77 (available at http://www.hematology.org).

Bloomfield CD, Lawrence D, et al. Frequency of prolonged remission duration after high-dose cytarabine intensification in acute myeloid leukemia varies by cytogenetic subtype. *Cancer Res* 1998; 58:4173–4179.

Byrd JC, Dodge RK, et al. Patients with t(8;21)(q22;q22) and acute myeloid leukemia have superior failure-free and overall survival when repetitive cycles of high-dose cytarabine are administered. *J Clin Oncol* 1999;17:3767–3675.

Camacho LH, Soignet SL, et al. Leukocytosis and the retinoic acid syndrome in patients with acute promyelocytic leukemia treated with arsenic trioxide. *J Clin Oncol* 2000;18:2620–2625.

Cassileth PA, Harrington DP, et al. Chemotherapy compared with autologous or allogeneic bone marrow transplantation in the management of acute myeloid leukemia in first remission. *N Engl J Med* 1998;339:1649–1656.

Cornelissen JJ, Carston M, et al. Unrelated marrow transplantation for adult patients with poor-risk acute lymphoblastic leukemia: strong graft-versus-leukemia effect and risk factors determining outcome. *Blood* 2001;97:1572–1577.

Druker BJ, Sawyers CL, et al. Activity of a specific inhibitor of the BCR-ABL tyrosine kinase in the blast crisis of chronic myeloid leukemia and acute lymphoblastic leukemia with the Philadelphia chromosome. *N Engl J Med* 2001;344:1038–1042.

Estey E. Treatment of refractory AML. *Leukemia* 1996;10:932–936.

Fenaux P, Chastang C, et al. A randomized comparison of all trans-retinoic acid (ATRA) followed by chemotherapy and ATRA plus chemotherapy and the role of maintenance therapy in newly diagnosed acute promyelocytic leukemia. The European APL Group. *Blood* 1999;94:1192–1200.

Giralt S, Thall PF, et al. Melphalan and purine analog-containing preparative regimens: reduced-intensity conditioning for patients with hematologic malignancies undergoing allogeneic progenitor cell transplantation. *Blood* 2001;97:631–637.

Grimwade D, Walker H, et al. The importance of diagnostic cytogenetics on outcome in AML: analysis of 1,612 patients entered into the MRC AML 10 trial. The Medical Research Council Adult and Children's Leukaemia Working Parties. *Blood* 1998;92:2322–2333.

Grimwade D, Walker H, et al. The predictive value of hierarchical cytogenetic classification in older adults with acute myeloid leukemia (AML): analysis of 1065 patients entered into the United Kingdom Medical Research Council AML11 trial. *Blood* 2001;98:1312–1320.

Harris NL, Jaffe ES, et al. World Health Organization classification of neoplastic diseases of the hematopoietic and lymphoid tissues: report of the Clinical Advisory Committee meeting—Airlie House, Virginia, November 1997. *J Clin Oncol* 1999;17:3835–3849.

Hoelzer D, Ludwig WD, et al. Improved outcome in adult B-cell acute lymphoblastic leukemia. *Blood* 1996;87:495–508.

Koller CA, Kantarjian HM, et al. The hyper-CVAD regimen improves outcome in relapsed acute lymphoblastic leukemia. *Leukemia* 1997;11:2039–2044.

Larson RA, Dodge RK, et al. A five-drug remission induction regimen with intensive consolidation for adults with acute lymphoblastic leukemia: cancer and leukemia group B study 8811. *Blood* 1995;85: 2025–2037.

Larson RA, Stock W, Hoelzer DF, et al. Acute lymphoblastic leukemia in adults. *Hematology 1998: the American Society of Hematology education program book*. Washington, D.C.: American Society of Hematology, 1988:44–62 (available at http://www.hematology.org).

Linker C, Damon L, et al. Intensified and shortened cyclical chemotherapy for adult acute lymphoblastic leukemia. *J Clin Oncol* 2002;20:2464–2471.

List AF, Kopecky KJ, et al. Benefit of cyclosporine modulation of drug resistance in patients with poor-risk acute myeloid leukemia: a Southwest Oncology Group study. *Blood* 2001;98:3212–3220.

Lowenberg B, Downing JR, et al. Acute myeloid leukemia. *N Engl J Med* 1999;341:1051–1062.

Mayer RJ, Davis RB, et al. Intensive postremission chemotherapy in adults with acute myeloid leukemia. Cancer and Leukemia Group B. *N Engl J Med* 1994;331:896–903.

Mortuza FY, Papaioannou M, et al. Minimal residual disease tests provide an independent predictor of clinical outcome in adult acute lymphoblastic leukemia. *J Clin Oncol* 2002;20:1094–1104.

Nguyen S, Leblanc T, et al. A white blood cell index as the main prognostic factor in t(8;21) acute myeloid leukemia (AML): a survey of 161 cases from the French AML Intergroup. *Blood* 2002;99: 3517–3523.

Ozer H, Armitage JO, et al. 2000 update of recommendations for the use of hematopoietic colony-stimulating factors: evidence-based, clinical practice guidelines. American Society of Clinical Oncology Growth Factors Expert Panel. *J Clin Oncol* 2000;18:3558–3585.

Pui CH, Evans WE. Acute lymphoblastic leukemia. *N Engl J Med* 1998;339:605–615.

Pui CH, Heslop HE, Hoelzer D. Advances in pediatric and adult acute lymphoblastic leukemia. In: *Oncology 2002: the American Society of Clinical Oncology 2002 education book*. Alexandria, VA: American Society of Clinical Oncology, 2002:32–57 (available at http://www.asco.org).

Secker-Walker LM, Prentice HG, et al. Cytogenetics adds independent prognostic information in adults with acute lymphoblastic leukaemia on MRC trial UKALL XA. MRC Adult Leukaemia Working Party. *Br J Haematol* 1997;96:601–610.

Sievers EL, Larson RA, et al. Efficacy and safety of gemtuzumab ozogamicin in patients with CD33- positive acute myeloid leukemia in first relapse. *J Clin Oncol* 2001;19:3244–3254.

Slovak ML, Kopecky KJ, et al. Karyotypic analysis predicts outcome of preremission and postremission therapy in adult acute myeloid leukemia: a Southwest Oncology Group/Eastern Cooperative Oncology Group Study. *Blood* 2000;96:4075–4083.

Stone RM. Postremission therapy in adults with acute myeloid leukemia. *Semin Hematol* 2001;38(suppl 6):17–23.

Tallman MS, Andersen JW, et al. Clinical description of 44 patients with acute promyelocytic leukemia who developed the retinoic acid syndrome. *Blood* 2000;95:90–95.

Tallman MS, Nabhan C, et al. Acute promyelocytic leukemia: evolving therapeutic strategies. *Blood* 2002;99:759–767.

Weick JK, Kopecky KJ, et al. A randomized investigation of high-dose versus standard-dose cytosine arabinoside with daunorubicin in patients with previously untreated acute myeloid leukemia: a Southwest Oncology Group study. *Blood* 1996;88:2841–2851.

Wetzler M, Dodge RK, et al. Prospective karyotype analysis in adult acute lymphoblastic leukemia: the Cancer and Leukemia Group B experience. *Blood* 1999;93:3983–3993.

19

Chronic Leukemias

Peter White

The chronic leukemias have traditionally been grouped together to underscore their differences from the more aggressive acute leukemias, but their course is not necessarily indolent; paradoxically, the possibility for achieving cure of these disorders has been more limited than with some acute leukemias. There is increasing optimism regarding both responsiveness and possible cure, however, due to the emergence of specific molecularly targeted therapy and improved techniques for stem cell transplantation (SCT).

I. Chronic myelogenous leukemia

A. Epidemiology and pathogenesis. Chronic myelogenous leukemia (CML) is a relatively uncommon disorder, accounting for 15% of adult leukemias in the United States. It is quite uncommon in childhood, but incidence increases throughout the succeeding decades, with median age at diagnosis 53 years. Approximately 30% of cases are over 60 years of age at diagnosis. Incidence in males is 1.3 times that in females.

The pathognomonic finding is the so-called Philadelphia (Ph) chromosome, involving translocation between chromosomes 9 and 22, t (9; 22) (q34;q11), resulting in a hybrid *BCR-ABL* gene. The fusion protein encoded by this gene, also known as the BCR-ABL protein, functions as a permanently switched-on tyrosine kinase in the signal transduction pathway for cellular proliferation. Thus, the Ph chromosome confers a proliferative advantage to the hematopoietic cells carrying this translocation. Evidence supports the notion that the Ph chromosome arises in a pluripotential stem cell so that progeny in all three myeloid series (erythroid, granulocytic, megakaryocytic) carry the Ph chromosome; in some cases, lymphoid precursors are also involved. The Ph chromosome can be identified by standard cytogenetic techniques in 95% of CML patients. In many of the remaining 5%, the *BCR-ABL* hybrid gene can be demonstrated utilizing molecular techniques such as fluorescence *in situ* hybridization (FISH), which can be performed on interphase (nonmitosing) cells in peripheral blood. Patients who are truly Ph⁻ constitute a heterogeneous group including those with chronic myelomonocytic leukemia (usually considered as one of the myelodysplastic syndromes; see Chapter 20) and chronic neutrophilic leukemia, a rare clonal myeloproliferative disorder of the elderly. In contrast to CML, these Ph⁻ patients lack basophilia and have elevated neutrophil alkaline phosphatase activity.

In addition to the proliferative advantages conferred by the Ph chromosome, there is also inhibition of apoptosis and altered adhesive properties of the Ph clone. Unlike acute leukemia, however, there is no apparent inhibition in cellular differentiation, so that the Ph progeny mature in an essentially normal fashion and exhibit essentially normal phagocytic and bactericidal function. For reasons that are not well understood, however, the Ph chromosome confers genomic instability, and virtually all CML cases undergo evolution to acute leukemia, usually accompanied by additional chromosomal abnormalities. This evolutionary process can be divided into three fairly distinct phases:

1. Chronic phase. Eighty-five percent of patients present at diagnosis with the so-called chronic phase. This is marked by immature myeloid cells in the peripheral blood and marked granulocytic hyperplasia in the marrow, but myeloblasts are less than 10% in both peripheral blood and bone marrow. Absolute eosinophilia and basophilia are typically present (in contrast to reactive leukocytosis). The chronic phase typically runs an indolent course of 3 to 5 years before progressing to the accelerated phase.

2. Accelerated phase. This is marked by one or more of the following: Peripheral blood blasts more than or equal to 15%, peripheral blasts plus promyelocytes greater than 30%, peripheral blood basophils greater than 20%, platelet count less than or equal to 100,000/µL, or new chromosomal abnormalities (in addition to persisting Ph chromosome). These laboratory findings are often accompanied by symptoms such as fever, bone pain, and fatigue, worsening splenomegaly and anemia, and less responsiveness to therapy.

3. Blast phase. The blast phase is defined by 30% or more blasts in marrow or peripheral blood. This is essentially acute leukemia, with 50% of cases showing myeloid phenotype (AML), 25% lymphoid (ALL), and 25% mixed. Persistence of the Ph chromosome again indicates evolution from the original clone, regardless of myeloid versus lymphoid morphology. Extramedullary tumor masses (chloromas) are not uncommon. Response to chemotherapy, using various acute leukemia regimens, is typically poor, and median survival in blast phase is 3 to 6 months.

Separation of these three stages is imprecise, and approximately 25% of patients progress directly from chronic phase to blast phase. Moreover, the duration of the chronic phase is difficult to predict, although a number of factors have been identified that indicate increased risk for progression. These include greater age, splenomegaly, elevated platelet counts, and higher numbers of peripheral blood myeloblasts, eosinophils, or basophils. One formulation of these factors to predict risk can be accessed on line at http://www.pharmacoepi.de/cmlscore.html (Hasford score). These scores are intended to predict survival based on findings at diagnosis. In addition, important prognostic information emerges (after hematologic remission has been achieved) by assessing cytogenetic response, that is, percentage decrease in Ph+ cells in marrow. With use of such formulations, low-risk groups have been identified with median survival of approximately 100 months versus high-risk groups with median survival of 45 months. Risk assessment is assuming increased importance in deciding between early and delayed SCT.

B. Diagnosis. CML patients presenting in chronic phase characteristically have leukocytosis of greater than 25,000/µL, with granulocytes in all stages of maturation, but with blasts at less than 10%. Increased eosinophils and basophils are also almost invariably present. Absolute lymphocyte count is often modestly elevated, owing to increased T cells. Platelet count is increased in approximately 50% of patients, and platelet dysfunction is occasionally seen. Mild to moderate anemia is common, with normal red cell morphology except for occasional nucleated red blood cells (RBCs). Bone marrow is markedly hypercellular owing to myeloid hyperplasia, but dysplastic features are minimal. Maturation proceeds in an orderly fashion, and blasts are less than 10%. A minor increase in reticulin fibrosis is common, but when severe, confusion with agnogenic myeloid metaplasia may result (see Chapter 20). In older reports, splenomegaly has been present in 90% of patients with diagnosis, but this is less often so in asymptomatic cases picked up on routine blood counts.

Leukocyte alkaline phosphatase score is usually markedly decreased in contrast to secondary leukocytosis ("leukemoid reactions") seen in infections and inflammatory stores; basophilia and eosinophilia are also lacking in the latter states. A key element for diagnosis is demonstration of the Ph chromosome, either by cytogenetics, FISH, or molecular techniques utilizing polymerase chain reaction (PCR) to confirm the presence of the BCR-ABL fusion protein.

C.   Therapy. Treatment of CML is currently in a state of flux, following the dramatic results of imatinib mesylate (Gleevec; formerly known as STI-571), the newly developed selective inhibitor of BCR-ABL tyrosine kinase activity. While early results are highly promising, it remains to be demonstrated that durable remissions and survival benefits are achieved, and it seems likely that optimal therapy will involve combinations of imatinib mesylate with other agents such as interferon (IFN).

1.   Stem cell transplants. Allogeneic SCT (allo-SCT) offers the only documented avenue for cure of CML at the present time. Graft-versus-leukemia effect appears crucial in eradicating the Ph clone and achieving cure; autologous SCT has thus far shown uncertain benefit but may prolong life for patients in chronic phase. It is not clear whether donor stem cells harvested directly from bone marrow are preferable to "mobilized" peripheral blood stem cells. The latter tend to produce more severe graft-versus-host disease but a lower relapse rate. Unfortunately, owing to lack of appropriate human leukocyte antigen (HLA)–matched donors (sibling or unrelated) and the advanced age of many patients (older than 55 years), only 20% of CML patients are suitable candidates for allo-SCT. Nonmyeloablative SCT holds some promise in allowing older patients to survive the rigors of transplantation but is still investigational, as is the use of umbilical cord blood stem cells from unrelated donors.

Timely referral of patients for transplant is important, since optimal results and minimal risk of relapse are seen with transplants performed in the chronic phase within 12 months following diagnosis. Survival and risk of relapse are significantly worse for patients transplanted in accelerated phase or blast crisis. Other important risk factors for survival that have proved useful in devising a prognostic score for SCT include patient age (under 20 years optimal), sex (female donor for male recipient unfavorable), and donor type (HLA-identical sibling better than unrelated donor). For chronic-phase patients who relapse following SCT, infusion of T lymphocytes from the original donor will re-establish complete remission (CR) in up to 75% of cases. Long-term leukemia-free survival rates are 60% to 80% for sibling SCT versus 40% to 60% with unrelated donors. Transplant-related mortality has been as low as 10% in certain highly favorable prognostic groups. Older patients in accelerated phase or blast crisis have transplant-related mortality in the 60% to 70% range, with high risk of subsequent relapse, and leukemia-free survival of less than 20% after 5 years.

2.   Imatinib mesylate (Gleevec). This agent, which is a selective inhibitor of the tyrosine kinase signal activity of BCR-ABL that blocks proliferation and induces apoptosis of Ph$^+$ progenitor cells, has been approved by the U.S. Food and Drug Administration (FDA) for use in Ph$^+$ CML in chronic phase and in accelerated phase or blast crisis of CML. Based on outstanding hemologic and cytogenic responses, its use as front-line therapy in newly diagnosed chronic-phase CML is now widely practiced. Prospective Phase III trials to more clearly define its role as first-line therapy are ongoing, with preliminary results showing superiority to IFN in rapidity of hematologic response, with higher rates of cytogenetic response as well. As imatinib mesylate's long-term efficacy, safety, and potential for cure become clarified, current treatment strategies for CML may well undergo dramatic revision. In chronic-phase CML patients failing IFN, imatinib mesylate has produced hematologic response in 91% of cases, with complete cytogenetic responses (i.e., 0% Ph$^+$ cells) in 36% and partial cytogenetic responses (35% or fewer Ph$^+$ cells) in an additional 19% of cases, with these responses durable in virtually all cases at 1 year. In accelerated phase and blast crisis, response rates have been significantly lower and relapses frequent, though cytogenetic responses (partial or complete) were achieved in roughly 20%.

The recommended starting dose is as follows:

*   **Imatinib mesylate** 400 mg PO daily for chronic phase and 600 mg PO daily for accelerated or blast phase, taken as a single daily dose with food.

There is no dose adjustment for age or weight. Safety in renal failure or hepatic dysfunction is uncertain, but there is negligible excretion via the kidney, and metabolism is primarily via hepatic enzymes of the cytochrome P-450 system. Interactions with other medications utilizing the P-450 system (e.g., warfarin, phenytoin) are a potential problem. Drugs with potential hepatotoxicity should also be avoided. Hepatotoxicity has been attributed to imatinib mesylate itself in a small percentage of cases, and liver chemistries should be monitored every 2 to 4 weeks. Imatinib mesylate is well tolerated symptomatically, but low-grade nausea, muscle cramps, edema, and diarrhea are relatively frequent. Tumor lysis syndrome is rare, but allopurinol coverage is advisable. Myelosuppression is common, with grade 4 neutropenia seen in 35%

to 50% of the patients in accelerated or blast phase. Complete blood counts (CBCs) should be checked weekly × 4, then every 2 to 4 weeks if the absolute neutrophil count (ANC) is over 1,500/µL and platelets over 100,000/µL. In patients with cytopenias due to previous therapy (e.g., IFN), imatinib mesylate should be deferred until counts have normalized. Imatinib mesylate should be discontinued in chronic-phase patients if ANC is less than 1,000/mL or platelets less than 50,000/mL; reduction in dosage to 300 mg daily can be considered if counts are slow to recover. Dose escalation to 800 mg daily can also be considered for patients not showing expected hematologic or cytogenetic response. Monitoring by conventional cytogenetics and FISH is recommended every 6 months.

3. Interferon-α. Its precise mechanism of action in CML is unknown, but IFN-α produces a hematologic response in approximately 80% of patients (complete in 50%) and major cytogenetic response (less than 35% Ph⁺ cells) in 10% to 20% of the cases. Responses are significantly better in low-risk patients than high risk (see above for risk scores). Meta-analysis of several IFN-α trials has shown 5-year survival of 57%, a significant improvement over the 46% survival seen with hydroxyurea, which rarely shows significant cytogenetic response. IFN-α patients who achieve complete cytogenetic response have been projected to have 70% 10-year survival. Optimal dose is not established, but a common dosage is as follows:

- **IFN-α** 5×10^6 U/m²/day. Lower doses may be given initially (e.g., 3×10^6 U three times per week) to lessen toxicity, and hydroxyurea (plus allopurinol) may be helpful at the outset for rapid control of markedly elevated white blood cell count (WBC).

Adverse effects are common and multiple and are detailed in Chapter 4. Fever, fatigue, nausea, and headache are seen early; premedication with acetaminophen and evening dosing may be helpful. Later effects include depression, insomnia, neurotoxicity, myelosuppression, and hepatic and renal dysfunction. Toxicities are more common in the elderly, for whom hydroxyurea may be more appropriate. Early reports suggest pegylated IFN is better tolerated and has similar efficacy in addition to the convenience of once-weekly injections.

There are no formal guidelines for duration of treatment, but it is reasonable to discontinue IFN-α if complete or near-complete hematologic response (normalization of CBC) is not achieved after 6 months or if there is no significant cytogenetic response after 12 months. For those who achieve complete or near-complete cytogenetic response, IFN-α can be continued indefinitely, utilizing a maintenance dose (e.g., 3×10^6 U three times per week). Monitoring cytogenetic response on a regular basis is recommended, utilizing both conventional cytogenetic and molecular techniques such as FISH or PCR for detection of *BCR-ABL.*

4. Interferon-α with low-dose cytosine arabinoside. In randomized French and Italian studies, greater cytogenetic response in CML patients has been reported when IFN-α is combined with cytosine arabinoside, given SC at either 20 or 40 mg/m^2/day for 10 consecutive days each month. Scheduled IFN-α dose was 5×10^6 U/m^2/day (though actual doses received were significantly lower). It seems reasonable to expect that increase in cytogenetic response will translate into improved survival, but this is not established. Adverse effects were somewhat higher with this two-drug combination but acceptable.

5. Hydroxyurea. Often referred to as "conventional" chemotherapy but largely replaced by IFN-α in the last decade, hydroxyurea provides rapid hematologic response and is useful for initial control of markedly elevated WBC. Starting doses can be as follows:

*   **Hydroxyurea** 3 to 5 g PO daily, with allopurinol.

It is also useful in patients who are intolerant or refractory to IFN-α and in the elderly. Usual maintenance dose is 500 to 2,000 mg/day, adjusted to keep WBC in the range of 5,000 to 15,000/μL. Hydroxyurea is well tolerated, with rapidly reversible myelosuppression as its major side effect. It rarely produces cytogenetic response and has only minimal impact on progression to accelerated phase or on survival.

6. Busulfan. Now used mostly as a second-line agent following IFN-α and/or hydroxyurea, busulfan has slow onset and can produce prolonged myelosuppression as well as pulmonary fibrosis and other chronic toxicities. Starting dose for *de novo* treatment of CML is as follows:

*   **Busulfan** 4 to 6 mg PO daily. Stop when WBC falls to 20,000 to 30,000/μL. Maintenance dose is variable—may be as low as 2 to 4 mg/week.

7. Algorithms for treatment. Overall strategies to optimize treatment for CML will undoubtedly undergo revision over the next several years, as data accrue on the durability of clinical and cytogenetic responses to imatinib mesylate. At present, it seems best to proceed on the assumption that allo-SCT offers the only realistic route to cure. The problem then is to balance the risk of progression to advanced phase (e.g., utilizing the Sokal or Hasford score) against the risks of transplant-related mortality as indicated by age, stage, donor type, etc. One tentative scheme proposes categorizing the patients into three groups:

*   **Group 1: early transplant recommended.** These include patients with the following characteristics:
    (a)   Age less than 35 years, favorable Hasford score, HLA-matched sibling donor available; or
    (b)   Age less than 25 years, favorable Hasford score, unrelated donor available (molecularly matched by deoxyribonucleic acid [DNA]–based techniques); or
    (c)   Age less than 45 years, unfavorable Hasford score with sibling donor; or
    (d)   Age less than 35 years, unfavorable Hasford score with unrelated donor.

*   **Group 2: delay recommended for transplant.** Patients perceived to be at higher risk for transplant-related mor-

tality, not meeting criteria for Group 1, can reasonably be placed on imatinib mesylate or IFN-α and assessed periodically for response. Those failing to achieve targeted goals of cytogenetic response would then be offered transplant. There is no precise definition of the appropriate target, but lack of major cytogenetic response at 6 or 12 months or relapse of Ph^+ cells following initial response would reasonably be called a failure.

- **Group 3: not a transplant candidate.** Patients without suitable donors (approximately 70% of CML patients, unfortunately) and those with unacceptable transplant risks due to age or co-morbidity should be treated with imatinib mesylate or IFN-α, ideally on trial protocols.

II. Chronic lymphocytic leukemia

Chronic lymphocytic leukemia (CLL) is marked by the accumulation of a clone of morphologically mature but immunologically incompetent B lymphocytes in the peripheral blood, bone marrow, spleen, and lymph nodes. Unlike CML, failure of apoptosis rather than increased proliferation accounts for this excess accumulation. Over 90% of CLL lymphocytes are in a quiescent G_0 stage of the cell cycle, and the doubling time for circulating lymphocytes is prolonged. The clinical course is indolent in the majority of patients, with the survival time in excess of 10 years for early-stage disease, but characteristics such as cytogenetics and immunoglobulin (Ig) gene rearrangements are now being identified that predict for much more rapid progression in some subsets of CLL.

CLL is the most common form of leukemia in Western societies (though not in Asia), with an annual incidence in the U.S.A. of 2.7 cases per 100,000 individuals. Incidence in males is twice that in females. There is a significant hereditary factor, as yet not elucidated: Relatives of CLL patients have a threefold increased risk of developing CLL or similar lymphoid neoplasms. CLL is primarily a disease of the elderly, with median age at diagnosis over 60 years; approximately 10% of patients are under 50 years.

  A. Diagnosis. Widely accepted diagnostic criteria require (1) sustained lymphocytosis greater than 5,000/μL; (2) marrow lymphocytosis greater than or equal to 30% of nucleated cells; and (3) phenotypic demonstration of monoclonality, with lymphocytes typically positive for CD5, CD19, CD20 (weak), and CD23; surface Ig is demonstrable but dim on flow cytometry, with monoclonality for kappa or lambda light chains; CD10 and FMC7 are negative. Marrow evaluation is not required if (1) and (3) are fulfilled but can provide a baseline in judging response to therapy. Moreover, the pattern of infiltration (nodular, interstitial, or diffuse) has prognostic import, and cytogenetics may give important prognostic information. The lymphocytes in CLL are morphologically mature and virtually indistinguishable from normal lymphocytes, although a few prolymphocytes with a prominent nucleolus may be found. Numerous prolymphocytes suggest transformation to prolymphocytic leukemia (seen in approximately 10% of advanced-stage CLL cases) or *de novo* prolymphocytic leukemia, a separate group of entities of either B-cell or T-cell lineage. Differential diagnosis of CLL involves a number of lymphoid neoplasms including hairy-cell leukemia, mantle-cell lymphoma, large granular lymphocytic leukemia, adult T-cell leukemia/lymphoma, follicle center-cell lymphoma, and Sezary syndrome. Characteristic morphology and/or phenotypic patterns on flow cytometry are crucial in separating these entities.

B.   Staging and prognosis. Two similar staging systems, developed by Rai (a five-tier system) and by Binet (three tiers), have proved valuable in relating overall tumor bulk to prognosis (see Tables 19.1 and 19.2). Other factors have also been recognized as prognostically important, independent of stage. These include marrow pattern (diffuse lymphocytic infiltrate unfavorable), doubling time of peripheral blood lymphocytes (less than 1 year unfavorable), CD38 (positive expression unfavorable—and frequently linked to the also unfavorable unmutated state of Ig variable-region genes), and karyotype ($17p^-$, trisomy 12, $11q^-$ unfavorable; 13 q^- favorable). Initial evaluation of patients should also include serum lactate dehydrogenase (LDH) and β_2-microglobulin (elevations unfavorable) and quantitation of Ig (hypogammaglobulinemia develops in 70% of CLL patients in advanced stage).

C.   Approach to therapy. A standard approach is to withhold treatment in asymptomatic early-stage patients. Conventional chemotherapy in this setting confers no survival advantage. Indications to initiate treatment include systemic symptoms (fatigue, weight loss, night sweats, etc.), significant cytopenias due to marrow suppression or autoimmune processes, symptomatic lymphadenopathy, marked splenomegaly, rapid lymphocyte-doubling time (less than 6 months), and hyperlymphocytosis. There is no agreed-upon treatment threshold for the absolute lymphocytosis, but a lymphocyte count of $150,000/\mu L$ is frequently used. (Hyperviscosity or leukostasis syndromes are rare under $500,000/\mu L$.) Duration of treatment depends on response, but in most cases treatment is discontinued after clinical control of the disease is achieved. There is no evidence that prolonged maintenance therapy improves survival.

Table 19.1.   Modified Rai Staging System for chronic lymphocytic leukemia

Stage (risk)	Criteria	Median survival time (yr)
0 (low risk)	Lymphocytosis only (in blood and bone marrow)	>10
I, II (intermediate risk)	Lymphocytosis plus adenopathy or lymphocytosis plus splenomegaly or hepatomegaly	6
III, IV (high risk)	Lymphocytosis plus anemia (hemoglobin <11 g/dL) or thrombocytopenia (platelets $<100 \times 10^3/\mu L$)	<2

Table 19.2.   Binet Staging System for chronic lymphocytic leukemia

Stage	No. of lymphoid areas involved[a]	Anemia or thrombocytopenia[b]	Median survival (yr)
A	0–2	No	>7
B	3–5	No	<5
C	0–5	Yes	<3

[a]Five areas are designated: cervical, axillary, inguinal, spleen, and liver. Bilateral involvement of regional nodes does not increase the number of areas designated.
[b]Anemia is defined as hemoglobin <10 g/dL, thrombocytopenia as platelets <100 × 10³/μL.

Criteria developed by a National Cancer Institute Working Group to classify response are as follows:

1. **Complete remission.** No evidence of clinical disease for longer than 2 months. Requires CBC with lymphocytes under 4,000/μL, neutrophils 1,500/μL or higher, platelets 100,000/μL or higher, hemoglobin 11 g/dL or higher, marrow 30% or lower lymphocytes, and no lymphoid nodules; no constitutional symptoms, hepatosplenomegaly, or palpable lymphadenopathy.

2. **Partial remission.** Reduction of 50% or more in peripheral blood lymphocyte count, 50% or more reduction in adenopathy and/or hepatosplenomegaly, plus at least one of the following: (a) 50% or more improvement in platelet and hemoglobin levels; (b) platelets 100,000/μL or more; or (c) hemoglobin 11 g/dL or more. Improvement in clinical stage (e.g., from Binet C to B) may also be considered a partial remission (PR). Patients who achieve CR except for persistence of lymphoid nodules in marrow are classified as "nodular PR."

3. **Stable disease.** Patients who fail to meet the criteria for PR but do not show evidence of progression (such as increasing lymphadenopathy) are considered to have stable disease.

D. **Specific regimens**

1. **Nucleosides**

    a. **Fludarabine.** This nucleoside analog is increasingly used as first-line therapy. In a large recent trial of intermediate- and high-risk (Rai stage I to IV) CLL patients, fludarabine gave 20% CR and 43% PR versus 4% CR and 33% PR for chlorambucil, formerly regarded as the standard agent. Time to progression was also longer for fludarabine: 25 versus 14 months. Importantly, however, there was no overall survival advantage for fludarabine, which also causes greater myelotoxicity and immunosuppression, with prolonged decreases in CD4 lymphocytes. Chlorambucil thus continues to be considered entirely appropriate for first-line treatment. For chlorambucil failures, fludarabine provides effective salvage treatments, with 46% response rate, in contrast to 7% response to chlorambucil given after

fludarabine failure. Patients with fludarabine-induced remissions lasting longer than 12 months show reasonable response rates when retreated with fludarabine upon relapse.
More recent data for fludarabine combinations with cyclophosphamide or rituximab as salvage therapy are given
below. The recommended dose is as follows:

- **Fludarabine** 25 mg/m^2/day IV (10- to 30-min infusion)
  days 1 to 5, q28 days, repeated for 6 to 10 cycles.

Patients who show no response after two cycles are
unlikely to benefit and should be considered for alternative therapies. Allopurinol is given for 10 to 14 days in
advanced-stage patients (tumor lysis syndrome may occur in
patients with exceptionally high tumor mass). Cytopenias
and immunosuppression are major side effects. To avoid
transfusion-related graft-versus-host disease, blood products should be irradiated. Prophylaxis against *Pneumocystis*
and *Mycobacterium tuberculosis* should be considered in selected patients. Reversible neurologic toxicity is occasionally
seen. Fludarabine may cause an increased incidence of autoimmune disorders such as Coombs-positive hemolytic anemia, and it is contraindicated in patients with prior history
of autoimmune hemolysis or idiopathic thrombocytopenic
purpura (ITP).

b.   Cladribine (2-chloro-deoxyadenosine). This is another nucleoside widely used in hairy-cell leukemia (see
below). Its efficacy in CLL is thought to be comparable with
that of fludarabine, with 40% to 60% response rates in
patients previously treated with alkylating agents. It is of
little benefit in fludarabine-refractory patients. The recommended dose is as follows:

- **Cladribine** 0.12 to 0.14 mg/kg (about 5 mg/m^2) IV as
  a 2-h IV infusion days 1 to 5; repeat q4 weeks. As with
  fludarabine, lack of response after two cycles is indication
  to discontinue. Toxicity is similar to that of fludarabine,
  with myelosuppression and prolonged immunosuppression to be expected.

2.   Alkylating agents

a.   Chlorambucil is still considered the first-line treatment of choice by many, despite the recent enthusiasm for
fludarabine. Well tolerated, with minimal nausea and no
alopecia, reversible myelotoxicity is the major side effect of
chlorambucil; prolonged use may lead to myelodysplastic
syndromes. Palliative responses will be seen in the majority of CLL patients, though not necessarily meeting the
criteria for PR as detailed above; CR occurs in a modest
percentage. It is not effective as salvage after fludarabine
or cladribine failure. Dosage may be either of the following:

- **Chlorambucil** 2 to 6 mg PO daily, with adjustments
  according to biweekly CBC (continuous schedule), *or*
- **Chlorambucil** 0.4 to 0.7 mg/kg (15 to 26 mg/m^2) PO
  given on day 1 or as divided doses spread out over 4 days,
  with repeat treatment 2 to 4 weeks depending on myelotoxicity (intermittent schedule).

Intermittent dosage may be less myelotoxic and have better patient compliance than the continuous daily schedule. Combination of chlorambucil with prednisone, formerly widely used, is of questionable benefit.

b. Cyclophosphamide (Cytoxan) is equally effective as chlorambucil but carries risks of nausea, alopecia, and hemorrhagic cystitis. **Continuous dose is 50 to 100 mg PO daily; intermittent dose is 500 to 750 mg/m^2 PO or IV q3 to 4 weeks.** To avoid cystitis, a.m. dosing and 2 to 3 L daily PO fluid intake are indicated.

c. Steroids. Prednisone may be useful in patients who cannot tolerate myelotoxic agents and is also used routinely for autoimmune complications. Hyperglycemia, psychiatric reactions, osteoporosis, and immunosuppression are hazards. **Preferred schedule is intermittent prednisone 40 to 80 mg daily for 5 to 7 days q4 weeks.** Continuous maintenance dosing is often needed for control of autoimmune hemolysis or thrombopenia. A transient initial rise in lymphocyte count is not unusual, followed by a fall, with subsequent improvement in lymphadenopathy and splenomegaly.

3. Monoclonal antibodies

a. Rituximab is a chimeric (mouse–human) monoclonal antibody specific against CD20, a surface glycoprotein antigen present on neoplastic and on mature normal B lymphocytes. It is thought to cause cell lysis via complement and antibody-dependent cellular cytotoxicity. CD20 expression on CLL lymphocytes is typically low compared with other lymphoid neoplasms, but responses (usually PR) have been reported in 25% of the patients previously treated with fludarabine or chlorambucil, utilizing standard rituximab doses. Escalated dosing may produce higher responses, but expense is significant. Rituximab is also being utilized in combination with fludarabine, cyclophosphamide, and other agents for salvage therapy. The standard dosage is as follows:

- **Rituximab** 375 mg/m^2 IV weekly $\times$ 4 (to 8). Infusions are started at 50 mg/h for the first hour and then escalated at 50-mg/h increments q30 min as tolerated up to 400 mg/h.

Infusion reactions are routinely seen, consisting of transient chills and fever, often accompanied by nausea, dyspnea, or flushing; hypotension occurs in approximately 10% of patients. Interrupting the infusion, while symptoms subside, will usually allow infusion to be resumed at half the previous rate, then slowly escalated to complete the scheduled dose. Subsequent infusions can usually be given at an initial rate of 100 mg/h, increasing by 100-mg/h increments at 30-min intervals, up to 400 mg/h. Pretreatment with acetaminophen and diphenhydramine is recommended, and epinephrine should also be on hand to treat rare anaphylactic reactions.

In patients with high tumor burden, a more ominous syndrome with vomiting, hypotension, and dyspnea has been described, related to massive release of tumor necrosis factor and other cytokines from damaged lymphocytes. Rarely, tumor lysis syndrome has also occurred. To minimize these problems, patients with lymphocyte counts higher than 50,000/μL may be given 50 mg of rituximab on day 1, 150 mg on day 2, and the remaining dose on day 3, to total 375 mg/m². When feasible, reduction in lymphocyte count with other agents should be undertaken prior to rituximab. Myelotoxicity with rituximab is minimal, although rare patients may develop severe cytopenias. Circulating normal B lymphocytes are depleted, but not T lymphocytes, and immunosuppression has not been a significant problem.

b. Alemtuzumab (Campath-1H). This chimeric (humanized) monoclonal antibody is targeted against CD52, a surface glycoprotein expressed on normal and neoplastic B and T lymphocytes as well as monocytes and macrophages but not on hematopoietic stem cells. Cell death results from apoptosis, complement activation, and antibody-dependent cell-mediated cytotoxicity. Alemtuzumab induces profound immunosuppression, with gradual return of CD4 lymphocytes over many months; opportunistic infections are common, including cytomegalovirus (CMV) and fungi. Severe anemia, neutropenia, and/or thrombocytopenia are seen in 50% to 70% of cases, with recovery typically in 3 to 4 weeks; rare cases of fatal pancytopenia are reported. As with rituximab, infusion-related chills, fever, and nausea are common; pretreatment with acetaminophen/diphenhydramine is recommended. Anti-infection prophylaxis with trimethoprim-sulfa DS b.i.d. 3 days/week and famciclovir 250 mg b.i.d. daily should be started with initiation of alemtuzumab treatment and continued until CD4 T-cell count is 200/μL or higher or for a minimum of 2 months after therapy. All blood transfusion products should be irradiated.

Alemtuzumab is indicated for use in patients with fludarabine-refractory CLL, where a response rate of 33% (31% PR, 2% CR) has been reported; median duration of response is 7 months. Recommended schedule is to give 2-h IV infusions with frequent monitoring of vital signs as follows: 3 mg on day 1; repeat 3 mg daily until well tolerated (infusion reaction minimal), then escalate to 10 mg; repeat 10 mg daily, then escalate to 30 mg when tolerated (30-mg level usually reached within 7 days); continue 30 mg three times weekly on alternate days (Monday, Wednesday, Friday). Total weekly dose should not exceed 90 mg. Continue up to 12 weeks depending on clinical response; discontinue after achieving CR or in presence of progressive disease or serious toxicity (cytopenias, major infection, etc.) or stable disease showing no improvement over a 4-week interval.

4. Combination chemotherapy. Enthusiasm has waned for the use of steroids combined with chlorambucil, and little advantage has been found utilizing lymphoma regimens such as cyclophosphamide/vincristine/prednisone with or without doxorubicin. There is currently great interest, however, in various combinations involving rituximab, alemtuzumab, fludarabine, and cyclophosphamide. Early indications are that these combinations provide significant improvement in the percentage of patients entering CR, both as first-line therapy and as salvage for relapsing or refractory CLL. There is currently no one regimen that can be considered a standard of care, but the following appear to be reasonable options:

a. **Fludarabine** 30 mg/m^2 IV days 1 to 3 and **cyclophosphamide** 250 mg/m^2 IV days 1 to 3 (both given as separate 30-min infusions); cycle repeated q28 days, up to six cycles, depending on response.

b. **Fludarabine** 25 mg/m^2 IV days 1 to 5 of each cycle plus **rituximab** 375 mg/m^2 IV on days 1 and 4 of cycle 1, but rituximab 375 mg/m^2 IV on day 1 only of cycles 2 to 6; repeat q28 days for six cycles, followed by consolidation (after 2-month observation interval) with rituximab 375 mg/m^2 IV once weekly × 4. This concurrent schedule appears preferable to sequential scheduling with rituximab given only after the completion of the fludarabine.

c. **Rituximab** 375 mg/m^2 IV day 1 plus **fludarabine** 25 mg/m^2 IV days 2 to 4 and **cyclophosphamide** 250 mg/m^2 IV on days 2 to 4 in cycle 1; in subsequent cycles (q28 days), rituximab dose is 500 mg/m^2 on day 1, with fludarabine 25 mg/m^2 days 1 to 3 and cyclophosphamide 250 mg/m^2 days 1 to 3. In previously untreated CLL, this combination has been reported to produce CR in 66%, nodular PR in 14%, and PR in 15%. In previously treated patients, CR was 23%, nodular PR 14%, and PR 36%. A significant percentage of patients in CR have no detectable residual neoplastic lymphocytes, as determined by molecular techniques. The impact of these responses on survival is unknown as yet.

5. **Transplantation.** As with CML, the role of SCT for CLL is in a state of flux. There is suggestive evidence that a significant fraction of patients may be cured following allo-SCT, since a survival plateau at 40% to 60% can be seen in various series, but transplant-related mortality, mostly due to graft-versus-host disease, has been in the 25% to 50% range. On the basis of limited evidence, it appears that success in SCT varies with age, extent and chemosensitivity of disease, and cytogenetics. Graft-versus-leukemia effect may lead to CR in chemoresistant patients, and detection of minimal residual disease after transplant does not necessarily predict for clinical relapse. The use of nonmyeloablative SCT allows for allografting at more advanced age and with low transplant-related mortality, but its role is not yet clearly defined. Autologous SCT appears feasible even in patients older than 70 years and achieves approximately 80% CR, with 40% to 70% overall survival at 4 years, but relapse rate is high and there is no plateau in the survival curve, suggesting cure is not achievable with current techniques. Improved purging methods to remove CLL cells contaminating the harvested stem cells may be helpful, but the absence of graft-versus-leukemia effect will likely remain an obstacle to long-term success for autografting.

6. **Radiation therapy.** For patients with refractory cytopenias or abdominal symptoms attributable to massive splenomegaly, low-dose radiation (e.g., 10 Gy delivered in multiple fractions) provides improvement in a majority of patients, though sometimes with significant worsening of cytopenias due to poorly understood remote suppression of bone marrow. Median duration of responses has been reported as 12 months. Radiation is also occasionally indicated for relief of compression of veins, nerve roots, ureters, etc.

7. Splenectomy. On rare occasions, splenectomy is indicated for relief of cytopenias or abdominal symptoms. Operative mortality is in the 10% range. Response is unpredictable, but significant improvement in platelet count is seen in the majority of patients.

E. Complications

1. Autoimmune syndromes. Despite the common development of hypogammaglobulinemia and the poor antibody response to vaccines exhibited by CLL patients, hemolytic anemia is seen in approximately 15% of CLL patients, and an equal number have positive Coombs test without overt hemolysis. The antibodies are typically polyclonal IgG warm antibodies of indeterminate antigen specificity. Hemolytic anemia constitutes an indication for chemotherapy of the CLL, regardless of stage. Alkylating agents are preferable to fludarabine, which may aggravate or precipitate autoimmune hemolysis. Steroids are also given (e.g., prednisone 1 mg/kg PO daily initially). Several recent reports indicate a role for rituximab as well.

In a small series, the following combination was highly effective:

Rituximab 375 mg/m^2 day 1, *and*
Cyclophosphamide 750 to 1,000 mg/m^2 IV day 2, *and*
Dexamethasone 12 mg IV days 1 and 2, then 12 mg PO days 3 to 7.
The cycle is repeated monthly.

Antibody-mediated thrombopenia occurs in approximately 2% of CLL patients. Steroids and an alkylating agent are recommended, with or without rituximab. Pure red cell aplasia is another autoimmune entity that is uncommon but increasingly recognized in CLL. Steroids and cyclosporine are recommended.

2. Infections. Hypogammaglobulinemia contributes to recurrent infections in CLL, typically with streptococci, staphylococci, and other pyogenic organisms. In patients further immunosuppressed by chemotherapy, fungi, *Pneumocystis, Listeria,* and other opportunistic organisms can pose formidable problems. Replacement therapy with pooled gamma globulin has been controversial, in part due to expense, but its use seems justifiable in patients who have experienced recurrent and/or life-threatening infections such as pneumococcal bacteremia. The dose is as follows:

- **Gamma globulin** 400 mg/kg IV q3 to 4 weeks; lower doses 200 to 250 mg/kg q4 weeks may provide protection at more acceptable costs.

Immunizations utilizing dead vaccines (e.g., antipneumo-coccal vaccine) are appropriate but usually elicit poor anti-body responses.

3.   Transformations. Unlike CML, CLL does not evolve to acute leukemia, except rarely. Instead, up to 10% of CLL patients develop an aggressive large-cell lymphoma or immunoblastic lymphoma, arising either *de novo* or from the original CLL clone. This is referred to as Richter's syndrome. Onset of fever and other systemic symptoms, rising LDH, and localized enlargement of lymph nodes often herald this omi-nous situation. Node biopsy is usually required to confirm the diagnosis. Chemotherapy utilizing regimens for intermediate- or high-grade lymphoma is appropriate but usually of marginal benefit. Median survival is approximately 5 months following recognition of Richter's syndrome.

Another 10% of CLL cases evolve into the picture of pro-lymphocytic leukemia, showing larger, less mature lympho-cytes with prominent nucleolus. Chemotherapy is generally unsatisfactory, with reported median survival of 9 months.

Distinction may be difficult between CLL patients under-going prolymphocytic transformation and patients with *de novo* prolymphocytic leukemia. The latter constitutes a heterogeneous group, of both B-cell and T-cell origin, distin-guishable by flow cytometry immunophenotype. By conven-tion, more than 55% prolymphocytes are required to establish the diagnosis. These patients are poorly responsive to chemo-therapy, although some success is achieved with nucleosides or cyclophosphamide, doxorubicin, vincristine, and prednisone (CHOP) as used in non-Hodgkin's lymphoma (see Chapter 22). Alemtuzumab shows promising response rates in T-cell pro-lymphocytic leukemia.

III.   Hairy-cell leukemia

Hairy-cell leukemia is an uncommon B-cell neoplasm charac-terized by mononuclear cells with villiform cytoplasmic projections, usually visible in peripheral blood smears or marrow aspirates, though increased marrow reticulin often results in a "dry tap" and "hairy cells" may be difficult to identify in peripheral blood. Pan-cytopenia is present in half the patients and cytopenia of at least one element in virtually all. Neutropenia can be profound, leading to recurrent infections. Splenomegaly is present in 90% of patients and may be massive; lymphadenopathy is uncommon.

Characteristic morphology, strongly positive staining for tartrate-resistant acid phosphatase (TRAP), and flow cytometry pattern (monoclonality for kappa/lambda light chains; strongly positive CD11c, CD20, CD22, CD25, and CD103) establish the diagnosis and distinguish hairy-cell leukemia from the similar en-tity of splenic lymphoma with villous lymphocytes. A variant form of hairy-cell leukemia may also cause confusion. This presents with cells that are negative for CD25 and CD103 and negative or weakly positive for TRAP and show prominent nucleoli; response to treat-ment is usually poor.

A.   Therapy. Some patients remain asymptomatic and do not require treatment. Indications for initiating chemotherapy include marked cytopenias, recurrent infections, symptomatic splenomegaly, vasculitis, or bony involvement.

1. Splenectomy will reverse cytopenias but is reserved for use in urgent situations such as uncontrolled infection, thrombopenic bleeding, and chemotherapy failure.

2. Interferon-α produces a response in the majority of patients, but CRs are uncommon, time to response is typically slow, and relapse is relatively frequent. IFN-α has largely been superseded by nucleosides.

3. Cladribine is currently considered the treatment of choice, with 75% to 90% CR following one cycle of treatment. Relapse rate is only 15% to 25%, but minimal residual disease can be detected in a substantial percentage of patients who are in apparent CR by morphologic criteria. It is not yet clear if permanent cure is achieved. Standard dosage is as follows:

- **A single cycle of cladribine** 0.1 mg/kg/day as continuous IV infusion over 7 days.

   Alternatively, a 5-day regimen may be used:

- **Cladribine** 0.12 to 0.14 mg/kg (about 5 mg/m²) IV as a 2-h IV infusion days 1 to 5.

   In addition to temporary exacerbation of cytopenias, many patients develop fever, perhaps due to the release of cytokines from damaged tumor cells. Prolonged immunosuppression is to be expected, with slow restoration of CD4 T cells over a number of months.

4. Pentostatin (2′-deoxycoformycin) is a nucleoside analog that seemingly acts through inhibition of adenosine deaminase. Pentostatin has response rates comparable with those of cladribine but requires multiple cycles of treatment. As with cladribine, cytopenias, fever, and prolonged immunosuppression are major side effects. Recommended dose is as follows:

- **Pentostatin** 4 mg/m² by IV bolus q2 weeks until CR is achieved (median of eight courses is required).

5. Rituximab. Hairy cells strongly express CD20. Early reports indicate respectable response rates in hairy-cell leukemia, in both relapsing and previously untreated patients. Four to eight infusions of rituximab 375 mg/m² weekly have been utilized.

SELECTED READINGS

Cheson BD, Bennett J, Grever M, et al. National Cancer Institute Sponsored Working Group guidelines for chronic lymphocytic leukemia: revised guidelines for diagnosis and treatment. *Blood* 1996;87: 4990–4997.

Druker BJ, Sawyers CL, Capdeville R, et al. Chronic myelogenous leukemia. In: *Hematology. American Society of Hematology education program book*. Washington, D.C.: American Socioety of Hematology, 2001:87–112 (available at http://www.asheducationbook.org).

Druker BJ, Talpaz M, Resta DJ, et al. Efficacy and safety of a specific inhibitor of the BCR-ABL tyrosine kinase in chronic myeloid leukemia. *N Engl J Med* 2001;344:1031–1037.

German CLL Study Group. *Br J Haematol* 2001;114:342–348.

Gratwohl A, Hermans J, Goldman JM, et al. Risk assessment for patients with chronic myeloid leukemia before allogeneic blood or marrow transplantation. *Lancet* 1998;352:1087–1092.

Hallek M, Schmitt B, Wilhelm M, et al. Fludarabine plus cyclophosphamide is an efficient treatment for advanced chronic lymphocytic leukaemia (CLL): results of a phase II study of the German CLL Study Group. *Br J Hematol* 2001; 114:342–8.

Ibrahim S, Keating M, Do Kim-Anh, et al. CD38 expression as an important prognostic factor in B-cell chronic lymphocytic leukemia. *Blood* 2001;98:181–186.

Kantarjian H, Sawyers C, Hochhaus A, et al. Hematologic and cytogenetic responses to imatinib mesylate in chronic myelogenous leukemia. *N Engl J Med* 2002;346:645–652.

Keating MJ, O'Brien S, Albitar M. Emerging information on the use of rituximab in chronic lymphocytic leukemia. *Semin Oncol* 2002; 29(suppl 2):70–74.

Kennedy B, Rawstron A, Carter C, et al. Campath-1H and fludarabine in combination are highly active in refractory chronic lymphocytic leukemia. *Blood* 2002;99:2245–2247.

Rai KR, Dohner H, Keating MJ, et al. Chronic lymphocytic leukemia: case-based session. In: *Hematology. American Society of Hematology education program book.* Washington, D.C.: American Society of Hematology, 2001:140–156 (available at http://www.asheducationbook.org).

Rai KR, Peterson BL, Appelbaum FR, et al. Fludarabine compared with chlorambucil as primary therapy for chronic lymphocytic leukemia. *N Engl J Med* 2000;343:1750–1757.

Sawyers CL. Chronic myeloid leukemia. *N Engl J Med* 1999;340: 1330–1340.

Myeloproliferative and Myelodysplastic Syndromes

Peter White

I. Myeloproliferative syndromes. The myeloproliferative syndromes are clonal disorders of the pluripotent hematopoietic stem cell or of lineage-committed progenitor cells. These syndromes are characterized by autonomous and sustained overproduction of morphologically and functionally mature granulocytes, erythrocytes, or platelets. The diagnostic label of the individual syndrome indicates the cellular element most strikingly increased, but it is not uncommon to have modest or even major elevations in other lineages (e.g., thrombocytosis and leukocytosis in polycythemia vera [P. vera]). Bone marrow aspirates and biopsy specimens show hyperplasia of megakaryocytes and of granulocytic and erythroid precursors, but maturation is normal. The progeny of the neoplastic lineages display essentially normal physiologic function in most respects, although it is not unusual for platelet dysfunction (reflected by prolonged bleeding time and abnormal aggregation studies) to contribute to bleeding. Chronic myelogenous leukemia is discussed in Chapter 19. The other myeloproliferative disorders are discussed here.

A. Polycythemia vera

1. Diagnosis. P. vera must be distinguished from relative or spurious polycythemia (normal red blood cell [RBC] mass, decreased plasma volume) and from secondary erythrocytosis (increased RBC mass due to hypoxia, carboxyhemoglobinemia, inappropriate erythropoietin syndromes with tumors or renal disease, etc.).

The proper formulation of major and minor criteria to establish the diagnosis of P. vera is a topic of some debate at present. Proposed modifications of the original criteria of the P. Vera Study Group incorporate the following elements:

A1. Increased RBC mass (may be inaccurate in laboratories performing the test infrequently; greater than 25% above mean predicted normal; may be inferred if hematocrit higher than 60% for males or higher than 56% for females or if multiple phlebotomies are required to lower hematocrit to normal range)

A2. Normal arterial O_2 saturation (higher than 92%)

A3. Splenomegaly

A4. Abnormal karyotype or other clonality marker

B1. Thrombocytosis greater than 400,000/µL

B2. Neutrophilic leukocytosis greater than 10,000/µL

B3. Hypercellular bone marrow with panmyelosis

B4. Subnormal serum erythropoietin level and/or no rise following phlebotomy

B5. Spontaneous growth of erythroid colonies *in vitro* in absence of erythropoietin (test is expensive and not widely available)

A1 + A2 + either A3 or A4 establishes diagnosis of P. vera
A1 + A2 + two or more B items establishes diagnosis of P. vera

An erythropoietin level in the low normal range showing no rise after phlebotomy is consistent with P. vera. An elevated erythropoietin level at diagnosis is strong evidence against P. vera. Splenomegaly is present in 70% of P. vera cases, but borderline enlargement on ultrasound is of questionable significance. Panmyelosis (hyperplasia of all nonlymphoid marrow elements) is present in 80% of cases but may be difficult to quantify; clusters of megakaryocytes strengthen the case for P. vera. Marrow karyotype is abnormal in 10% to 20% of patients at diagnosis; iron stores are typically absent.

2.   Aims of therapy. Thrombosis is a major cause of morbidity in P. vera, due primarily to increased blood viscosity and stasis. This may lead to stroke, myocardial infarct, and venous thromboembolism. Lowering the hematocrit to 40% to 45% reduces the risk of thrombosis; risk is best minimized by concomitant use of phlebotomy and hydroxyurea or other myelosuppressive agents, particularly if platelets are elevated. It is particularly important to maintain good control of hematocrit and platelets in the elderly and in others predisposed to thrombosis.

3.   Treatment regimens

   a.   Phlebotomy. Removal of 350 to 500 mL of blood every 2 to 4 days (less often in the elderly or in patients with cardiac disease) is the standard initial approach, with the aim of lowering the hematocrit to 40% to 45%. The blood cell count is then checked monthly, and phlebotomy is repeated as needed to maintain the hematocrit at less than 45%. Rapid lowering of the hematocrit may also be achieved in surgical or thrombotic emergencies by erythroapheresis. Elective surgery should be deferred for 2 to 4 months after stabilizing the hematocrit at 45% or less. Platelet function should be evaluated (using bleeding time, aggregation studies, or both) before surgery or invasive procedures.

   b.   Antithrombotic therapy. Concomitantly with phlebotomy, use of low-dose aspirin (81 mg daily) is regarded as appropriate, though evidence of efficacy is not established. Higher doses of aspirin (325 mg daily) carry risk of bleeding in patients with high platelet counts, who may have depletion of von Willebrand factor (this typically corrects with normalization of platelet count). Anagrelide may also be used to reduce platelet counts and reduce risk of thrombosis (see below and Chapter 4).

   c.   Myelosuppressive agents. Myelosuppressive agents are commonly indicated in conjunction with phlebotomy, particularly for persistent thrombocytosis, recurrent thrombosis, enlarging spleen, or similar problems. They may also reduce the risk of progression to myelofibrosis compared with phlebotomy alone. Alkylating agents such as chlorambucil carry a high risk of producing leukemia and are no longer recommended. Currently recommended choices are as follows:

      (1)   Hydroxyurea 600 to 800 mg/m^2 PO daily. This drug requires weekly blood cell counts initially and dosage adjustments to maintain the hematocrit at 40% to 45%, the platelet count at 100,000 to 500,000/µL, and the white blood cell (WBC) count at more than 3,000/µL. Side effects are usually minimal, but long-term use may cause painful leg ulcers and aphthous stomatitis; risk of leukemia is probably slightly increased as well.

For cases that are difficult to control with hydroxyurea, acceptable alternatives include the following:

(2)   Interferon-α is usually effective in controlling hematocrit, platelet count, and splenomegaly and in relieving pruritus. The starting dose is 1 to 3×10^6 U/m^2 three times weekly. Side effects include myalgia, fever, and asthenia, usually controlled with acetaminophen. Leukemogenic effects are presumably absent, but high cost is a deterrent to long-term use.

(3)   Radioactive phosphorus (^{32}P) 2.3 mCi/m^2 IV (5 mCi maximum single dose). Repeat in 12 weeks if the response is inadequate (25% dose escalation optional). Lack of response after a third dose mandates a switch to other forms of therapy. Use of ^{32}P entails about a 10% risk of leukemia by 10 years, and it is best reserved for use in the elderly and in patients refractory to other modalities. Supplemental phlebotomies may be required for patients with satisfactory platelet and WBC counts but with rising hematocrit levels.

(4)   Busulfan appears to have less leukemogenic potential than other alkylating agents and is appropriate in patients whose disease is not controlled by other treatments or in the elderly. It is best given in short courses over several weeks (to avoid prolonged marrow suppression) at 2 to 4 mg/day.

(5)   Anagrelide selectively inhibits platelet production, and a decrease in the platelet count is seen after 7 to 14 days. The WBC count is unaffected, and the hemoglobin level may fall slightly. Responses to anagrelide have been reported in more than 80% of patients with all myeloproliferative syndromes. The recommended starting dose is 0.5 mg PO q.i.d. Average dose needed to control platelet count is 2.4 mg daily. Side effects include headache (44%), palpitations, diarrhea, asthenia, and fluid retention. It should be used with caution in patients with cardiac disease. Anagrelide appears to reduce risk of thrombosis.

d.   Ancillary treatments. Allopurinol 300 mg/day is commonly needed to control hyperuricemia. Pruritus is a frequent problem in P. vera but usually abates with myelosuppressive therapy. Cyproheptadine 5 to 20 mg/day and cimetidine 900 mg/day may be helpful. Interferon-α is also frequently effective. Aspirin and similar antiplatelet agents are often helpful for erythromelalgia (hot, red, painful digits) and are commonly used to prevent thrombosis, although their efficacy is unclear.

4.   Evolution and outcome. The median survival time for patients with P. vera is about 10 years. One-third of deaths are caused by thrombosis. The risk of leukemia is small in patients treated by phlebotomy alone. Many patients progress to a "spent phase," with increasing splenomegaly and stable or falling hematocrit. A substantial number show extensive myelofibrosis (see Section I.C). Splenectomy or splenic irradiation may be indicated for massive splenomegaly in such patients.

B. Essential thrombocythemia

1. Diagnosis. Diagnosis of essential thrombocythemia requires a persistent elevation of the platelet count above 600,000/μL plus the absence of other known causes of reactive or secondary thrombocytosis (e.g., iron deficiency, malignancy, or chronic inflammatory disease). The hematocrit level and RBC mass should not be elevated; differentiation from "bled-out" P. vera may be difficult. Moderate leukocytosis is common. Marrow aspiration and biopsy should be performed to assess hyperplasia of megakaryocytes, evaluate iron stores, and exclude myelofibrosis and myelodysplasia. Overall cellularity is clearly increased in approximately 70%, and marked megakaryocytic hyperplasia is seen in 65%. Marrow chromosome studies are desirable to exclude the Philadelphia chromosome, *BCR/ABL* gene rearrangements, and myelodysplastic syndrome (MDS; notably, 5q⁻ syndrome), but an abnormal karyotype is found in less than 10% of patients. Palpable splenomegaly is present in less than 50% of patients. Platelet function studies may show either spontaneous aggregation or impaired response to agonists. Microvascular occlusion may cause digital gangrene, transient ischemic attacks, visual complaints, and paresthesias. Large-vessel occlusion (myocardial infarct, cerebrovascular accident) and hemorrhagic manifestations due to platelet dysfunction are also seen. Deep venous thrombosis is uncommon.

2. Treatment regimens. Observation alone is considered a reasonable course in younger, symptom-free patients with less than 1×10^6 platelets/μL. Therapy to lower platelet count should be undertaken in patients at increased risk for hemorrhagic or thrombotic complications and in the elderly. Options include the following:

a. Hydroxyurea 600 to 800 mg/m² PO daily, with dosage adjustments on the basis of the weekly complete blood cell count, should achieve satisfactory response in 2 to 6 weeks. Protection against thrombosis has been shown. Possible teratogenic and leukemogenic effects are pertinent to bear in mind.

b. Anagrelide can now be considered a reasonable alternative to hydroxyurea, with demonstrated protection against thrombosis (see Section I.A.3.c.5). This agent should not be used in pregnancy.

c. Interferon-α. Most thrombocythemic patients respond to this agent, at an initial dose of 3×10^6 U/day SC. Maintenance doses of 3×10^6 U three times weekly usually suffice. Its use in pregnancy is considered safe. As noted in Section I.A.3.c.2, side effects and expense are potential problems, and its effectiveness in reducing thrombotic and hemorrhagic complications remains uncertain.

d. Platelet apheresis. Platelet apheresis may be indicated in emergent situations (e.g., cerebral ischemia), but the effect is usually short-lived. On occasion, platelet trans-fusion may be indicated to control hemorrhage despite high platelet count.

e. ^{32}P and alkylating agents. These agent are effective but carry increased risk of secondary leukemia. Nitrogen mus-tard (mechlorethamine 0.15 to 0.3 mg/kg [6 to 12 mg/m^2] IV) can be helpful when rapid reduction in platelet count is needed. Busulfan 2 to 4 mg/day initial dose is appropriate in selected patients resistant to other agents, particularly the elderly.

f. Aspirin 325 mg/day may control erythromelalgia and similar vaso-occlusive problems but is contraindicated in pa-tients with a history of hemorrhagic symptoms or platelet dysfunction (e.g., prolonged bleeding time). Aspirin may be useful in the management of pregnant patients, in whom the preceding agents are contraindicated.

3. Evolution and outcome. The course of essential throm-bocytopenia is often indolent, particularly in young patients. The median survival time probably exceeds 10 years, and some patients appear to have normal life expectancy. In a few patients, the disease transforms to other myeloproliferative disorders or to acute leukemia.

C. Agnogenic myeloid metaplasia

1. Diagnosis. This disorder of the stem cell, also called idio-pathic myelofibrosis, is marked by an intense reactive fibrosis of the marrow; splenomegaly (frequently massive), reflecting ectopic hematopoiesis in the spleen and portal hypertension; and the presence of immature granulocytes, nucleated RBCs, and teardrop RBCs in the peripheral blood (leukoerythrob-lastic blood picture). An abnormal karyotype is demonstrable in 30% to 60% of patients and connotes shortened survival time. Other adverse prognostic factors include advanced age, anemia, WBC less than 4,000/μL or greater than 30,000/μL, thrombopenia, blasts in peripheral blood, and hypercatabo-lic symptoms (weight loss, night sweats, fever). Major causes of death in agnogenic myeloid metaplasia (AMM) include marrow failure, infection, portal hypertension, and leukemic transformation. Causes of secondary marrow fibrosis, such as metastatic carcinoma, hairy-cell leukemia, and granuloma-tous infections, must be excluded. Cases of MDS with mar-row fibrosis are easily confused with AMM. Postpolycythemic myelofibrosis is clinically indistinguishable but carries a poor prognosis, evolving to acute leukemia in 25% to 50% of patients (compared with 5% to 20% for *de novo* AMM). Acute myelofi-brosis is also distinct from AMM and may be identical or closely related to acute megakaryoblastic leukemia.

2. Treatment regimens. The median survival time is 5 years, but symptom-free patients may do well without treatment for a number of years. Intervention is indicated in the following situations:

a. Anemia. Androgens (e.g., testosterone enanthate 600 mg IM weekly or oxymetholone 50 mg PO q.i.d. for men; danazol 600 mg PO daily for women) are recommended and may reduce transfusion requirements. Corticosteroids (e.g., prednisone 40 mg/m^2 PO daily) should be tried if overt hemolysis is present. Erythropoietin is helpful in a minority of patients but requires large doses. It is unlikely to be effective if serum erythropoietin level is greater than 200 mU/mL.

b. Splenomegaly. Massive splenomegaly may lead to cytopenias, portal hypertension, variceal bleeding, abdominal pain, or compression of adjacent organs. Anorexia, fatigue, and hypercatabolic complaints may be prominent. Options for control include myelosuppressive therapy with hydroxyurea as for P. vera (see Section I.A.3.c) or busulfan 2 mg/day in older patients. Interferon-α produces responses in a significant percentage of cases, but its role is not clearly established in AMM. In a recent single report, low-dose melphalan (2.5 mg PO three times weekly, with escalations up to 2.5 mg daily as tolerated) improved splenomegaly in 50% and improved hemoglobin or platelet counts in over 50%. Low-dose thalidomide has also been advocated, but results are preliminary.

Radiation 50 to 200 cGy is effective in improving splenomegaly but causes cytopenias in 40% of patients. Radiation occasionally is indicated for extramedullary hemopoietic tumors causing compression syndromes or for bone pain. Splenectomy is indicated in carefully selected cases but carries significant perioperative mortality and morbidity from bleeding, sepsis, and postoperative thrombocytosis. Splenectomy may also increase the risk of blast formation.

c. Curative intent. Allogeneic marrow or stem cell transplantation (SCT) from appropriately matched donors appears to be potentially curative but remains controversial. While experience is limited, complete hematologic remission is reported in 70%, with 47% 5-year survival, but there is also a 27% transplant-related mortality. Marrow fibrosis does not prevent successful engraftment. Autologous transplants may provide palliation by improving cytopenias and splenomegaly.

II. Myelodysplastic syndromes. This represents another group of neoplastic disorders of hematopoietic stem cells, with an apparently increasing incidence that is now comparable with that of CLL (chronic lymphocytic leukemia) in persons older than 70 years. Distinctive features include the following:

- **Clonality.** An abnormal karyotype with clonal pattern is demonstrable in 50% to 80% of patients, especially in cases with increased marrow blasts and in patients with secondary MDS, arising after exposure to radiation, alkylating agents, topoisomerase inhibitors, or other cytotoxic drugs (this group comprises 10% to 20% of all MDS cases). A multitude of cytogenetic abnormalities has been reported, involving various chromosomes, most commonly 5, 7, 8, 11, 12, and 20. Karyotype is of major prognostic import, with anomalies of 7 (e.g., monosomy 7, 7q⁻) or complex abnormalities involving three or more chromosomes, connoting very poor outlook.

- **Dysplastic morphology.** The dysplastic morphologic features that characterize MDS may include any of the following: Megaloblastoid precursors in any lineage, budding and irreg-

ular nuclear outline of normoblasts, hypochromia and baso-
philic stippling of RBCs, iron-laden sideroblasts, and hyposeg-
mentation (bilobed Pelger–Huet–like forms are characteristic)
and hypogranularity of neutrophils, hypolobular and/or micro-
megakaryocytes, and hypogranular platelets. Variable numbers of marrow blasts are present (see Table 20.1). Marrow
hypercellularity is the rule, but 10% to 20% may be normo- or
hypocellular, leading to diagnostic confusion with aplastic
anemia.

- **Cytopenias.** Impaired maturation and apoptosis of precursor
  cells in the marrow result in cytopenia involving one or more cellular elements in peripheral blood, including low reticulocyte
  counts, despite the hypercellular marrow (the picture of ineffective hematopoiesis). In contrast to myeloproliferative disorders, functional abnormalities of platelets and neutrophils
  are common, contributing to bleeding and infection.
- **Evolution to acute myeloblastic leukemia.** MDS cases frequently evolve to acute myeloblastic (nonlymphocytic) leukemia, though the risk varies widely, from less than 10% for
  refractory anemia with ringed sideroblasts to more than 50% for
  patients with 10% or more blasts. Karyotype is also an important predictor. Scoring systems have been devised to help
  assess this risk (see Table 20.2.)

A.   Diagnosis and classification. The typical picture is an
elderly patient (80% are over 60 years of age at diagnosis) with
macrocytic anemia with or without thrombopenia and neutropenia. Studies of marrow morphology and cytogenetics are essential. Differential diagnosis includes vitamin B_{12} and folate
deficiency, lead poisoning, and alcohol abuse in patients with
sideroblastic anemia, aplastic anemia, and AMM in patients
with hypoplastic or fibrotic marrow. Distinction from incipient
acute myeloblastic leukemia may be quite difficult in patients
with increased blasts, and controversy exists over whether
cases with 20% to 30% blasts should be classified as MDS or
acute leukemia. Despite these uncertainties, the joint French–
American–British (FAB) classification for MDS put forth in
1982 continues to be useful (see Table 20.1). Together with the
more recently developed International Prognostic Scoring System
(IPSS) for MDS, this provides the framework for understanding
the literature and arriving at management decisions.

B.   Prognosis. As indicated in Table 20.1, survival correlates
with FAB subtype of MDS. Deaths are most commonly due to
marrow failure, infections, bleeding, and evolution to acute leukemia. The latter in turn correlates strongly with percentage of
blasts and karyotype. The IPSS incorporates these factors plus
the number of cytopenias to stratify risk for both overall survival
and evolution to acute leukemia (Table 20.2). Not included in
IPSS is patient age, which also is of major prognostic import (e.g.,
median survival for low-risk patients is 11.8 years for age under
60 years versus 3.9 years for age over 70 years).

C.   Treatment.

    1.   Transplantation. Allogeneic SCT offers the only realis-
tic approach to cure and should be considered in younger patients in IPSS high-risk or intermediate-2-risk category with

Table 20.1. MDS subtypes: FAB classification

FAB subtype	% marrow blasts	% peripheral blood blasts	Other findings	Median survival (mo)
Refractory anemia (RA)	<5	≤1	—	43
Refractory anemia with ring sideroblasts (RARS)	<5	≤1	≥15% ring sideroblasts	73
Refractory anemia with excess blasts (RAEB)	5–20	<5	—	12
Refractory anemia with excess blasts in transformation (RAEBt)[a]	20–30 or	≥5 or	Presence of Auer rods	5
Chronic myelomonocytic leukemia (CMML)	≤20	<5	Monocytes >1,000/μL	20

[a] In a recent revised scheme, RAEBt cases are reclassified as acute leukemia.

Table 20.2. International prognostic scoring system for MDS

Prognostic factor	Score value				
	0	0.5	1.0	1.5	2.0
% marrow blasts	<5	5–10	—	11–20	21–30
Karyotype[a]	Good	Intermediate	Poor	—	—
Cytopenias[b]	0–1	2–3	—	—	—

Risk category	Total score	Median survival (yr)
Low	0	5.7
Intermediate—1	0.5–1.0	3.5
Intermediate—2	1.5–2.0	1.2
High	2.5	0.4

[a] Good, normal karyotype, –Y, 5q⁻, or 20q⁻. Poor, chromosome 7 abnormal (monosomy, 7q⁻, etc.); or complex (three separate abnormalities). Intermediate, all other abnormal karyotypes.

[b] Cytopenias defined by hemoglobin <10 g/dL, neutrophils <1,500/μL, and platelets <100,000/μL.

suitable sibling donors. While some series report 40% disease-free survival at 3 to 6 years, results vary markedly depending on age, percentage blasts, karyotype, etc. Relapse rates and transplant-related mortality are high in older patients. Those over 50 years of age or with more than 5% blasts are likely to have less than 20% long-term survival; favorable outcomes with SCT are less than 10% in patients with abnormalities of chromosome 7 or complex cytogenetic abnormalities. Autologous SCT carries low transplant-related mortality, but relapse rate is greater than 50% and possibility of cure is uncertain. Nonmyeloablative SCT, with programmed reinfusion of donor lymphocytes, appears to carry promise for use in older patients, but results are very preliminary.

2. Chemotherapy. There is no clear consensus regarding the role of chemotherapy in MDS. Its use is typically restricted to patients in IPSS intermediate- and high-risk groups. Supportive care is more appropriate for most patients with refractory anemia or refractory anemia with ring sideroblasts. Induction chemotherapy utilizing acute leukemia-type regimens (e.g., anthracycline/cytosine arabinoside) can induce complete responses in 50% to 60% of MDS patients, but remissions tend to be brief and outcomes correlate strongly with karyotype. Quinine (30 mg/kg/day, given as continuous IV infusion) may enhance response to anthracyclines by inhibiting P-glycoprotein (mediator of multidrug resistance); side effects appear to be minor but include tinnitus, vertigo, and bradycardia or prolongation of QT interval on electrocardiogram. Topotecan, a topoisomerase I inhibitor, has been postulated to have selectively favorable effectiveness in MDS, but its role is not well established. In hopes of minimizing toxicity, low-dose chemotherapy has been utilized, most notably with cytosine arabinoside at doses of 5 to 20 mg/m^2 daily, as a q12 h SC injection, continued for 10 to 20 days. Hematologic responses are seen in 20 to 30% of patients, but without any significant survival benefit, and serious marrow suppression may result. Melphalan given at a dose of 2 mg PO daily, continued until progressive disease, toxicity, or response is seen, has been recently reported to give 40% response rate with minimal side effects, though patients with hypercellular marrow (the majority of MDS) or complex cytogenetic abnormalities do poorly. Still investigational is the use of two deoxyribonucleic acid (DNA)–hypomethylating agents, 5′-azacytidine and decitabine, which have shown promising results.

3.   Immunomodulating agents. Immune mechanisms, both humoral and cell mediated, have been postulated to contribute to pathogenesis in MDS. Evidence indicates that tumor necrosis factor-α may enhance apoptosis in marrow precursor cells, for example. A number of immunosuppressive agents have accordingly been tried, with mixed success. Prednisone is occasionally helpful in improving cytopenias (about 10% response rate overall), particularly in those patients with evidence of hemolysis.

Antithymocyte globulin (40 mg/kg/day × 4 days, given as a 4-h infusion with steroid coverage to minimize serum sickness) has been reported to improve cytopenias in 40% of MDS patients with refractory anemia and refractory anemia with excess blasts. Cyclosporine has shown high response rates in limited studies, utilizing 5 to 6 mg/kg/day initially, then monitored with dose adjustments to maintain serum levels of 100 to 300 ng/mL.

Amifostine is an organic thiophosphate with antioxidant and cytoprotective properties. It is postulated to reduce apoptotic cell death in MDS, and it has been reported to improve cytopenias in approximately 30% of MDS patients in Phase II studies, though its efficacy is not yet well established. Dosage is 200 mg/m^2 IV as a 15-min infusion three times weekly. Nausea and transient hypotension are the main side effects.

Thalidomide, a drug with both immunosuppressive and antiangiogenic effects, has produced partial responses, including conversion to transfusion independence, in 30% of MDS patients, though responses were low in patients with increased blasts. Dosage used was 100 mg PO daily, escalating to 400 mg PO daily as tolerated. Side effects were frequent and included fatigue, constipation, dyspnea, and fluid retention; 16% of patients discontinued treatment owing to side effects.

4.   Differentiating agents. Low-dose cytosine arabinoside was initially postulated to work by enhancing differentiation and maturation. This notion has been dispelled, but the concept remains appealing, strengthened by the success of growth factors such as erythropoietin and neupogen (granulocyte colony-stimulating factor [G-CSF]). Numerous studies have looked at agents such as retinoids, vitamin D analogs, butyrates, interferon, and 5'-azacytidine. To date, none of these agents has an established role in MDS.

5.   Treatment of anemia. Maintaining an adequate hemoglobin level is crucial to quality of life in the typical elderly MDS patient. Transfusions will be needed in most patients as the disease evolves. Iron loading becomes a problem, and chelation therapy with desferrioxamine is indicated when serum ferritin levels exceed 1,500 to 2,000 ng/mL or after 20 to 30 RBC U (200 mg of iron/U of RBC) have been transfused.

For patients with sideroblastic anemia, a trial of pyridoxine 100 to 200 mg daily is reasonable, though responses are rare. Steroids may be tried if hemolysis is suspected.

Erythropoietin is effective in approximately 20% of MDS patients overall but requires large doses, 20,000 to 60,000 U/week or more, and expense becomes a problem. Response rate is less than 10% in patients whose serum erythropoietin level is greater than 200 U/L. Sadly, poor response is also seen in patients requiring transfusion on a regular basis prior to starting erythropoietin. Response rates are doubled by adding G-CSF (e.g., 300 μg SC two to three times weekly). Late responses are occasionally seen, but it is reasonable to discontinue erythropoietin if there is no response after 2 months.

6.   Treatment of neutropenia. G-CSF is effective in 90% of MDS patients in raising the neutrophil count. Neutrophil bactericidal activity may also be enhanced by generation of more oxygen radicals. Short-term use of G-CSF may be appropriate in infected, severely neutropenic patients. It has no impact on the evolution of MDS, and indications for long-term use are quite limited.

SELECTED READINGS

Bennett JM, Catovsky D, Daniel MT, et al. Proposals for the classification of the myelodysplastic syndromes. *Br J Haematol* 1982;51: 189–199.

Deeg HJ, Shulman HM, Anderson JE. Allogenic and syngeneic marrow transplantation for myelodysplastic syndrome in patients 55 to 66 years of age. *Blood* 2000;95:1188–1194.

Friedburg JW, Neuberg D, Stone RM, et al. Outcome in patients with myelodysplastic syndrome after autologous bone marrow transplantation for non-Hodgkin's lymphoma. *J Clin Oncol* 1999;17: 3128–3135.

Greenberg P, Cox C, LeBeau MM. International Scoring System for evaluating prognosis in myelodysplastic syndromes. *Blood* 1997;89: 2079–2088.

Hellström-Lindberg E, Willman C, Barrett AJ, et al. Achievements in understanding and treatment of myelodysplastic syndromes. In: *Hematology. American Society of Hematology program book.* Washington, D.C.: American Society of Hematology, 2000:110–132 (available at http://www.asheducationbook.org).

Jonasova A, Neuwirtova R, Cermak J, et al. Cyclosporin A therapy in hypoplastic MDS patients and certain refractory anaemias without hypoplastic bone marrow. *Br J Haematol* 1998;100:304–309.

Molldrem JJ, Caples M, Mavroudis D. Antithymocyte globulin for patients with myelodysplastic syndrome. *Br J Haematol* 1997;99: 699–705.

Pearson, TC, Messinezy M, Westwood N, et al. A polycythemia vera update: diagnosis, pathobiology, and treatment. In: *Hematology. American Society of Hematology education program book.* Washington, D.C.: American Society of Hematology, 2000:51–68 (available at http://www.asheducationbook.org).

Spivak JL. The optimal management of polycythemia vera. *Br J Haematol* 2002; 116:243–254.

Tefferi A. Myelofibrosis with myeloid metaplasia. *N Engl J Med* 2000; 342:1255–1265.

21

Hodgkin's Disease

Richard S. Stein and David S. Morgan

Hodgkin's disease (HD) is a lymphoproliferative malignancy that accounts for approximately 1% of cancers in the U.S.A. HD almost always presents as solitary or generalized lymphadenopathy, and as documented by clinical observation and by data collected during staging laparotomies, HD generally spreads in a contiguous fashion. Most patients present with disease limited to lymph nodes or to lymph nodes and the spleen. The average age at presentation is 32 years with a bimodal incidence curve: One peak occurs at age 25, the other at age 55.

Patients with limited disease can be cured by radiation therapy; patients with advanced disease can be cured by combination chemotherapy. One of the major issues in HD therapy over the last two decades is where to draw the line between limited and advanced disease. Over time, the trend has been to consider chemotherapy for lesser stages of disease.

While HD is highly curable at presentation, patients who relapse following initial treatment may be cured by salvage therapy. Salvage chemotherapy may produce cures in patients initially treated with radiation therapy. Readministration of standard-dose chemotherapy or, more commonly, the administration of high-dose chemotherapy in conjunction with autologous stem cell transplantation may produce cures in patients initially treated with combination chemotherapy. Nevertheless, the potential for cure should not lead clinicians and patients to lose sight of the fact that HD is a malignancy and that approximately 20% to 25% of patients initially diagnosed with HD eventually die of the disease.

The success in the salvage therapy of HD makes it difficult to offer definitive recommendations regarding initial treatment. For most malignancies, disease-free survival is a valuable surrogate marker for overall survival. However, for HD, the success of salvage therapy means that the treatment options that are associated with superior disease-free survival may not necessarily produce superior overall survival when the results of salvage therapy are considered. Additionally, when therapies have significant long-term consequences such as secondary malignancies associated with larger radiation therapy fields or acute leukemia associated with combined-modality therapy, disease-free survival may overestimate the value of a specific therapy. Nevertheless, for each stage of HD, a number of rational therapeutic options exist.

I. Diagnosis and pathology. Diagnosis of HD requires biopsy of an involved node and review of the material by a hematopathologist. Lymph node biopsy is recommended for any patient with lymphadenopathy greater than 1 cm in diameter and persisting for more than 4 weeks. HD and other types of lymphoma may be suspected when the nodes are freely movable and rubbery rather than stony hard. However, these clinical features are not totally specific. Whenever the diagnosis of HD is made in a patient presenting at an extranodal site or at a nodal site below the diaphragm, the diagnosis should be subjected to greater than usual scrutiny.

HD has generally been subclassified into one of four subtypes: lymphocyte-predominant subtype (approximately 5% of cases), nodular sclerosis subtype (approximately 70% of cases), mixed cellularity subtype (approximately 20% of cases), and lymphocyte-depleted subtype (less than 5% of cases). With the demonstration that lymphocyte-predominant HD is a B-cell neoplasm that is positive for CD20 and negative for CD30, the recent World Health Organization (WHO) classification of HD divides HD into two groups. The first group is nodular lymphocyte-predominant HD; the second group is "classical" Hodgkin's lymphoma, which includes nodular sclerosis HD, lymphocyte rich classical HD, mixed cellularity HD, and lymphocyte depletion HD. Stage co-varies with histology as patients with lymphocyte-depleted HD usually present with stage III or IV disease (retroperitoneal disease and/or bone marrow involvement). The average patient with mixed cellularity HD usually presents at a more advanced stage than the average patient with the nodular sclerosis subtype of HD. The presentation with cervical, supraclavicular, and mediastinal adenopathy in a young adult is classical for the nodular sclerosis type of HD. Because of this association of stage with histologic subtype, it is generally true that patients with the nodular sclerosis subtype of HD do better than patients with mixed cellularity HD, who in turn do better than patients with lymphocyte-depleted HD. However, whenever one stratifies patients by stage of disease, the impact of histopathology on prognosis is minimal.

   II.   Staging. In determining therapy for the patient with HD, the critical variable is the stage of the patient. Accurate staging also provides a baseline so that the completeness of a response can be determined when therapy has been completed.

   A.   Cotswold staging system. The Cotswold modification of the Ann Arbor Staging System (Table 21.1) is used for patients with HD. Clinically, patients are placed in one of four stages and are further classified as to the absence "A" or presence "B" of symptoms. In addition, the subscript E (e.g., II_E) may be used to denote involvement of an extralymphatic site primarily or, more commonly, by direct extension, such as a large mediastinal mass extending into the lung. Stage III HD is often subdivided into stages III_1 and III_2 based on the extent of intra-abdominal disease.

   B.   Staging tests. Staging must be performed with consideration of therapeutic options, and not just to complete a checklist. When performing staging tests, one should remember that HD tends to spread in a contiguous manner. Considering that the thoracic duct makes the left supraclavicular area and the abdomen contiguous sites, it is not surprising that abdominal disease is found in 40% of patients with left supraclavicular presentations and in only 8% of patients with right supraclavicular presentations. Procedures used in the staging of HD are as follows:

      1.   History taking. As with any patient, the staging of the patient with HD begins with a history and a physical exam. Special attention should be given to symptoms such as bone pain that might signal a specific extranodal site of disease.

Table 21.1.   Cotswold modification of the Ann Arbor Staging System for Hodgkin's disease

Stage I	Involvement of a single lymph node region
Stage II	Involvement of two or more lymph nodes regions on the same side of the diaphragm
Stage III$_1$	Involvement of lymph node regions on both sides of the diaphragm. Abdominal disease is limited to the upper abdomen, i.e., spleen, splenic hilar, celiac, and/or porta hepatis nodes.
Stage III$_2$	Involvement of lymph node regions on both sides of the diaphragm. Abdominal disease includes para-aortic, mesenteric, iliac, or inguinal nodes, with or without disease in the upper abdomen.
Stage IV	Diffuse or disseminated involvement of one or more extralymphatic tissues or organs, with or without associated lymph node involvement
A	No symptoms
B	Fever, drenching sweats, weight loss
X	Bulky disease greater than one-third widening of the mediastinum
E	Involvement of a single extranodal site contiguous to a nodal site

The symptoms that are considered "B symptoms" are fever, night sweats, and weight loss greater than 10% of body weight. Fever in HD can have any pattern, but the pattern of days of high fever separated by days without fever, so-called "Pel–Ebstein fever," has been associated with HD for over a century. Pain at the site of HD in association with alcohol ingestion is a rare finding but may give hints as to visceral sites of involvement.

2.   Complete physical examination. Attention must be paid to all lymph node regions and the spleen. Splenomegaly is seen at presentation in approximately 10% of patients with HD and does not necessarily indicate splenic involvement by HD.

3.   Laboratory tests. Complete blood counts, erythrocyte sedimentation rate, serum alkaline phosphatase, and tests of liver and kidney function should be obtained. Hepatic enzymes may be elevated "nonspecifically" in patients with HD and do not necessarily indicate hepatic involvement by HD.

4.   Chest x-ray and computed tomography scans. A chest x-ray and computed tomography (CT) scans of the chest, abdomen, and pelvis are routinely obtained in patients with HD.

5.   Lymphangiogram. The lymphangiogram is useful in that it can detect normal-sized nodes in which the internal architecture has been obliterated by HD. These nodes may be too small to be detected by CT of the abdomen. However, performance of lymphangiography is dependent on the availability of a radiologist who can perform the test and interpret the results. As a result, clinical staging of the abdomen is often limited to performance of an abdominal CT scan.

Since lymphangiography can be associated with embolization of lipid dye to the lungs, the procedure should not be performed in patients with pulmonary HD or with a large mediastinal mass. Omission of the lymphangiogram is of no clinical consequence in these patients since they are candidates for chemotherapy, anyway.

6. Gallium scan and positron emission tomography scan. These tests are not part of routine staging. However, in patients presenting with a large mediastinal mass, it is difficult to distinguish between residual disease and persistent scar. These tests may be helpful in making that distinction and in guiding further therapy.

7. Bone marrow biopsy. The test is rarely positive except in patients who are found to have at least stage III disease by other tests. However, because of the potential use of autologous bone marrow transplantation (ABMT) or stem cell transplantation as salvage therapy, a bone marrow biopsy is a reasonable baseline study in all patients with HD. Alternatively, if chemotherapy is planned and if blood counts are normal, the test may be omitted until the time that stem cell transplantation is considered.

8. Staging laparotomy. Staging laparotomy is the most accurate means of determining the extent of abdominal involvement with HD. However, staging laparotomy is rarely performed, as most clinicians are willing to make clinical decisions on the basis of radiologic staging and to compensate for uncertain clinical staging by administering chemotherapy. If performed, staging laparotomy should include inspection, liver biopsies (wedge biopsy of the left lobe plus needle biopsy of both lobes), and biopsies of the splenic hilar, celiac, porta hepatis, mesenteric, paraaortic, and iliac lymph nodes.

III. Therapy of Hodgkin's disease

A. General considerations. Therapy of HD must be considered on a stage-by-stage basis. The incidence of various stages of HD is presented in Table 21.2, which also presents an estimated cure rate for each stage. In general, limited stages of HD (stages IA and IIA) are generally treated with radiation therapy, while advanced stages (IIIB, IVA, and IVB) are generally treated with combination chemotherapy. Therapy of the intermediate stages (IIB, IIIA) remains somewhat controversial, and while radiation therapy can be considered for these patients, the tendency of most oncologists is to treat these patients with combination chemotherapy. Despite the success in the treatment of HD, decisions regarding the optimal choice of therapy for all stages of HD have become more complex.

Late complications of radiation therapy for HD include breast cancer, lung cancer, hypothyroidism, thyroid cancer, coronary artery disease, and valvular heart disease. While the incidence of each of these complications is fairly low, the cumulative risk of all of these complications may be as much as 15% at 15 years following treatment. It is therefore reasonable to consider chemotherapy or chemotherapy plus involved field radiation

Table 21.2.   Hodgkin's disease: incidence of stages and results of therapy

Stage	Relative incidence (%)	Potential cure rate (%)
IA	10	95
IIA	35	85
IB, IIB	13	70
III$_1$A	12	85
III$_2$A	8	65
IIIB	12	60
IVA, IVB	10	60

therapy as an approach to limited-stage HD. Unfortunately, there are no data showing that the overall survival of patients with limited-stage HD can be improved with this alteration of therapy. Thus, after decades of "knowing" that radiation therapy was the optimal approach to limited HD, there is now uncertainty as to whether or not this is the case.

While chemotherapy has clearly been established as the optimal therapy for advanced-stage disease, clinical trials have not resolved the question as to which regimen represents optimal treatment. Regardless of which chemotherapy regimen is chosen, standard regimens should not be altered arbitrarily as dose reductions may decrease the possibility of cure. Although most patients receive six cycles of chemotherapy, the data actually support the policy of administering a minimum of six cycles, with therapy being given until a complete remission (CR) has been achieved and then administered for an additional two cycles. While the tumor lysis syndrome has not been reported in HD, it is prudent to administer allopurinol during the first cycle of chemotherapy or during the first 2 weeks of radiation therapy.

B.   Radiation therapy. Studies conducted in the 1960s established that the optimal dose for local control is 36 to 40 Gy given over 3.5 to 4.0 weeks. Standard radiation therapy ports are illustrated in Fig. 21-1.

With modern equipment, adequate radiation can be administered to involved areas while shielding adjacent tissues. As a result, radiation pneumonitis and radiation pericarditis occur only rarely. Because of the common occurrence of hypothyroidism and the less common occurrence of thyroid cancer in patients who receive radiation to the thyroid gland, thyroid-stimulating hormone (TSH) levels should be monitored yearly in these patients starting at 8 to 10 years following administration of radiation therapy. Patients with elevated levels of TSH, even if clinically euthyroid, should be placed on thyroid hormone replacement to limit stimulation of the radiated thyroid gland by elevated levels of TSH. While radiation therapy alone has not been associated with an increased risk of acute leukemia, the use of radiation therapy in conjunction with combination chemotherapy has been associated with a risk of acute nonlymphocytic leukemia as high as 7% to 10% in the decade following therapy.

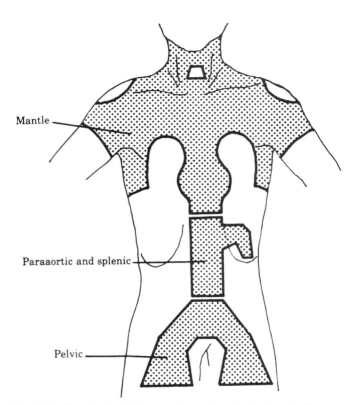

Fig. 21-1.   Standard radiation ports used for the treatment of Hodgkin's disease. For disease presenting above the diaphragm, the mantle plus para-aortic and splenic ports would be regarded as extended-field radiation therapy. The use of all three ports would be considered total nodal irradiation. (Reprinted by permission from Salzman JR, Kaplan HS. Effect of prior splenectomy on hematologic tolerance during total lymphoid radiotherapy of patients with Hodgkin's disease. *Cancer* 1972;27:472).

Women receiving radiation therapy for HD are at higher risk of developing breast cancer, and the risk is higher the younger the woman is at the time radiation therapy is administered. Women who receive radiation therapy for HD should receive yearly mammograms starting 8 years following the completion of therapy.

C.   Treatment by stage of disease

    1.   Stages IA and IIA. Patients with stage IA disease are most commonly treated with mantle irradiation when the disease occurs above the diaphragm (as it does in 90% of cases) or with pelvic radiation therapy when the disease presents in an inguinal node. Patients with stage IIA disease presenting above the diaphragm are most commonly treated with mantle plus para-aortic–splenic radiation therapy. While the use of more extensive radiation fields has been associated with a significantly lower rate of relapse, overall survival has not been shown to be significantly improved by the use of more extensive radiation ports. Additionally, the increased incidence of late malignancies with extended field radiation therapy suggests that results that are superior at 10 years may not necessarily be superior at 15 or 20 years.

Alternatively, clinicians may treat patients with stage IA or IIA disease with radiation therapy plus chemotherapy to cover the possibility that occult disease is present outside the radiation port. While the use of chemotherapy in limited-stage disease has been shown to decrease the rate of relapse, as with the use of more extensive radiation therapy fields, this approach has not been associated with superior overall survival. This is due in large part to the fact that patients who relapse after radiation therapy alone may be salvaged by chemotherapy.

In attempts to limit long-term toxicity, investigators at Stanford have studied the use of involved field radiation in conjunction with a combination regimen less toxic than usually employed, specifically, vinblastine, bleomycin, and methotrexate (VBM). Early results have been encouraging, but long-term follow-up will be needed to determine if late complications are significantly decreased by this approach. At this time, the following treatment options can be justified for patients with stage IA or IIA disease:

- Involved field radiation therapy (for stage IA only),
- Extended field radiation therapy,
- Involved field radiation therapy with combination chemotherapy, and even
- Combination chemotherapy alone.

2. Stage II$_X$ disease with bulky mediastinal mass. Patients with bulky mediastinal masses (disease diameter greater than 10 cm or greater than one-third of the chest diameter) present a special problem. When these patients, who are generally at stage II$_X$, are treated with radiotherapy alone, the risk of relapse approaches 50%. Combination chemotherapy with radiation therapy is most commonly employed in these patients. However, it is not clear that radiation therapy is necessary for all patients. Clearly, disease-free survival is superior when combined-modality therapy is given. However, combined-modality therapy is associated with an increased risk of acute leukemia, as high as 7% to 10% in the decade following therapy, and the addition of radiation therapy to chemotherapy creates a long-term risk of lung cancer and breast cancer. Therefore, it is not clear that overall survival is superior using a combined-modality approach.

One approach is to treat these stage II$_X$ patients with combination chemotherapy and to give low-dose radiation therapy (20 Gy) only to patients who have residual disease upon completion of chemotherapy. When this is done, radiation is administered only to the area of residual disease. If one chooses to use this approach, it seems rational to use a positron emission tomography (PET) scan to document completeness of response in order to select patients who will not receive radiation therapy. Unfortunately, there are no long-term follow-up data to confirm that excellent clinical results can be achieved using PET scans to select patients who will not receive radiation therapy.

3.   Stages IB and IIB. In view of the limited number of patients with these stages of disease, available data do not allow firm treatment recommendations to be made. These patients are most commonly treated with extended-field radiation therapy or radiation therapy in conjunction with combination chemotherapy such as MOPP, ABVD, or MOPP/ABV (Table 21.3). A discussion of the relative merits of the chemotherapy options for advanced-stage disease HD is found in the discussion of stage IIIB, IVA, and IVB disease.

4.   Stage IIIA. Therapy for stage IIIA disease has become less controversial in the last 10 to 15 years, although consensus regarding the optimal therapy for these patients has not been achieved. Therapeutic options include total nodal radiation therapy alone, combination chemotherapy alone, or combined-modality therapy, that is, radiation therapy plus chemotherapy.

With the demonstration that combined-modality therapy was associated with a high risk of acute leukemia, combined modality therapy fell from favor. Additionally, studies in the early 1980s established that total nodal radiation therapy without chemotherapy was adequate therapy only for patients with limited stage III disease, that is, III_1 disease. For patients with III_2 disease, the use of radiation therapy alone was associated with a significant increase in mortality due to unacceptably high relapse rates and the inability of these patients to tolerate salvage chemotherapy at the time of relapse. If one decides to use different approaches to stage III_1 and stage III_2 disease, a staging laparotomy is necessary to definitively stage these patients. As a result, the simplest approach to clinical stage III disease is to treat all stage III patients with combination chemotherapy.

5.   Stages IIIB, IVA, and IVB. Combination chemotherapy is the standard approach to these stages of HD, although there remains some controversy as to which chemotherapy approach is optimal.

D.   Chemotherapy. In 1970, the demonstration by investigators at the National Cancer Institute (NCI) that MOPP (mechlorethamine, Oncovin [vincristine], procarbazine, and prednisone) chemotherapy could cure advanced HD was one of the major milestones of the modern chemotherapy era as it was the first demonstration that a previously incurable advanced disease could be cured by combination chemotherapy. This has provided the rationale for the use of combination chemotherapy in medical oncology. However, more recent studies have indicated that the classic MOPP regimen is probably not the optimal regimen for patients with advanced HD.

Table 21.3.   Chemotherapy regimens used in the treatment of Hodgkin's disease

Regimen	Drugs and dosages
MOPP	Mechlorethamine 6 mg/m^2 IV on days 1 and 8 Vincristine (Oncovin) 1.4 mg/m^2 IV on days 1 and 8 (not to exceed 2.5 mg) Procarbazine 100 mg/m^2 PO on days 1–14 Prednisone 40 mg/m^2 PO on days 1–14, cycles 1 and 4 only Repeat cycle every 28 days.
ABVD	Doxorubicin (Adriamycin) 25 mg/m^2 IV on days 1 and 15 Vinblastine 6 mg/m^2 IV on days 1 and 15 Bleomycin 10 U/m^2 IV on days 1 and 15 Dacarbazine 375 mg/m^2 IV on days 1 and 15 Repeat cycle every 28 days
MOPP/ABV	Mechlorethamine 6 mg/m^2 IV on day 1 Vincristine (Oncovin) 1.4 mg/m^2 IV on day 1 (not to exceed 2.5 mg) Procarbazine 100 mg/m^2 PO on days 1–7 Prednisone 40 mg/m^2 PO on days 1–14 Doxorubicin (Adriamycin) 25 mg/m^2 IV on day 8 Vinblastine 6 mg/m^2 IV on day 8 Bleomycin 10 U/m^2 IV on day 8 Repeat cycle every 28 days
VBM	Vinblastine 6 mg/m^2 IV on days 1 and 8 Bleomycin 10 U/m^2 IV on days 1 and 8 Methotrexate 30 mg/m^2 IV on days 1 and 8 Repeat cycle every 28 days
Stanford V	Vinblastine 6 mg/m^2 IV weeks 1, 3, 5, 7, 9, and 11 Doxorubicin 25 mg/m^2 IV weeks 1, 3, 5, 7, 9, and 11 Vincristine 1.4 mg/m^2 IV (not to exceed 2 mg) weeks 2, 4, 6, 8, 10, and 12 Bleomycin 5 U/m^2 IV weeks 2, 4, 6, 8, 10, and 12 Mechlorethamine 6 mg/m^2 IV weeks 1, 5, and 9 Etoposide 60 mg/m^2 IV daily × 2 weeks 3, 7, and 11 Prednisone 40 mg/m^2 PO every other day on weeks 1–10, with tapering weeks 11 and 12 (No repeat)

1.   Dose and duration of therapy. Arguments regarding selection of the "best" regimen should not obscure the following principles:

- Drugs should be administered in accordance with prescribed doses and schedules and not modified for toxicities such as nausea and vomiting (which should be controlled symptomatically).
- Full doses should be given when cytopenias are due to bone marrow involvement with HD.

- Vincristine should be decreased only in the presence of ileus, motor weakness, or numbness involving the whole fingers, not just the fingertips.
- Patients should be treated for a minimum of six cycles, but also until a CR is documented, and then for another two cycles. If tests are equivocal, it is better to treat with additional cycles rather than to prematurely discontinue therapy.

2. Classical MOPP therapy. When MOPP was initially administered, 81% of patients achieved a CR. Of these patients, 66% (representing 53% of the total series) remained in CR for 5 years, and an identical percentage remained in CR for 10 years. Thus, while late relapses have been seen on occasion, 5-year disease-free survival probably represents cure for most patients. Since salvage therapy can cure patients who are not cured by initial chemotherapy, the figure of 53% represents a minimal estimate for the cure of advanced HD.

3. Alternatives to MOPP induction therapy. Many efforts have been made to develop combination regimens that are more effective and less toxic than the standard MOPP regimen. Some regimens represent minimal modifications of MOPP, but the regimen that has attracted the most interest is ABVD (Adriamycin [doxorubicin], bleomycin, vinblastine, dacarbazine), a regimen composed of agents not cross-resistant to MOPP. In a large randomized trial, ABVD was shown to be superior to MOPP with respect to remission rates and survival. Defenders of the MOPP regimen have noted that in the MOPP-versus-ABVD trial, MOPP was administered at doses less than used in the initial NCI trial. Since the MOPP dose modifications reflect problems that clinicians and patients have with the classical MOPP regimen as originally designed, this argument may be of limited value. In any case, ABVD has been established as an alternative to MOPP therapy.

An additional approach to advanced HD is to integrate MOPP and ABVD into a single-chemotherapy regimen. Based on kinetic models of tumor resistance, initial studies alternated 1 month of MOPP with 1 month of ABVD. That alternating regimen has been shown to produce results equivalent to those achieved with ABVD. However, for the last decade, one of the standard approaches to advanced HD has been to integrate both effective regimens into a hybrid regimen, MOPP/ABV, in which all drugs are given during each cycle. With use of the MOPP/ABV hybrid, a CR rate of 84% has been achieved. This CR rate was elevated to 97% by administration of radiation therapy to areas of residual adenopathy. At a median follow-up approaching 4 years, 90% of complete responders remained free of disease for a projected disease-free survival of 88%.

In a randomized trial comparing hybrid MOPP/ABV with sequential MOPP and ABVD, the hybrid regimen was found to be superior to the sequential regimen. The MOPP/ABV hybrid produced CRs in 83% of patients with a failure-free survival rate of 64%. Whether MOPP/ABV is superior to

ABVD will not be known until ongoing trials are completed and analyzed.

Thus, standard MOPP, ABVD, MOPP/ABVD (alternating months), as well as the hybrid regimen MOPP/ABV are reasonable choices for the initial chemotherapy of patients with HD. In patients who are concerned about fertility, ABVD is the treatment of choice.

Although some investigators have combined chemotherapy with radiation therapy as treatment of advanced disease, there is no evidence that the standard use of this approach can improve results enough to compensate for the leukemogenic risk of that practice. In selected patients with bulky disease, however, it is reasonable to consider supplementing combination chemotherapy with local radiation therapy to sites of bulky disease.

Also, as high-intensity therapy in conjunction with stem cell transplantation has been shown to be effective salvage therapy of HD, more intense induction regimens have been studied in HD. Favorable results have been reported by German investigators using BEACOPP and by investigators at Stanford using Stanford V. Doses of the latter regimen are included in Table 21.3.

4.   Salvage therapy. Salvage therapy may produce cures in patients with HD who relapse following initial therapy. However, the chance of curing a patient with relapsed HD is greater if the relapse is nodal than if the relapse is visceral. Additionally, the chance of cure is greater when the initial stage of disease was limited than when the initial stage was advanced.

For patients with limited nodal relapses following radiation therapy, additional radiation therapy may be considered. If the recurrence represents a marginal miss at the edge of a radiation field, this may be feasible. However, if the recurrence is within a treatment field, further irradiation of the area is usually contraindicated and chemotherapy is needed.

For patients who relapse following chemotherapy, the variable that best predicts the chance of cure is the disease-free interval. Among patients initially treated with MOPP therapy, patients whose first CR lasted less than 1 year had a second CR rate of 29%, and only 14% of these second remissions lasted more than 4 years. Among patients whose first CR lasted more than 1 year, 93% achieved a second CR, and 45% of second CRs were projected to last more than 20 years. While the drugs used to obtain the first CR may be successful as salvage therapy, the general trend is to use drugs to which the patient has not been exposed. Thus, for patients treated with MOPP, the ABVD combination is the most commonly used salvage therapy.

While the use of combination chemotherapy, using drugs to which the patient has not been exposed, is a rational therapeutic approach to salvage therapy, the widespread use of MOPP/ABV renders this policy moot. The general approach to salvage therapy is therefore to use high-dose chemotherapy in conjunction with ABMT or peripheral blood stem cell transplantation (PBSCT).

High-dose therapy in conjunction with ABMT or PBSCT is based on the rationale that bone marrow toxicity limits the dosages of the drugs that are most effective in HD. When autologous marrow or stem cells are stored and reinfused following chemotherapy, drug doses can be escalated to levels that would ordinarily be fatal. A number of standard preparative regimens exist for use in conjunction with ABMT and PBSCT, and these regimens are presented in Table 21.4.

Controlled trials comparing preparative regimens for autologous transplantation have not been conducted, and in view of the heterogeneity of relapsed patients with respect to prior therapy, sensitivity to therapy, site of relapse, and disease-free interval, it is impossible to compare regimens across studies. Nevertheless, as improvements in supportive care, such as the use of granulocyte colony-stimulating factor (G-CSF; filgrastim) or granulocyte–macrophage colony-stimulating factor (GM-CSF; sargramostim), have lowered treatment-related mortality to approximately 5%, it appears that long-term disease-free survival may occur in approximately 50% of patients treated with ABMT or PBSCT. Patients who achieved long disease-free intervals with standard treatment, especially if they have good performance status and remain sensitive to standard chemotherapy, have an even better chance for long-term disease-free survival.

E.   Treatment of symptoms. Fever, and occasionally pruritis, may be disabling for some patients with HD. The basic approach to these problems is to treat the disease. However, if disease is drug resistant, that approach may be an oversimplification. Indomethacin 25 to 50 mg PO t.i.d. may be helpful in these patients. Anecdotal experience also supports the use of other nonsteroidal anti-inflammatory agents in these patients.

IV.   Follow-up. HD patients who achieve a complete remission and who later relapse usually do so at a site of previous disease. Our policy for follow-up is to see the patient every 2 months for the first year, every 3 months for the second year, every 4 months during the third year, every 6 months during the fourth year, and every year thereafter. Follow-up evaluation for possible relapse is limited to physical examination (the most important tool for detecting relapse) and chest x-ray films (for patients with mediastinal involvement at presentation). If the chest x-ray is indeterminate for relapse, a chest CT scan can be obtained. Some investigators have found gallium scanning to be useful in monitoring patients for relapse. However, it has not been proven that the routine use of gallium scanning is cost effective in detecting relapses that would otherwise go undetected. Furthermore, if a gallium scan is used to detect relapse, it is necessary to obtain a baseline gallium scan to document that the tumor is positive for gallium uptake.

If a patient who presented with B symptoms develops recurrent symptoms while in apparent remission, an abdominal CT scan should be performed, even though the ability of CT scanning to detect retroperitoneal disease is limited. Areas suspicious for relapse should be biopsied to confirm the diagnosis of recurrent HD prior to proceeding with treatment.

Because of the risk of acute leukemia following therapy, we obtain complete blood counts at the time of each visit in patients who

Table 21.4.   Regimens used as preparative regimens for autologous transplantation in Hodgkin's disease

Regimen	Drugs and dosages
CBV	Cyclophosphamide 1,800 mg/m^2 IV on days −7, −6, −5, −4 BCNU 600 mg/m^2 IV on day −3 Etoposide (VP-16) 800 mg/m^2 IV on days −7, −6, −5
CBV	Cyclophosphamide 1,500 mg/m^2 IV on days −5, −4, −3, −2 BCNU 300 mg/m^2 IV on day −5 Etoposide (VP-16) 300 mg/m^2 IV on days −5, −4, −3
BEAM	BCNU 300 mg/m^2 IV on day −6 Etoposide (VP-16) 100–200 mg/m^2 IV on days −5, −4, −3, −2 Cytosine arabinoside 200–400 mg/m^2 IV on days −5, −4, −3, −2 Melphalan 140 mg/m^2 IV on day −1

Day 0 is the day of reinfusion of progenitor cells. Therefore, day −5 would be 5 days before reinfusion.

have received combination chemotherapy. Monitoring for hypothyroidism was discussed in the section on radiation therapy. While elevated sedimentation rates and lactic dehydrogenase (LDH) levels may provide hints of relapse, we have not routinely used these tests for follow-up monitoring in our practice.

SELECTED READINGS

Andrieu JM, Ifrah N, Payen C, et al. Increased risk of secondary leukemia after extended field radiation combined with MOPP chemotherapy for Hodgkin's disease. *J Clin Oncol* 1990;8:1148–1154.

Canellos GP, Anderson JR, Propert KJ, et al. Chemotherapy of advanced Hodgkin's disease with MOPP, ABVD, or MOPP alternating with ABVD. *N Engl J Med* 1992;327:1478–1484.

Crnkovich MJ, Leopold K, Hoppe RT, et al. Stage I to IIB Hodgkin's disease: the combined experience at Stanford University and the Joint Center for Radiation Therapy. *J Clin Oncol* 1987;5:1041–1049.

DeVita VT Jr, Serpick AA, Carbone PP. Combination chemotherapy in the treatment of advanced Hodgkin's disease. *Ann Intern Med* 1970;73:881–895.

DeWit M, Baumann D, Beyer W, et al. Whole body positron emission tomography (PET) for diagnosis of residual mass in patients with lymphoma. *Ann Oncol* 1997;8(suppl 1):57–60.

Diehl V, Franklin J, Hasenclever D, et al. BEACOPP, a new dose-escalated and accelerated regimen, is at least as effective as COPP/ABVD in patients with advanced stage Hodgkin's lymphoma: interim report from a trial of the German Hodgkin's Lymphoma Study Group. *J Clin Oncol* 1998;16:3810–3821.

Glick JH, Young ML, Harrington D, et al. MOPP/ABV hybrid chemotherapy for advanced Hodgkin's disease significantly improves failure-free and overall survival: the 8-year results of the intergroup trial. *J Clin Oncol* 1998;16:19–26.

Hancock SL, Cox RS, McDougall IR. Thyroid diseases after treatment of Hodgkin's disease. *N Engl J Med* 1991;325:599–605.

Horning SJ, Hoppe R, Hancock SL, et al. Vinblastine, bleomycin, and methotrexate. An effective regimen in favorable Hodgkin's disease. *J Clin Oncol* 1988;6:1822–1831.

Horning SJ, Williams J, Bartlett NL, et al. Assessment of the Stanford V regimen and consolidative radiotherapy for bulky and advanced Hodgkin's disease: Eastern Cooperative Oncology Group pilot study E1492. *J Clin Oncol* 2000;18:972–980.

Klimo P, Connors JM. An update on the Vancouver experience in the management of advanced Hodgkin's disease treated with MOPP/ABV hybrid regimen. *Semin Hematol* 1988;25(suppl 2):34–40.

Lister TA, Crowther D. Staging for Hodgkin's disease. *Semin Oncol* 1990;17:696.

Longo DL, Duffey PL, Young RC, et al. Conventional-dose salvage combination chemotherapy in patients relapsing with Hodgkin's disease after combination chemotherapy: the low probability of cure. *J Clin Oncol* 1992;10:210–218.

Mauch P, Larson D, Osteen R, et al. Prognostic factors for positive surgical staging in patients with Hodgkin's disease. *J Clin Oncol* 1990;8:257–265.

Mauch P, Tarbell N, Weinstein H, et al. Stage IA and IIA supradiaphragmatic Hodgkin's disease: prognostic factors in surgically staged patients treated with mantle and paraaortic irradiation. *J Clin Oncol* 1988;6:1576–1583.

Salzman JR, Kaplan HS. Effect of prior splenectomy on hematologic tolerance during total lymphoid radiotherapy of patients with Hodgkin's disease. *Cancer* 1972;27:472.

Specht L, Gray RG, Clarke MJ, et al. Influence of more extensive radiotherapy and adjuvant chemotherapy on long-term outcome of early stage Hodgkin's disease: a meta-analysis of 23 randomized trials involving 3,888 patients. International Hodgkin's Disease Collaborative Group. *J Clin Oncol* 1998;16:830–848.

Stein S, Golomb HM, Wiernik PH, et al. Anatomic substages of stage IIIA Hodgkin's disease. *Cancer Treat Rep* 1982;66:733–741.

Vose JM, Bierman PJ, Armitage JO. Hodgkin's disease: the role of bone marrow transplantation. *Semin Oncol* 1990;17:749–757.

Non-Hodgkin's Lymphoma

Richard S. Stein and John P. Greer

The non-Hodgkin's lymphomas (NHLs) are a diverse group of malignancies in which the cell of origin is a lymphocyte. If the site of origin is the bone marrow, the disorder may be classified as a form of lymphocytic leukemia, but when disease is present in both nodes and marrow, the distinction between leukemia and lymphoma is somewhat arbitrary. The disorders included in NHL differ in many basic characteristics. At the time of presentation, some types of lymphoma such as small cleaved cell lymphoma—nodular are almost always disseminated and the bone marrow is usually involved by lymphoma. By contrast, patients with large noncleaved cell lymphoma—diffuse type (diffuse large B-cell lymphoma) may present with disease limited to one or two lymph node areas in approximately one-third of cases; in this histologic type of lymphoma, bone marrow involvement is seen at presentation less than 20% of the time.

Some types of lymphoma, primarily those lymphomas with a nodular pattern under the microscope, have a slow indolent course. Patients with small cleaved cell lymphoma—nodular, the most common nodular lymphoma, may initially do well with no treatment at all or with minimal therapy. Median survival for these patients is between 8 and 12 *years,* with patients experiencing a series of responses and relapses before the disease becomes refractory to further therapy and terminates fatally. In contrast, other types of lymphoma such as diffuse large cell lymphomas are fatal in 4 to 12 *months* in the absence of therapy but may be cured by combination chemotherapy in 40% to 50% of cases. For the majority of patients with NHL, including the types previously discussed, the cell of origin is a B lymphocyte; for a minority of cases, the cell of origin is a T lymphocyte.

In view of this clinical diversity, accurate classification of NHL is essential for scientific and clinical purposes. Ideally, a classification system would identify types of NHL that were both scientifically and clinically meaningful. A classification system should define entities that are relatively homogeneous from a morphologic, immunologic, and clinical point of view. One would also want a classification system that was associated with concordance among pathologists regarding the classification of individual cases. Unfortunately, such an ideal classification system does not exist, and since confusion over pathology has compromised the generation of meaningful clinical data regarding NHL, it is reasonable to start a review of NHL with a consideration of the pathologic classification of lymphoma.

I. Pathologic classification of lymphoma

Problems related to the pathologic classification of NHL can best be appreciated from a historical perspective. In the 1960s, Rappaport proposed a classification of NHL that divided the disorders on the basis of whether the predominant cell was small ("poorly differentiated lymphocytic lymphoma"), large ("histiocytic lymphoma"), or a mixture of small and large cells ("mixed cell lymphoma"). Lymphomas were also categorized as nodular or diffuse. This system was easy to use, and concordance between pathologists was high. Studies conducted using this system demonstrated that nodular lymphomas composed of small lymphocytes were generally indolent disorders, while so-called "histiocytic" lymphoma was curable with combination chemotherapy. However, the **Rappaport system** predated the understanding that lymphocytes were B cells or T cells and that many adult lymphomas were composed of the cells found in normal follicular centers. Rappaport's use of the term "nodular" was specifically chosen to emphasize the fact that it had not been proven that the nodules of nodular lymphoma were similar to the follicles normally seen in lymph nodes. The demonstration that the nodules of nodular lymphoma are composed of the same cells found in germinal follicles rendered this distinction irrelevant. Additionally, studies eventually established that so-called "histiocytic lymphoma" was actually composed of many disorders, the majority of which were B-cell disorders (large noncleaved cell lymphoma, large cleaved cell lymphoma, immunoblastic sarcoma of B cells) and a minority of which were T-cell disorders (anaplastic large cell lymphoma, peripheral T cell lymphoma). These findings established the need for better terminology and for a more scientific classification system.

In the 1970s, therefore, a large number of classification systems were created, each trying to define immunologically homogeneous entities. In the United States, the most prominent of these systems was the **Lukes–Collins classification system.** While the Lukes–Collins system represented a scientific step forward, several problems limited its adoption. First, several systems considering immunologic features were simultaneously advocated by various hematopathologists worldwide, creating a chaos of competing terminologies. Second, while the Lukes–Collins system attempted to define entities on the basis of their immune origin, Lukes and Collins developed their system at a time when flow cytometry and studies of surface markers were in their infancy. As a result, while Lukes and Collins used immunologic studies to help in developing their system, they originally defined their entities based on morphologic appearance under light microscopy (on the assumption that not all pathologists would have access to "sophisticated" immune technology). As a result, as many as 25% of lymphomas were considered unclassified by pathologists using the Lukes–Collins system. With the widespread use of immune markers and the routine study of fresh tissue, these problems in classification diminished, but before these problems could be solved, a classification system based on empirical clinical utility rather than scientific principles became the standard of the day.

In the 1980s, in the face of competition among classification systems, the lack of concordance among pathologists, and major clinical advances in the treatment of lymphoma, the National Cancer Institute assembled a working panel of hematopathologists who created the **New Working Formulation.** This classification considered many of the concepts of the Lukes–Collins system (and other immunologically oriented systems). However, instead of defining entities based on their "cell of origin," the New Working Formulation (Table 22.1) defined broad categories of

Table 22.1. New working formulation for non-Hodgkin's lymphoma

Low-grade lymphomas
  Small lymphocytic consistent with CLL or plasmacytoid cell
    lymphoma
  Follicular, predominantly small cleaved cell
    Diffuse areas
    Sclerosis
  Follicular, mixed, small cleaved cell and large cell
    Diffuse areas
    Sclerosis
Intermediate-grade lymphomas
  Follicular, predominantly large cell
    Diffuse areas
    Sclerosis
  Diffuse small cleaved cell
  Diffuse mixed, small cleaved cell and large cell
    Sclerosis
    Epithelioid cell component
  Diffuse large cell
    Cleaved cell
    Noncleaved cell
    Sclerosis
High-grade lymphomas
  Large cell, immunoblastic
    Plasmacytoid
    Clear cell
    Polymorphous
    Epithelioid cell component
  Lymphoblastic
    Convoluted cell
    Nonconvoluted cell
  Small noncleaved cell
    Burkitt's
    Follicular areas
Miscellaneous
    Composite
    Mycosis fungoides
    Histiocytic
    Extramedullary plasmacytoma
    Unclassifiable
    Other

Modified from the Non-Hodgkin's Lymphoma Pathologic Classification Project.
National Cancer Institute sponsored study of classification of non-Hodgkin's
lymphomas: summary and description of a working formulation for clinical
usage. *Cancer* 1982;49:2112.

lymphoma based on general clinical prognosis. Specifically, the New Working Formulation defined low-grade lymphoma, intermediate-grade lymphoma, and high-grade lymphoma. The idea of this classification was to use the pathologic appearance of the lymphoma to tell the clinician how the lymphoma needed to be treated.

In the context of the New Working Formulation, **low-grade lymphomas** are indolent lymphomas such as chronic lymphocytic leukemia (also known as small B-cell lymphoma) and follicular nodular small cleaved cell lymphoma. In asymptomatic patients, even in patients with widespread disease, watchful waiting (i.e., no initial treatment) may be appropriate management. These disorders are associated with a high response rate to single-agent or combination chemotherapy, but after a prolonged clinical course (8 to 12+ years), these diseases are invariably fatal.

Intermediate-grade lymphomas were defined by the New Working Formulation as more aggressive lymphomas, associated with a fatal course within months to years in the age of single-agent chemotherapy but curable 40% to 50% of the time in the era of combination chemotherapy. This category includes diffuse large noncleaved cell lymphoma (the most common so-called histiocytic lymphoma) as well as diffuse forms of small cleaved cell lymphoma. Mixed cell lymphomas were considered intermediate grade when diffuse and low grade when nodular, a policy that is compromised by the fact that more than 70% of mixed cell lymphomas are both nodular and diffuse. While the majority of intermediate-grade lymphomas are B-cell lymphomas, this category also includes T-cell lymphomas.

High-grade lymphomas as defined by the New Working Formulation are those lymphomas associated with a very high growth fraction and a rapidly lethal clinical course in the absence of effective therapy. This category includes small noncleaved cell lymphoma, a term that is equivalent to Burkitt's and Burkitt's-like NHL. At the time the New Working Formulation was designed, the complete remission rate in patients with high-grade lymphoma was only 20%. However, in the intervening years, as response rates in "intermediate-grade NHL" maintained a plateau of 40% to 50%, complete response rates in "high-grade lymphoma" rose from the 20% range to the 40% to 50% range with the use of more aggressive chemotherapy. Nevertheless, while response rates for intermediate- and high-grade lymphoma have come together, this distinction is still relevant as high-grade lymphomas will not achieve such results if treated with standard CHOP therapy, a regimen that is acceptable for intermediate-grade NHL.

While the New Working Formulation provided a framework for clinical trials, at the time of its promulgation, it represented a scientific step backward. As additional information was discovered regarding the cell of origin of lymphomas, it became clear that grouping diverse entities together creates concordance among pathologists at the price of defining entities that are heterogeneous and potentially of limited biologic meaning. Based on the assumption that the scientific study of lymphomas requires the delineation of meaningful entities, the **REAL (Revised European–American Classification of Lymphoid Neoplasms) classification system** was developed to delineate the entities that hematopathologists, immunologists, and molecular biologists have defined in the last 15 years. It has since been adopted and modified by the World Health Organization (WHO) as the REAL/WHO classification system.

The **REAL/WHO classification system** (Table 22.2) has the advantage of recognizing lymphomas that can be defined at the pathologic and molecular level but that are obscured by the use of the New Working Formulation. Entities such as mantle cell lymphoma, with its specific t(11;14) translocation, and anaplastic large cell lymphoma are recognized as distinct entities in this system. However, in the REAL classification system (Table 22.2), the largest entity, diffuse large B-cell disease (31% of cases), is likely a heterogeneous disease, and the division of follicular lymphoma (22% of cases) into three grades does not clarify the classification of those entities. Thus, the REAL/WHO classification may have the advantage of delineating uncommon lymphomas while neglecting the lymphomas most commonly encountered in clinical practice. Only time will tell if this approach leads to a more scientific clinical analysis of lymphoma.

II.   Staging of lymphoma

The Cotswold modification of the Ann Arbor classification is generally used for patients with NHL as well as for patients with Hodgkin's disease. Despite the widespread use of this model, the clinical applicability of the four-stage model to NHL is uncertain. For practical purposes, many clinicians believe that there may be only two stages of NHL: limited disease (stage I) and advanced disease (stages II, III, and IV). In contrast to Hodgkin's disease, it has been established that radiation therapy has no role in the curative treatment of stage II NHL. In fact, in the case of intermediate-grade lymphomas, for stage I disease, radiation therapy alone has been supplanted by chemotherapy plus radiation therapy as the treatment of choice. Additionally, in contrast to Hodgkin's disease, which arises at an extranodal site in less than 1% of cases, approximately 10% to 20% of NHLs have an extranodal presentation.

Perhaps as important as the staging of lymphoma in general is the **International Prognostic Index** (IPI) for use in patients with intermediate-grade lymphoma. This prognostic index (Table 22.3) predicts the probability of cure in intermediate-grade NHL based on the age, stage, performance status, number of extranodal sites of disease, and lactate dehydrogenase (LDH) level. For patients of all ages, 5-year survival was 73% for low-risk patients, 51% for low intermediate-risk patients, 43% for high/intermediate-risk patients, and 26% for high-risk patients. For patients under the age of 60, a similar prognostic system was developed (see Table 22.3). For patients younger than 60, 5-year survival was 83% for low-risk patients, 69% for low/intermediate-risk patients, 46% for high/intermediate-risk patients, but only 32% for high-risk patients.

The evaluation of the patient with NHL begins with a history and a physical examination. When performing the physical examination, special care must be given to examining Waldeyer's ring, epitrochlear nodes, femoral nodes, and popliteal nodes, sites that are almost never involved in Hodgkin's disease but that may be involved in a small percentage of cases of NHL. The bone marrow biopsy is generally regarded as a key diagnostic procedure in the staging of NHL, owing to the high incidence of involvement,

Table 22.2.   REAL/WHO classification of lymphoid neoplasms

B-Cell lymphomas

Precursor B-cell neoplasms
  Precursor B lymphoblastic

Mature (peripheral) B-cell neoplasms
  **Small lymphocytic lymphoma/(chronic lymphocytic
    leukemia) (7%)**
  B-Cell prolymphocytic leukemia
  Lymphoplasmacytic (1.2%)
  Splenic marginal zone B-cell lymphoma
  Hairy cell leukemia
  Plasma cell myeloma/plasmacytoma
  **Extranodal marginal zone B-cell lymphoma of mucosa-
    associated lymphoid tissue (MALT) type (8%)**
  Nodal marginal zone B-cell lymphoma with or without
    monocytoid B cell
  Mantle cell (6%)
  Follicle center, follicular (22.1%)
    Grade I (10%)
    Grade II (6%)
    Grade III (6%)
  Diffuse large B cell (31%)
  Mediastinal large B cell (2.4%)
  Primary effusion lymphoma
  Burkitt's lymphoma/Burkitt's cell leukemia (<1%)

T- and NK-cell lymphomas

Precursor T-cell neoplasms
  Precursor T-lymphoblastic lymphoma/leukemia precursor T-cell
    acute lymphoblastic leukemia (1.7%)

Mature (peripheral) T-cell neoplasms
  T-Cell prolymphocytic leukemia
  T-Cell granular lymphocyte leukemia
  Aggressive NK-cell leukemia
  Adult T-cell lymphoma/leukemia (human T-cell lymphotropic
    virus type I positive) (1%)
  Extranodal NK/T-cell lymphoma nasal type (1.4%)
  Enteropathy-type T-cell lymphoma (<1%)
  Hepatosplenic $\gamma\delta$ T-cell lymphoma (<1%)
  Subcutaneous panniculitis-like T-cell lymphoma
  Mycosis fungoides/Sezary syndrome (<1%)
  Anaplastic large-cell lymphoma T cell/null cell, primary
    cutaneous type
  Peripheral T cell, not otherwise specified (7%)
  Angioimmunoblastic T-cell lymphoma (1.2%)
  Anaplastic large-cell lymphoma T cell/null cell, primary systemic
    type

Percentages represent the data presented after an international review of cases
of NHL. Entities that represent ≥5% of cases are in boldface.

Table 22.3.   International Prognostic Index for NHL

Variable	0 points	1 point
All patients[a]		
Age (yr)	≤60	>60
Stage	I or II	III or IV
No. of extranodal sites	≤1	>1
Performance status	0 or 1	≥2
LDH	Normal	Elevated
Patients aged <60 yr[b]		
Stage	I or II	III or IV
Performance status	0 or 1	≥2
LDH	Normal	Elevated

[a] Low risk, 0 or 1; low intermediate risk, 2; high intermediate risk, 3; high risk, 4 or 5.
[b] Low risk, 0; low intermediate risk, 1; high intermediate risk, 2; high risk, 3.

especially in small cleaved cell lymphoma. In other histologic types of NHL, the test is important as a baseline test because of the possible use of autologous bone marrow or stem cell transplantation at the time of relapse. Nevertheless, if a patient with NHL is going to be treated with chemotherapy, omitting the baseline bone marrow evaluation clearly does not compromise care.

Baseline computed tomography (CT) scans are an essential part of the staging of patients with NHL as much to establish a baseline for evaluating the response to treatment as for determining the actual extent of disease. In Hodgkin's disease, involved nodes are often small and may be missed by CT scanning. However, in NHL, retroperitoneal masses, if present, are often large and easily detected by CT scans. In addition, whereas mesenteric nodes are rarely involved in Hodgkin's disease, they are involved in the majority of cases of nodular NHL and can be detected by CT scan.

Gallium scans may be helpful in the baseline evaluation of the patient with NHL, especially when bulky disease is present. These patients with bulky disease often have residual disease after treatment with chemotherapy, and the hope has been that the gallium scan might be able to distinguish between residual disease (requiring further treatment) and residual scar. Among patients who have positive CT scans after treatment, patients in whom the residual areas are "gallium positive" are at greater risk of relapse than are patients who are "gallium negative." However, the gallium scan is clearly not 100% sensitive or specific for residual NHL. Additionally, the gallium scan is of very limited value in evaluating abdominal disease since the isotope may pool in the gut.

Preliminary studies have suggested that the positron emission tomography (PET) scan may be extremely well suited to evaluating residual masses detected by CT scanning and separating scar from active disease. In a study of patients completing therapy for Hodgkin's disease and NHL, 17 had negative PET scans, and all remained free of disease with a median follow-up of 62 weeks. Seventeen patients were PET positive; seven of these patients were not evaluable because biopsies were not performed and they received additional therapy after the results of the PET scan were noted. However, of the other 10 patients with positive PET scans, 7 were confirmed to have persistent disease either at the time of the PET scan or shortly thereafter. The predictive value of PET scans has been confirmed in other studies. If the PET scan is going to be used upon completion of therapy in a patient with a residual mass, it is rational to get a baseline PET scan to document that the tumor is PET positive.

Peripheral blood counts are an insensitive measure of bone marrow involvement. The majority of patients with small cleaved cell lymphoma have focal marrow involvement, and almost all of these patients have normal peripheral blood counts. Abnormal blood counts may suggest marrow infiltration by lymphoma but may also occur when the spleen is infiltrated by lymphoma and extensively enlarged. Since the vast majority of patients with NHL will receive chemotherapy, evaluation of the blood counts is a basic part of staging of NHL. The serum LDH is an important prognostic indicator and is one of the variables considered in the IPI. Other molecular markers such as bcl-2, bcl-6, p53, and markers for multidrug resistance are under active investigation as prognostic indicators but are not part of standard staging systems.

III. Radiation therapy of non-Hodgkin's lymphoma

Because most patients with NHL have disseminated disease, radiation therapy plays a more limited role in NHL than in Hodgkin's disease. However, the value of radiation therapy should not be overlooked. With most histologic types of nodular lymphoma, doses of 44 Gy can achieve control of local disease. Because disease occurs outside of treatment fields, such as in the bone marrow, radiation therapy is rarely curative. However, when patients with nodular lymphoma have large masses, local radiation therapy may be the most effective means of palliation. A dose–response curve for radiation therapy of large cell lymphoma is less well established, although radiation therapy may play a role in palliating patients with large cell lymphoma who have become refractory to chemotherapy.

Although 30% of patients with large cell lymphoma have stage I or II disease, the role of radiation therapy, as the sole treatment in these patients, has not been supported by clinical studies. Radiation therapy has been associated with cure rates exceeding 80% in stage I large cell lymphoma *only* when patients have been staged by laparotomy. Rather than subjecting these patients to a laparotomy, the usual approach is to treat clinical stage I and II intermediate-grade NHL patients with either six cycles of a chemotherapy regimen such as CHOP or three cycles of CHOP in conjunction with involved-field radiation therapy. In a randomized clinical trial, combined-modality therapy was associated with a projected 5-year progression-free survival of 77% as compared with a projected 5-year progression-free survival of 64% in patients receiving chemotherapy alone. However, with further follow-up, the survival curves have become almost overlapping, putting in doubt the superior value of combined-modality therapy in limited-stage patients.

IV. Therapy of low-grade non-Hodgkin's lymphomas

Follicular small cleaved cell lymphomas (follicle center, follicular B-cell lymphoma) represent the majority of cases

of low-grade lymphoma. The following discussion relates to the management of that disease entity. While the terms "follicular small cleaved cell lymphoma" and "low-grade lymphoma" are used somewhat interchangeably in the medical literature, it must be recognized that other disorders are included in the category "low-grade lymphoma." Most studies of low-grade lymphoma involve patient populations in which follicular small cleaved cell lymphomas are a majority, but not the totality, of the cases.

Follicular small cleaved cell lymphomas are associated with widespread disease at presentation. Bone marrow involvement is the most easily demonstrated site of advanced disease as it is found in 55% to 65% of cases on routine bone marrow biopsy. In patients whose bone marrow is negative by light microscopy, sensitive molecular techniques have often shown bone marrow involvement. This suggests that the true incidence of bone marrow involvement is at least 90% and may actually be close to 100%.

A. Watchful waiting. Nevertheless, despite the advanced stage of disease at presentation, median survival in the majority of series ranges from 5 to 10 years. Patients are often "treated" initially with "watchful waiting," a strategy of watching the patient until the tumor burden is substantial or until symptoms develop. This is, in essence, the strategy used in chronic lymphocytic leukemia, when patients with elevated blood counts and moderate adenopathy are simply observed until the disease becomes more advanced, as indicated by the development of anemia and/or thrombocytopenia. Often, patients can be followed for years without treatment. In a randomized trial, overall survival was similar for patients initially receiving combination chemotherapy as compared with those receiving no initial treatment.

B. Initial chemotherapy. Alternatively, patients may be treated with single-agent chlorambucil, single-agent fludarabine, antibody therapy (such as rituximab), combination chemotherapy, or a combination of chemotherapy and rituximab.

- **Chlorambucil** is generally employed at a dose of 2 to 4 mg PO daily or 30 to 60 mg PO every 2 weeks.
- **Fludarabine** is generally administered at a dose of 25 mg/m^2 IV daily for 5 days every 4 weeks.

Combination-chemotherapy regimens have produced complete remissions in up to 80% of patients. However, such remissions are not durable, and the administration of combination chemotherapy may be associated with myelotoxicity, nausea, vomiting, and neurotoxicity. In general, clinicians tend to avoid anthracyclines in these patients since therapy is palliative and in view of the age of the patients, the toxicity of anthracyclines may be disproportionate to the relative benefit of using a regimen such as CVP (see Table 22.4 for definitions and regimens).

C. Secondary chemotherapy. For patients who relapse following initial therapy, several options are available. If initial therapy has been low-dose chlorambucil, a regimen such as CHOP or CNOP would be reasonable, although clinicians tend to avoid anthracyclines in low-grade lymphoma. If a regimen such as CHOP or CNOP has been used initially, one can consider fludarabine 25 mg/m^2/day IV daily for 5 days.

Table 22.4.   Combination chemotherapy regimens for non-Hodgkin's lymphoma

CVP[a]
  Cyclophosphamide 400–600 mg/m^2 IV day 1
  Vincristine (Oncovin) 1.4 mg/m^2 IV day 1 (maximum 2 mg)
  Prednisone 100 mg PO days 1–5
    Repeat every 21 days.
CHOP
  Cyclophosphamide 750 mg/m^2 IV day 1
  Doxorubicin (Adriamycin) 50 mg/m^2 IV day 1
  Vincristine (Oncovin) 1.4 mg/m^2 IV day 1 (maximum 2 mg)
  Prednisone 100 mg PO days 1–5
    Repeat every 21 days.
CNOP
  As above for CHOP, with mitoxantrone (Novantrone) 10 mg/m^2 IV day 1 substituted for doxorubicin

[a] Primarily used in low-grade lymphoma.

- **Rituximab** 375 mg/m^2/week × 4 to 8 weeks has become a popular choice for the therapy of low-grade lymphoma as the drug is effective in approximately one-half of patients and has minimal toxicity.
  Additional antibody therapies with conjugated radioisotopes are under investigation, and some recently have been approved by the U.S. Food and Drug Administration (FDA).
  Another alternative for patients relapsing after initial treatment or failing to respond to initial therapy is the use of one of the salvage regimens designed for use in intermediate-grade lymphoma, that is, a regimen such as DHAP, ESHAP, MINT, or ICE (Table 22.5). Since low-grade lymphomas are associated with prolonged survival despite multiple recurrences, there is no single clinical algorithm to be applied to all patients. Palliative treatments should be individualized based on extent of disease, clinical pace of disease, and age of the patient.

D.   High-dose chemotherapy with stem cell transplantation. Another approach to low-grade NHL involves the use of very-high-dose chemotherapy, with or without total-body radiation therapy, in conjunction with autologous bone marrow or stem cell transplantation. This approach is limited by the fact that the bone marrow and presumably the peripheral blood are frequently involved in low-grade lymphoma. Even when genetic markers such as *bcl-2* are used to confirm successful purging of tumor cells, lymphoma may not be completely removed from the reinfused stem cell product. Autologous transplantation has produced long-term disease-free survival in patients whose disease remains sensitive to chemotherapy at the time of transplantation. However, as with other therapies for low-grade lymphoma, there is no evidence that these results represent cures. Additionally, the optimal timing of such therapy (after one, two, or three chemotherapy regimens), the optimal preparative regimen (with or without total-body irradiation),

Table 22.5. Combination chemotherapy regimens useful as salvage regimens in non-Hodgkin's lymphoma

ESHAP
   Etoposide 60 mg/m^2 IV days 1–4
   Methylprednisolone 500 mg IV days 1–4
   Cytarabine 2 g/m^2 over 2 h on day 5[a]
   Cisplatin 25 mg/m^2/d continuous infusion days 1–4
      Repeat every 28 days.
DHAP
   Dexamethasone 40 mg PO or IV days 1–4
   Cytarabine 2 g/m^2 IV over 2 h on every 12 h for 2 doses on day 2[a]
   Cisplatin 100 mg/m^2 continuous infusion over 24 h, day 1
      Repeat every 3–4 weeks.
MINT
   Ifosfamide 1.3 g/m^2 IV over 1 h days 1, 2, 3
   Mesna 1.3 g/m^2 IV with ifosfamide days 1, 2, 3
   Mesna 1.3 g/m^2 IV over 1 h, 6 h after ifosfamide
   Mitoxantrone 8 mg/m^2 IV day 1 only
   Taxol 27.5 mg/m^2/day IV by continuous infusion × 4 days
      Repeat every 3–4 weeks.
ICE (one of several regimens with these three agents)
   Ifosfamide 1,000 mg/m^2 IV over 1 h (hours 0–1) days 1 and 2
   VP-16 150 mg/m^2 IV b.i.d. (hours 1–11 and 12–24) days 1 and 2
   Carboplatin 200 mg/m^2 IV (hour 11–12) days 1 and 2
   Mesna 333 mg/m^2 IV 30 min prior to ifosfamide and 4 and 8 h
      after each dose of ifosfamide
      Repeat every 3–4 weeks.

[a] If age is > 70 years, reduce to 1 g/m^2.

and the value of purging are issues that have not been resolved. The best results have been obtained in patients with sensitive disease who have received minimal therapy. However, since lead-time and selection bias confound these observations, it is impossible to state that autologous transplantation is part of standard therapy for low-grade lymphoma. While allogeneic transplantation eliminates the risk of reinfusing tumor cells, allogeneic transplantation is associated with intrinsic risks such as graft-versus-host disease. Clinical results using allogeneic transplantation in this disorder have been highly variable, and the value of allogeneic transplantation in this disease requires further investigation. Nevertheless, it appears that allogeneic transplantation is the one approach to low-grade lymphoma that has a potential to achieve cure.

V.   Therapy of intermediate-grade non-Hodgkin's lymphomas
   The most common intermediate-grade lymphoma is large non-cleaved cell lymphoma, a B-cell lymphoma. Also included in this category are diffuse mixed cell lymphomas, diffuse small cleaved cell lymphoma, mantle cell lymphoma, immunoblastic lymphoma of B-cell origin, T-cell rich B-cell lymphomas, anaplastic large cell lymphoma (generally a T-cell disease), and peripheral T-cell lymphoma. While recommendations can be made for intermediate-

grade lymphomas as if they were a single entity, one must recognize that some of the entities behave in a distinct fashion. Specifically, while it is said that intermediate-grade lymphomas have a response rate between 70% and 80% and a cure rate between 40% and 50%, patients with peripheral T-cell lymphoma have a slightly lower response rate and are rarely cured (with the exception of the small minority of peripheral T-cell lymphoma patients with low IPI). Additionally, patients with mantle cell lymphoma have a high response rate but almost always relapse and die within a few years of diagnosis.

The clinical progress in treating intermediate-grade lymphoma not only represents one of the major success stories of modern oncology, it represents a major caution regarding the problems associated with overinterpreting uncontrolled clinical observations. In the 1960s, patients were routinely treated with single-agent therapy, usually chlorambucil. The median survival was 6 months; the 2-year survival rate was only 5% to 10%; cures were rare. In the early 1970s, parallel to the observation that MOPP (nitrogen mustard, Oncovin, procarbazine, and prednisone) could cure Hodgkin's disease, workers at the National Cancer Institute reported that COPP (a regimen that substituted cyclophosphamide for nitrogen mustard) could produce complete remissions in 41% of patients with "histiocytic lymphoma" and long-term disease-free survival in 35%. This result was confirmed and slightly improved with investigators who used the CHOP regimen, a regimen that further substituted doxorubicin (hydroxydaunorubicin, Adriamycin) for procarbazine.

The studies with COPP and CHOP established the basic principles regarding the chemotherapy of intermediate-grade lymphoma. First, the studies established that this group of lymphomas is curable with combination chemotherapy, although, with further data collection, we have come to realize that some subsets, such as peripheral T-cell lymphoma, may be less curable than other subsets of intermediate-grade lymphoma. Second, the studies demonstrated that depending on how a complete remission is defined, from 60% to 80% of complete remissions represent cures. Many patients with lymphoma have residual masses upon completion of therapy. These residual masses may represent "scar" or may represent persistent disease. If the term "complete remission" is used only for patients who have no progression of residual masses for 3 months following completion of therapy, up to 80% of complete remissions may represent cures. Third, while complete remissions do not necessarily represent cures, complete remissions that persist for 2 years represent cures almost 95% of the time; that is, relapses after 2 years of remission are uncommon, although they do occur.

In the decade following the publication of the results of the CHOP regimen, a number of more intense combination-chemotherapy regimens were studied in uncontrolled, single-institution, Phase II studies. These regimens, shown in Table 22.6, suggested that long-term complete remission might be achieved in up to 75% of patients as compared with the 40% to 45% range observed with CHOP. However, even before randomized trials were conducted, there were several reasons to suspect that the improvement might be less than was suggested by uncontrolled Phase II studies.

Table 22.6.   Combination chemotherapy regimens useful as primary treatment of intermediate-grade lymphoma

CHOP
  Cyclophosphamide 750 mg/m^2 IV day 1
  Doxorubicin (Adriamycin) 50 mg/m^2 IV day 1
  Vincristine (Oncovin) 1.4 mg/m^2 IV day 1 (maximum 2 mg)
  Prednisone 100 mg PO days 1–5
    Repeat every 21 days.

CHOP plus rituximab
  Rituximab 375 mg/m^2 IV day 1
  Cyclophosphamide 750 mg/m^2 IV day 3
  Doxorubicin (Adriamycin) 50 mg/m^2 IV day 3
  Vincristine (Oncovin) 1.4 mg/m^2 IV day 3 (maximum 2 mg)
  Prednisone 100 mg PO days 3–7
    Repeat every 21 days.

BACOP
  Bleomycin 5 U/m^2 IV days 15 and 22
  Doxorubicin (Adriamycin) 25 mg/m^2 IV days 1 and 8
  Cyclophosphamide 650 mg/m^2 IV days 1 and 8
  Vincristine (Oncovin) 1.4 mg/m^2 IV days 1 and 8 (maximum 2 mg)
  Prednisone 60 mg/m^2 PO days 15–28
    Repeat every 28 days.

m-BACOD
  Methotrexate 200 mg/m^2 IV on days 1 and 8
  Leucovorin 10 mg/m^2 PO q6 h for 8 doses, start 24 h after
    methotrexate
  Bleomycin 4 U/m^2 IV day 1
  Doxorubicin (Adriamycin) 45 mg/m^2 IV day 1
  Cyclophosphamide 600 mg/m^2 IV day 1
  Vincristine (Oncovin) 1 mg/m^2 IV day 1 (maximum 2 mg)
  Dexamethasone 6 mg/m^2 PO days 1–5
    Repeat every 21 days.

MACOP-B
  Methotrexate 400 mg/m^2 IV weeks 2, 6, 10; one-fourth of dose as
    IV bolus, then three-fourths of dose over 4 h
  Leucovorin 15 mg/m^2 PO q6 h for 6 doses, start 24 h after each
    methotrexate dose
  Doxorubicin (Adriamycin) 50 mg/m^2 IV weeks 1, 3, 5, 7, 9, 11
  Cyclophosphamide 350 mg/m^2 IV weeks 1, 3, 5, 7, 9, 11
  Vincristine (Oncovin) 1.4 mg/m^2 IV (maximum 2 mg), weeks 2, 4,
    6, 8, 10, 12
  Bleomycin 10 U/m^2 IV weeks 2, 4, 6, 8, 10, 12
  Prednisone 75 mg/day PO for 12 weeks, taper to zero during
    weeks 10–12

First, as regimens became more dose intense, older patients, who generally do worse than younger patients, were selectively excluded on the grounds that they would be unable to tolerate the more intense therapy. The median age in the early CHOP study was 58 years; the median age in the MACOP-B study was 44 years. Second, with the demonstration that stage II disease was not routinely curable with radiation therapy, stage II patients became eligible for new chemotherapy regimens. By contrast, the early CHOP study contained only stage III and IV patients. Since patients with lesser stages of disease would be expected to do better, including them in studies of newer regimens would favorably bias the results achieved with those regimens. Third, in the 1970s when the CHOP regimen was first studied, mixed cell lymphoma as defined by Rappaport was considered separately from "histiocytic" lymphoma. In the 1980s, studies using the New Working Formulation included these patients in studies of intermediate-grade lymphoma. While mixed cell lymphoma may be a heterogeneous group, it is probable that these cases were primarily large cleaved cell lymphoma, a disease in which there is a high response rate but also a high relapse rate. However, since these patients may stay in remission for many years, their inclusion might favorably bias early results in studies in which they were included.

The key study regarding the role of chemotherapy in intermediate-grade lymphoma was the Intergroup Study, which randomly assigned patients with intermediate-grade lymphoma to CHOP, m-BACOD, MACOP-B, and ProMACE-CYtaBOM. Contrary to the expectations of clinicians who felt these regimens were clearly better than CHOP, there were no significant differences among the regimens with respect to survival or disease-free survival. For all regimens, actuarial survival was between 40% and 45%.

   A.   Initial chemotherapy. Thus, CHOP remains the standard-of-care chemotherapy regimen for patients with intermediate-grade lymphoma. Recently, randomized clinical trials have found higher remission rates to be associated with adding rituximab to CHOP chemotherapy. However, long-term follow-up of these studies will be necessary to establish the role of this therapy in the management of intermediate-grade lymphoma. Nevertheless, given the minimal toxicity of antibody therapy, it seems reasonable to combine rituximab therapy with CHOP therapy when treating intermediate-grade lymphoma.

   B.   Secondary chemotherapy. The fact that only 40% to 45% of patients with intermediate-grade lymphoma are cured with standard combination chemotherapy means that the majority of patients are candidates for second-line treatment. Salvage chemotherapy regimens (Table 22.5) can produce responses in 50% to 60% of patients, with 20% to 30% of patients achieving a complete remission. However, cures with salvage chemotherapy are uncommon and occur in approximately 5% of patients.

   C.   High-dose chemotherapy with stem cell transplantation. For this reason, the standard approach to patients with relapsed or refractory intermediate-grade lymphoma has been to initiate salvage chemotherapy and to proceed to autologous stem cell transplantation in patients who respond to salvage therapy. The optimal preparative regimen for autologous transplantation has not been determined. Although some studies have suggested that results are equivalent whether or not total-body irradiation is included in the preparative regimen, even this point has not been firmly established.

1.   Salvage chemotherapy. In a randomized clinical trial, patients with intermediate-grade lymphoma who were responding to salvage chemotherapy were randomized to continue on salvage chemotherapy or to switch over to high-dose therapy in conjunction with stem cell transplantation. **Five-year event-free survival was significantly higher in the group assigned to autologous transplantation (46%) as compared with 5-year event-free survival in the nontransplant group (12%) ($p = 0.001$).** Survival was also significantly better in the patients undergoing autologous transplantation than in patients receiving conventional salvage chemotherapy (53% versus 32%, respectively; $p < 0.05$).

2.   Consolidation chemotherapy. With autologous transplantation shown to be effective as salvage treatment in intermediate-grade NHL, a logical issue to pursue is whether or not such therapy might be effective as consolidation of complete remission. Haioun and associates (1994,1997) randomized patients with intermediate- and high-grade NHL who were in first complete remission to receive either high-dose chemotherapy and autologous transplantation or consolidation chemotherapy. In the initial report of this trial, disease-free survival was not significantly better in the patients receiving autologous transplantation than in patients receiving consolidation chemotherapy (59% versus 52%); 3-year survival was also similar for the two treatment groups (69% versus 71%, respectively). With additional follow-up of the same series of patients, disease-free survival and survival were again similar for patients receiving consolidation chemotherapy and for patients receiving autologous transplantation as consolidation. However, among patients with intermediate- and high-grade lymphoma classified as high risk and high/intermediate risk by the age-adjusted IPI, 5-year disease-free survival was significantly better in patients receiving autologous transplantation than in patients receiving consolidation chemotherapy (59% versus 39%, respectively; $p = 0.01$). Five-year survival was also better in the transplant arm than the consolidation chemotherapy arm (65% versus 52%, respectively); however, this difference only approached statistical significance ($p = 0.06$). Since this evaluation was a retrospective subset analysis and recent studies have failed to find a survival benefit of transplantation as consolidation of complete remission, the role of this approach is not established.

D.   Advanced age and co-morbid disease. The incidence of lymphoma increases with age. Thus, a common clinical problem involves the selection of appropriate therapy for a patient with intermediate-grade NHL over the age of 70 or older than 60 with significant co-morbid disease. Clearly, elderly patients should not be denied a chance of cure on the basis of age alone, and elderly patients with good performance status and well-controlled co-morbid disease are good candidates for curative therapy. Despite considerable efforts to design less intensive, better tolerated therapies for older patients, there is no firm evidence that any of these regimens is equivalent to CHOP. The best strategy, therefore, is to attempt to administer CHOP therapy and use growth factors such as granulocyte colony-stimulating factor (G-CSF) or granulocyte–macrophage colony-stimulating factor (GM-CSF) starting with cycle 1 to limit marrow toxicity.

VI.   Therapy of high-grade non-Hodgkin's lymphomas
The most commonly seen high-grade lymphomas are Burkitt's and Burkitt's-like lymphoma, lymphoblastic lymphoma, and peripheral T-cell lymphomas (excluding anaplastic large cell lymphoma, which has a prognosis similar to other intermediate-grade lymphomas). Because these diseases have different clinical manifestations, it is most reasonable to consider them separately.

A.   Burkitt's lymphoma and Burkitt's-like lymphoma. These diseases have similar morphologic features and a similar prognosis. They are both B-cell lymphomas of small noncleaved cells, and both have been associated with a t(8;14) translocation. In the United States, Burkitt's lymphoma tends to occur in younger patients and to be associated with a higher incidence of gastrointestinal disease and a lower incidence of bone marrow involvement. Both diseases are relatively resistant to standard chemotherapy regimens such as CHOP as that therapy is generally associated with a median survival between 6 and 10 months. More intense therapy such as the high-intensity brief-duration regimen and the hyper-CVAD regimen presented in Table 22.7 has been associated with long-term disease-free survival in almost 50% of patients, but these results are dependent on stage. Patients with disease involving the central nervous system (CNS) or bone marrow or with marked elevation of LDH have an especially poor prognosis. Salvage therapy with or without stem cell transplantation is less effective in high-grade lymphoma as compared with intermediate-grade lymphoma. This provides a rational basis for using high-dose therapy and stem cell transplantation as routine consolidation therapy of remission in patients with Burkitt's and Burkitt's-like lymphoma. However, the validity of this approach has not been established by clinical trials.

B.   Lymphoblastic lymphoma. Lymphoblastic lymphoma is a T-cell malignancy that can be regarded as a variant of T-cell acute lymphoblastic leukemia (ALL). This disorder commonly presents with a mediastinal mass and bone marrow involvement. Patients may be treated with any of the regimens used to treat ALL, and ALL-type therapy is most commonly employed (see Chapter 18). However, excellent results have been reported with a regimen devised at Stanford University, which includes a CHOP-like induction, CNS prophylaxis, and consolidation that includes methotrexate and 6-mercaptopurine. In the initial report of this regimen, patients with marrow involvement, CNS involvement, and elevated LDH had a 5-year survival of only 19%, while patients without these features had a 5-year survival of 94%. Unfortunately, further studies of other regimens have not established that marrow involvement, CNS involvement, and LDH are the sole reliable prognostic factors in lymphoblastic lymphoma. As with Burkitt's lymphoma, high-

Table 22.7.   Therapy for high-grade lymphoma

High-intensity brief-duration therapy
  Cyclophosphamide 1,500 mg/m^2 IV days 1, 2, and 29
  Etoposide 300 mg/m^2 IV days 1, 2, and 3
  Etoposide 100 mg/m^2 IV days 29, 30, and 31;
  Cisplatin 30 mg/m^2 IV days 1, 2, 3, 29, 30, and 31
  Doxorubicin 45 mg/m^2 IV days 29 and 30
  Prednisone 60 mg/m^2 PO days 1–7 and days 29–35
  Vincristine 1.4 mg/m^2 IV days 8, 22, 36, and 50 (capped at 2 mg)
  Bleomycin 10 U/m^2 IV days 8, 22, 36, and 50
  Methotrexate 200 mg/m^2 IV days 15, and 43
  Leucovorin rescue 15 mg/m^2 IV or PO every 6 h for 6 doses,
    starting 24 h after methotrexate.
Hyper-CVAD[a]
  Cycles 1, 3, 5, and 7
    Cyclophosphamide 300 mg/m^2 IV over 2 h, every 12 h, for 6 doses
    Mesna 600 mg/m^2 IV daily, days 1–3, starting 1 h before
      cyclophosphamide and completed 12 h after the last
      cyclophosphamide dose
    Vincristine 2 mg IV days 4 and 11
    Doxorubicin 50 mg/m^2 IV over 2 h on day 4
    Dexamethasone 40 mg/day IV or PO days 1–4 and 11–14
  Cycles 2, 4, 6, and 8
    Methotrexate 1 g/m^2 IV over 24 h on day 1, *and*
    Leucovorin 50 mg IV to start 12 h after methotrexate, then
      15 mg IV every 6 h until serum methotrexate <1 × 10^{-8} *M, and*
    Cytarabine 3 g/m^2 IV infusion over 1 h every 12 h × 4 doses on
      days 2 and 3 (reduce cytarabine dose to 1 g/m^2 for patients
      over 60 years old)

[a] Filgrastim (G-CSF) should be administered starting on day 4 and again on day 32, and continued until granulocyte recovery occurs.

dose therapy in conjunction with stem cell transplantation is a rational but unproven form of consolidation therapy.

C.   Peripheral T-cell lymphomas. For many years, controversy has existed over whether the T-cell lymphomas included in intermediate-grade lymphoma have the same prognosis or a worse prognosis as the B-cell lymphomas that make up the majority of intermediate-grade lymphomas. Over the last several years, clinical pathologic studies have shed some important light on this issue. First, the entity of T-cell–rich B-cell lymphomas has been identified. These lymphomas are B-cell lymphomas, with a prognosis similar to that of other B-cell lymphomas. However, since the majority of cells in the lymphoma are nonmalignant T cells, these lymphomas may have been included in studies of T-cell lymphoma, falsely improving the prognosis of T-cell lymphoma. Second, the category of T-cell lymphomas includes anaplastic large cell lymphoma, a group of lymphomas that have a prognosis similar to that of B-cell lymphomas. Once these lymphomas are excluded, the remaining T-cell lymphomas have a prognosis that is worse than that of B-cell intermediate-grade lymphomas, and as a result, the category of peripheral T-cell lymphomas may be considered as high-grade lymphomas, although this is not accepted by all investigators.

Peripheral T-cell lymphomas are a heterogeneous group of lymphomas that constitute approximately 5% to 7% of adult NHLs (Table 22.2). CHOP therapy is generally associated with long-term survival in 0% to 20% of patients with these disorders. With the exception of infrequent cases of peripheral T-cell lymphoma with low IPI, which do relatively well with CHOP, no optimal therapy for these patients have been defined, and the most rational course seems to be the use of one of the regimens employed for Burkitt's or Burkitt's-like lymphoma (Table 22.7).

VII.   Therapy of other lymphomas

The classification of NHL into low grade, intermediate grade, and high grade is, as shown by Tables 22.1 and Table 22.2, an oversimplification of this complex group of disorders. While a consideration of every entity is beyond the scope of this chapter, a number of subtypes of lymphoma have specific features that are worth noting.

A.   Mantle cell lymphomas are composed of small B lymphocytes. The cell of origin is the mantle zone cell, which surrounds the lymphoid follicle and not the follicular center cell of follicular lymphoma. These lymphomas have a diffuse pattern, are generally CD5 positive and CD23 negative, and are associated with a t(11;14) chromosomal translocation. These lymphomas used to be included in low-grade lymphoma and were often regarded as diffuse forms of small cleaved cell follicular lymphoma. However, in contrast to small cleaved cell lymphoma, median survival in this type of lymphoma is from 3 to 4 years. While responses are seen with CHOP, relapses are the rule rather than the exception, and cure is rarely, if ever, seen. The high incidence of marrow involvement limits the use of autologous stem cell transplantation, and early encouraging results using that approach as consolidation or salvage therapy have not been confirmed. This has led some investigators to advocate aggressive chemotherapy followed by allogeneic transplantation as consolidation therapy in this group of lymphomas. However, further data will be necessary to establish the role of that approach in mantle cell lymphoma.

B.   Maltomas are *m*ucosal-*a*ssociated *l*ymphoid *t*umors, which are low-grade B-cell lymphomas that can occur at a number of sites including conjunctiva, thyroid, salivary gland, and gastrointestinal tract. Maltomas tend to be localized and are associated with a better survival than other low-grade lymphomas. Maltomas of the stomach have been associated with infection by *Helicobacter pylori,* and cures have been achieved with eradication of *H. pylori* by the use of antibiotics. This suggests that certain lymphomas may require continued antigenic stimulation in order to persist.

C.   Anaplastic large cell lymphomas (ALCLs) are usually T-cell lymphomas, though null cell forms of ALCL exist. The lymphomas are usually associated with a t(2;5) translocation and are generally CD30 positive. However, CD30 is not pathognomonic for ALCL as it may also be seen in Hodgkin's disease, other B-cell and T-cell lymphomas, embryonal carcinoma, and seminoma. ALCL is commonly seen in young patients, usually involves multiple lymph node groups, and has the prognosis of other intermediate-grade lymphomas. A form of ALCL limited to the skin also exists and is associated with a more indolent prognosis than nodal-based ALCL. ALCL limited to the skin is generally negative for t(2;5), ALK negative ALCL, suggesting a different etiology for these tumors.

VIII. Special considerations

   A. Central nervous system prophylaxis. Involvement of the CNS by NHL is almost exclusively limited to small non-cleaved cell lymphoma (Burkitt's and Burkitt's-like) and lymphoblastic lymphoma. Since marrow involvement has been present in most cases with CNS involvement, a rational policy is to give intrathecal methotrexate and cranial irradiation to patients with these high-grade lymphomas and bone marrow involvement. Whether patients with intermediate-grade lymphoma and bone marrow involvement should receive CNS prophylaxis is not known. Since low-grade lymphomas do not involve the CNS unless transformation to intermediate-grade lymphoma has occurred, CNS prophylaxis is not needed for low-grade lymphoma despite the high incidence of bone marrow disease in these patients.

   B. Lymphomas in patients with human immunodeficiency virus infection. (Also see Chapter 25.) Among patients with human immunodeficiency virus (HIV) infection, 3% to 6% develop lymphoma. Lymphoma is an acquired immune deficiency syndrome (AIDS)–defining illness, and it is estimated that approximately one-fourth of new cases of NHL occur in patients with HIV. The lymphomas are generally intermediate-grade lymphoma (diffuse large B-cell lymphoma) and high-grade lymphoma (small noncleaved cell lymphoma). Over the last 15 years, there has been a diagnostic shift, and large B-cell lymphoma is now the most common lymphoma seen in these patients. Additionally, with the use of highly active antiretroviral therapy (HAART), the incidence of primary CNS lymphoma has decreased.

   Despite more effective treatment of HIV, median survival of patients with HIV who develop NHL has not improved since the early days of the AIDS epidemic and has remained 6 months for patients with systemic lymphoma and 2 months for patients with CNS lymphoma. In patients with HIV infection, NHL is associated with advanced disease and a low CD4 count. Over the years, the median CD4 count at presentation has decreased from 177/μL (during the interval 1982 to 1986) to 53/μL (during the interval 1995 to 1998). In view of the poor prognosis of these patients and their underlying immunosuppression, chemotherapy regimens characterized by dose reductions (such as half-dose or three-quarter–dose CHOP) have become somewhat standard for these patients. Large-scale randomized studies to determine the optimal regimen for these patients have not been performed. While more intense therapies might be more effective in controlling the lymphoma, it is doubtful that they would uniformly improve results in all patients, and the criteria for selective use of more aggressive treatments have not been defined. Patients with NHL and HIV infection should be evaluated for the presence of CNS disease including the presence of meningeal disease. If symptomatic CNS disease is present, therapy is indicated with an aim of improving quality, if not quantity, of life.

C. Extranodal lymphomas. NHLs arise at extranodal sites in approximately 10% to 20% of cases. In the past, these patients were often treated with radiation therapy alone. However, with extensive evidence that chemotherapy with or without radiation therapy can produce excellent results in patients with stage I lymphomas, these patients are rarely treated with radiation therapy alone. Certain extranodal sites present special considerations for which specific comments are needed.

1. Stomach. The most common site for extranodal lymphoma is the stomach. About one-half of all gastric lymphomas are maltomas, and the next most common histology is large B-cell lymphoma (intermediate-grade lymphoma). As noted previously, gastric maltomas may respond to treatment for *H. pylori*. For gastric lymphomas, chemotherapy is the treatment modality of choice. In the past, surgery was part of the standard therapy for gastric lymphomas owing to the risk of perforation during therapy. However, with most tumors diagnosed by endoscopic biopsy, surgery is rarely a part of the management of this disease.

2. Primary central nervous system lymphoma is commonly seen in patients with HIV but is also observed without HIV infection as a predisposition. All patients presenting with primary CNS lymphoma should be evaluated for possible HIV infection. In patients without HIV infection, the most common histologic types of lymphoma are large B-cell lymphoma and immunoblastic lymphoma. Treatment with radiation therapy alone is generally associated with a median survival of less than a year. Recent trials employing chemotherapy, specifically high-dose methotrexate, prior to radiation have produced superior results, with a median survival approaching 5 years. While combined-modality therapy produces the best results, in patients over the age of 60, combined-modality therapy (chemotherapy plus radiotherapy) has been associated with clinical deterioration due to brain necrosis. Accordingly, an alternative approach is to give chemotherapy alone and reserve radiotherapy until the time of disease progression.

3. Testicular lymphomas represent the most common testicular tumor seen in elderly men, with large B-cell lymphoma being the most common histologic type. Therapy consists of orchiectomy, chemotherapy, and radiation of the contralateral testis. Additionally, since testicular lymphoma is associated with CNS disease, prophylactic treatment of the CNS is indicated.

4. Nasopharyngeal lymphomas are more commonly seen in Asia than in the United States. The most common histologic type of NHL is angiocentric lymphoma of T cell or natural killer (NK) cell origin. Formerly known as lethal midline granuloma, this highly lethal lymphoma is often treated with radiation therapy and chemotherapy as well as with CNS prophylaxis. However, despite aggressive therapy, survival of greater than a year is uncommon.

5. Cutaneous lymphomas include a wide variety of diseases of both B-cell and T-cell origin. The most common cutaneous lymphoma is cutaneous or cerebriform T-cell lymphoma (CTCL), also known as mycosis fungoides. When there is generalized erythroderma and involvement of the peripheral blood, the syndrome is known as Sezary syndrome. CTCL is an indolent but lethal disease. The disease may exist as plaques in the skin for many years before progressing to involve skin tumors, adenopathy, or visceral disease. Often, this clinical progression occurs in association with a pathologic transformation to a large cell lymphoma. If disease is limited to the skin, topical therapy such as topical nitrogen mustard, electron beam radiotherapy, or psoralen in conjunction with ultraviolet radiation may be employed. Combination chemotherapy as employed for intermediate-grade lymphoma may be used for tumor stage of disease or for disease involving nodes or viscera. Unfortunately, such therapy may lead to simultaneous necrosis of skin tumors as well as the development of neutropenia, leading to fatal sepsis. Other approaches to this disease include the use of denileukin diftitox (Ontak), an antibody to CD25, and bexarotene (Targretin), a novel retinoid X receptor (RXR)–selective retinoid, or rexinoid.

IX.   Posttransplant lymphomas

Following organ transplantation and the associated immunosuppression, the most common tumors are skin cancer and NHL. Extranodal sites of disease including the CNS and gastrointestinal tract are commonly observed, and the histologic appearance is that of an intermediate- or high-grade lymphoma. These tumors are associated with Epstein–Barr virus (EBV), and if disease is limited in extent, one can employ therapy designed at increasing the host response to EBV, such as withdrawing or decreasing immunosuppression, administering interferon, or giving lymphocytes from individuals who have had EBV infection. Such therapy is most effective in limited disease and in patients in whom the lymphocytes are polyclonal. For more advanced disease and for disease in which the lymphocytes are monoclonal, chemotherapy is necessary, although rituximab has also been shown to be effective in this setting. Unfortunately, response rates are lower for transplant-associated lymphomas than for *de novo* lymphomas, and long-term survival is seen in less than 20% of patients.

SELECTED READINGS

Abrey L, Yahalom J, DeAngelis LM. Treatment for primary CNS lymphoma: the next step. *J Clin Oncol* 2000;18:3144–3150.

Banks PM, Chan J, Cleary ML, et al. Mantle cell lymphoma: a proposal for unification of morphologic, immunologic, and molecular data. *Am J Surg Pathol* 1992;16:637–640.

Coleman CN, Picozzi VJ, Cox RS, et al. Treatment of lymphoblastic lymphoma in adults. *J Clin Oncol* 1986;4:1628–1637.

Czuczman MS, Grillo-Lopez AJ, White CA, et al. Treatment of patients with low grade B-cell lymphoma with the combination of chimeric anti CD20 monoclonal antibody and CHOP. *J Clin Oncol* 1999;17:268–276.

DeVita VT Jr, Canellos GP, Chabner B, et al. Advanced diffuse histiocytic lymphoma, a potentially curable disease. *Lancet* 1975;1: 248–250.

DeWit M, Bumann D, Beyer W, et al. Whole-body positron emission tomography (PET) for diagnosis of residual mass in patients with lymphoma. *Ann Oncol* 1997;8(suppl 1):57–60.

Fisher RI, Gaynor ER, Dahlberg S, et al. Comparison of a standard regimen (CHOP) with three intensive chemotherapy regimens for advanced non-Hodgkin's lymphoma. *N Engl J Med* 1993;328: 1002–1006.

Greer JP, Kinney MC, Collins RD, et al. Clinical features of 31 patients with Ki-1 anaplastic large-cell lymphoma. *J Clin Oncol* 1991;9: 539–547.

Haioun C, Lepage E, Gisselbrecht C, et al. Comparison of autologous bone marrow transplantation with sequential chemotherapy for intermediate-grade and high grade non-Hodgkin's lymphoma in first complete remission; a study of 464 patients. *J Clin Oncol* 1994; 12:2543–2551.

Haioun C, Lepage E, Gisselbrecht C, et al. Benefit of autologous bone marrow transplantation over sequential chemotherapy in poor-risk aggressive non-Hodgkin's lymphoma: updated results of the prospective study LNH87-2. *J Clin Oncol* 1997;15:1131–1137.

Harris NL, Jaffe ES, Stein H, et al. A revised European–American classification of malignant lymphoid neoplasms: a proposal from the International Lymphoma Study Group. *Blood* 1994;84:1361–1392.

International Non-Hodgkin's Lymphoma Prognostic Factors Project. A predictive model for aggressive non-Hodgkin's lymphoma. *N Engl J Med* 1993;329:987–994.

Levine AM, Seneviratne L, Espina BM, et al. Evolving characteristics of AIDS related lymphoma. *Blood* 2000;96:4084–4090.

Maloney D, Grillo-Lopez A, White C, et al. IDEC-C2B8 (Rituxan AB) anti-CD20 monoclonal antibody therapy in patients with relapsed low grade non-Hodgkin's lymphoma. *Blood* 1997;90:2188–2195.

McKelvey EM, Gottleib JA, Wilson HE, et al. Hydroxyldaunomycin (adriamycin) combination chemotherapy in malignant lymphoma. *Cancer* 1976;38:1484–1493.

McMaster, ML, Greer, JP, Greco FA, et al. Effective treatment of small non-cleaved cell lymphoma with high intensity, brief duration chemotherapy. *J Clin Oncol* 1991;9:941–946.

Miller TP, Dahlberg S, Cassady JR, et al. Chemotherapy alone compared with chemotherapy plus radiotherapy for localized intermediate and high-grade non-Hodgkin's lymphoma. *N Engl J Med* 1998;339:21–26.

Non-Hodgkin's Lymphoma Pathologic Classification Project. National Cancer sponsored study of classification of non-Hodgkin's lymphomas: summary and description of a working formulation. *Cancer* 1982;49:2112–2135.

Thomas DA, Cortes J, O'Brien S, et al. Hyper-CVAD program in Burkitt's type adult acute lymphoblastic lymphoma. *J Clin Oncol* 1999;17:2461–2470.

Young RC, Longo DL, Glatstein E, et al. The treatment of indolent lymphomas: watchful waiting v aggressive combined modality treatment. *Semin Hematol* 1988;25(suppl 2):11–16.

Multiple Myeloma and Other Plasma Cell Dyscrasias

Martin M. Oken

I. Introduction

A. Types of plasma cell dyscrasias. Plasma cell dyscrasias, or plasma cell neoplasms, are a group of conditions characterized by unbalanced proliferation of cells that normally synthesize and secrete immunoglobulins. They range from malignant neoplasms such as multiple myeloma to monoclonal gammopathy of undetermined significance, a usually benign condition that is sometimes termed *benign monoclonal gammopathy.* Associated with the abnormal cellular proliferation in nearly all instances is the production of homogeneous monoclonal immunoglobulin, referred to either as *myeloma protein* or *M protein,* or of excessive quantities of homogeneous polypeptide subunits of a monoclonal protein. The latter usually appear as monoclonal free light chains excreted into the urine but can be detected by special assay in the serum as well. Frequently, both whole-immunoglobulin M protein and free light chains are produced. The plasma cell dyscrasias discussed in this chapter are multiple myeloma, macroglobulinemia (Waldenström's macroglobulinemia), heavy-chain diseases, amyloidosis, and monoclonal gammopathy of undetermined significance.

B. M protein. Unlike most neoplastic diseases, which are followed objectively by serial evaluation of palpable or radiographically measurable tumor masses, most plasma cell dyscrasias are best followed by serial measurements of the monoclonal protein (M protein) elaborated by the tumor. Effective use of this tumor marker is important for the proper evaluation of the disease course of most plasma cell dyscrasias and is usually essential to the determination of response to treatment. The basic immunoglobulin unit comprises two identical heavy chains with a molecular mass of 55,000 Da linked to two identical light chains with molecular masses of 22,500 Da. The heavy chains are either γ, α, μ, δ, or ϵ, corresponding to immunoglobulin IgG, IgA, IgM, IgD, and IgE, respectively. The light chains exist as either κ or λ subtypes. Serum M protein is a monoclonal whole immunoglobulin and therefore possesses only one heavy-chain type and one light-chain type. Urine M protein consists of free light chains or, in the case of some heavy-chain diseases, free heavy-chain fragments of single specificity. Serum M protein may be quantitatively evaluated by either serum protein electrophoresis or determining the concentration of the individual immunoglobulins (particularly IgG, IgA, and IgM). Urinary M protein, usually in the form of free light chain, may be characterized by immunoelectrophoresis as monoclonal κ or λ light chain and then followed sequentially, expressed as urinary light-chain excretion in grams per 24 h. This characterization requires determination of 24-h urine protein excretion and scanning the urine protein electrophoresis to determine the percentage of urine protein present as free monoclonal immunoglobulin light chain.

II.   Multiple myeloma

A.   General considerations and aims of therapy

1.   Diagnosis. Multiple myeloma is a neoplasm of malignant plasma cells invading bone and bone marrow, causing widespread skeletal destruction, bone marrow failure, and problems related to quantitatively abnormal serum or urinary M proteins. The diagnosis of multiple myeloma requires histologic documentation by the demonstration of increased numbers (usually over 10%) or abnormal, atypical, or immature plasma cells in the bone marrow in addition to finding serum or urinary M protein or characteristic osteolytic bone lesions. Some patients have multiple plasmacytomas of bone with intervening normal areas of bone marrow. In these patients, a random bone marrow aspirate and biopsy may fail to reveal the tumor, and biopsy of specific bone lesions may be necessary to establish the diagnosis. One variant is the polyneuropathy, organomegaly, endocrinopathy, monoclonal gammopathy syndrome (POEMS). Patients with POEMS have a better survival than do those with multiple myeloma.

2.   Incidence. The annual incidence of multiple myeloma is 4 per 100,000 population, with a peak occurrence between ages 60 and 70 years. Although as many as 4% of patients with myeloma have indolent or smoldering disease at diagnosis, and an additional 5% have an isolated plasmacytoma of bone, most patients with multiple myeloma require chemotherapy of their disease soon after diagnosis.

3.   Effect of treatment. The goals of therapy are to improve the duration of survival and to diminish or prevent the serious manifestations of this disease, such as bone pain, pathologic fractures, severe anemia, renal failure, and hypercalcemia. Treatment produces an objective response in at least half of patients as determined by a sustained 50% decline in the levels of serum or urine M protein. Temporary, sometimes longlasting, alleviation of symptoms occurs in nearly all patients exhibiting an objective response to treatment and in some additional patients with lesser degrees of objective improvement. Median survival times usually reported for treated patients range from 2 to 3 years and are influenced by response to treatment and by the initial tumor load.

4.   Prognostic factors. Table 23.1 presents a clinical staging system developed to estimate myeloma tumor cell mass using readily obtained clinical findings. Severe anemia, hypercalcemia, advanced osteolytic lesions, and extremely high M-protein production rates are all associated with a high tumor burden and a poor survival prognosis. Renal failure, although not well correlated with tumor burden, is associated with poor prognosis. Advanced age, poor performance status, high serum lactate dehydrogenase level, and plasmablastic subtype have also been established as adverse prognostic signs.

The serum level of β_2-microglobulin correlates with the myeloma tumor burden but is of little value for serially monitoring patients with myeloma. Serum β_2-microglobulin usu-

Table 23.1.   Clinical staging system for myeloma

Stage	Criteria	Myeloma cell mass (cells/m^2)

I	All of the following:
	1. Hemoglobin >10 g/dL
	2. Serum calcium value normal (≤12 mg/dL)
	3. On radiograph, normal bone structure or solitary bone plasmacytoma only
	4. Low M-component production rates
	  a. IgG value <5 g/dL
	  b. IgA value <3 g/dL
	  c. Urine light-chain M component on electrophoresis <4 g/24 h
		<0.6 × 10^{12} (low)

II	Fitting neither stage I nor stage III	0.6 × 10^{12} to 1.2 × 10^{12} (intermediate)

III	One or more of the following:
	1. Hemoglobin <8.5 g/dL
	2. Serum calcium value >12 mg/dL
	3. Advanced lytic bone lesions
	4. High M-component production rates
	  a. IgG value >7 g/dL
	  b. IgA value >5 g/dL
	  c. Urine light-chain M component on electrophoresis >12 g/24 h
		>1.2 × 10^{12} (high)

Subclass of any stage
  A Serum creatinine <2 mg/dL
  B Serum creatinine ≥2 mg/dL

Modified from Durie BGM, Salmon SE. A clinical staging system for multiple myeloma: correlation of measured myeloma cell mass with presenting clinical features, response to treatment and survival. *Cancer* 1975;36:842.

ally falls during response to therapy and may increase during relapse, but it has been inconsistent in detecting fulminant progression in which the serum or urinary M proteins may fail to reflect the increasing tumor mass. The plasma cell–labeling index is a reflection of the proportion of myeloma cells that are synthesizing deoxyribonucleic acid (DNA). Patients with a labeling index higher than 3% who have a high cell mass have a particularly poor survival prognosis. A low labeling index has been associated with more indolent disease and particularly with a stable plateau phase during an objective response to therapy.

When the pretreatment plasma cell–labeling index is combined with serum β_2-microglobulin, one can assign half the patients either to a very favorable prognostic group in which both values are low and the prognosis approaches 6 years or to a very poor prognostic group in which both values are high and the survival prognosis is less than 2 years. The remaining patients have an intermediate and less well defined prognosis. Others have used serum levels of C-reactive protein as a reflection of interleukin-6 (IL-6) activity and have combined this with the β_2-microglobulin level to produce an index that divides myeloma patients into low-, intermediate-, and high-risk groups with observed median survival times of 54, 27, and 6 months, respectively. Recently, deletions of chromosome 13 have been shown to convey an adverse prognosis in multiple myeloma. Other adverse prognostic factors include low circulating CD19 B lymphocytes and high serum levels of the IL-6 receptor.

B. Initial treatment

1. General measures. Complications of myeloma (e.g., hypercalcemia and renal failure) may be present at the time of diagnosis (see Section II.C). These complications should be promptly identified and treated before the start of chemotherapy. Patients who present with smoldering or indolent asymptomatic stage IA disease may be followed with observation alone until evidence of progression appears. Most patients have more advanced or progressive disease at diagnosis and require chemotherapy. Patients should be maintained on allopurinol 300 mg/day PO through the first 2 months of chemotherapy to prevent urate nephropathy. A general supportive care regimen emphasizing ambulation and hydration should be maintained throughout the initial treatment. Bisphosphonates, either pamidronate or zoledronic acid, are recommended for nearly every myeloma patient with normal renal function, particularly those with bone disease (see Section II.C.5).

2. Approach to primary therapy (see Sections II.B.3 to 5 for specific regimens). The goal of primary treatment for myeloma is to extend the patient's life and to protect comfort and functionality. For patients under age 70, the possibility of high-dose therapy with autologous stem cell transplant should be discussed. With mortality from this procedure down to 1% in qualified centers, the decision to proceed with transplant in first remission is based on convenience, patient preference, and availability of an excellent transplant facility experienced in multiple myeloma. It is not based on expectation of cure or survival advantage, neither of which is yet proven. A reasonable alternative is to proceed with standard chemotherapy and resort to high-dose therapy and stem cell transplant after first relapse.

If high-dose therapy is a possibility at any time, stem cells sufficient for at least one transplant should be harvested prior to exposing the patient to alkylating agents. The preferred induction therapy is usually two to four cycles of vincristine, Adriamycin, and dexamethasone (VAD) (see Section II.B.5) or dexamethasone alone or the recently described thalidomide–dexamethasone regimen. Patients should receive prophylactic antibiotics or enter a study evaluating them during this induction phase.

High-dose therapy usually is in the form of melphalan. Total-body radiation is usually not used in this setting, and tandem transplants should be reserved for clinical trials until their efficacy is more clearly demonstrated. Maintenance therapy with interferon (IFN) should be considered after recovery.

For patients not undergoing transplant in first remission, stem cell harvest should be followed by standard chemotherapy. In this setting, combination chemotherapy with a regimen such as vincristine, carmustine (BCNU), melphalan, cyclophosphamide, and prednisone (VBMCP) is well tolerated and offers a higher response rate than melphalan and prednisone (MP) and a longer time to progression (TTP). IFN maintenance is reasonable for those who tolerate it.

For patients over age 70, some remain excellent candidates for stem cell transplant and should by treated as those younger than 70 years described above. For the majority, however, standard chemotherapy should be used. Patients with an Eastern Cooperative Oncology Group (ECOG) performance status (PS) of 2 or greater or with serious co-morbidity do not tolerate intensive combination chemotherapy and should be treated with MP instead. Relatively healthy patients with PS of 0 to 1 tolerate chemotherapy better and should be considered for VBMCP, although MP is a reasonable alternative. In the following paragraphs, the elements of primary therapy are discussed in greater detail.

3.   High-dose therapy with bone marrow or peripheral blood stem cell transplantation. Allogeneic bone marrow transplantation after high-dose therapy can cure myeloma, but this happens in fewer than 17% of patients, according to recent updates. At present, suitable candidates represent only a small portion of patients with myeloma. Early transplantation-related mortality rates of 25% to 45% further limit its usefulness at this time. However, in carefully selected patients under 55 years of age, with a matched-related donor and with poor prognostic factors, some feel that it is reasonable to consider allotransplantation in first remission.

High-dose therapy followed by autologous transplantation with bone marrow or peripheral blood stem cells as rescue is unlikely to be curative but, with growth factor support, can be carried out with relative safety and merits consideration as consolidation therapy in first remission or after relapse in patients with responsive disease. Its precise role is yet to be determined and is still the subject of ongoing clinical trials. One reported trial shows a 52% 5-year survival, with about half of the patients surviving 5 years still in their first remission. Other major trials are still accruing patients. It has been well demonstrated that patients who would be candidates for transplantation therapy have a better prognosis than the average myeloma patient and that this explains part of the improvement in survival seen in many uncontrolled transplantation reports. The most commonly used preparative regimens include high-dose melphalan 200 mg/m^2 without total-body radiation. A role for purging the graft of potentially malignant cells seems intuitively likely, but proof of its efficacy in preventing recurrence remains an unmet challenge.

Future treatments will target the minimal residual disease that virtually always remains after a successful autologous transplantation.

4. Standard induction chemotherapy recommendations. These recommendations are based in part on an ECOG prospective, randomized clinical trial comparing moderate MP therapy with the more intensive VBMCP regimen. In that study, VBMCP yielded an objective response rate of 72% in contrast to a 51% objective response rate with MP. Median survival time was similar for the two treatments at 28 to 30 months, but 26% of VBMCP patients survived 5 years compared with a 19% 5-year survival rate with MP. A meta-analysis of a wide variety of studies comparing various combinations with MP or M alone failed to demonstrate a survival difference, although response rates were higher with the combinations.

   a.   Most patients can receive VBMCP. With this regimen, the prednisone schedule is frequently individualized so that slowly responding patients with persistent generalized bone pain or severe anemia may receive low-dose prednisone each day of the first two or three cycles in addition to the higher scheduled prednisone dose on days 1 to 14.

   The VBMCP regimen consists of the following:

Vincristine 1.2 mg/m² IV on day 1 (up to 2 mg), *and*
Carmustine (BCNU) 20 mg/m² IV on day 1, *and*
Melphalan 8 mg/m² PO on days 1 to 4, *and*
Cyclophosphamide 400 mg/m² IV on day 1, *and*
Prednisone 40 mg/m² PO on days 1 to 7 (all cycles), 20 mg/m²
   PO on days 8 to 14 (cycles 1 to 3 only).
Repeat cycle of VBMCP every 35 days for at least 1 year
   and until maximal response is reached.

   b.   Patients over 70 years old who have poor performance status, defined as partially or completely bedridden (ECOG grades 2 to 4), do not tolerate VBMCP. These high-risk patients, who comprise 10% to 15% of myeloma patients, should instead be treated with MP according to the following schedule:

Melphalan 8 mg/m² PO on days 1 to 4, *and*
Prednisone 60 mg/m² PO on days 1 to 4.
Repeat cycle every 28 days for at least 1 year.

   Because of the similarity in median survival data between VBMCP and MP, the latter regimen can also be considered an alternative to VBMCP for some patients not in the above high-risk group if a less aggressive approach is required. Because of erratic absorption of melphalan in most patients, some investigators recommend cautiously escalating the dose of melphalan on subsequent cycles of chemotherapy until a dose is reached that produces moderate nadir leukocyte counts of 2,000 to 3,000 cells/µL. For reliable absorption, melphalan should be taken on an empty stomach.

5.   Alternative induction chemotherapy
   a.   VBMCP + recombinant interferon-α₂ represents an alternative approach to induction therapy. With this regi-

men, two initial cycles of VBMCP are given, followed by alternating 3-week cycles of recombinant IFN-α_2 (rIFN-α_2) with 3-week cycles of VBMCP. The rIFN-α_2 is administered in a dosage of 5×10^6 U/m^2 SC three times a week for 10 doses each cycle, for a total treatment duration of 2 years. The advantages of this regimen over VBMCP are a higher complete response rate and longer response duration. The disadvantages are the expense and toxicity of IFN. The latter is a minor problem for some, but for others, the fatigue is dose limiting.

b.   VAD. High-dose dexamethasone, either alone or as part of the VAD regimen, is useful as a pre–bone marrow harvest induction regimen or as a salvage regimen in patients previously treated with alkylating agents. The three-drug VAD regimen is constructed as follows:

Vincristine 0.4 mg/day as a continuous IV infusion on days 1 to 4, *and*

Doxorubicin (Adriamycin) 9 mg/m^2/day as a continuous IV infusion on days 1 to 4, *and*

Dexamethasone 40 mg PO on days 1 to 4, 9 to 12, and 17 to 20.

Repeat cycle every 28 to 35 days until four cycles beyond occurrence of maximum reduction in myeloma protein. Maximum cumulative doxorubicin dose is 540 mg/m^2. To avoid problems related to adrenal steroid excess, the frequency of dexamethasone courses should be decreased after two or three VAD cycles. One approach is to administer the dexamethasone only days 1 to 4 on the even-numbered cycles but to give it days 1 to 4, 9 to 12, and 17 to 20 on all odd-numbered cycles. VAD is associated with response rates of 70% or more in previously untreated patients.

c.   DVD. A new alternative to VAD uses pegylated liposomal doxorubicin (Doxil) 40 mg/m^2 IV day 1 (over one hour for first dose, then over 30 minutes), vincristine 2 mg IV day 1, and Dexamethasone 40 mg IV or PO daily × 4 days. Repeat cycle every 4 weeks.

d.   Thalidomide. High-dose dexamethasone may also be combined with thalidomide 200 mg/day (thal-dex), which is a marrow-sparing regimen reported to yield response rates of at least 60%. This regimen is currently under evaluation as an induction therapy prior to stem cell harvest. It is also an effective regimen in patients who have relapsed from prior chemotherapy. Patients may require gradual escalation of the thalidomide from 50 to 200 mg/day to avoid excessive somnolence. Doses above 200 mg/day are not usually needed in myeloma and are associated with an increased frequency of neurotoxicity. In patients who achieve remission, doses should be adjusted to patient tolerance, frequently as low as 50 mg daily. Dexamethasone, when combined with thalidomide, is administered in varying schedules. One schedule begins with dexamethasone 40 mg daily on days 1 to 4, 9 to 12, and 17 to 20. In subsequent cycles (of 3 weeks), dexamethasone 40 mg daily is given only on days 1 to 4 of the entire 21-day period.

6.   Duration of therapy and role of maintenance therapy. Although no study has conclusively demonstrated benefit by continuing chemotherapy beyond 1 year in responding patients, several investigators have noted earlier re-emergence of active myeloma after early cessation of therapy. Therefore, one acceptable approach is to continue the induction regimen for a total duration of 1 year or to maximal response but to decrease its frequency to one cycle every 6 to 8 weeks during the second year while continuing to follow M-protein production carefully. It is probably safe to stop treatment at 1 year in patients who started therapy with stage I disease and whose disease has remained stable, in plateau phase, for at least 6 months. These patients should be observed carefully, with re-evaluation of serum and urine M protein once every 3 months.

Several randomized trials evaluated maintenance therapy with IFN after at least 1 year of induction chemotherapy. Most of these showed significant improvement in response duration but no significant difference in survival. Intriguingly, the nonsignificant survival trends tended to favor the IFN maintenance. A meta-analysis evaluating all controlled trials randomizing for the use of IFN in maintenance or induction in myeloma is to be reported soon and could well resolve this issue. At present, it is reasonable to employ IFN maintenance for those who tolerate its side effects. A preferred regimen is rIFN-α_2 2×10^6 U/m^2 SC three times a week to relapse. This regimen can also be used following transplantation.

7.   Role of radiotherapy. Solitary plasmacytoma of bone is best treated by local radiation therapy and may not require chemotherapy for months to years. Radiotherapy is also useful as palliative therapy for patients with extraskeletal plasmacytomas, large lytic lesions threatening fracture of long bones, spinal cord or root compression by plasma cell tumor, and certain pathologic fractures. Repeated local irradiation should be avoided when possible in patients with disseminated myeloma because chemotherapy is the only treatment demonstrated to improve survival while controlling systemic manifestations of the disease. Excessive use of radiation therapy can impair marrow reserves and render the patient less able to tolerate subsequent chemotherapy.

C.   Complications of disease or therapy. Chemotherapy for multiple myeloma typically causes myelosuppression, and packed red blood cell transfusions are often required during the early weeks of treatment and the late refractory period. Toxicity of each chemotherapeutic agent is described in Chapter 4. In addition to these problems, several complications characteristic of multiple myeloma may occur.

1.   Hypercalcemia. This common complication of multiple myeloma is believed to result from the liberation of bone calcium stimulated by osteoclast-activating factors, especially receptor activator of nuclear factor-κB (RANK) ligand produced by bone marrow stromal cells and acting in consort with cytokines produced by myeloma cells. Presenting symptoms may include anorexia, nausea, vomiting, constipation, and polyuria, progressing to lethargy, confusion, coma, and death. Dehydration and potentially reversible renal failure frequently occur during hypercalcemic crises. Control of hypercalcemic crises of multiple myeloma is usually accomplished with saline hydration (initially, 200 mL/h IV), furosemide (20 mg every 4 to 6 h × 2 to 3 doses) once the hypovolemia has been corrected, and prednisone (60 mg PO daily for 3 to 7 days). When hypercalcemia occurs in previously untreated patients, prompt initiation of chemotherapy of the myeloma, in addition to these measures, usually produces effective, durable control. In some patients, bisphosphonates (pamidronate or zoledronic acid) may be needed.

    a. Bisphosphonates

        (1) Pamidronate 90 mg given as a 2-h IV infusion that can be repeated at 7- to 30-day intervals if needed, **or**

        (2) Zoledronic acid 4 mg IV over 15 to 30 min.

    b. Calcitonin 100 to 300 U SC every 8 to 12 h for up to 2 to 3 days. Calcitonin is usually given with prednisone 10 to 20 mg PO two or three times daily to prolong its effectiveness.

    c. Hemodialysis is effective but seldom needed for hypercalcemia with the availability of highly effective bisphosphonates.

2. Infection. Myeloma patients are highly susceptible to respiratory and urinary tract infections with common gram-positive and gram-negative bacterial pathogens. Deficiency of normal immunoglobulins, diminished bone marrow reserves, and immobilization due to skeletal disease are important predisposing factors. The weeks immediately following initiation of chemotherapy are a particularly high-risk period for infection. Prompt evaluation of fever or other manifestations of infection is essential. Antibiotic coverage for gram-positive and gram-negative organisms should be instituted while awaiting culture results from patients whose clinical picture suggests infection. Infection prophylaxis with antibiotics during the first 2 months of chemotherapy may be of help. Use of trimethoprim-sulfamethoxazole (1 double-strength tablet b.i.d.) or ciprofloxacin (500 mg b.i.d.) is under study in this setting. Granulocyte colony-stimulating factor (G-CSF; filgrastim) 5 μg/kg/day SC hastens neutrophil recovery by 1 to 3 days in neutropenic febrile patients. More dramatic reduction in the duration of neutropenia may be seen when this agent is used from 24 h after cytotoxic therapy until full recovery from nadir neutropenia has occurred. Such prophylactic use of G-CSF is justified in patients with prior prolonged neutropenia or infection or who are at exceptionally high risk of infection due to age, intercurrent illness, chemotherapy regimen, or prior history of infection during chemotherapy.

3. Hyperviscosity may present as central nervous system impairment, congestive heart failure, ischemia, or bleeding tendency. It is more characteristic of Waldenström's macroglobulinemia than of multiple myeloma, but it may be seen in patients with extremely high IgG or IgA concentrations or in patients whose M protein tends to form aggregates. Treatment of symptomatic hyperviscosity is with plasmapheresis.

4. Renal dysfunction may be caused by myeloma kidney, amyloidosis, pyelonephritis, hypercalcemia, hyperuricemia with urate nephropathy, hyperviscosity syndrome, plasma cell infiltration of both kidneys (rare), and renal tubular acidosis. Most of these problems are at least partially reversible if recognized and treated promptly. Renal failure may also result from radiographic contrast material, particularly in a patient whose renal function is already compromised or who is dehydrated. Hypercalcemia and hyperuricemia are especially common potential causes of reversible renal failure and should be ruled out at the onset of the evaluation of a patient with myeloma. In patients with severe renal failure, hemodialysis should be considered as long as chemotherapy offers the potential for a prolonged remission.

5.   Skeletal destruction is a major cause of disability and immobilization in multiple myeloma. Radiation therapy, surgery, or both may be needed to treat fractures or to prevent impending fractures of weight-bearing bones. In patients who exhibit lytic disease, monthly infusions of pamidronate 90 mg given over 2 to 4 h can decrease or delay destructive skeletal events and improve the patient's comfort. Zoledronic acid 4 mg IV over 15 to 30 min can be substituted for pamidronate. It is necessary to follow the serum creatinine sequentially to rule out progressive bisphosphonate-induced renal impairment.

6.   Anemia. For patients with refractory disease and chronic symptomatic anemia, treatment with recombinant human erythropoietin frequently diminishes or eliminates the transfusion requirement and returns the hemoglobin to asymptomatic levels. A schedule of 150 to 250 U/kg SC two times a week may be used. Alternatively, 40,000 U weekly may be given empirically.

7.   Leukemia. Acute nonlymphocytic leukemia (ANLL; acute myelogenous leukemia) develops in about 4% of myeloma patients who receive chemotherapy. The incidence of ANLL is appreciably greater in patients surviving 4 years or more after the start of chemotherapy. Leukemia in this setting appears to be caused by the interaction of a carcinogenic drug with a predisposed host. ANLL complicating multiple myeloma is usually preceded by sideroblastic anemia as part of a myelodysplastic syndrome.

D.   Recurrence and treatment of refractory disease. Objective responses to chemotherapy have a median duration of about 2 years. Response duration is influenced by the degree of reduction of tumor burden as reflected by the degree of reduction of myeloma proteins in the serum and urine. Eventually, virtually all patients develop recurrent or refractory disease. These patients pose a difficult clinical problem because of the small number of chemotherapeutic agents with proved activity in myeloma. In patients who relapse months or years after last receiving chemotherapy, remission can frequently be reinduced with the original regimen.

1.   Treatment of disease refractory to melphalan. Disease that is refractory to melphalan or melphalan plus prednisone regimens may still respond to other alkylating agents. Two regimens that may be considered are as follows:

a.   VBMCP. (See Section II.B.4.a.)

b.   BCP may be effective in patients who absorb oral melphalan poorly.

Carmustine (BCNU) 75 mg/m² IV on day 1, *and*
Cyclophosphamide 400 mg/m² IV on day 1, *and*
Prednisone 75 mg PO on days 1 to 7.
Repeat every 4 weeks.

Treatment with these alkylating agent–based regimens can be expected to yield objective responses in about 20% of patients refractory to prior MP therapy. These regimens remain useful as conservative treatment choices for patients in their first relapse or for some patients who have failed initial MP therapy.

2. Alternative regimens not based on standard dose alkylating agents include the following:

a. VAD or DVD. (See Section II.B.5.b. and c.)

b. High-dose cyclophosphamide. Cyclophosphamide 600 mg/m² IV is given on days 1 to 4, with this dosage repeated in 1 to 2 months. This aggressive regimen effectively produces pain relief of more than 1 month's duration and yields short-term objective responses in more than 30% of patients with disease that was refractory to prior treatments. Because the regimen is highly myelotoxic (it is employed without dose modification), its use should generally be limited to patients with active, markedly symptomatic refractory disease in institutions equipped to render intensive support, including platelet transfusion and infectious disease consultation. The prophylactic use of filgrastim (G-CSF) is reasonable with this regimen. A recommended schedule is filgrastim 5 µg/kg SC daily starting 24 h after chemotherapy and continuing through the nadir until the granulocyte count exceeds 8,000 to 10,000/µL.

c. Thalidomide at a dose of 200 mg PO daily may be effective in producing objective responses in 30% to 35% of patients with refractory myeloma. Sometimes, careful escalation of the dose to 400 to 600 mg may be needed. It may also be combined with high-dose dexamethasone (see Section II.B.5.d). Side effects of constipation, somnolence, and neuropathy can be dose limiting and may occur even at the 200-mg level.

d. High-dose methylprednisolone. Methylprednisolone 2 g IV three times weekly for 8 weeks, followed by 2 g weekly, produces clinical benefits in about one-third of patients. It is particularly useful in patients whose marrow status is severely impaired.

III. Waldenström's macroglobulinemia

A. General considerations and aims of therapy. This neoplasm is characterized by the proliferation of plasmacytoid lymphocytes that elaborate a monoclonal IgM. In contrast to multiple myeloma, skeletal destruction does not occur, but hepatosplenomegaly and lymphadenopathy are common. The major problems are hyperviscosity syndrome, severe anemia, and occasionally pancytopenia. The median survival time is only about 5 years from diagnosis, owing partly to the advanced age of most affected patients (60 to 75 years old) as well as to the common association with second neoplasms (20% of patients) and chronic or recurrent infections (25% of patients). The primary aims of therapy are to control complications and to decrease their incidence. Although response to chemotherapy has been associated with a more favorable median survival, the actual role of chemotherapy in prolonging survival in this disease has not been fully defined.

B.   Treatment

1.   Anemia. Most patients with macroglobulinemia are anemic; however, erythropoietin or transfusions should generally be reserved for those with symptomatic anemia. Overtransfusion is dangerous because of the important contribution of red blood cells to whole-blood viscosity.

2.   Hyperviscosity. Hyperviscosity syndrome requires plasmapheresis for acute management and chemotherapy with alkylating agents for long-term control.

3.   Chemotherapy. In general, chemotherapy is withheld until symptomatic disease or progressive cytopenia occurs.

a.   Standard chemotherapy

Chlorambucil 2 to 6 mg PO daily, *or*

Cyclophosphamide 50 to 100 mg PO daily.

(Prednisone 40 to 60 mg PO on days 1 to 4 every 4 weeks may be added.)

b. Alternatively, a **high-dose intermittent chlorambucil plus prednisone regimen** may be used every 2 to 3 weeks.

Chlorambucil 30 mg/m^2 PO on day 1, *and*

Prednisone 40 mg/m^2 PO on days 1 to 4.

c.   VBMCP. (See Section II.B.4.a.)

d.   Fludarabine 25 mg/m^2 IV days 1 to 5 every 3 to 4 weeks is effective in up to 40% of patients but may cause prolonged CD4 lymphocyte suppression. This agent is yet to be compared with standard regimens such as intermittent chlorambucil.

4.   Disease variants. Some patients with IgM monoclonal proteins have clinical chronic lymphocytic leukemia or lymphoma and should have their treatment directed at that disease. Rare patients with macroglobulinemia have prominent skeletal disease, and their disease should be approached as IgM myeloma and treated similarly to other multiple myelomas.

IV.   Heavy-chain diseases. Heavy-chain diseases comprise a group of rare plasma cell dyscrasias in which the abnormal clone of plasma cells or B lymphocytes elaborates an abnormal polypeptide consisting of anomalous γ, α, or μ heavy chains with deleted segments.

A.   γ heavy-chain disease presents as a lymphoma usually with lymphadenopathy, hepatosplenomegaly, and involvement of Waldeyer's ring. The latter may lead to characteristic palatal edema. Bone marrow involvement is the rule. Treatment by local radiotherapy or lymphoma-directed chemotherapy regimens is sometimes effective.

B.   α heavy-chain disease appears to be the most common of the heavy-chain diseases and occurs mainly in people under the age of 50 years. Its most common clinical presentation is in the enteric form, with chronic diarrhea, malabsorption syndrome, and marked lymphoplasmacytic infiltration of the small bowel mucosa. Remissions have been reported using lymphoma chemotherapy regimens and occasionally antibiotics alone.

C.   μ heavy-chain disease is rare, usually presenting as chronic lymphocytic leukemia, and it should be managed as such.

V.   Amyloidosis. Only primary amyloidosis with or without associated plasma cell or lymphoid neoplasms is considered in this section. With these disorders, the amyloid substance consists of fragments of immunoglobulin light chains and is therefore termed an *amyloid L-chain protein.* This type of amyloid characteristically infiltrates the tongue, heart, skin, ligaments, and muscle and occasionally the kidney, liver, and spleen. In patients with documented lymphomas or plasma cell neoplasms, treatment is of the underlying neoplasm, but the decline in the amount of amyloid is often minimal. With primary amyloidosis without a demonstrable underlying neoplasm, treatment with MP has been shown to be of moderate benefit when tested in a randomized double-blind study, although the exact role of chemotherapy for this disease is not yet clear. High-dose therapy with stem cell rescue is also under investigation.

VI.   Monoclonal gammopathy of undetermined significance. This disease has been found in up to 3% of people over 70 years of age. It has been termed *benign monoclonal gammopathy;* however, because about 20% of patients with this finding progress to more severe plasma cell dyscrasias, the term *monoclonal gammopathy of undetermined significance* has been introduced as more appropriate. With this condition, patients usually have an M spike of less than 2 g/dL, no bone lesions, no conclusive evidence of myeloma on bone marrow aspirate or biopsy, no anemia or bone marrow failure, and stability of the clinical picture and M-protein studies over a period of follow-up. The serum β_2-microglobulin and the plasma cell–labeling index are both low. Once initial stability has been demonstrated, these patients should be followed at yearly intervals with evaluation of hemoglobin levels and M-protein status. No treatment is indicated unless progression to myeloma or symptomatic macroglobulinemia occurs.

SELECTED READINGS

Attal M, Harousseau J-L, Stoppa A-M, et al. A prospective randomized trial of autologous bone marrow transplantation and chemotherapy in multiple myeloma. *N Engl J Med* 1996;335:91–97.

Barlogie B, Smith L, Alexanian R. Effective treatment of advanced multiple myeloma refractory to alkylating agents. *N Engl J Med* 1984;310:1353–1356.

Bataille R, Boccadoro M, Klein B, et al. C-reactive protein and beta 2-microglobulin produce a simple and powerful myeloma staging system. *Blood* 1992;80:733–737.

Berenson JR, Lichtenstein A, Porter L, et al. Efficacy of pamidronate in reducing skeletal events in patients with advanced multiple myeloma. *N Engl J Med* 1996;334:488–493.

Blade J, San Miguel JF, Fontanillas M, et al. Survival of multiple myeloma patients who are potential candidates for early high-dose therapy intensification/autotransplantation and who were conventionally treated. *J Clin Oncol* 1996;14:2167–2173.

Case DC, Lee BJ, Clarkson BD. Improved survival times in multiple myeloma treated with melphalan, prednisone, cyclophosphamide, vincristine and BCNU: M-2 protocol. *Am J Med* 1977;68:897–903.

Durie BG, Dixon DO, Carter S, et al. Improved survival duration with combination chemotherapy induction for multiple myeloma: a Southwest Oncology Group Study. *J Clin Oncol* 1986;4:1227–1237.

Durie BGM, Salmon SE. A clinical staging system for multiple myeloma: correlation of measured myeloma cell mass with presenting clinical features, response to treatment and survival. *Cancer* 1975;36:842–854.

Durie BGM, Salmon SE, Moon TE. Pretreatment tumor mass, cell kinetics and prognosis in multiple myeloma. *Blood* 1980;55:364–372.

Fernand JP, Ravaud P, Chevret S, et al. High-dose therapy and autologous peripheral blood stem cell transplantation in multiple myeloma: up-front or rescue treatment? Results of a multicenter sequential randomized clinical trial. *Blood* 1998;92:3131–3136.

Fonseca R, Harrington D, Oken MM, et al. Biological and prognostic significance of interphase fluorescence in situ hybridization detection of chromosome 13 abnormalities in multiple myeloma: an Eastern Cooperative Oncology Group study. *Cancer Res* 2002;62:715–720.

Gahrton G, Tura S, Ljungman P, et al. Allogeneic bone marrow transplantation in multiple myeloma. *N Engl J Med* 1991;325:1267–1273.

Greipp PR, Katzmann JA, O'Fallon WM, et al. Value of beta-2 microglobulin level and plasma cell labeling indices as prognostic factors in patients with newly diagnosed myeloma. *Blood* 1988;72:219–223.

Greipp PR, Lust JA, O'Fallon WM, et al. Plasma cell labeling index and beta 2-microglobulin predict survival independent of thymidine kinase and C-reactive protein in multiple myeloma. *Blood* 1993;81:3382–3387.

Hussein MA, Wood L, Hsi E, et al. A Phase II trial of pegylated liposomal doxorubicin, vincristine, and reduced-dose dexamethasone combination therapy in newly diagnosed multiple myeloma patients. *Cancer* 2002; 95:2160–8.

Kyle RA, Therneau TM, Rajkkumar SV, et al. A long-term study of prognosis in monoclonal gammopathy of undetermined significance. *N Engl J Med* 2002;346:564–569.

Mandelli F, Avvisati G, Amadori S, et al. Maintenance treatment with recombinant interferon alfa-2b in patients with multiple myeloma responding to conventional induction chemotherapy. *N Engl J Med* 1990;322:1430.

Mirallis GD, O'Fallon JR, Talley NJ. Plasma-cell dyscrasia with polyneuropathy. *N Engl J Med* 1992;327:1919–1923.

Oken MM. Standard treatment of multiple myeloma. *Mayo Clin Proc* 1994;69:781–787.

Oken MM, Harrington DP, Abramson N, et al. Comparison of melphalan and prednisone with vincristine, carmustine, melphalan, cyclophosphamide and prednisone in the treatment of multiple myeloma. Results of Eastern Cooperative Oncology Group Study E2479. *Cancer* 1997;79:1561–1567.

Oken MM, Pomeroy C, Weisdorf D, et al. Prophylactic antibiotics for the prevention of early infection in multiple myeloma. *Am J Med* 1996;100:624–628.

Samson D, Gaminara E, Newland A, et al. Infusion of vincristine and doxorubicin with oral dexamethasone as first-line therapy for multiple myeloma. *Lancet* 1989;2:882–885.

Metastatic Cancer of Unknown Origin

Martin M. Oken

In about 5% of patients with newly diagnosed cancer (excluding nonmelanoma skin cancer), the primary site remains unknown despite a detailed history and physical examination, routine blood chemistries, complete blood count, urinalysis, chest radiograph, and histologic evaluation of the biopsy. The problem of metastatic cancer of unknown origin raises difficult questions for both diagnosis and treatment. Although the median survival time of patients with cancer of unknown origin has been reported to be less than 6 months, subgroups of patients have been defined who have a far better outlook with proper management. With modern therapy, the overall survival of these patients appears to be improving. A major responsibility of the clinician is to identify those patients with a characteristic presentation who might benefit from a specific strategy and to identify the increasingly large group of patients that might benefit from a trial of chemotherapy.

I. General considerations and aims of therapy
A. Histology and presenting clinical manifestations.
Adenocarcinoma and undifferentiated carcinoma each comprise up to 40% of all cancers of unknown origin. Fewer than 15% of cancers of unknown origin are squamous cell carcinomas (SCCs), and at most 2% to 5% are malignant melanoma. Other histologies that may present as cancer of unknown origin include lymphomas, germ cell tumors, and neuroendocrine carcinomas. These histologies are particularly important to identify because they represent tumors that may be effectively managed with systemic chemotherapy. Nearly half of all patients with unknown primaries and well over half of those with adenocarcinoma present with hepatomegaly, abdominal mass, or other abdominal symptoms. Lymphadenopathy is the presenting clinical manifestation in 15% to 25% of patients. Lower cervical or supraclavicular lymph nodes usually contain adenocarcinoma or undifferentiated carcinoma, and middle to high cervical adenopathy generally represents SCC. Between 10% and 20% of patients present with manifestations of bone, lung, or pleural involvement, whereas fewer than 10% present with evidence of central nervous system disease. Most of the latter group are eventually found to have either lung or gastrointestinal tract primaries.

Two presentations of advanced carcinoma of unknown primary site have been recognized as more treatable than others: poorly differentiated carcinoma or adenocarcinoma, especially with predominant sites of involvement in the mediastinum, retroperitoneum, lymph nodes, or lungs; and adenocarcinoma in women predominantly involving the peritoneal surfaces. In these instances, platinum-based chemotherapy regimens designed for germ cell or ovarian cancers have produced many useful objective responses and occasional long-term disease-free survival.

B. Sites of origin. It is sometimes possible to predict the most likely primary sites from the histology and location of the metastatic lesion of unknown origin. Pancreas and lung are the most common ultimately determined sites of origin. Together they represent more than 40% of the adenocarcinomas of unknown origin. Colorectal, gastric, and hepatobiliary carcinoma each represents about 10% of the cancers of unknown origin.

In general, adenocarcinomas or undifferentiated carcinomas presenting with hepatic metastases or left supraclavicular adenopathy are eventually demonstrated to be of gastrointestinal origin. SCCs that present in the supraclavicular or low cervical lymph nodes are usually from lung primaries, whereas similar lesions of higher cervical nodes are more likely to have originated from occult primary lesions in the head and neck region.

The pattern of metastatic involvement associated with occult primary tumors differs from that associated with overt primaries. For example, occult lung cancer rarely involves bone, a common site of metastasis from overt lung cancer; however, bone metastases appear to be more common in patients with gastrointestinal cancer who have occult primaries than in those who have overt primaries.

C. Aims of diagnostic evaluation. The first objective in the management of a patient newly diagnosed with cancer of unknown origin is to plan the appropriate diagnostic evaluation. There are three chief aims of this evaluation:

1. Identify a tumor in which cure or effective disease control is possible.
2. Determine if the tumor is regionally confined or widely metastatic.
3. Identify any complication for which immediate local therapy is indicated.

D. Goal of treatment. In patients with tumors for which effective systemic therapy is available and in patients with disease regionally confined to peripheral lymph nodes alone, active management with the goal of prolongation of life through extended disease control or cure should be considered. These patients represent about 25% of patients with occult primaries. For the remaining patients, the chance of prolonging life has been less likely, but with newer therapy, it might be improving. Treatment should also address palliation of symptoms and preservation of the best possible quality of life.

II. Diagnostic evaluation

A. Analysis of the biopsy specimen. If possible, the pathologist should receive fresh, unfixed material to allow electron microscopy, histochemistry, immunohistology, and hormone receptor studies to be done, if needed, after routine examination. Careful review of the biopsy material should be undertaken to classify the tumor conclusively as SCC, adenocarcinoma, or other identifiable histology. Up to 40% of cancers of unknown origin are undifferentiated or poorly differentiated tumors based on evaluation of hematoxylin and eosin–stained material. Electron microscopy, when available, may be useful for the further classification of these tumors through the identification of desmosomes and intercellular bridges (SCC); tight junctions, microvilli, and acinar spaces (adenocarcinoma); premelanosomes (amelanotic melanoma); neurosecretory granules (small cell or neuroendocrine carcinoma); and absence of junctions (lymphoma). Immunohistology is an indispensable part of the evaluation of carcinoma of unknown primary site. Immunohistochemical studies on the tumor may be used to demonstrate the presence of prostatic acid phosphatase or prostate-specific antigen (PSA; prostate carcinoma), human chorionic gonadotropin (β-hCG; germ cell tumors), α-fetoprotein (germ cell tumors or hepatocellular carcinoma), or monoclonal immunoglobulin (lymphoma, plasmacytoma). Immunoglobulin or T-cell receptor gene rearrangements may be helpful in identifying tumors of lymphoid origin. Undifferentiated carcinomas or adenocarcinomas in women should be evaluated for estrogen and progesterone receptors. Mucin positivity is helpful in eliminating the possibility of renal cell carcinoma.

Clearly, the use of many of these specialized studies must be balanced against their expense. If judiciously applied, they can aid in the identification of some of the undifferentiated or poorly differentiated tumors of unknown origin and help to focus their subsequent diagnostic evaluation and management.

One exception to the policy of seeking a definitive histologic diagnosis as the first step in evaluating a tumor of unknown origin is when the patient presents with a potentially resectable neck mass (other than supraclavicular adenopathy) and no other apparent lesion. In these patients, a head and neck primary should be sought by detailed head and neck examination, radiographs of the sinuses, and, if necessary, panendoscopy under general anesthesia to include laryngoscopy, bronchoscopy, esophagoscopy, and nasopharyngoscopy with blind biopsy of the base of the tongue, piriform sinuses, nasopharynx, and tonsillar fossae if no gross primary is found. A computed tomography (CT) scan of the head and neck may also be of value. [18F]Fluorodeoxyglucose positron emission tomography (FDG-PET) scanning has also been utilized in this setting. If this work-up is not diagnostic, biopsy of the neck mass is undertaken. This order of evaluation is chosen so that if a resectable SCC of the head and neck is found, the neck mass can be removed as part of the curative procedure.

B.   Squamous cell carcinoma. For SCCs with apparent involvement of only one lymph node group, the possibility of long-term survival exists if proper treatment is carried out. The diagnostic evaluation depends on the lymph node region involved. The most common lymph node presentation for SCCs of unknown origin is in the cervical or supraclavicular region. Cervical lymph node metastases above the supraclavicular region usually originate from head and neck primary lesions. The diagnostic approach to these lesions is discussed in the preceding section. Because surgery, irradiation, or both, with curative intent, are employed if disease is localized to this region, distant metastases should be excluded with a bone scan, a chest radiograph, and, in some instances, a chest CT scan. SCC of supraclavicular lymph nodes is usually of lung or esophageal origin and seldom represents regionally confined disease. Evaluation is the same as that for disease that extends beyond regional lymph nodes.

SCC in axillary or inguinal lymph nodes is rarely associated with an occult primary. Regional skin and lung should be examined as possible primary sites with axillary disease, whereas the skin, anus, and genitalia should be carefully examined when the presentation is SCC in the inguinal nodes.

SCC with generalized lymphadenopathy or, more commonly, with disease that extends beyond the lymph nodes represents disease that cannot be satisfactorily controlled by present-day techniques. The search for the primary lesions should be done mainly by a chest radiograph and careful physical examination of the appropriate organs. Serum chemistries, including the calcium level, should be determined. Further diagnostic studies are needed only if indicated by signs, symptoms, or abnormalities on the initial studies.

C. Adenocarcinoma and poorly differentiated carcinoma. Women with adenocarcinoma or poorly differentiated carcinoma of unknown origin should undergo mammography, careful pelvic examination, and hormone receptor evaluation of the tumor. In men, serum acid phosphatase, PSA, β-hCG, and α-fetoprotein should be determined to help exclude prostate and germ cell tumors, respectively. An elevated CA 27.29 level would point toward a breast primary. All patients should have stools and urine examined for occult blood, and the serum should be tested for abnormalities in the liver chemistries, creatinine, and electrolytes. With disease apparently confined to axillary lymph nodes, mammography is particularly important in women and should be considered in some men as well. If there is a strong suspicion of breast cancer and the mammogram is negative, magnetic resonance imaging (MRI) should be considered. Undifferentiated carcinoma found only in middle to high cervical lymph nodes should be evaluated in the same manner as described in Section II.B for cervical node SCC.

Traditional contrast studies such as intravenous pyelogram, barium enema, and upper gastrointestinal series are not indicated unless specifically suggested by signs or symptoms (e.g., occult blood in the stool). Abdominal CT scan with intravenous contrast medium is a reasonable option in view of the frequency with which it detects carcinoma of the pancreas or hepatobiliary cancer in this setting.

D. Malignant melanoma. The finding of malignant melanoma confined to a single lymph node group and without a detectable primary lesion represents stage II disease and is associated with a 30% 5-year survival rate after lymphadenectomy. Evaluation to exclude more extensive disease should include a history, physical examination (emphasizing skin and ophthalmoscopic examination), chest radiograph, liver chemistries, liver scan, and brain CT scan.

III. Treatment

A. General strategy. The importance of identifying tumors that may be treated effectively, such as lymphomas, germ cell tumors, trophoblastic tumors, and breast, prostate, ovarian, and neuroendocrine carcinomas, is readily apparent. Once identified, these lesions should be treated as described in their respective chapters. In patients whose primary lesion remains obscure, a therapeutic distinction must be made between those with disease confined to one lymph node region and those with more widespread disease or involvement of visceral organs. In the former, some may be treated with curative intent, whereas in the latter, the aims of treatment are palliative.

B. Squamous cell carcinoma. Patients with SCC confined to the cervical lymph nodes above the supraclavicular region should receive full-course radiotherapy to a field extending from the base of the skull to the clavicles. Alternatively, they may be treated with radical lymph node dissection followed by radiation therapy. In either case, the irradiation is designed to include any possible head and neck primary carcinoma. Survival of patients so treated is at least as good as that for patients with known head and neck primaries. More limited lymph node dissection or regional irradiation may also be indicated for SCC confined to unilateral involvement of the axillary or inguinal nodes.

More widespread SCCs of unknown origin are treated with a palliative intent. No treatment except for local radiotherapy to symptomatic lesions is the standard approach. In patients with symptomatic or progressive disease who desire chemotherapy, regimens designed mainly for head and neck or non–small cell lung cancer should be considered.

1. CF

Cisplatin 100 mg/m^2 IV on day 1, *and*
Fluorouracil 1,000 mg/m^2 as a continuous 24-h IV infusion for 4 days (days 1 to 4).
Repeat every 3 weeks.

2. MBP

Methotrexate 40 mg/m^2 IM on days 1 and 15, *and*
Bleomycin 10 U IM on days 1, 8, and 15, *and*
Cisplatin 50 mg/m^2 IV on day 4.
Repeat every 3 weeks.

3. Various combinations of cisplatin or carboplatin with paclitaxel as outlined in Chapter 7 on lung cancer can also be used.

Do not use regimens 1 or 2 if the serum creatinine level is more than 1.5 mg/dL. The cumulative dose of bleomycin should not exceed 300 U. Use proper hydration with cisplatin as described elsewhere in this text.

C. Adenocarcinoma and poorly differentiated carcinoma. In women, if these carcinomas are confined to the unilateral axillary lymph nodes, they should be considered possible breast cancer and treated accordingly as stage II disease (see Chapter 10). A woman with adenocarcinoma or poorly differentiated carcinoma predominantly confined to the peritoneal surface should be considered for a cisplatin-based ovarian cancer regimen. Undifferentiated carcinoma confined to the middle or high cervical lymph nodes should be treated actively as SCC (see Section II.B). Men with adenocarcinoma of unknown primary and a positive tumor or serum PSA should have a trial of hormonal therapy.

Patients with more advanced adenocarcinoma or poorly differentiated carcinoma in whom the evaluation previously described in Section II.C does not suggest breast, prostate, or other highly treatable primary should be managed according to the histology. Cisplatin-based combination chemotherapy is valuable in the treatment of poorly differentiated carcinoma and poorly differentiated adenocarcinoma. In these patients, the germ cell regimen of bleomycin, etoposide, and cisplatin (BEP) or EP (BEP without the bleomycin) has been studied in a series of 220 patients. This combination may produce more than a 60% objective response rate and more than a 20% complete response rate with up to a 13% long-term survival rate. This regimen is fully described in Chapter 12.

Patients with widespread adenocarcinoma that is well or moderately well differentiated may be more responsive to systemic therapy than previously thought. The combination of paclitaxel, carboplatin, and oral etoposide (PCE) yields objective responses in 45% of patients, and the doxorubicin and mitomycin (DM) regimen may produce partial responses in about one-third of patients.

1. PCE

Paclitaxel 200 mg/m² as a 1-h IV infusion on day 1, *and*
Carboplatin at an area under the curve (AUC) of 6 IV over 30 to 60 min on day 1, *and*
Etoposide 50 and 100 mg PO on alternate days for days 1 to 10.
Repeat every 3 weeks.
Follow the usual paclitaxel toxicity prophylaxis regimen with dexamethasone and H1- and H2-histamine receptor antagonists (Chapter 4).

2. DM

Doxorubicin (Adriamycin) 50 mg/m² IV on days 1 and 22, *and*
Mitomycin 20 mg/m² IV on day 1.
Repeat every 42 days.
Do not exceed a 540-mg/m² cumulative dose of doxorubicin.

Both regimens are worthy of consideration in patients with good performance status because occasional durable responses have occurred. Both reports are based on limited accrual Phase II studies. Responding patients show improvement within two cycles, and chemotherapy should be stopped after two cycles if no improvement is seen. PCE is also effective in patients with poorly differentiated adenocarcinoma and poorly differentiated carcinoma and may be considered as an alternative to BEP.

D. Malignant melanoma. For disease confined to a single lymph node group, radical lymph node dissection yields long-term survival in 30% of treated patients. Treatment of disseminated melanoma is discussed in Chapter 14.

E. Neuroendocrine carcinoma. Poorly differentiated neuroendocrine carcinoma may represent up to 13% of cases of poorly differentiated carcinoma or adenocarcinoma. The diagnosis is secured by recognition of neurosecretory granules on electron microscopy. Localized lesions are uncommon and should be treated with surgery or radiation therapy. Metastatic disease frequently responds to platinum-based chemotherapy such as etoposide plus cisplatin.

SELECTED READINGS

Abbruzzese JL, Abbruzzese MC, Hess KR, et al. Unknown primary carcinoma: natural history and prognostic factors in 657 consecutive patients. *J Clin Oncol* 1994;12:1272–1284.

Altman E, Cadman E. An analysis of 1539 patients with cancer of unknown primary site. *Cancer* 1986;57:120–124.

Greco FA, Burris HA III, Litchy S, et al. Gemcitabine, carboplatin, and paclitaxel for patients with carcinoma of unknown primary site: a Minnie Pearl Cancer Center Research Network Study. *J Clin Oncol* 2002;20:1651–1656.

Greco FA, Vaughn WK, Hainsworth JD. Advanced poorly differentiated carcinoma of unknown primary site: recognition of a treatable syndrome. *Ann Intern Med* 1986;104:547–556.

Hainsworth JD, Erland JB, Kalman LA, et al. Carcinoma of unknown primary site: treatment with one-hour paclitaxel, carboplatin, and extended schedule etoposide. *J Clin Oncol* 1997;15:2385–2393.

Hainsworth JD, Greco FA. Treatment of patients with cancer of an unknown primary site. *N Engl J Med* 1993;329:257–263.

Hainsworth JD, Johnson DH, Greco FA. Poorly differentiated neuroendocrine carcinoma of unknown primary site: a newly recognized clinicopathologic entity. *Ann Intern Med* 1988;109:364–371.

Hainsworth JD, Johnson DH, Greco FA. Cisplatin-based combination chemotherapy in the treatment of poorly differentiated carcinoma and poorly differentiated adenocarcinoma of unknown primary site: results of a 12-year experience. *J Clin Oncol* 1992;10:912–922.

Lenzi R, Hess KR, Abbruzzese MC. Poorly differentiated carcinoma and poorly differentiated adenocarcinoma of unknown origin: favorable subsets of patients with unknown-primary carcinoma. *J Clin Oncol* 1997;15:2056–2066.

Moertel CG. Adenocarcinoma of unknown origin. *Ann Intern Med* 1979;91:646–647.

Neumann KH, Nystrom JS. Metastatic cancer of unknown origin: nonsquamous cell type. *Semin Oncol* 1982;9:427.

Stokkel MP, Terhoard CH, Hordij KFJ, et al. The detection of unknown primary tumors in patients with cervical metastases by dual-head positron emission tomography. *Oral Oncol* 1999;35:390–394.

Strnad CM, Grosh WW, Baxter J, et al. Peritoneal carcinomatosis of unknown primary site in women: a distinctive subset of adenocarcinoma. *Ann Intern Med* 1989;11:213–217.

Woods RL, Fox RM, Tattersall MH, et al. Metastatic adenocarcinomas of unknown primary site: a randomized study of two combination chemotherapy regimens. *N Engl J Med* 1980;303:87–89.

25

Human Immunodeficiency Virus–Associated Malignancies

Diely A. Pichardo and Jamie H. Von Roenn

I. Introduction. Four malignancies are considered acquired immunodeficiency syndrome (AIDS)–defining illnesses: Kaposi's sarcoma (KS), primary central nervous system lymphoma (PCNSL), non-Hodgkin's lymphoma (NHL), and cervical cancer. Although other malignancies appear to have an increased incidence in human immunodeficiency virus (HIV)–infected patients (e.g., squamous cell anal cancer and Hodgkin's disease), their precise relationship to HIV infection has not yet been established. The management of any cancer in an HIV-infected patient requires an integrated team approach. Treatment of the underlying HIV infection must be incorporated into the overall treatment plan, in addition to aggressive prophylaxis and treatment of opportunistic infections, maintenance of general health and nutrition, and psychosocial support.

II. Kaposi's sarcoma

A. Epidemiology. KS is one of the most common HIV-associated malignancies. The incidence of KS in both developed and developing countries rose steadily in the 1970s and 1980s, peaked around 1994, and has declined dramatically since the introduction of highly active antiretroviral therapy. As an AIDS-defining illness, the incidence of KS has decreased from about 33% of patients in the early 1980s to 14% in the early 1990s to only 6.4% in 1998. In recent years, KS most often presents as a late, non-AIDS-defining manifestation of HIV infection. In developing counties, however, the incidence of KS remains high. In some parts of Africa, KS is the most common cancer in men, accounting for up to 50% of all cancers in men. Significant evidence points to the importance of human herpes virus type 8 (HHV-8) in the pathogenesis of KS. HHV-8 DNA is identified in more than 90% of KS biopsies. Serologic studies demonstrate detectable antibodies to HHV-8 in a high percentage of KS patients. Furthermore, antibodies to HHV-8 have been associated with the subsequent development of KS.

B. Presentation and detection. The natural history of KS is extremely variable. KS most often presents as a pink or brown–purple papule or plaque on the skin or mucous membranes. Lesions are frequently symmetric and follow Langer's lines. KS can present anywhere but has a predilection for the retroauricular areas, soles of the feet, extremities, genitalia, and face. In addition to their cosmetic unacceptability, KS lesions can cause significant morbidity and organ dysfunction. Dermal lymphatic involvement, most commonly involving the lower extremities, genitalia, and periorbital area, can cause painful and disfiguring lymphedema. The edema is often out of proportion to the visible skin involvement. Oral cavity lesions occur in about 45% of patients with cutaneous KS, and the oral cavity is the first site of disease in 15% of patients. Oral lesions can interfere with speech and eating. Gastrointestinal involvement, present in up to half of patients, is often asymptomatic but can cause pain, diarrhea, and bleeding. Pulmonary involvement is the most common life-threatening manifestation of KS. It may be difficult to differentiate from opportunistic infection because the chest radiograph may show a reticulonodular or nodular infiltrate, with or without pleural effusions. Bronchoscopy is useful to visualize the characteristic erythematous plaque-like bronchial lesions of KS. However, biopsy is rarely done because of the risk of bleeding from these highly vascular tumors. Thallium and gallium scans may be useful to differentiate KS from an opportunistic pulmonary infection.

C.   Staging. KS is a multicentric tumor and hence does not easily fit the usual TNM categorization. Because the overall prognosis is more closely related to the degree of underlying immune dysfunction than to sites of disease involvement, the AIDS Clinical Trials Group (ACTG) developed a staging system that reflects various prognostic factors (Table 25.1). Patients are defined as good or poor risk on the basis of tumor burden, sites of involvement, CD4 lymphocyte count, history of opportunistic infections, systemic symptoms, and performance status. A recent study validating the ACTG staging system identified tumor burden as a significant predictive factor only in patients with a CD4 count of at least 200 cells/µL. The presence of systemic symptoms was not a predictor of outcome, and a CD4 count of 150 cells/µL, rather than 200 cells/µL, was a better discriminant of outcome.

The initial evaluation of a patient with KS should include a careful physical examination, including a rectal examination with Hemoccult testing. The history should focus on the rate of

Table 25.1.   AIDS Clinical Trials Group staging for epidemic Kaposi's sarcoma[a]

Disease status	Relative risk	
	Good risk (0) (all of the following)	Poor risk (1) (any of the following)
Tumor (T)	Confined to skin, minimal oral disease, or both	Edema; extensive oral ulcers; visceral and gastrointestinal disease
Immune status (I)[a]	CD4 count ≥150/µL	CD4 count <150/µL
Systemic illness (S)	No prior opportunistic infection or thrush; no B symptoms	Prior opportunistic infection or thrush; B symptoms; performance status <70%; other HIV-related illness

[a]Modified by recent validation study.

progression of KS, lesion-associated symptoms (pain, edema, disfigurement), as well as the history of HIV treatment, HIV-related opportunistic infections, the rate of decline in CD4 lymphocyte counts, and viral load. Even though the lesions are characteristic, a biopsy should be done to exclude other cutaneous processes. A baseline chest radiograph is important to look for asymptomatic visceral disease. Computed tomography (CT) scans are not indicated unless the patient's symptoms suggest abdominal disease. Upper endoscopy and colonoscopy are not indicated in the absence of unexplained gastrointestinal bleeding or symptoms. Medications should be reviewed to ensure that patients are receiving appropriate highly active antiretroviral therapy and prophylaxis for opportunistic infections as well as to identify potentially myelosuppressive drugs that may complicate the use of chemotherapeutic agents (e.g., trimethoprim-sulfamethoxazole, sulfadiazine, zidovudine).

D. Treatment. Effective treatment of KS is dependent on clear communication between the doctor and patient with regard to the risks and benefits of the proposed therapy, its interaction with HIV treatment, and the patient's overall expectations. **KS is not a curable tumor. Treatment has not clearly been shown to prolong survival.** The first decision to be made is whether to initiate therapy. Indications to initiate treatment for KS include prevention of disease progression, cosmesis, palliation of symptoms, and visceral disease. In general, local therapies are used for minimal, primarily cosmetically disturbing KS or for patients with severe multisystem compromise who may not tolerate systemic treatment. Systemic therapy is indicated for bulky, rapidly progressing, symptomatic, or life-threatening disease (Table 25.2). The determination of appropriate therapy is based on an evaluation of both tumor and immune status. Regardless of the extent of KS, effective HIV suppression tends to improve both the response to KS treatment and the durability of the response.

1. **Local therapy.** Limited numbers of small lesions can be treated by radiotherapy, topical therapy, cryotherapy, or intralesional injection. Surgery is occasionally useful for an isolated pedunculated lesion. Cryotherapy with liquid nitrogen can lead to hypopigmentation, which may be cosmetically unacceptable to dark-skinned patients. Intralesional therapy with vinblastine or interferon (IFN) can be effective but is limited by the need for multiple injections (Table 25.3). After the injection of oral lesions, patients typically slough the oral mucosa in 24 to 48 h, for which narcotic analgesics should be empirically provided. Intralesional IFN-α is occasionally effective even in patients who have failed systemic IFN. Topical alitretinoin has been approved for the local therapy of KS. The 0.1% retinoic acid gel is applied initially twice a day with escalation to three or four daily doses as tolerated. Overall response rates for individual lesions range from 27% to 49%. The main adverse effect is local skin irritation and local pain. There is no evidence of systemic absorption. Radiation therapy is effective for local control of KS. Depending on the dose and schedule, radiation therapy results in the

Table 25.2.   Treatment guidelines for Kaposi's sarcoma[a]

Disease status of KS	HIV disease status	Treatment options
Minimal cutaneous disease	CD4 count <200/μL; prior OI; B symptoms	Local therapy
	CD4 count ≥200/μL; no prior OI; no B symptoms	Interferon and antivirals or local therapy
Isolated, cosmetically disturbing disease	Any	Local therapy
Extensive cutaneous disease	CD4 count <200/μL; prior OI; B symptoms	Chemotherapy
	CD4 count ≥200/μL; no prior OI; no B symptoms	Interferon and antivirals or chemotherapy
Localized bulky or painful disease	Any	Radiation therapy or chemotherapy
Tumor-associated edema	Any	Chemotherapy
Symptomatic visceral disease	Any	Chemotherapy

KS, Kaposi's sarcoma; OI, opportunistic infection.
[a] Best antiviral therapy is always a component of KS therapy.
Adopted with permission from Susan Krown, M.D.

most satisfying cosmetic result and longest duration of benefit of all the available local interventions.

2.   Systemic therapy

   a.   Biologic response modifiers. IFN-α is the best-studied biologic response modifier. A clear-cut dose–response relationship has not been established. Responses have been reported with doses ranging from 1×10^6 U/day to 36×10^6 U three times per week (see Table 25.4 for recommended dosing). Immune function, as measured by CD4 lymphocyte counts, is the best predictor of response to IFN as a single agent. Patients with CD4 lymphocyte counts of more than 400 cells/μL have an overall response rate of 45%, whereas patients with CD4 lymphocyte counts of less

Table 25.3.   Intralesional chemotherapy for Kaposi's sarcoma

Chemotherapy regimen[a]	
Vinblastine (0.2 mg/mL)	0.1 mL/0.5 cm of surface area of lesion (maximum 4 mL)
Interferon-α	$3–5 \times 10^6$ U 3 ×/wk for 4 wk

[a] Appropriate local anesthesia should be given before injection.

Table 25.4. Selected systemic treatment regimens for Kaposi's sarcoma

Regimens	
Biologic response modifier	
Interferon-α	$1–10 \times 10^6$ U/d SC
Chemotherapy	
Liposomal doxorubicin (Doxil)	20 mg/m^2 IV every 3 wk
Liposomal daunorubicin (DaunoXome)	40 mg/m^2 IV every 2 wk
Paclitaxel	100 mg/m^2 IV every 2 wk, *or* 135 mg/m^2 IV every 3 wk

than 100 cells/μL respond less than 10% of the time. Although it may take more than 8 weeks to respond, the responses are often durable, with median response duration of 1 to 2 years. IFN is best prescribed in combination with antiretroviral agents. IFN plus azidothymidine (AZT) results in a response rate of greater than 40%, with responses seen even in patients with CD4 counts below 100 cells/μL. Ongoing trials are evaluating IFN in combination with other less myelosuppressive antiretroviral agents. Most practitioners begin with antiretroviral therapy and relatively low-dose IFN-α, 1 to 5×10^6 U SC daily.

b. Chemotherapy. Chemotherapy provides rapid palliation of KS-related symptoms for most patients (see Table 25.4). Liposomal anthracyclines (e.g., daunorubicin [DaunoXome], liposomal doxorubicin [Doxil]) are currently considered the chemotherapeutic agents of choice for advanced KS. Multiple randomized trials of bleomycin and vincristine, with or without doxorubicin (Adriamycin), compared with one of the liposomal anthracyclines have consistently demonstrated less toxicity and equal or better response rates and response durations with the liposomal anthracyclines. For second-line therapy, paclitaxel 100 mg/m^2 every 2 weeks or 135 mg/m^2 every 3 weeks has produced response rates of 50% to 70% associated with significant palliation of tumor-related symptoms.

Patients often require growth factor support between cycles. Granulocyte colony-stimulating factor 5 μg/kg SC given days 7 to 12 of a 14-day (or 21-day) treatment cycle is often sufficient to preserve adequate neutrophil counts to prevent infection and allow timely administration of therapy. An absolute neutrophil count of 750/μL is adequate to deliver therapy with liposomal anthracyclines.

The duration of treatment is variable. Treatment should be continued until the maximal response is obtained; however, intercurrent illness may interrupt therapy. Although lesions may progress after therapy is discontinued, an effective maintenance therapy has not yet been defined. Recent data suggest, however, that maximal viral suppression with highly active antiretroviral therapy (HAART) may suppress KS tumor regrowth after discontinuation of chemotherapy. Several studies have reported improved survival and an increase in the median time to treatment failure for patients with KS treated with HAART. Furthermore, HAART alone has been anecdotally reported to lead to complete resolution of cutaneous and visceral KS lesions. This appears to be related to immune reconstitution, as an antiviral effect on HHV-8 has not been demonstrated *in vitro*.

III. Non-Hodgkin's lymphoma

A. Background. HIV-seropositive patients have a 5% to 10% lifetime risk of developing NHL. In a small proportion of patients (2% to 3%), NHL is the AIDS-defining event; but for most, NHL is a late manifestation of HIV infection, arising in the milieu of prolonged immunosuppression. HIV-associated NHLs are high-grade B-cell lymphomas similar to those seen in other immunocompromised patients.

B. Presentation and detection. The most common presentations for HIV-associated NHL are constitutional symptoms (fevers, night sweats, and weight loss) or an enlarging mass. Extranodal presentations, while once common, have become less frequent since the introduction of HAART. Primary CNS lymphoma accounts for less than 15% of the new AIDS-associated NHL. Nodal presentations occur in 60% of patients, and the remainder present with extranodal disease, most commonly involving the gastrointestinal tract, bone marrow, and liver. Very unusual sites of NHL have been seen, including the ear lobe, heart, and bile ducts. Seventy-five percent of patients present with advanced disease (stage III or IV).

C. Staging. The Ann Arbor staging classification is commonly used to stage HIV-related NHL (see Chapter 22); however, the correlation between stage and prognosis is weaker with HIV-associated cases. Prognosis is more closely related to immune function. In a recent study, four important adverse prognostic factors were identified for HIV-associated NHL: CD4 lymphocyte counts of less than 100 cells/µL, age older than 35 years, stage III or IV, and use of IV drugs. The presence of three or four of these indicators was associated with a median survival of only 18 weeks compared with 46 weeks for patients with one or none of these indicators. Similarly, in a retrospective review of 60 patients, two prognostic subgroups were identified based on immune function, performance status, and bone marrow involvement (Table 25.5).

Complete staging evaluation should include CT scans of the head, chest, abdomen, and pelvis; bilateral bone marrow biopsies; and lumbar puncture with cerebrospinal fluid (CSF) sent for protein and cytologic evaluation. Prior to the availability of HAART, 40% of patients had CNS involvement; therefore, all patients should undergo CSF evaluation regardless of clinical stage. The incidence of CNS involvement at presentation in the HAART era is unknown but appears to be decreasing.

D. Treatment

1. General approach. The best therapy for HIV-associated NHL remains to be defined. As is the case for KS, aggressive treatment of the underlying HIV infection is an important component of treatment. Fortunately, many clinical trials

Table 25.5. Prognostic stratification for HIV-associated non-Hodgkin's lymphoma (NHL)

From Levine	From Strauss
Good prognosis: median survival = 11.3 mo	Good prognosis: median survival = 18 wk
No prior AIDS diagnosis, *and* Karnofsky performance status >70%, *and* No bone marrow involvement	Good prognosis: presence of 0–1 indicator
Poor prognosis: median survival = 4.0 mo	Poor prognosis: median survival = 46 wk
Prior AIDS diagnosis, *or* Karnofsky performance status <70%, *or* Bone marrow involvement	Poor prognosis: presence of 3–4 indicators • Age <35 • CD4 <100 • Stage III or IV • Use of IV drugs

From Levine AM, Sullivan-Halley J, Pike MC, et al. Human immunodeficiency virus-related lymphoma: prognostic factors predictive of survival. *Cancer* 1991;68:2466–2472; and Strauss, with permission.

are ongoing to improve our understanding and treatment of this disease. Therapy must be tailored to the overall condition of each individual patient.

2. Systemic therapy. Before the availability of HAART, patients with AIDS-related NHL had a high incidence of opportunistic infections, limited bone marrow reserve, and poor outcomes with dose-intensive treatment. Because of this, the ACTG compared standard m-BACOD (Table 25.6) with low-dose (50% doses of cyclophosphamide and doxorubicin) m-BACOD in patients with HIV-associated NHL. There was no difference in the complete response rate or median survival between the two groups, but the low-dose group had significantly less hematologic toxicity. This led to the recommendation of low-dose treatment, particularly for patients with CD4 counts of less than 200 cells/μL.

In the HAART era, standard chemotherapy should be recommended for patients with well-controlled HIV infection. The optimal treatment recommendation for patients with poorly controlled HIV infection is unclear. French/Italian randomized studies have shown that for patients with good performance status and relatively preserved immune function, treatment with standard-dose CHOP is feasible and leads to a complete response (59%) and event-free survival rates (33% at 2 years) significantly higher than those obtained with low-dose CHOP.

Based on data suggesting that longer exposure of tumor cells to drugs may enhance drug efficacy, a 4-day infusional regimen of cyclophosphamide, etoposide, and doxorubicin (CDE) has been evaluated in HIV-associated NHL. Phase II

Table 25.6. Selected chemotherapy regimens for HIV-associated non-Hodgkin's lymphoma

Low-dose m-BACOD

Bleomycin	4 mg/m^2 IV day 1
Doxorubicin	25 mg/m^2 IV day 1
Cyclophosphamide	300 mg/m^2 IV day 1
Vincristine	1.4 mg/m^2 IV day 1 (not to exceed 2 mg total)
Dexamethasone	3 mg/m^2 PO days 1–5
Methotrexate	500 mg/m^2 IV day 15
Leucovorin	25 mg PO every 6 h for four doses, day 16 beginning exactly 24 h after methotrexate

CHOP

Cyclophosphamide	750 mg/m^2 IV day 1
Doxorubicin	50 mg/m^2 IV day 1
Vincristine	1.4 mg/m^2 IV day 1, not to exceed 2 mg total
Prednisone	100 mg/m^2 PO days 1–5

CDE chemotherapy

Cyclophosphamide	200 mg/m^2/24 h CIV days 1–4
Doxorubicin	12.5 mg/m^2/24 h CIV days 1–4
Etoposide	60 mg/m^2/24 h CIV days 1–4

Infusional EPOCH regimen (repeated q3 wk × 6 cycles)

Etoposide	50 mg/m^2/d CIV × 4 days
Vincristine	0.4 mg/m^2/d CIV × 4 days
Doxorubicin	10 mg/m^2/d CIV × 4 days
Cyclophosphamide	187 mg/m^2 IV on day 5 for CD4+ count <100, *or* 375 mg/m^2 IV on day 5 for CD4+ count ≥100
Prednisone	60 mg/m^2 PO days 1–5
G-CSF	Starting on day 6

CIV, continuous IV infusion.

studies demonstrated a complete remission (CR) rate (46%) similar to that obtained with standard regimens but with prolongation of the median time to progression to 17 months and a near doubling of the 1-year survival rate (48%). Randomized trials comparing infusional versus bolus chemotherapy are underway.

While HIV suppression is consistently associated with improved overall survival for patients with HIV-associated malignancies, it is not clear that HAART and NHL therapy must be delivered concurrently. A potential downside of chemotherapy plus HAART is the potential for enhanced toxicity. Protease inhibitors interfere with the excretion of drugs metabolized through hepatic cytochrome P-450, and indinavir, in particular, decreases cyclophosphamide clearance by 40%. Recommendations for dose modifications based on these pharmacologic interactions are not yet available. Saquinavir has been associated with significant mucositis in patients receiving myelosuppressive chemotherapy.

Little and colleagues treated patients with infusional EPOCH treatment (Table 25.6) and withheld HAART until the completion of chemotherapy. The observed CR rate was 77% with overall survival 74%, after nearly 30 months median follow-up. The median survival has not yet been reached. Resumption of HAART after chemotherapy leads to rapid repopulation of CD4+ cells and suppression of HIV viral load within 3 months.

For patients with well-controlled HIV infection, who are not eligible for a randomized clinical trial, standard-dose CHOP plus or minus rituximab, infusional EPOCH, or infusional CDE are reasonable therapeutic options (see Table 25.6). Careful observation for increased or unusual toxicities is essential. Growth factor support is frequently needed. Aggressive prophylaxis against opportunistic infections is important. Regardless of CD4 lymphocyte count, all patients should receive prophylaxis for *Pneumocystis carinii* pneumonia during treatment of a high-grade lymphoma (Table 25.7).

3. Central nervous system prophylaxis. CNS prophylaxis is recommended for patients with small noncleaved cell tumors or epidural, bone marrow, or paranasal sinus involvement. CNS prophylaxis should include four weekly treatments of either preservative-free methotrexate (12 mg) or cytosine arabinoside (50 mg). In patients with documented meningeal disease, intrathecal therapy should be given three times per week until the CSF clears, then weekly for 8 weeks and monthly for 10 months. An Ommaya reservoir should be placed to facilitate therapy.

4. Follow-up. In this era of cost containment, repeat staging studies are often controversial. Despite this zeal to minimize testing, documentation of a complete response as early as clinically warranted is important to minimize the duration of therapy in this already-immunocompromised group of patients. Treatment should be continued for a minimum of four cycles or for two cycles after attainment of complete response.

5. Salvage therapy. Some patients who relapse after initial treatment have been successfully treated with an alternative NHL regimen. There are currently no specific recommendations for salvage therapy.

IV. Primary central nervous system lymphoma

A. Background. PCNSL represents about 10% of all cases of HIV-associated NHL. Unlike systemic HIV-associated NHL,

**Table 25.7. Prophylaxis regimens for
Pneumocystis carinii pneumonia**

Trimethoprim-sulfamethoxazole (Bactrim DS) 1 tablet PO, Monday,
  Wednesday, Friday, *or*

Dapsone 100 mg PO daily[a]

---

[a] Exclude glucose-6-phosphatase deficiency by quantitative spectrophotometry in high-risk patients before initiating therapy.

which can occur at earlier stages of HIV infection, PCNSL typically occurs in profoundly immunocompromised patients with CD4 lymphocyte counts of less than 50 cells/μL. The Epstein–Barr virus (EBV) genome is identified in virtually all investigated cases of HIV-associated PCNSL. This supports the belief that EBV may have a direct etiologic role in the development of this disease.

B.   Presentation and detection. The diagnosis of PCNSL is often difficult to make. Most patients present with a focal neurologic deficit. CT scan or magnetic resonance imaging (MRI) of the head typically shows single or multiple contrast-enhancing masses with surrounding edema. These lesions are often in a periventricular location and may be difficult to distinguish from those of toxoplasmosis. CSF cytology is rarely diagnostic, and stereotactic biopsy is often recommended to establish a tissue diagnosis. Because 95% of HIV-positive patients with toxoplasmosis have serologic evidence of *Toxoplasma* sp. infection, the *Toxoplasma* titer can be useful to determine a course of action.

- If the *Toxoplasma* titer is negative, stereotactic biopsy should be considered.
- If the *Toxoplasma* titer is positive and the patient is either clinically unstable or the clinician feels uncomfortable without a tissue diagnosis based on the clinical scenario, stereotactic biopsy should be considered.
- If, however, the *Toxoplasma* titer is positive and the patient is clinically stable, a 1- to 2-week trial of empiric therapy for a presumptive diagnosis of toxoplasmosis may be appropriate. If there is no evidence of clinical or radiologic improvement or if there is evidence of clinical decompensation, stereotactic biopsy should be considered.

This approach requires close and frequent monitoring for signs of neurologic deterioration or progression. A newer potential alternative to the above is the use of EBV polymerase chain reaction (PCR) in the spinal fluid as a diagnostic clue. The presence of EBV by PCR in the CSF is highly specific for primary PCNSL. This, in the context of both a suggestive MRI or CT of the brain and a positive thallium scan, may be considered highly suggestive of PCNSL in the absence of a tissue diagnosis.

C.   Treatment. Whole-brain radiation therapy is the standard therapy. Temporary control and improvement of neurologic deficits occur in 70% of patients. A range of radiation doses (2,000 to 6,000 cGy) has been used. In one retrospective review, survival was found to be a function of performance status, not the total radiation dose administered. **Median survival is only 2 to 5 months.** Treatment with combined-modality therapy (CHOP plus radiation therapy) based on the experience in non–HIV-related PCNSLs was evaluated and did not demonstrate superior results to radiation therapy alone. High-dose methotrexate, with or without intrathecal chemotherapy, has been reported to lead to prolongation of median survival to as much as 40 months; however, studies done to date have been very small. Small clinical trials evaluating preradiation chemotherapy with CHOD/BVAM (cyclophosphamide, doxorubicin, vincristine, and dexamethasone alternated with BCNU, vincristine, ara-C, and methotrexate) have reported prolonged survival but with significant toxicity including dementia and leukoencephalopathy.

V.   Cervical cancer

A.   Background. It was not until 1993 that cervical cancer became an AIDS-defining illness. As in non–HIV-infected women, the development of cervical squamous carcinoma has been directly linked to prior infection with human papilloma virus (HPV). Although both HIV and HPV are sexually transmitted diseases, other immunosuppressed populations also have an increased incidence of HPV infection, suggesting that immune competence is a deterrent to the development of HPV co-infection. The presence of HPV, especially types 16, 18, and 31, is correlated with a higher incidence of cervical intraepithelial neoplasia (CIN).

B.   Presentation and detection. Presentation is similar to that of non–HIV-related cervical cancer, except the disease is often more aggressive in HIV-infected patients and advanced disease is more common. Routine Papanicolaou's (Pap) smears may not be sensitive enough to detect this aggressive neoplasm. It has been recommended that colposcopy, not Pap smears, be the standard for following HIV-infected women at high risk of CIN. Because CIN may progress at a faster rate in HIV-infected women, annual screening may not detect "curable" disease. Women with rapidly progressing CIN should probably be tested for HIV.

C.   Staging. The FIGO staging system, used for non–HIV-infected patients, is used in this population as well (see Chapter 11). Stage for stage, however, the prognosis appears worse in HIV-infected women owing to their compromised immune function.

D.   Treatment. In a small study, women with CD4 lymphocyte counts of less than 500 cells/μL did significantly worse than women with intact immune function. Until these results are confirmed in larger trials, HIV-positive women with invasive cervical cancer should be treated in the same manner as women without HIV infection.

VI.   Other malignancies. Hodgkin's lymphoma, testicular carcinoma, and anal cancers are also seen frequently in HIV-infected patients. Anecdotally, these malignancies appear more aggressive than their usual counterpart in immunocompetent patients, but no large trial has yet confirmed either increased virulence or increased incidence. It is interesting to speculate that EBV may play a role in the development of Hodgkin's disease. The role of HPV in the development of anal cancers has been well described. We recommend treatment of these malignancies with standard therapy. However, close attention should be paid to the prophylaxis and treatment of opportunistic pathogens as well as to the appropriate use of antiretroviral agents.

SELECTED READINGS

Formenti SC, Gill PS, Lean E, et al. Primary central nervous system lymphoma in AIDS: results of radiation therapy. *Cancer* 1989;63: 1101–1107.

Forsyth PA, DeAngelis LM. Biology and management of AIDS-associated primary CNS lymphomas. *Hematol Oncol Clin North Am* 1996;10:1125–1134.

Gill PS, Wernz J, Scadden DT, et al. Randomized phase II trial of liposomal daunorubicin (DaunoXome) versus doxorubicin, bleomycin, vincristine (ABV) in AIDS-related Kaposi's sarcoma. *J Clin Oncol* 1996;14:2353–2364.

Goldstein JD, Dickson DW, Moser FG, et al. Primary central nervous system lymphoma in acquired immune deficiency syndrome: a clinical and pathologic study with results of treatment with radiation. *Cancer* 1991;67:2756.

Kaplan L, Strauss D, Testa M, et al. Low-dose compared with standard dose m-BACOD chemotherapy for non-Hodgkin's lymphoma associated with human immunodeficiency virus infection. *N Engl J Med* 1997;336:1164–1648.

Knowles DM. Etiology and pathogenesis of AIDS-related non-Hodgkin's lymphoma. *Hematol Oncol Clin North Am* 1996;10:1081–1109.

Krown SE, Testa MA, Huang J. AIDS-related Kaposi's sarcoma: prospective validation of the AIDS Clinical Trials Group staging classification. *J Clin Oncol* 1997;15:3085–3092.

Levine AM, Sullivan-Halley J, Pike MC, et al. Human immunodeficiency virus-related lymphoma: prognostic factors predictive of survival. *Cancer* 1991;68:2466–2472.

Levine AM, Wernz JC, Kaplan L, et al. Low-dose chemotherapy with central nervous system prophylaxis and zidovudine maintenance in AIDS-related lymphoma. *JAMA* 1991;266:84–88.

Maiman M, Fruchter RG, Guy L, et al. Human immunodeficiency virus infection and invasive cervical carcinoma. *Cancer* 1993;71:402–406.

Maiman M, Tarricone N, Vieira J, et al. Colposcopic evaluation of human immunodeficiency virus-seropositive women. *Obstet Gynecol* 1991;78:84–88.

Miles SA. Pathogenesis of AIDS-related Kaposi's sarcoma: evidence of a viral etiology. *Hematol Oncol Clin North Am* 1996;10:1011–1021.

Mitsuyasu RT. Interferon alpha in the treatment of AIDS-related Kaposi's sarcoma. *Br J Haematol* 1991;79(suppl 1):69–73.

Northfelt DW. Treatment of Kaposi's sarcoma. *Drugs* 1994;48:569–582.

Robinson WR, Morris CB. Cervical neoplasia: pathogenesis, diagnosis and management. *Hematol Oncol Clin North Am* 1996;10:1163–1176.

Saville MW, Lietzau J, Pluda JM, et al. Treatment of HIV-associated Kaposi's sarcoma with paclitaxel. *Lancet* 1995;346:26–28.

Schafer A, Friedmann W, Mielke M, et al. The increased frequency of cervical dysplasia–neoplasia in women infected with the human immunodeficiency virus is related to the degree of immunosuppression. *Am J Obstet Gynecol* 1991;164:593–599.

Sparano JA, Wiernik PH, Strack M, et al. Infusional cyclophosphamide, doxorubicin and etoposide in HIV-1 and HTLV-1-related non-Hodgkin's lymphoma: a highly active regimen. *Blood* 1993;81:2810–2815.

Stelzer KJ, Griffin TW. A randomized prospective trial of radiation therapy for AIDS-associated Kaposi's sarcoma. *Int J Radiat Oncol Biol Phys* 1993;27:1057–1061.

IV

Selected A
Supportive
Patients w

26

Side Effects of Cancer Chemotherapy

Janelle M. Tipton

Systemic cancer chemotherapy agents are valuable in their role as cancer treatment; however, there are undesirable effects to normal replicating cells. Rapidly dividing normal cells that are vulnerable to damage include cells of the bone marrow, hair follicles, and mucous membranes. Other toxicities may occur that are unrelated to cell growth and are particular to individual agents. The side effects of cancer chemotherapy agents may be acute, self-limited, and mild or can be chronic, permanent, and potentially life threatening in nature. Many advances have been made in the last 10 to 15 years in the management of side effects of chemotherapy. Although much progress has been made, the management of side effects continues to be of utmost importance for the tolerability of therapy and effect on overall quality of life.

I. Acute reactions

A. Extravasation. Extravasation is defined as the leakage or infiltration of drug into the subcutaneous tissues. *Vesicant* drugs that extravasate are capable of causing tissue necrosis or sloughing. *Irritant* drugs cause inflammation or pain at the site of extravasation. Common vesicant and irritant agents and potential antidotes are listed in Table 26.1.

1. Risk factors for peripheral extravasation include small, fragile veins, venipuncture technique, site of venipuncture, drug administration technique, presence of superior vena cava syndrome, peripheral neuropathy, and concurrent use of medications that may cause somnolence, altered mental status, excessive movements, vomiting, and coughing.

2. Incidence of extravasation for vesicant chemotherapy is recorded as 1% to 6% in the literature for peripheral chemotherapy. Extravasation may also occur with central venous catheters. Potential causes for central venous catheter extravasation include backflow secondary to fibrin sheath or thrombosis in the central venous catheter, needle dislodgement from a venous access port, central venous catheter damage, breakage, or separation, and displacement or migration of the catheter from the vein.

3. Common signs and symptoms of extravasation are pain or burning at the IV site, redness, swelling, inability to obtain a blood return, and change in the quality of the infusion. Any of these complaints or observations should be considered a symptom of extravasation until proven otherwise.

4. Procedures for peripheral extravasation are imperative to have in place, including guidelines or orders for extravasation management of vesicant and irritant agents before administration. If an extravasation is suspected, the following actions should be taken:

Table 26.1. Common vesicant and irritant drugs and potential antidotes

Chemotherapy agent	Pharmacologic antidote	Nonpharmacologic antidote	Method of administration
Mechlorethamine HCl (nitrogen mustard)	Sodium thiosulfate	None	Prepare 1/6 M solution: If 10% Na thiosulfate solution, mix 4 mL with 6 mL sterile water for injection. Through existing IV line, inject 2 mL for every 1 mL extravasated. Inject SC if needle is removed.
Cisplatin (Platinol)	Sodium thiosulfate	None	For large extravasations only (>20 mL of cisplatin solution with 0.5 mg/mL). Use 2 mL 10% sodium thiosulfate solution for each 100 mg cisplatin. Administer as with mechlorethamine.
Doxorubicin (Adriamycin), daunorubicin (Cerubidine), idarubicin (Idamycin)	None	Topical cooling	Apply cold pad with circulating ice water, ice pack, or cryogel pack for 15–20 min at least 4 ×/d for first 24–48 h. Some research studies suggest benefit of 99% dimethyl sulfoxide (DMSO) 1–2 mL applied to site every 6 h.
Vincristine (Oncovin), vinblastine (Velban), vinorelbine (Navelbine)	None	Warm compresses	Apply heat for 15–20 min at least 4 ×/d for first 24–48 h.
Etoposide (VP-16)	None	Warm compresses	Treatment necessary only if large amount of concentrated solution extravasates.
Paclitaxel (Taxol)	None	Topical cooling	Apply ice pack for 15–20 min at least 4 ×/d for first 24 h.

1. Stop administration of the chemotherapy agent.
2. Leave the needle/catheter in place and immobilize the extremity.
3. Attempt to aspirate any residual drug in the tubing, needle, or suspected extravasation site.
4. Notify the physician.
5. Administer the appropriate antidote, as shown in Table 26.1. This may include instillation of a drug antidote or application of heat or cold to the site.
6. Provide the patient and/or caregiver with instructions, including the need to elevate the site for 48 h and the continuation of antidote measures as appropriate.
7. Discuss the need for further intervention with the physician and photograph if indicated.
8. Document extravasation occurrence according to institutional guidelines.
9. Continued monitoring of extravasation site at 24 h, 1 week, 2 weeks, and additionally as guideline recommends. Secondary complications such as infection and pain may occur. Follow-up photographs at these time periods, if possible, are helpful in monitoring extent of injury and progress in healing.

5. Procedures for central extravasation are also critically important to follow, as extravasation of chemotherapy agents in the upper torso or neck area is difficult to manage and may result in extensive defects, requiring reconstructive surgery. Extreme caution should be taken by nurses administering chemotherapy by this route. Procedures followed in central extravasation are similar to peripheral extravasation. Assessment of lack of blood return, patient reports in changes of sensation, pain, burning, or swelling at the central venous catheter site or chest warrant immediate discontinuation of chemotherapy. Prompt administration of the appropriate antidote is recommended, but if the extravasation has been extensive, the actions may not prevent damage. Collaboration with the physician regarding the need for further studies to identify the cause of the extravasation will be necessary as well as other decisions for future plans for venous access.

B. Hypersensitivity and anaphylaxis. Specific drugs with the potential for hypersensitivity with or without an anaphylactic response should be administered under constant supervision of a competent and experienced nurse and with a physician readily available, preferably during the daytime hours. Important preassessment data to be documented include the patient's allergy history, though this information may not predict an allergic reaction to chemotherapy. Drugs with the highest risk of immediate hypersensitivity reactions are asparaginase, murine monoclonal antibodies (e.g., ibritumomab tiuxetan [Zevalin]), and paclitaxel. Drugs with a low to moderate risk include the anthracyclines, bleomycin, cisplatin, carboplatin, docetaxel, IV melphalan, etoposide, and humanized (e.g., trastuzumab) or chimeric (e.g., rituximab) monoclonal antibodies. Test doses or skin tests may be performed if there is an increased suspicion for hypersensitivity. In specific occasions, this is generally done with bleomycin and asparaginase.

1.   Type I hypersensitivity reactions are the most common chemotherapy-induced type of reactions. These reactions characteristically occur within 1 h of receiving the drug; however, with paclitaxel, the hypersensitivity reactions often occur within the first 10 min of the start of the infusion. Common manifestations of a type I reaction include urticaria, respiratory distress, bronchospasm, hypotension, angioedema, flushing, chest and back pain, and anxiety. With appropriate premedication, the incidence of the hypersensitivity reactions has markedly decreased with paclitaxel. Commonly used premedications include dexamethasone, diphenhydramine, and an H_2-histamine antagonist such as cimetidine, ranitidine, or famotidine. Emergency equipment should be immediately accessible, including oxygen, an Ambu respiratory assist bag, and suction equipment. The following parenteral drugs should also be stocked in the treatment area: epinephrine 1:1,000 or 1:10,000 solution, diphenhydramine 25 to 50 mg, methylprednisolone 125 mg, and dexamethasone 20 mg. The development of a clinical guideline for hypersensitivity reactions, with or without true anaphylaxis, may be helpful in preparing for a potential reaction, reducing delays in response time to a reaction, and standardizing the management of a reaction with standing orders. Table 26.2 provides a sample preprinted/standing order for the management of hypersensitivity and anaphylactic reactions.

Table 26.2.   Sample standing orders for hypersensitivity reactions to chemotherapy agents

1. Have the following medications available:
   a. Diphenhydramine (Benadryl) 50 IV
   b. Methylprednisolone (Solumedrol) 125 mg IV or equivalent hydrocortisone
   c. Epinephrine (1:10,000) 10-mL single-dose vial (or 1 mL of 1:1,000, 1-mg vial)
2. If signs/symptoms of hypersensitivity occur (such as urticaria [hives], respiratory distress, bronchospasm, hypotension, angioedema, flushing, chest/back pain, anxiety), stop infusion of chemotherapy/biotherapy agent.
3. Maintain IV access with IVF normal saline at 200 mL/h until blood pressure stabilizes.
4. Administer oxygen at 2–4 L/min and measure pulse oximetry.
5. Administer methylprednisolone 125 mg IVP.
6. Administer diphenhydramine (Benadryl) 50 mg IVP.
7. Continuously monitor blood pressure, pulse, and oxygen saturation.
8. Notify physician immediately for further orders.
9. If symptoms do not resolve or worsen, administer epinephrine as directed by MD.
10. Initiate a code if airway patency is not maintained or cardiopulmonary arrest occurs.

2. Retreatment and rechallenge of patients who have experienced paclitaxel-associated hypersensitivity reactions are supported in the literature. If rechallenge is considered, the paclitaxel should be administered in the appropriate setting where immediate emergency situations may be handled. The decision to reinstitute the paclitaxel should be based on the clinical importance of using the drug in the particular disease setting. Patients have been successfully retreated within hours to days of the initial paclitaxel reactions at full doses.

   a. Reinstitution of paclitaxel after experiencing a hypersensitivity reaction includes immediate discontinuation of the paclitaxel infusion at the onset of symptoms and rapid administration of additional diphenhydramine and methylprednisolone. Following stabilization of the patient and waiting approximately 30 min, the paclitaxel infusion is reinitiated, with initial infusion rates 10% to 25% of the total infusion rate. If tolerated, the rate can be gradually increased over the next several hours. Nursing care would also include vital signs every 5 min or continuous observation for the first 15 min, then every 15 min through the first hour, then hourly until completed. An alternative is to pretreat the patient for 24 h with dexamethasone 10 mg $\times$ 3 orally and to restart the infusion at the rate indicated above on the second day.

   b. Rechallenge after a severe hypersensitivity reaction of the second episode of hypersensitivity reaction is documented in the literature; however, planning for the "densensitization" is necessary. Regimens including dexamethasone 20 mg orally at 36 and 12 h before chemotherapy and the morning of chemotherapy have been studied. A full 30 min before the chemotherapy, other IV premedications such as dexamethasone 20 mg, diphenhydramine 50 mg, and H_2-histamine antagonist are given. The desensitization procedure continues with administration of a test dose of paclitaxel 2 mg in 100 mL of normal saline over 30 min. If no reaction, 10 mg in 100 mL of normal saline is given over 30 min, followed by the remaining full dose in 500 mL of normal saline over 3 h if still no reaction. If a reaction is experienced, the usual diphenhydramine and methylprednisolone medications are given.

II. Nausea and vomiting. Patients who are about to begin chemotherapy are often concerned and apprehensive about nausea and vomiting. Nausea and vomiting can be distressing enough to the patient to cause extreme physiologic and psychological discomfort, culminating in withdrawal from therapy. With the advent of more effective antiemetic regimens in the last 10 years, many improvements in the prevention and control of nausea and vomiting have led to a better quality of life for patients receiving chemotherapy. The goal of therapy is to prevent the three phases of nausea and vomiting: that which occurs before the treatment is administered (anticipatory), that which follows within the first 24 h after the treatment (acute), and that which occurs more than 24 h after the treatment (delayed). It is also important to assess nausea and vomiting separately because they are different events and may have different causes. Factors related to the chemotherapy that can affect the likelihood and severity of symptoms include the specific agents used, the doses of the drugs, and the schedule and route of administration. Other patient characteristics that may effect emesis include history of poor emetic control, history of alcoholism, age, gender, and history of motion sickness.

A.   Emetic potential of the drug. To plan an effective approach to control nausea and vomiting, the chemotherapeutic agents are grouped according to their emetic potential (Table 26.3). This type of categorization is helpful in making decisions regarding possible antiemetics to be used and how aggressive the antiemetic regimen should be for patients receiving chemotherapy for the first time or in subsequent treatments.

B.   Antiemetic drugs. Agents that have been effective in preventing and treating nausea and vomiting (Table 26.4) come from various pharmacologic classes. They work by different mechanisms that may relate to the pathophysiologic processes causing nausea and vomiting. For many years, the mainstays of antiemetic therapy have been agents that block dopamine receptors. These agents have been somewhat effective but have limited value for highly emetogenic agents and, in escalating doses, have caused problematic side effects. Within the last 10 years, it was discovered that agents that block predominately the serotonin (5-hydroxytryptamine) subtype 3 (5-HT3) receptors, rather than the dopamine receptors, have greater efficacy in the prevention of nausea and vomiting. More recent research indicates that the tachykinins, including a peptide called substance P, may play an important role in emesis. Substance P binds to the neurokinin type 1 (or NK-1) receptor. Thus, the NK-1-receptor antagonists are now being studied in their role in inhibiting emesis. Oral NK-1-receptor antagonists are thought to improve acute nausea and vomiting associated with chemotherapy when combined with standard regimens (i.e., dexamethasone) and to have additional effect during the period of delayed nausea and vomiting, alone or in combination with dexamethasone. With use of agents from various classes, it is important to use an antiemetic regimen sufficient to prevent nausea and vomiting to the greatest degree possible to avoid the development of conditioned responses and failure of antiemetic therapy.

C.   Combination antiemetic therapy. Several antiemetic regimens are effective, but their design should be based on several general principles:

1.   Combinations of antiemetics have been shown to be more effective than single agents. It is common to use two or more antiemetics to prevent or manage nausea and vomiting.

2.   Preemptive treatment and scheduled administration are also necessary to prevent nausea and vomiting early in therapy and to manage potential delayed nausea and vomiting for several hours or days. Table 26.5 shows examples of antiemetic regimens that may be used when the chemotherapy has a high, moderate, and low emetic potential.

D.   Nonpharmacologic interventions. Patients who are likely to experience or who have experienced anticipatory nausea and vomiting related to chemotherapy may benefit from the use of nonpharmacologic interventions in addition to the pharmacologic agents taken. The use of guided imagery, massage

Table 26.3. Emetogenic potential for commonly used chemotherapeutic agents[a]

Highly emetogenic agents (≥75% potential for nausea, vomiting, or both)	Moderately emetogenic agents (50%–75% potential for nausea, vomiting, or both)	Mildly emetogenic agents (25%–50% potential for nausea, vomiting, or both)
Carmustine	Carboplatin	Asparaginase
Cisplatin (>40 mg/m^2)	Cisplatin (<40 mg/m^2)	Bleomycin
Cyclophosphamide (>1 g/m^2)	Cyclophosphamide (200 mg/m^2 to 1 g/m^2)	Busulfan
Cytarabine (>1 g/m^2)	Cytarabine (200 mg/m^2 to 1 g/m^2)	Capecitabine
Dacarbazine (days 1 and 2)	Daunorubicin	Chlorambucil
Dactinomycin	Doxorubicin (<60 mg/m^2)	Cladribine
Doxorubicin (>60 mg/m^2)	Etoposide	Cyclophosphamide (<200 mg/m^2)
Epirubicin	Gemcitabine	Cytarabine (<200 mg/m^2)
Ifosfamide (>1.2 g/m^2)	Idarubicin	Docetaxel
Mechlorethamine	Ifosfamide (<1.2 g/m^2)	Fludarabine
Methotrexate (>1 g/m^2)	Irinotecan	Fluorouracil
Mitomycin (>15 mg/m^2)	Methotrexate (50 mg/m^2 to 1 g/m^2)	Hydroxyurea
Oxaliplatin	Mitomycin (<15 mg/m^2)	Imatinib (Gleevec)
Streptozocin	Mitoxantrone	Liposomal doxorubicin
	Procarbazine	Melphalan
	Topotecan	Methotrexate (<50 mg/m^2)
	Vinorelbine	Paclitaxel
		Rituximab
		Thioguanine or mercaptopurine (6-MP)
		Thiotepa
		Trastuzumab
		Vinblastine
		Vincristine

[a]High-dose therapy requiring progenitor cell support is not included in this table.

therapy, music therapy, and self-hypnosis shows some effectiveness in preventing nausea and vomiting. These forms of distraction assist patients in maintaining a feeling of control over their treatment effects. Acupressure, acupuncture, and transcutaneous electrical nerve stimulation have also had pilot testing and may have a role in combination with antiemetic drugs. With increasing attention to complementary therapies, it is hoped that more clinical studies will determine their value in patient care. Patients who are able to have little or no nausea and vomiting with their first chemotherapy treatment often assert that positive thinking is helpful as well. Patients may also prepare for their chemotherapy treatments by eating foods that do not

Table 26.4.   Agents used for chemotherapy-induced nausea and vomiting

Agent	Route of administration	Dose	Comments
Phenothiazines			
Prochlorperazine (Compazine)	PO PO (sustained release) IM or IV PR	10 mg q4–6 h 15–30 mg q12 h 2–10 mg q4–6 h 25 mg q8–12 h	Some EPS; potential for postural hypotension when given IV
Thiethylperazine (Torecan)	PO, IM, or PR	10 mg q6–8 h	Some EPS
Trimethobenzamide (Tigan)	PO IM or PR	250 mg q4–6 h 200 mg q4–6 h	Some EPS
Butyrophenones			
Haloperidol (Haldol)	IM, PO, or IV	2–5 mg q2–4 h	Some EPS
Droperidol (Inapsine)	IV or IM	0.5–2.5 mg q4 h	Causes sedation, cardiac arrhythmias, EPS, hypotension. Not recommended.
Substituted benzamide			
Metoclopramide (Reglan)	PO or IV	10–40 mg q.i.d. to 1- to 2-mg/kg dose at 2-h intervals	EPS common in higher doses which should be given with diphenhydramine; EPS worse with younger patients; may have diarrhea in higher doses

	Route	Dose	Comments
Benzodiazepines			
Lorazepam (Ativan)	PO or SL IV	1–2 mg q4–6 h 0.5–2 mg q4–6 h	Causes sedation, amnesia, and confusion
Corticosteroids			
Dexamethasone (Decadron)	IV	4–20 mg (10–20 mg ×1), otherwise q4–6 h	Potential for agitation, delirium
	PO	4–8 mg q4 h	
Serotonin (5-HT$_3$) antagonists			
Ondansetron (Zofran)	IV	8–32 mg ×1 0.15 mg/kg, q4 h ×3	For highly emetogenic chemotherapy; lower doses effective for less emetogenic regimens
	PO	8 mg b.i.d.	
Granisetron (Kytril)	IV PO	1 mg ×1 1–2 mg ×1	Similar to ondansetron
Dolasetron (Anzemet)	IV or PO	100 mg before (once daily)	Similar to above
Cannabinoids			
Dronabinol (Marinol)	PO	2.5–10 mg q4–6 h	Causes sedation, may be habit forming, a controlled substance

EPS, extrapyramidal symptoms.

Table 26.5.   Examples of regimens for antiemetic prevention and management of chemotherapy-induced nausea and vomiting

Level I: patients receiving a mildly emetogenic agent

Dexamethasone 10 mg PO before chemotherapy

With or without

Prochlorperazine 10 mg PO before chemotherapy, then 10 mg PO q4–6 h p.r.n., *or*

Lorazepam 1 mg PO q4–6 h p.r.n., *or both*

Level II: patients receiving a moderately emetogenic agent or patients receiving a mildly emetogenic agent who have failed to respond to or are intolerant of at least two level 1 regimens

Granisetron[a] 1 mg PO (or 0.5–1 mg IV) before chemotherapy, *and*

Dexamethasone 20 mg PO (or IV) before chemotherapy

With or without

Lorazepam 1 mg PO or IV before q4–6 h p.r.n., *or*

Prochlorperazine 10 mg PO q4–6 h p.r.n., *or both*

Level III: patients receiving a highly emetogenic agent or patients receiving two or more moderately emetogenic agents or patients who have failed a level 2 regimen

Granisetron[b] 1 mg IV or 2 mg PO before chemotherapy, *and*

Dexamethasone 20 mg PO or IV before chemotherapy, *and*

Lorazepam 1 mg PO or IV before chemotherapy, then q4–6 h p.r.n.

In addition, for delayed nausea and vomiting:

Metoclopramide 40 mg PO q6 h × 4 days, *or*

Compazine spansules 15–30 mg PO q12 h × 4 days, *with*

Dexamethasone 4 mg PO q6 h × 3 days, then 4 mg PO q12 h × 1 day

---

Give antiemetics 20 min prior to chemotherapy when using the IV route and 1 h prior to chemotherapy when using the PO route. Given in this fashion, oral medication as usually as effective as the same medication IV, and the cost is considerably less.

[a] Alternatives (5-HT$_3$): ondansetron 10 mg IV × 1 before chemotherapy, *or* dolasetron 100 mg PO or IV before chemotherapy.

[b] Alternatives (5-HT$_3$ antagonists): ondansetron 32 mg IV before chemotherapy; dolasetron 100 mg PO or IV before chemotherapy.

have offensive odors or spicy taste. Clear liquids, foods served at room temperature, soda crackers, and carbonated beverages are sometimes good suggestions. Following chemotherapy, smaller, more frequent meals are less likely to promote the development of nausea and vomiting.

III.   Other short-term complications related to cancer chemotherapy

   A.   Stomatitis and other oral complications. The oral mucosa is vulnerable to the effects of chemotherapy and radiotherapy because of its rapid growth and cell turnover rate. Radiotherapy also interferes with the production of saliva and may increase oral complications because of a consequent reduction in the protective effect of the saliva. It is crucial to manage oral complications effectively because patients may experience considerable discomfort or develop secondary infections from the disruption of the oral mucosa. The likelihood of the development of stomatitis from a drug is dependent on the agent, the dose, and the schedule of administration. Continuous rather than intermittent administration is more likely to cause stomatitis with the antimetabolites.

   1.   Specific chemotherapy agents that may cause stomatitis include the following:

   Antimetabolites: methotrexate, fluorouracil, capecitabine, cytarabine, irinotecan
   Antitumor antibiotics: doxorubicin, idarubicin, dactinomycin, mitomycin, bleomycin
   Plant alkaloids: vincristine, vinblastine, vinorelbine
   Taxanes: docetaxel, paclitaxel
   Alkylating agents: high doses of busulfan, cyclophosphamide
   Biologic agents: interleukins, lymphokine-activated killer cell therapy

   2.   Prevention and early detection. If oral complications are anticipated, it is important to implement a good oral hygiene program before the initiation of therapy. Maintaining good nutrition and dental hygiene are also primary preventive measures. Systematic oral assessments should be integrated into the physical examination at regular intervals. Special attention should be given to the tongue, the gingiva, the buccal mucosa, the soft palate, and the lips. It is also important to assess the patient for soreness, functional ability to swallow, and any effects on eating.
   3.   Management of oral complications. Although the primary goal is prevention, once oral complications develop, the focus of care should shift to the continuation of good oral hygiene and treatment of symptoms. Agents used for oral care are categorized according to function: cleansing agents, lubricating agents, analgesic agents, and preventive agents. Table 26.6 lists several commonly used agents. Commercial mouthwashes and lemon glycerin swabs are not recommended for use because of their irritating and drying effects. A common oral care agent used is chlorhexidine 15 mL, which is swished and expectorated twice a day. If painful ulcerations do develop, topical relief may be obtained by using a stomatitis mixture containing diphenhydramine (Benadryl) elixir 5 mL, antacid (Maalox) 30 mL, and viscous lidocaine (Xylocaine) 5 mL. Systemic pain control measures such as oral or parenteral narcotics should be implemented if topical analgesics are ineffective.
   4.   Xerostomia that follows radiation therapy to the mouth area may require treatment with artificial saliva. It may also be benefited by the administration of pilocarpine 5 to 10 mg PO t.i.d. before meals. Before the initiation of radiation therapy to the head and neck area, dental consultation is necessary to evaluate oral hygiene, the state of repair of the teeth, and the health of the gums. Amifostine shows promise as a

Table 26.6.   Agents for oral care

Agent	Indications and comments
Cleansing Agents	
Normal saline solution ($\frac{1}{2}$ tsp salt in 8 oz water)	Economical, nondamaging
Hydrogen peroxide (mix with normal saline or tap water)	Germicidal, debriding
Sodium bicarbonate	Nonirritating, debriding
Chlorhexidine (15 mL swish and spit b.i.d.)	May decrease infection
Lubricating agents	
Saliva substitutes	Decreases dryness
Water- or oil-based lubricants	Useful emollient; oil-based lubricants should not be used in mouth because of danger of aspiration
Analgesic agents	
a. ***Healing and coating agents***	
Sulcralfate	Binds to mucosa, forms protective coating
Vitamin E	Protection to mucosa, healing properties
Antacids	Enhance comfort, coat mucosa
Allopurinol	May decrease intensity of mucositis with fluorouracil
b. ***Topical anesthetics***	
Lidocaine viscous	Transient pain relief, absorbed systemically
Diclonime hydrochloride	Transient pain relief
Benzocaine	Transient pain relief
Zilactin	Burns on application
Capsaicin	Active ingredient in chili peppers; given in candy vehicle will decrease pain
c. ***Systemic analgesics***	
Nonsteroidal anti-inflammatory drugs Narcotic analgesics	Take before meals and as needed
Prevention agents— hematologic growth factors	
Filgrastim, Sargramostim	Less severe mucositis experienced by patients receiving growth factors

protective agent for xerostomia and is used concurrently with
radiation to the head and neck.

5.   Secondary oral infections should be treated promptly
and as accurately as possible. Fungal infections may be treated
with nystatin suspension, clotrimazole troches, or oral fluconazole. Viral infections may be reactivated after chemotherapy and are commonly treated with oral or IV acyclovir. The
benefit of prophylactic use of antiviral agents or antifungal
agents is not well established. However, in patients with a
known history of cold sores or positive herpes simplex virus
titers, it may be advantageous to administer prophylactic
acyclovir.

Patients with dentures may be encouraged to remove them
during the period after chemotherapy when they are at risk for
infection, except at mealtime. In addition, the dentures should
be cleansed before use. Although removal of the dentures may
be detrimental to the patient's self-esteem, irritation of the
dentures may lead to inflammation, ulceration, and secondary
infection.

B.   Alopecia. Chemotherapy-induced hair loss is not necessarily a serious physiologic complication, but psychologically, it can
be one of the most devastating side effects. Partial or total hair
loss can contribute to a perceived negative body image owing to
the emphasis placed on the hair and overall appearance in society. The hair loss from chemotherapy, which often occurs 2 to
3 weeks after chemotherapy, is usually temporary. Hair growth
returns in about 1 to 2 months after the treatment is completed,
but it may take approximately 4 to 5 months before the patient
will feel comfortable not wearing a wig. The new hair may have
a different texture or color from its pretreatment characteristics.
In addition to scalp hair loss, it is important to remind patients
of the hair loss that may occur in other areas such as the eye-
brows, eyelashes, axilla, pubis, and other fine hair.

1.   Specific chemotherapy agents with a high potential
of causing alopecia include doxorubicin, cyclophosphamide,
ifosfamide, vincristine, and paclitaxel. Other drugs capable
of causing alopecia include bleomycin, dactinomycin, daunorubicin, etoposide, vinblastine, methotrexate, and mitoxantrone.
The extent of alopecia depends on the mechanism of the drug,
the dose, the serum half-life, the infusion technique (bolus versus continuous infusion), and the use of combinations of drugs.

2.   Nursing interventions start with informing and preparing the patient for the possibility of alopecia. It is helpful to
encourage purchasing wigs and other headwear before the
alopecia occurs so that the hair color and style may be used in
selecting a wig as well as allowing time for adjustment. It is
important to encourage discussion of feelings regarding the
hair loss for both men and women and to recognize their concerns and fears. The American Cancer Society's program "Look
Good, Feel Better" is helpful in providing guidance about wigs,
make-up, and skin care. Scalp hypothermia has been used in
the past as an attempt to restrict the circulation to the scalp,
with the goal of minimizing alopecia. Because of the concern
for scalp metastases and sanctuary sites, scalp hypothermia is
no longer recommended.

C.   Diarrhea. Among the many causes of diarrhea in patients with cancer are chemotherapy, radiotherapy, the cancer itself, medications, supplemental feedings, and anxiety. Osmotic diarrhea refers to that caused by chemotherapy agents, where the actively dividing epithelial cells of the gastrointestinal tract are destroyed. Unabsorbable substances draw water into the intestinal lumen by osmosis, resulting in increased stool volume and weight. Secretory diarrhea may result from infectious causes (e.g., *Clostridium difficile* or other enterocolitis-causing bacteria), with or without concurrent neutropenia. The opportunistic infection may intensify the inflammatory reaction in the gut, causing excessive intestinal mucosal secretion of electrolytes and fluids from the bacterial toxins. Prolonged diarrhea can lead to discomfort, severe electrolyte imbalances and dehydration, altered social life, and poor quality of life. In the past, little attention has been paid to the prompt evaluation and management of diarrhea, but with increasing use of agents such as irinotecan, the observation of severe and potentially life-threatening problems has heightened awareness of this side effect. The elderly, in particular, may be at increased risk for treatment-related diarrhea and may require close monitoring.

1.   Chemotherapy and biologic agents may contribute to the development of diarrhea and most commonly include the antimetabolites such as fluorouracil, capecitabine, methotrexate, cytarabine, and irinotecan. In addition, agents such as dactinomycin, floxuridine, hydroxyurea, idarubicin, the nitrosoureas, and paclitaxel relatively frequently cause diarrhea. When diarrhea from fluorouracil, floxuridine, or irinotecan is present while on therapy, it is a sign of toxicity that must be monitored closely and that could escalate to severe levels at which the drug might need to be held or discontinued. With the increased use of biologic agents, diarrhea has been noted with interferon-α and interleukin-2. High-dose chemotherapy regimens used in stem cell transplantation may also be associated with severe diarrhea and may be caused by acute graft-versus-host disease.

2.   Assessment of a patient experiencing diarrhea should begin with a baseline history of usual elimination patterns, pattern of symptoms, and concurrent medications. The duration of the diarrhea and frequency of stool passage should be noted with reference to a stool diary if indicated. The physical examination may disclose abdominal tenderness, signs of dehydration, and disruption in perianal or peristomal skin integrity. Laboratory data may be obtained to assess serum chemistries, complete blood count, and stool samples for *C. difficile* toxin and other enteropathic bacteria.

3.   Management of treatment-related diarrhea is often symptomatic and requires little or no alteration in cancer therapy. Agents that decrease bowel motility should not be used for longer than 24 h unless significant infections have been excluded. In the absence of obvious inflammation and infection, it is appropriate to treat most patients with nonspecific treatment for diarrhea, including opioids (loperamide, diphenoxylate, and codeine), anticholinergics (atropine, scopolamine), or both. More recently, it has been recognized that octreotide is often effective in controlling chemotherapy-related diarrhea and diarrhea associated with the carcinoid syndrome. Table 26.7 lists common agents used to treat diarrhea. Nonpharmacologic measures that may also assist in the prevention and management of diarrhea are a low-residue diet and increased fluids. If the diarrhea is severe, IV hydration is necessary to prevent serious hypovolemia, electrolyte disturbances, and shock. In patients who experience severe irinotecan-associated diarrhea, antibiotic therapy such as ciprofloxacin is recommended because of a high incidence of infectious contribution to the gastrointestinal problems, including functional ileus, which may be associated.

D. Constipation. In patients whose cancer has resulted in debility or immobility or in those who require narcotic analgesics, constipation can be a particular problem. Constipation may also develop in patients who have received neurotoxic chemotherapy agents including the vinca alkaloids, etoposide, and cisplatin, each of which may cause autonomic dysfunction. Decreased bowel motility due to intra-abdominal disease, hypercalcemia, or dehydration can also contribute to constipation. Chronic constipation in patients with cancer is a problem that is more easily prevented than treated. A diet high in bulk fiber, fresh fruits and vegetables, and adequate fluid intake may help to minimize constipation. Patients started on narcotic analgesics should also begin a bowel regimen, first with mild stool softeners and bulk laxatives and then proceeding to stimulants or osmotic laxatives if the milder regimen is not effective. A bowel regimen example for a patient at risk for constipation is as follows:

1. Docusate sodium 100 mg b.i.d. alone or with casanthranol (Peri-Colace), 1 capsule b.i.d.

Table 26.7. Pharmacologic management strategies for diarrhea

Agent	Comments
Kaolin pectin (Kaopectate)	30–60 mL PO after each loose stool
Loperamide (Imodium)	2 capsules (4 mg) PO 4 h initially, then add 1 capsule (2 mg) after each loose stool; should not exceed 16 capsules daily
Diphenoxylate hydrochloride, atropine sulfate (Lomotil)	1–2 tablets PO 4 h; should not exceed 8 tablets daily; there may be anticholinergic effects due to atropine
Paregoric	1 tsp PO 4 ×/d; may alternate with Lomotil
Octreotide	May be useful for fluorouracil-induced diarrhea; starting dose: 0.05–0.1 mg SC t.i.d; may be increased to 1.8 mg/d in refractory diarrhea

2. If no bowel movement, add:
    a. Senna at bedtime (dose varies with the preparation), *or*
    b. Milk of magnesia 30 mL at bedtime
3. If no bowel movement with the above, may add:
    a. Biscodyl 1 to 3 tablets or 1 10-mg suppository, at bedtime, *or*
    b. Lactulose 1 to 4 tablespoons daily
4. Other more aggressive alternatives, if there is no impaction, include:
    a. Fleet enema
    b. Magnesium citrate 1 bottle
    c. Tap-water enema

E.   Altered nutritional status. Patients with cancer often experience progressive loss of appetite and sometimes severe malnutrition during the course of the disease and treatment. Malnutrition may result from a side effect of the therapy or a direct effect of the cancer (e.g., gut obstruction or hepatic or brain metastases). The resulting effects of malnutrition are a poorer response to therapy, increased incidence of infections, and an overall worsening of patient well-being. Many times, one of the presenting signs that leads to the diagnosis of cancer is weight loss; therefore, the patient is most likely already experiencing some alteration in nutritional status. Malnutrition is reported to occur in 50% to 80% of patients with advanced disease. Nutritional management of the patient with cancer involves early intervention using a supportive health care team.

1.   Effects of chemotherapy and radiation therapy on nutrition. Chemotherapy has a major effect on nutritional status because of the direct insult on the gastrointestinal tract. Among the gastrointestinal effects are anorexia, nausea, vomiting, taste alterations, stomatitis, esophagitis, colitis, constipation, and diarrhea. Not only are the effects physiologic in nature, but also the added psychologic impact of the disease and therapy can result in anxiety and depression, which can contribute to the lack of interest in food.

2.   Nutritional assessment. Early in the patient's treatment, a thorough nutritional assessment should be completed by the health care team. The assessment should include diet history, nutrient intake, anthropometric measurements (height, weight, and skin-fold thickness and midarm circumference, if possible), laboratory tests for anemia and serum albumin, and an evaluation of activity and functional status. A good nutritional assessment may help to identify patients who are already at risk of malnutrition or those who may be prone to develop problems during the course of the illness and treatment.

3.   Nutritional intervention. Nutritional intervention should be considered during the initial and ongoing assessments. Situations that warrant nutritional intervention include involuntary weight loss (more than 10% within the last 6 months, especially when combined with weakness and fatigue), history of recent physiologic stress, serum albumin below 3.2 g/dL, or severe immunocompromise. Nurses, dietitians, and even family members can identify problems and may be the first to act to promote weight gain. Various approaches to help increase weight are changes in diet; symptomatic treatment of nausea and vomiting, stomatitis, and other gastrointestinal effects of chemotherapy, and supplemental nutrition.

    a. Nutritional supplements. Several nutritional supplements are commercially available for oral use. One benefit of nutritional supplements is that they are a concentrated form of nutrition for protein and calories. Some of the disadvantages are the unappealing taste and the high cost to the consumer. Some patients and their families are able to develop some creative high-protein and -calorie supplements using household items with some suggestions from the health care team.

    b. Tube feedings. Enteral nutrition through a nasogastric or gastrostomy tube may be an alternative if oral intake is not possible. Enteral feedings are the recommended route if the gastrointestinal tract is functional. Advantages of enteral feeding include lower cost and fewer complications than with parenteral feedings and maintenance of normal gastrointestinal function. Some care and maintenance are involved with feeding tubes, and patients and their families need to be given information regarding available options for feeding.

    c. Total parenteral nutrition. Parenteral nutrition should be considered in patients who do not have a functioning gastrointestinal tract or in those for whom supplemental nutrition is anticipated for a short period of time. Patients who receive total parenteral nutrition (TPN) usually require the insertion of a central venous catheter, which may result in other iatrogenic complications such as pneumothorax, vein thrombosis, and catheter-related infections. In many situations, TPN used in the patient with cancer increases morbidity, especially from infection, without improving survival. Thus, TPN has considerable economic, ethical, and medical consequences that must be evaluated in conjunction with the patient's overall prognosis.

    4. Pharmacologic interventions. A recent area of interest is pharmacologic appetite stimulation. One of the agents currently used is megestrol acetate oral suspension 800 mg/day (20 mL/day). Agents such as megestrol acetate have documented evidence in promoting increased weight gain in some patients and at least a decreased weight loss in others.

F. Neurotoxicity. The incidence of neurotoxicity associated with chemotherapy is increasing, potentially because of the greater use of high-dose chemotherapy and newer drugs causing neurotoxicity used in combination. In many cases, early detection and treatment of neurotoxicity (i.e., reduction of drug dose or discontinuation) allow for the reversal of symptoms. The neurotoxic symptoms may manifest as altered level of consciousness or coma, cerebellar dysfunction, ototoxicity, or peripheral neuropathy, which may be temporary but can cause significant changes in functional ability that persist as a long-term effect. It is also important to assess renal function because poor renal function may reduce clearance of the chemotherapy agent, leading to increased neurotoxicity.

1. Chemotherapy and biologic agents with known potential for neurotoxicity include high-dose cytarabine, high-dose methotrexate, vincristine, vinblastine, vinorelbine, ifosfamide, cisplatin, carboplatin, paclitaxel, docetaxel, procarbazine, thalidomide, interleukin-2, and the interferons.

2. Prevention and early detection of neurotoxicity is key to prevention of permanent neurologic damage. Assessment of symptoms of neurotoxicity should be documented on a routine basis. In certain treatment regimens, altering the drug sequence can markedly decrease the symptoms.

3. Management of peripheral neurotoxicity is being studied, with the goal of slowing, halting, and reversing the neuropathy. One agent that has shown promise in early trials is the cytoprotectant amifostine. Pyroxidine or vitamin B_6 may also be used, 100 mg b.i.d., in attempt to minimize the peripheral neuropathy. If pain becomes a major concern, anticonvulsants (gabapentin or carbamazepine) or tricyclic antidepressants (amitriptyline) may also be used.

G. Palmar–plantar erythrodysesthesia or hand–foot syndrome. Palmar–plantar erythrodysesthesia (PPE) is not a new side effect due to cancer chemotherapy. It has been seen with continuous-infusion fluorouracil in the past but has captured recent attention with newer chemotherapy drugs with high incidence. PPE is a toxic drug reaction that begins as a cutaneous eruption of the integument on the palms of the hands and plantar surfaces of the feet. Theories postulate that PPE occurs because of drug extravasation in the microcapillaries of the hands and feet due to local everyday trauma or by drug concentration and accumulation in sweat glands found in the palms and soles with resultant tissue damage. PPE is time exposure dependent and occurs with protracted, chronic exposure over long periods (i.e., more than 3 to 4 weeks).

1. Chemotherapy agents with a known potential for the development for PPE include fluorouracil (primarily with continuous infusions), capecitabine, doxorubicin, and liposome-encapsulated doxorubicin.

2. Clinical findings of PPE include tingling, numbness, pain, dryness, erythema, swelling, rash, blister formation, and pruritis of the hands and feet. Clinical knowledge of the potential for PPE and early assessment is imperative for adjustments of dose or withholding of therapy. Table 26.8 shows a staging scale that can be utilized to evaluate functional and clinical criteria for dose modification.

3. Management of PPE and symptomatic treatment result from prompt identification of symptoms. At the first sign of PPE, the drug should be stopped, or the interval between doses should be increased, or the drug dose should be reduced. If identified at grade 2 toxicity, symptoms typically improve within a few days of stopping the drug. If untreated, grade 2 side effects may quickly progress to grade 3 or 4, requiring more intense medical concern and intervention. Depending on the drug used, recommendations are available for dose modifications. Education on preventative measures

Table 26.8.   Hand–foot syndrome (palmar–plantar erythrodysesthesia) grading scale

Grade 1	Grade 2	Grade 3	Grade 4
Painless erythema, or welling, numbness, dysesthesia/paresthesia, and tingling that do not disrupt activities of daily living	Painful erythema with swelling that affects activities of daily living	Moist desquamation, ulceration, blistering, and severe pain	Not applicable

Based on National Cancer Institute of Canada CTG Expanded Common Toxicity Criteria.

should be given to patients before beginning the drug where PPE is likely. Patients should be counseled to avoid tight-fitting shoes and rings or repetitive rubbing pressure to the hands or feet. Other precautionary measures include avoiding excessive pressure and heat on the skin for 3 to 5 days after treatment, avoidance of hot baths, showers, or hot tubs (hot water for 24 h prior to and 72 h after treatment), and friction-causing activities such as exercise for 3 to 5 days after treatment. Patients should also be advised to use emollients such as Bag Balm (Dairy Association Co., Lyndonville, VT), Udderly Smooth (Redex Industries, Salem, OH), or other petroleum- or lanolin-containing creams liberally and frequently. Patients should also be instructed to notify their health care providers at the first signs or symptoms of PPE. If the grade of toxicity worsens, supportive care related to analgesia and prevention of infection is important. COX = 2 non-steroidal anti-inflammatory agents (e.g., celecoxib, 100–200 mg b.i.d.) lessens PPE in many patients. Other anecdotal interventions include topical steroids and oral premedication with steroids, application of a nicotine patch, and oral administration of pyridoxine. Further studies need to be done to evaluate which interventions are helpful for PPE and do not exacerbate the skin toxicity.

SELECTED READINGS

Bender CM, McDaniel RW, Murphy-Ende K, et al. Chemotherapy-induced nausea and vomiting. *Clin J Oncol Nurs* 2002;6:94–102.

Brown KA, Esper P, Kelleher LO, et al., eds. *Chemotherapy and biotherapy: guidelines and recommendations for practice.* Pittsburgh: Oncology Nursing Society, 2001.

Campos D, Periera JR, Reinhardt RR, et al. Prevention of cisplatin-induced emesis by the oral neurokinin-1 antagonist, MK-869, in combination with granisetron and dexamethasone or with dexamethasone alone. *J Clin Oncol* 2001;19:1759–1767.

Gralla RJ, Osoba D, Kris MJ, et al. Recommendations of the use of antiemetics: evidence-based, clinical practice guidelines. *J Clin Oncol* 1999;17:2971–2994.

Hallquist P, Yamamoto DS, Geyton JE. Extravasation of infusate via implanted ports: two case studies. *Clin J Oncol Nurs* 1999;3:145–151.

Hesketh PJ, Kris MG, Grunberg SM, et al. Proposal for classifying the acute emetogenicity of cancer chemotherapy. *J Clin Oncol* 1997;15: 103–109.

Hoff PM, LoRusso P, Lokich JJ, et al. Chemotherapy associated hand–foot syndrome: a clinician's guide to diagnosis and management. Nutley, NJ: Roche Laboratories, 2000.

Kornblau S, Benson AB, Catalano R, et al. Management of cancer treatment-related diarrhea: issues and therapeutic strategies. *J Pain Symptom Manage* 2000;19:118–129.

Markman M, Kennedy A, Webster K, et al. Paclitaxel-associated hypersensitivity reactions: experience of the gynecologic oncology program of the Cleveland Clinic Cancer Center. *J Clin Oncol* 2000; 18:102–105.

Mrozek-Orlowski ME, Frye DK, Sanborn HM. Capecitabine: nursing implications of a new oral chemotherapeutic agent. *Oncol Nurs Forum* 1999;26:753–762.

Myers JS. Hypersensitivity reaction to paclitaxel: nursing interventions. *Clin J Oncol Nurs* 2000;4:161–163.

Rogers BB. Mucositis in the oncology patient. *Nurs Clin North Am* 2001;36:745–760.

Infections: Etiology, Treatment, and Prevention

Neeraja L. Varanasi and Rodger D. MacArthur

Infection is a major source of morbidity and mortality among patients with cancer, despite recent advances in prevention and treatment. In many series, infection is the most frequent cause of death, exceeding all other causes combined. Granulocytopenia, cellular immune dysfunction, humoral immune dysfunction, and splenectomy can each predispose patients to certain types of infections. In addition, mucosal or integumentary damage, prolonged hospitalization, lack of ambulation, malnutrition, neurologic dysfunction, and local tumor effect all contribute to the risk of infection. The presence of intravascular catheters, stents, and other diversionary procedures can further predispose the immuno-compromised host to infections.

Most bacterial and fungal infections in patients with cancer arise from the patients' own flora. Environmental reservoirs may also contribute to infection in certain circumstances. Prolonged hospitalization and antibiotic use tend to favor the acquisition of resistant strains of organisms. Careful hand washing by health care workers is the most important means of reducing the occurrence of infection. Reverse isolation of patients can be justified only rarely. The prompt initiation of therapy with broad-spectrum antibiotics in documented and suspected bacterial infections is essential. The addition of antifungal therapy should be considered in patients who do not respond within a reasonable period of time to antibiotics. Daily re-evaluation of all patients is critical. Appropriate diagnostic studies (e.g., computed tomography [CT] scans, bronchoscopy, cultures) should be obtained earlier, rather than later, in the evaluation of any febrile patient with cancer.

I. Reasons for infection
A. Granulocytopenia
1. **General comments.** Acute leukemias or lymphomas after chemotherapy are prototypic malignancies in which infection resulting from granulocytopenia is seen. Virtually all cytotoxic drugs and radiation therapy used in the treatment of malignant diseases have a deleterious effect on the proliferation of the hematopoietic progenitor cells. An increase in the incidence of infection can be expected when the granulocyte count is less than 500/μL. A substantial increase in both the incidence and the severity of infection occurs when there are fewer than 100 granulocytes/μL. Infection early in the course of granulocytopenia typically is caused by relatively nonresistant endogenous bacteria. Fungal infections and infection with resistant bacteria most often occur during prolonged periods of granulocytopenia. Factors that increase the susceptibility to infection in neutropenic patients are rapid onset, prolonged (longer than 10 days) and profound neutropenia, severe mucositis, presence of renal failure, and intravascular catheters.

2.   Sites of infection. Damage to skin and mucosal membranes (e.g., from venipuncture or chemotherapy) greatly increases the risk of infection in granulocytopenic patients. Thus, the integument, periodontium, oropharynx, colon, and perianal area are common foci from which organisms can seed the bloodstream and disseminate. Pneumonia typically is caused by bacteria that have colonized the oropharynx.

3.   Sequence of events during neutropenia. Ten days from the day of administration of intensive cytotoxic chemotherapy, neutropenia develops and is often accompanied by severe mucositis. The first fever during a neutropenic episode often represents bacteremia by pathogens originating from the gastrointestinal tract and occurs about 10 days after chemotherapy. The risk of infections related to a central venous catheter increases with the length of time that the catheter is left in place, with signs and symptoms usually manifest during the third week after chemotherapy. Pulmonary infiltrates tend to occur beyond this period. The major factor that influences immunologic reconstitution after allogenic bone marrow transplantation is acute graft-versus-host disease (GVHD) and its treatment, with cytomegalovirus (CMV), adenovirus, fungi, and *Pneumocystis carinii* being the major pathogens. Chronic GVHD develops 3 months from transplantation and places the patient at risk for varicella zoster virus (VZV) reactivation and pulmonary infections with *P. carinii* and CMV (see Table 27.1).

4.   Microbiology

    a.   General comments. The epidemiology of organisms causing infections in cancer patients has changed in the last 10 to 15 years. The number of infections caused by gram-positive bacteria and fungi has increased markedly; the number of infections caused by gram-negative bacteria has remained constant but has decreased as a percentage of all infections. Gram-positive bacteria now account for about 60% to 70% of microbiologically documented infections. The most likely explanation for the increase in gram-positive infections is the increased use of indwelling venous catheters and the prompt use of empirical and prophylactic therapy against gram-negative rods, which results in a selective pressure. The specific bacteria most commonly associated with infections tend to vary from institution to institution and often vary within institutions over time. The classic microorganisms associated with a high mortality rate are still the *Enterobacteriaceae* (*Escherichia coli, Klebsiella* species) and *Pseudomonas aeruginosa.* An alarming increase in the incidence of multiresistant *Enterobacter* species has been reported, attributed to induced chromosomal β-lactamases due to the frequent use of the third-generation cephalosporins. Enterococci are becoming an increasing cause of nosocomial bacteremia, with *Enterococcus faecium* being more common than *E. faecalis.* Vancomycin-resistant enterococci (VRE) are also increasing in incidence, occurring more commonly in patients with gastrointestinal tract colonization and thought to occur after use of antibiotics with antianaerobic activity. Newer bacteria like *Lactobacillus, Leuconostoc, Corynebacterium jeikium, Rhodo-*

Table 27.1. Common pathogens in different immunocompromised conditions

Condition	Gram positive	Gram negative	Fungi	Viruses
First 10 days of neutropenia	*Streptococcus viridans, Staphylococcus* spp.	*E. coli, K. pneumoniae, P. aeruginosa, Enterobacter, Serratia*		
3 wk of neutropenia	*S. epidermidis, S. aureus, C. jeikium,* VRE	*E. coli, K. pneumoniae*	*Aspergillus, C. albicans* and non–*C. albicans* spp.	
Acute GVHD			*Aspergillus,* PCP, *Fusarium, Curvularia* PCP	CMV, adenovirus
Chronic GVHD >3 mo from transplant				VZV reactivation, CMV
Cellular immune dysfunction; Hodgkin's, ALL, corticosteroids	*Legionella pneumophila, Nocardia, Salmonella, Listeria, M. tuberculosis, M. kansasii*		*Cryptococcus neoformans, Histoplasma capsulatum, coccidiomycosis,* PCP	VZV, HSV, CMV
Humoral immune dysfunction	*Streptococcus pneumoniae, H. influenzae, Neisseria meningitides, E. coli*			

coccus equi, and *Pediacoccus* and fungi-like *Fusarium, Alternaria, Pseudoallescheria,* and *Scopulariopsis* can be pathogens in this setting. The sensitivity patterns of bacteria to antibiotics also vary widely among institutions. Hospital-specific organism sensitivity and resistance data are typically updated at least yearly and can be invaluable in selecting an appropriate initial antibiotic regimen.

b.   Gram-negative bacteria. *E. coli, K. pneumoniae,* and *P. aeruginosa* predominate, although the incidence of infection with *P. aeruginosa* has decreased in recent years for unknown reasons. *Enterobacter* species, *Acinetobacter* species, *Serratia marcescens, Burkholderia (Pseudomonas) cepacia,* and *Stenotrophomonas (Xanthomonas) maltophilia* are less common, but still important, pathogens.

c.   Gram-positive bacteria. Coagulase-negative staphylococci are the most common cause of catheter-acquired sepsis. In the presence of intravascular devices, caution is required in interpreting coagulase-negative staphylococci as a contaminant in the blood cultures. Infection with either *Staphylococcus epidermidis* or *Staphylococcus aureus* is now almost as common as infection with gram-negative bacteria. *C. jeikeium* and VRE are occasionally found in association with catheter infections.

d.   Fungi. *Candida* species (primarily *albicans* and *tropicalis*), *Aspergillus* species, and the agents of mucormycosis are the important pathogens. Recently, the incidence of infection with *C. krusei* has increased at many centers. *Pseudallescheria boydii, Fusarium, Curvularia,* and *Alternaria* species, *Trichosporon* species, and other "unusual" fungi are seen less frequently but should not be assumed to be contaminants when isolated.

B.   Cellular immune dysfunction

1.   General comments. Cellular immune dysfunction and its associated infections can result either from the underlying disease or from antineoplastic agents and corticosteroids. Hodgkin's disease and acute lymphocytic leukemia (ALL) in long-term remission are characteristic malignancies in which cellular immune dysfunction–related infection is encountered.

2.   Microbiology

a.   Bacteria. *Legionella pneumophila* is of special concern, as are the *Nocardia* species. Nocardiosis typically presents with one or more lesions in the lung, skin, and brain. Infections caused by *Salmonella* species and *Listeria monocytogenes* are considerably less common.

b.   Mycobacteria. *Mycobacterium avium–intracellulare* is being seen with increasing frequency in patients with non-Hodgkin's lymphomas receiving intensive cytotoxic therapy. The incidence of infection with *M. kansasii* is increased in patients with hairy-cell leukemia. *M. tuberculosis* is surprisingly unusual in patients with cancer with altered cell-mediated immunity. Recently, there have been reports of increased occurrence of *M. tuberculosis* associated with the use of infliximab.

c.   Fungi. *Candida* and *Aspergillus* species are the most common causes of nosocomial fungal infections. *Cryptococcus* *neoformans* is seen frequently. Meningitis is the most common presentation, but pulmonary and cutaneous infections also occur. The incidence of *Histoplasma capsulatum* and *Coccidioides immitis* is geographically dependent. Infections caused by the former are seen in the Central River Valley regions of the United States, whereas infections caused by the latter are seen in the Southwest. Pneumonia is the most common presentation with each of these fungi. *P. carinii,* which is genotypically more similar to fungi than to protozoa, is a common cause of pneumonia, especially in children with ALL and following tapering doses of corticosteroids. The use of trimethoprim-sulfamethoxazole (TMP-SMX) has effectively reduced the incidence of infections with *P. carinii.*

   d.   Viruses. VZV, causing either varicella or zoster, is particularly common in this group of patients. Varicella can be life threatening in children with ALL, causing pneumonitis, purpura fulminans, and encephalitis. Oropharyngeal or esophageal lesions due to herpes simplex virus (HSV) can predispose to infection with bacterial or fungal pathogens. CMV is seen most often in patients undergoing bone marrow transplantation and typically results from reactivation of virus previously acquired by either donor or recipient. Interstitial pneumonia is the most common disease manifestation of CMV infection. The current incidence of CMV disease in CMV-seropositive bone marrow transplant recipients is between 2% and 10%. In CMV-seronegative recipients, the incidence of disease approximates 0% if the donor is also CMV seronegative and CMV-seronegative blood product support is used. Respiratory syncytial virus (RSV), adenovirus, parainfluenza virus, and influenza virus occasionally cause pneumonia in bone marrow transplant recipients.

   e.   Protozoa and helminths. Infection with *Toxoplasmosis gondii* presents as either chorioretinitis or cerebral abscesses. *Strongyloides stercoralis* can cause diarrhea or life-threatening disseminated infections. Diffuse pulmonary infiltrates, shock, and sepsis from enteric gram-negative bacilli are the typical features of disseminated strongyloidiasis.

C.   Humoral immune dysfunction

   1.   General comments. Agammaglobulinemic or hypogammaglobulinemic patients are susceptible to infections because they often lack opsonizing antibodies to the common encapsulated pyogenic bacteria. Many of these patients are also deficient in functional complement activity. Multiple myeloma and chronic lymphocytic leukemia are prototypic neoplasms with humoral immune dysfunction.

   2.   Microbiology. *Streptococcus pneumoniae* predominates. In addition, decreased complement activity increases the risk of infection by *Haemophilus influenzae, Neisseria meningitidis,* and *E. coli.*

D.   Splenectomy

   1.   General comments. The spleen is the organ most efficient at removing nonopsonized bacteria. Specific opsonizing antibodies are required for effective killing of the encapsulated bacteria. Thus, splenectomized patients are at risk of overwhelming sepsis when infected with a strain of encapsulated bacteria against which they have never had an opportunity to make antibodies.

2. Microbiology. Infections are usually caused by *S. pneumoniae* and, to a lesser extent, by *H. influenzae* and *N. meningitidis*. Fulminant sepsis can occur following dog bites and scratches with *Capnocytophaga canimorsus*.

E. Other factors

1. Indwelling vascular catheters increase the risk of bacterial and fungal infections. The risk increases with the length of time they have been in place. Concurrent granulocytopenia magnifies the infection risk.

2. Nonambulation and length of stay have been identified as independent risk factors for infection in most studies. Other factors such as previous antibiotic use and the presence of a Foley catheter are correlated with nonambulation and length of stay but are not independent risk factors for infection.

3. Malnutrition and neurologic dysfunction. It is controversial whether malnutrition is an independent risk factor for immunosuppression. On the other hand, malnourished patients who require enteral feedings are certainly at increased risk for aspiration. Loss of the gag reflex also increases the risk of aspiration. Loss of sensation facilitates the development of cutaneous ulcers.

4. Local tumor effect. Complete or partial obstruction by tumor may lead to infection behind the obstruction. Two examples of this phenomenon are postobstructive pneumonia in a patient with bronchogenic cancer and ascending cholangitis in a patient with an intra-abdominal lymphoma.

II. Treatment of infection

A. Clinical findings that suggest the diagnosis of infection

1. Symptoms

a. General. Malaise, fatigue, confusion, and other nonspecific or subtle symptoms may be the first indication of infection. Any unexplained change in the patient's condition should be evaluated clinically and microbiologically.

b. Localizing. Symptoms referable to a particular organ system are particularly worrisome and demand an immediate and thorough evaluation.

2. Signs

a. Fever is the single most important indicator of infection in cancer patients. Often, it is the only abnormal finding. It is dangerous to assume that an unexplained fever is due to the underlying malignancy. Similarly, it is unwise to rely exclusively on fever to diagnose infection: Debilitated or elderly patients occasionally are afebrile in the presence of infection. In general, a single oral temperature reading of more than 38.5°C or two or three oral temperature readings higher than 38.0°C within a 24-h period strongly suggest the presence of infection.

b. Hypotension and shock occur with a variety of infections; they are not specific for infections caused by gram-negative bacteria.

c. Tachycardia, especially if new or unexplained, can also suggest infection.

   d. Inflammation, if present, suggests underlying infection. Note, however, that granulocytopenic patients often fail to show a normal inflammatory response to infection. Consequently, bacterial pneumonia can present without an identifiable infiltrate on chest radiograph or even without significant sputum production. Similarly, abscess formation is often minimal or absent despite significant local or systemic infection.

   e. Leukocytosis, especially when accompanied by an increase in neutrophils or band-form neutrophils, suggests infection. Of course, patients who are leukopenic from chemotherapy do not show this response. Toxic granulation of neutrophils also suggests infection.

B. Evaluation of patients with suspected infection

   1. General. A thorough, daily evaluation of all hospitalized patients with cancer is necessary to diagnose and treat infections properly. Areas that should not be overlooked include the retinae, ears and sinuses, mouth, skin, catheter sites, axillae, perineum, perianal region, and extremities. Diminished inflammatory response to infections in a neutropenic host can result in a cutaneous infection without typical cellulitis, pneumonia without an infiltrate on a radiograph, meningitis without pleocytosis in the cerebrospinal fluid (CSF), and a urinary tract infection without pyuria.

   2. Cultures

   a. General approach. Multiple cultures from multiple sites need to be obtained whenever infection is suspected. All culture material needs to be delivered promptly to the microbiology laboratory. Any change in a patient's condition suggestive of new infection should warrant repeat culturing, even if a pathogen had been isolated previously. Blood, urine, and respiratory cultures typically are obtained with each evaluation. Specimens from other sources are obtained depending on specific circumstances.

   b. Blood

   (1) Technique. Two sets (aerobic and anaerobic bottles) should be drawn in every 24-h period in which infection is suspected to be present, until a diagnosis is made. At least 5 mL of blood should be injected into each culture bottle.

   (2) Central venous catheters. If these indwelling devices are present, it is important to obtain additional cultures through each port of the device in addition to obtaining peripheral specimens in the usual manner.

   (3) Resin bottles. Culture bottles containing an antibiotic-binding resin or other antibiotic-binding substance should be included with each culture set for patients who are receiving antibiotics at the time of evaluation.

   c. Urine. Clean-catch or straight-catheterization specimens are preferred. Urine that has been present in a closed collection system for more than 1 h should not be sent for culture. If necessary, urine can be obtained from the catheter tubing using a syringe and a small-gauge needle.

   d. Respiratory specimens

   (1) Spontaneously expectorated sputum and endotracheal aspirates. A good specimen should have fewer than 10 squamous epithelial cells per low-power (100×) field.

(2)   Induced sputum. Using 3% saline delivered to the patient's respiratory tract through an ultrasonic nebulizer can increase the yield on bacterial culture of respiratory specimens. *P. carinii* infection is often diagnosed by this technique in centers experienced with its use, thereby sparing patients the need for bronchoscopy. Three percent saline can cause significant bronchospasm and should be administered cautiously only by trained personnel.

(3)   Transtracheal aspiration. This procedure is used rarely. More commonly, patients undergo bronchoscopy or open-lung biopsy if pulmonary pathology is suspected and the first two techniques fail to provide an answer.

(4)   Nasal washings. Nonbacteriostatic fluid (e.g., saline) delivered to the nares through a bulb syringe and then quickly aspirated back into the syringe is an effective way to obtain virus for culture. The fluid can be transported to the laboratory in any closed container but needs to be done so promptly. It is important to let the laboratory know which viruses are suspected. Unfortunately, the yield of nasal washings is often much lower than that of bronchoscopy-obtained fluid, primarily because of physician inexperience with the nasal washing technique.

e.   Cerebrospinal fluid

(1)   Criteria. A lumbar puncture should be performed in any patient who has an abnormal or a changed neurologic examination. A lumbar puncture should be strongly considered in any patient in whom no other source can be found to explain the suspected infection.

(2)   Studies. CSF should always be sent for gram stain, bacterial cultures, cell count with differential, glucose, and protein. A cryptococcal antigen titer should be performed if the patient has reasons for cellular immune dysfunction. Acid-fast bacillus (AFB) stains and cultures are not indicated routinely.

f.   Stool

(1)   Clostridium difficile. This toxin-producing anaerobic bacterium is a common cause of diarrhea in patients who have been on antibiotics. A mild to moderate leukocytosis as well as a temperature reading above 38.0°C typically are part of the syndrome. All patients with diarrhea should have stool sent for a cytotoxic assay for *C. difficile* toxin. It is important to test the stool for cytotoxin A and B as a significant number of infections are caused by cytotoxin B–producing organisms. Rapid antigen detection tests are not as reliable.

(2)   Bacterial cultures. A stool culture should be sent to the microbiology laboratory from patients in whom the diagnosis of infectious diarrhea is suspected. Occasionally, *Salmonella* species and *L. monocytogenes* are causes of nosocomial diarrhea or sepsis.

(3)   Fecal leukocytes. The presence of white blood cells in the stool suggests an invasive inflammatory process of the colon. Fecal leukocytes are seen with *Shigella* species,

Campylobacter species, invasive *E. coli,* and, variably, *Salmonella* species and *C. difficile.* A methylene blue stain of the stool should be ordered routinely along with the culture.

(4)   Ova and parasites. Diarrhea that develops more than 3 days after the patient's hospitalization almost never has a parasitic cause. The routine ordering of this test should be discouraged. The important exception is in geographic regions in which *S. stercoralis* is endemic (e.g., southeastern United States).

g.   Viral cultures

(1)   Herpes simplex virus and varicella zoster virus. Suspicious vesicular lesions need to be cultured for HSV or VZV. Fluid-filled lesions should be carefully unroofed. A swab should then be rubbed on the base of the lesion and sent in viral transport medium to the laboratory within 30 min. These specimens need to be promptly inoculated into tissue culture or stored at 4 to 9°C for no more than 18 h. A direct fluorescent antibody test is also available for HSV 1 and 2.

(2)   Cytomegalovirus. Blood and urine cultures frequently are positive in bone marrow transplant patients who have CMV interstitial pneumonia but are not synonymous with disease. Isolation (culture) of CMV from pulmonary specimens is suggestive of disease if a concurrent chest radiograph or CT scan reveals an interstitial pattern. Evidence of tissue invasion by histologic and histochemical techniques confirms the diagnosis of CMV disease.

h.   Other. Biopsy or aspirate cultures from any accessible suspected site of infection should be obtained as soon as possible. The risk of complications from such procedures (e.g., infection, bleeding) must be weighed against the possible gains.

3.   Imaging studies

a.   Radiographs. A chest radiograph should be obtained routinely in any patient suspected of having an infection. Sinus films are also frequently important.

b.   Computed tomography. CT scans of the chest, abdomen, brain, head and neck, spine, and other areas can add considerable information to the diagnostic work-up. The ordering of these tests needs to be individualized to the specific clinical situation.

c.   Ultrasonography. An echocardiogram should be obtained when endocarditis is suspected. Ultrasonography is also good at detecting ascites and biliary, hepatic, and pancreatic pathology. A portable (bedside) ultrasound can be useful in critically ill patients who are too sick to be transported to the radiology department.

d.   Nuclear medicine. Unfortunately, radionuclide scanning using indium-labeled granulocytes or gallium is often nondiagnostic. False-positive and false-negative results occur too frequently to recommend these tests on a routine basis.

4. **Invasive studies**
    a. **Bronchoscopy.** Bronchoalveolar lavage (BAL) for *P. carinii* and other fungi and for CMV, RSV, and other viruses should be considered for patients at risk for one of these organisms. The adequacy of the specimen can be ascertained by noting the presence of alveolar macrophages on subsequent stains. Specimens also should be sent for gram stain, AFB stain and culture, and fungal and bacterial cultures.
    b. **Skin biopsy.** Suspicious dermatologic lesions should be sampled and sent for bacterial, fungal, and AFB cultures and for methenamine silver staining for fungi.
    c. **Open-lung biopsy.** A persistent unexplained infiltrate on chest radiograph is often evaluated best with this approach. Morbidity is low in patients with adequate platelets and normal coagulation indexes.
    d. **Bone marrow biopsy.** Specimens should be sent for AFB stains and culture.
    e. **Percutaneous liver biopsy.** Occasionally, this procedure is helpful in diagnosing bacterial or fungal pathogens (e.g., *Candida* species) if abnormalities referable to this organ are suspected based on imaging studies or serum chemistries.
    f. **Exploratory laparotomy.** Even multiple imaging studies sometimes fail to reveal intra-abdominal abscesses. A positive blood culture and abdominal tenderness should be clues to this diagnosis. An exploratory laparotomy might be required if symptoms persist. Alternatively, surgery may need to be considered if intra-abdominal abnormalities detected by other studies fail to resolve with therapy.
5. **Miscellaneous studies**
    a. **A complete blood count** with differential should be performed on every patient suspected of having an infection.
    b. **Liver function tests** are often abnormal in generalized sepsis or during infections involving the organ itself.
    c. **Urinalysis** can help differentiate infection from contamination. The absence of white blood cells suggests the latter diagnosis. Note, however, that white blood cells may be absent in neutropenic patients.
    d. **Sedimentation rate.** This nonspecific test is rarely useful and is seldom indicated.
    e. **Serology.** In general, serologic tests are of little value in diagnosing acute infections.
    f. **Antigen and antibody rapid-detection tests.** Direct fluorescent antibody testing of sputum for *L. pneumophila* and other *Legionella* species can provide a diagnosis more rapidly than culture, although the sensitivity of this test is somewhat lower than that of culture at most large centers. A urine antigen detection test for *L. pneumophila* serogroup 1 has sensitivity that rivals culture but detects only the most common serogroup of *L. pneumophila* and not other *Legionella* species. Urine and serum antigen tests also are available in some centers for *H. capsulatum* and may be useful both for diagnosis and for following response to therapy. Antigen tests for other fungi lack sufficient sensitivity

to be clinically useful at this time. An enzyme-linked immunosorbent assay (ELISA) test is available for detecting influenza A and B from nasal washings.

g. Deoxyribonucleic acid probes. Deoxyribonucleic acid (DNA) hybridization tests for ribosomal ribonucleic acid (RNA) that is genus specific exist for *Legionella* species, *H. capsulatum,* various mycobacteria, and other organisms. The sensitivity of these tests equals but does not exceed that of other diagnostic techniques. The major advantage of the DNA probes is their ability to determine the identity of organisms growing in culture sooner than is possible by traditional methods.

h. Polymerase chain reaction. Quantitative polymerase chain reaction (PCR) for CMV is being investigated as a means of determining which patients are at greatest risk of developing disease. PCR techniques have also been used to diagnose HSV encephalitis because the yield of CSF culture for this virus is extremely poor.

C. Therapy

1. Empiric therapy

a. Timing. Two or three oral temperature elevations above 38°C or one elevation above 38.5°C during a 14-h period suggest infection. Patients with fewer than 500 neutrophils/μL should be started on antibiotics at this time. Nonneutropenic patients may also require antibiotics, but that decision should be individualized based on other findings.

b. Neutropenic coverage (antibiotics). Prompt initiation of empiric antibiotic therapy has been shown to reduce mortality. Three different regimens of IV antibiotic therapy with similar efficacy are considered here.

(1) Single-drug therapy (monotherapy). Several randomized controlled trials have shown no difference between monotherapy and combination therapy for empirical treatment of uncomplicated febrile neutropenic patients. Monotherapy is generally preferred in patients with moderately severe neutropenia (more than 100/mm³ and less than 1,000/mm³), duration less than 10 days, and no other complications. A third- or fourth-generation cephalosporin (ceftazidime or cefepime) or a carbapenem (imipenem-cilastin or meropenem) may be used. Presence of extended-spectrum β-lactamases has reduced the utility of ceftazidime for monotherapy. It must be kept in mind that these drugs do not usually cover coagulase-negative staphylococci, methicillin-resistant *Staphylococcus aureus* (MRSA), VRE, some strains of penicillin-resistant *Streptococcus pneumoniae,* and viridans streptococci. Studies evaluating quinolones for monotherapy have favorable and unfavorable outcomes and thus cannot be recommended for monotherapy.

(2) Two-drug therapy without a glycopeptide antibiotic (vancomycin) combination therapy is preferred in cases with severe neutropenia (less than 100/mm³), duration more than 10 days, complications such as hypotension, adult respiratory distress syndrome (ARDS), sepsis, mucositis, inflamed IV site, and recurrent febrile neutropenia. Two antipseudomonal antibiotics should be included (Fig. 27-1). The most commonly used two-drug combination is an aminoglycoside (gentamicin, tobramycin, or amikacin) with an antipseudomonal carboxypenicillin or ureidopenicillin (ticarcillin-clavulanic acid or piperacillin-tazobactam); an aminoglycoside with an antipseudomonal cephalosporin (cefepime or ceftazidime); and an aminoglycoside plus a carbapenem (imipenemcilastin or meropenem). Other regimens are possible; the one that is chosen should reflect local sensitivity patterns. Advantages of combination therapy are potential synergistic effects against some gram-negative bacilli and minimal emergence of drug-resistant strains during treatment. The major disadvantages are the nephrotoxicity and ototoxicity associated with aminoglycosides. Single daily dosing of aminoglycosides has resulted in a decrease of the nephrotoxicity.

A loading dose of 2 mg/kg of tobramycin or 7.5 mg/kg of amikacin should be given initially. High peak serum levels (e.g., 7 to 8 μg/mL of tobramycin) have been shown to be beneficial in treating infections in neutropenic patients. To avoid unacceptably high trough levels, it is often necessary to decrease the dosing frequency and increase the amount given with each dose. A reasonable approach is to give slightly less than a loading dose (e.g., 1.7 to 2 mg/kg of tobramycin every 8 h) with each dose and to adjust only the dosing interval by monitoring peak and trough levels. Alternatively, once-daily dosing of tobramycin (5 mg/kg/day) and amikacin (15 mg/kg/day) has been shown to be as effective as traditional dosing schedules, with no increase in nephrotoxicity or ototoxicity in patients with normal renal function.

(3)   Therapy with glycopeptide (vancomycin) plus one or two drugs. Addition of vancomycin to the initial empiric therapy is prudent in the following clinical conditions: clinically suspected serious catheter-related infections, known colonization with penicillin- and cephalosporin-resistant pneumococci or MRSA, positive blood culture results for gram-positive bacteria before final identification, and hypotension. Linezolid, an oxazolidinone, has activity against drug-susceptible gram-positive bacterial infections, MRSA, and VRE. Thrombocytopenia is a side effect of this drug. Quinupristindalfopristin has also been recently approved by the U.S. Food and Drug Administration (FDA) and is effective against vancomycin-resistant *E. faecium*. The drug is to be administered via a central line only and can cause severe myalgias.

(4)   Duration. Antibiotics should be continued for a full 14-day course in patients who remain neutropenic, even if they become afebrile during therapy. This approach is a compromise: Stopping antibiotics too quickly in neutropenic patients results in an unacceptably high percentage of the patients requiring subsequent courses of antibiotics, whereas continuing the antibiotics until

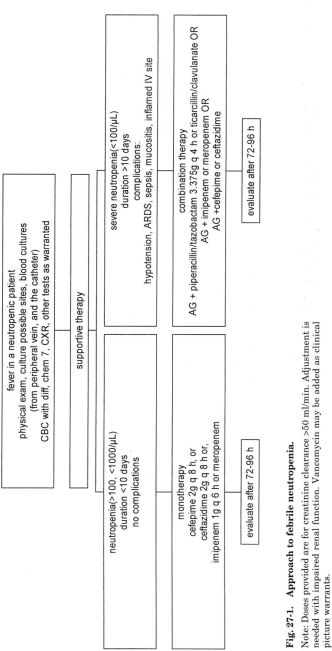

Fig. 27-1. Approach to febrile neutropenia.

Note: Doses provided are for creatinine clearance >50 ml/min. Adjustment is needed with impaired renal function. Vancomycin may be added as clinical picture warrants.

granulocyte counts are more than 500/µL may increase the risk of antibiotic-associated toxicities and the development of resistance. Patients who show recovery of their granulocyte counts to more than 500/µL before completion of a 14-day course of antibiotics can have their antibiotics discontinued after they have been afebrile for at least 72 h.

(5)   Antifungal therapy. Indications for addition of empiric antifungal therapy in the febrile neutropenic host include persisting fever after 1 week of being on antibiotic therapy, recurrence of fever after 1 week of neutropenia, sinus tenderness and facial swelling, nasal ulcerative lesions with black eschars, pulmonary infiltrates on radiograph or CT scan, and presence of pleurisy or pericardial rub. Amphotericin B at a dose of 0.5 to 0.7 mg/kg/day should be started if neutropenic patients remain febrile despite broad-spectrum antibiotic coverage for more than 5 to 7 days (Table 27.2). Although the optimal total dose and duration of antifungal therapy are unknown, it seems prudent to continue antifungal therapy to a total dose of 500 mg, assuming that the patient responds to therapy by becoming afebrile. If the patient does not become afebrile within several days of initiating antifungal therapy, the dose of amphotericin should be increased to at least 0.8 mg/kg/day to cover fungi such as *Aspergillus* species. Two recent prospective randomized trials have demonstrated that fluconazole is an acceptable alternative to amphotericin B for use as empirical antifungal therapy at institutions where mold infections (*Aspergillus* species) and drug-resistant *Candida* species (*C. kruseii* and *C. glabrata*) are uncommon. *C. krusei, Aspergillus, Mucor,* and some other non-*albicans* species of *Candida* are resistant to fluconazole. The lipid complex (Ambisome) formulations of amphotericin B have been shown to have less nephrotoxicity than amphotericin B, with similar efficacy in a multicenter randomized trial. In a recent controlled study of febrile neutropenic patients with cancer, itraconazole and amphotericin B were equivalent in efficacy as empirical antifungal therapy. Caspofungin, an echinocandin, has been recently FDA approved for the treatment of invasive aspergillosis refractory to amphotericin B and itraconazole. Newer-generation azoles are being developed that have a broader spectrum of action against the various *Candida* species, *Aspergillus,* and other filamentous fungi. One such drug is voriconazole, which has less

Table 27.2.   Antifungal therapy with amphotericin

For candidiasis and initial empiric therapy: 0.5–0.7 mg/kg/d
For cryptococcosis or histoplasmosis: 0.6–0.8 mg/kg/d
For resistant candidiasis or persistent fever: 0.8–1.2 mg/kg/d
For aspergillosis: 1.0–1.5 mg/kg/d

nephrotoxicity and equal efficacy when compared with amphotericin B in the treatment of invasive aspergillosis.

(6) Additional coverage. Patients at risk for pneumonia caused by *P. carinii* or *Legionella* species should have TMP-SMX and erythromycin, respectively, included in their antibiotic regimens, if evidence for pulmonary infection exists. Anaerobic coverage (e.g., metronidazole or clindamycin) should be considered in patients with necrotizing gingivitis, perianal tenderness, and acute abdominal pain suggestive of typhlitis.

2. **Definitive therapy**
   a. **Antibiotics**
      (1) General. Re-evaluation of the empiric antibiotic regimen is mandatory when the identity and sensitivity pattern of an isolated pathogen become available.

      (2) Gram-negative infections. Neutropenic patients should be treated with two antibiotics, each effective against the isolated organism. Nonneutropenic patients with *P. aeruginosa* pneumonia also should receive therapy with two antibiotics, at least initially.

      (3) Gram-positive infections. One antibiotic is sufficient, but coverage against gram-negative organisms should be continued in neutropenic patients, as discussed previously.

   b. **Specific infections**
      (1) Catheter-related sepsis. Staphylococcal infections predominate. Removal of infected indwelling intravascular devices is optimal but not always possible. Eradication of infection can often be accomplished with long-term antibiotics alone. There is about a 70% to 80% chance of curing an *S. epidermidis* infection with 3 to 4 weeks of antibiotics administered through each port of the device. The chance of success drops to 30% to 50% for gram-negative and *S. aureus* infections. Fungal infections require immediate removal of the catheter. Tunnel infections also generally require catheter removal.

      (2) <u>Candida</u> species infections
         (a) Significance. Isolation of *Candida* species from sputum, urine, stool, or drainage fluid is not necessarily synonymous with infection. On the other hand, isolation of *Candida* species from three or more nonblood sites has been shown to correlate with disseminated candidiasis in neutropenic patients. Isolation of this organism from the blood is always significant. The presence of macronodular skin lesions shown on biopsy to be consistent with candidal infection is synonymous with dissemination.

         (b) Therapy. Amphotericin B remains the treatment of choice. The optimum dose and duration are unknown, especially in patients who remain neutropenic. Most centers use doses of 0.5 to 0.7 mg/kg/day, to a total dose of at least 500 mg for documented infections. The addition of 5-fluorocytosine (flucytosine) at doses of 25 mg/kg every 6 h is often synergistic and may increase response rates. This agent is potentially bone marrow suppressive, and serum levels should be monitored. Fluconazole at doses of 400 to 800 mg/day shows promise against *C. albicans* infection but is ineffective against *C. krusei* and certain other non-*albicans* species of *Candida*. A higher dose of fluconazole, 800 mg/day, is required to treat *C. glabrata* fungemia.

(c) Dissemination. Candidemia or other evidence of dissemination should prompt a search for deep organ involvement. Weekly funduscopic examinations are essential in such circumstances. When deep organ involvement is present, therapy with amphotericin B should be continued to a total of at least 1 to 2 g. Surgery, when feasible, may improve survival in selected cases of deep organ involvement.

(3) Aspergillus species infections. Even a single positive culture for one of the *Aspergillus* species warrants the initiation of therapy. Pulmonary involvement is the most common disease manifestation, but thrombosis of major blood vessels and widespread dissemination occur in neutropenic patients. Aggressive therapy is necessary to reduce mortality: Early initiation of amphotericin B at doses of 1 to 1.5 mg/kg/day is recommended. A total course of 2 g is typical. Itraconazole, studied in a large open multicenter study of proven and probable invasive aspergillosis, showed a response rate of 41%. Caspofungin is approved for aspergillosis refractory to amphotericin B and itraconazole. The other new agent approved for the treatment of invasive aspergillosis is voriconazole.

(4) Herpes simplex virus and varicella zoster virus infections. Early initiation of therapy helps to prevent dissemination. The dose of acyclovir for HSV infections in immunocompromised patients with normal renal function is 6.25 mg/kg every 8 h, administered IV. VZV infections require 12.5 mg/kg of acyclovir every 8 h. Serum levels following an oral dose average about 25% of levels obtained after an IV dose; for this reason, oral acyclovir typically is not used for acute HSV or VZV infections in cancer patients. High-dose oral regimens (800 mg five times daily) have been tried with some success, but gastrointestinal distress is a common side effect. Neither valacyclovir nor famciclovir has been studied adequately in cancer patients. Foscarnet is the choice of therapy in acyclovir-resistant herpes virus infections.

(5) Cytomegalovirus interstitial pneumonia. CMV interstitial pneumonia occurs at a median of 50 to 60 days after bone marrow transplantation. The 6-month mortality rate still exceeds 30%, despite recent improvements in therapy. The current treatment of choice is the combination of ganciclovir at a dose of 5 mg/kg IV every 12 h plus immune globulin 500 mg/kg IV every other day for 21 days, followed by the combination of ganciclovir 5 mg/kg IV every day (5 days/week) plus immune globulin 500 mg/kg IV once weekly for the duration of major immunosuppressive therapy. Significant bone marrow toxicity can occur with ganciclovir use, and CMV resistance to ganciclovir has been reported. Unfortunately, the use of foscarnet, with its associated nephrotoxicity, causes problems in these patients, who typically are on concomitant cyclosporin A. Valganciclovir has been approved and studied for the treatment of CMV retinitis in human immunodeficiency virus (HIV) patients.

(6) Respiratory syncytial virus pneumonia. The mortality rate for this difficult-to-treat infection in bone marrow transplant recipients exceeds 50% in many centers. The combination of aerosolized ribavirin administered as a small-particle aerosol into a tent or mask continuously for 18 h/day for 2 to 5 days plus immune globulin 500 mg/kg IV every other day for the duration of ribavirin therapy may be more effective than ribavirin alone. Amantadine or rimantadine can decrease illness if begun in the first 48 h of influenza A. Neither of them is effective against pneumonia caused by influenza B. Oseltamivir is effective against influenza A and B.

(7) Nocardia species infections. Altered cell-mediated immunity, whether intrinsic or corticosteroid induced, is the main risk factor for infection with these organisms. The treatment of choice remains oral sulfadiazine 6 to 8 g/day. Therapy should be continued for at least 3 months, and regimens of 6 to 12 months are not uncommon. TMP-SMX (IV or oral), sulfisoxazole, and triple-sulfonamide combinations are likely to be as efficacious as sulfadiazine. Minocycline is an alternative for patients with sulfa allergies, and imipenem has shown impressive *in vitro* activity.

c. Biologic response modifiers

(1) Granulocyte transfusions. Beneficial results have not been seen consistently in controlled trials and hence are not routinely recommended. Transfusion reactions, allosensitization to human leukocyte antigens (HLAs), and transfusion-associated CMV infection occur frequently and further limit the usefulness of this approach. An increased incidence of severe pulmonary reactions, especially when transfusions are given to patients receiving amphotericin B, has also been noted.

(2) Colony-stimulating factors. Controlled trials with granulocyte–macrophage and granulocyte colony-stimulating factor have shown that these products can shorten the duration of neutropenia, but these agents have not reduced the duration of fever, use of anti-infectives, or costs of management of febrile neutropenic episodes. The 2001 update of the American Society of Clinical Oncology Guidelines recommends against the routine use of hematopoietic growth factors in uncomplicated cases of fever and neutropenia. Their use is indicated in the following conditions with worsening of course predicted and long delay in recovery of the marrow: pneumonia, hypotensive episodes, severe cellulitis or sinusitis, systemic fungal infections, and multiorgan dysfunction secondary to sepsis.

(3) Passive immunization. Passive immunization is not routinely recommended.

(a) Monoclonal antibodies. Immunization with high-titer antibody directed against the core glycolipid of gram-negative organisms (J-5 antisera) appears to reduce mortality from infection, presumably by neutralizing endotoxin. Preparation of the antisera is difficult and expensive, and the technique remains primarily a research tool at this time. Successful immunization with a "cocktail" of antibodies directed against different antigenic determinants of gram-negative bacilli has not been achieved.

(b) Pooled immunoglobulin preparations. These preparations contain antibodies to many potential pathogens. Results of controlled trials have been disappointing.

(c) Tumor necrosis factor-α antiserum. Tumor necrosis factor-α (TNF-α) has been shown to be a central mediator of endotoxic shock. However, antibody to TNF-α has failed to reduce mortality in multiple large randomized clinical trials. Newer data suggest that TNF-α might even have a beneficial effect on host defenses as an activator of macrophages. Better targeting of patients likely to benefit from blocking TNF-α (e.g., those with elevated serum levels of interleukin-6) has been suggested as a way of reducing mortality from the sepsis syndrome.

(d) Interleukins and interferon. Activation of monocytes and neutrophils by these substances might be expected to reduce mortality from certain kinds of infections. Unfortunately, systemic side effects limit the usefulness of this approach.

(e) Activated protein C. A recent trial has demonstrated a decrease in mortality rate in patients with severe sepsis on activated protein C compared with placebo. The use of this agent is strictly restricted to severe sepsis and is associated with intracranial bleeding in some patients.

III. Prevention of infection

A. Environmental manipulations

1. Hand washing. Numerous studies have confirmed that scrupulous adherence to good hand-washing technique reduces infections. Patients should be told to remind their physicians to wash their hands before allowing them to proceed with the examination. In addition, neutropenic patients should have hand-washing signs placed outside of their rooms as a reminder to all personnel.

2. Protective isolation

a. Definition. The concept of a "total protected environment" includes the use of laminar airflow rooms; sterilization of all objects placed in those rooms; gowning, masking, and gloving of personnel before entering the rooms; decontamination of the skin and gut with antimicrobials; and special food preparation to reduce the number of microorganisms present on the food.

b. Disadvantages. This approach is expensive; is cumbersome for patients, their families, and hospital personnel; and decreases perceived quality of life. It is also difficult to justify: Recent studies have not shown a significant advantage of protective isolation when compared with other preventive techniques.

3. Reservoir recognition and removal

   a. Foods. Fresh fruits, vegetables, and nonprocessed dairy products are frequently contaminated with gram-negative bacteria, especially *P. aeruginosa, E. coli,* and *K. pneumoniae.* Adherence to a cooked diet during periods of neutropenia helps to reduce the risk of infection with these organisms.

   b. Objects. Faucet aerators, sinks, shower heads, and flowers are known to harbor bacteria. However, most epidemiologic studies have not found these objects to be significant causes of infection. No special precautions, except for good hand-washing technique, are necessary.

   c. Construction. The incidence of infections caused by *Aspergillus* species is increased in areas of construction. Patients at risk should be moved to other areas of the hospital during periods of renovation.

B. Surveillance cultures. Routine bacterial surveillance cultures are rarely of benefit. In centers where *Aspergillus* species infection is a significant problem, periodic fungal cultures of the nares for this fungus might be useful for early detection.

C. Prophylaxis

1. Antibiotics

   a. Nonabsorbable agents

   (1) Rationale. Oral vancomycin, gentamicin, and nystatin have been used in attempts to suppress gut flora and lessen the importance of this reservoir of infection.

   (2) Disadvantages. The combination of antibiotics is poorly tolerated by patients; increased bacterial resistance develops, especially to gentamicin; the regimens do not provide protection against bacteria originating from other body sites; and some controlled studies have failed to demonstrate decreased infection rates.

   (3) Recommendations. These oral nonabsorbable antibiotics should not be used at this time.

   b. Quinolones

   (1) Efficacy. Both norfloxacin and ciprofloxacin have been shown to reduce the incidence of infection (but not mortality) in neutropenic cancer patients. Comparative studies of ofloxacin or ciprofloxacin versus TMP-SMX suggest that the effectiveness of quinolones is equal or superior to that of TMP-SMX for the prevention of febrile episodes of infectious origin. Bacteremia due to methicillin-resistant staphylococci may occur more frequently in neutropenic patients who receive quinolone prophylaxis than in those who do not. Newer floroquinolones with improved activity against gram-positive bacteria are available, but clinical experience in neutropenic patients is limited.

   (2) Mechanism of action. The quinolones suppress gram-negative and gram-positive aerobic gut flora and also achieve therapeutic serum and tissue levels against many bacteria.

(3)   Recommendations. Side effects have been minimal, and resistance has been slow to develop. Some cancer centers now routinely place patients on a regimen of 400 mg of norfloxacin twice daily before beginning chemotherapy when prolonged neutropenia is anticipated. The quinolones are not approved for use in children.

c.   Trimethoprim-sulfamethoxazole. The use of this agent has fallen out of favor for bacterial prophylaxis because of its potential for bone marrow suppression and other side effects. Increased bacterial resistance and break-through infections have also been observed. It is recommended for *P. carinii* pneumonia (PCP) prophylaxis in patients at risk.

2.   Antifungals. Prophylaxis, usually against *Candida* species, has been attempted with a number of antifungal agents. Fluconazole has been shown to reduce the frequency of both superficial and systemic infections in patients who undergo bone marrow transplantation. Efficacy of fluconazole is limited by its lack of activity against *C. kruseii,* some strains of *C. glabrata,* and the molds. The 2000 Guidelines from the Centers for Disease Control and Prevention (CDC), Infectious Disease Society of America (IDSA), and American Society of Blood and Bone Marrow Transplantation recommend administration of fluconazole at a dose of 400 mg/day from the day of hematopoietic stem cell transplantation until engraftment.

3.   Antivirals. Both IV (6.25 mg/kg twice daily) and oral (400 to 800 mg two or three times daily) acyclovir can prevent recurrences of HSV infections. Acyclovir is ineffective for treatment of CMV infection but may have some limited prophylactic efficacy against CMV. Ganciclovir 5 mg/kg IV twice daily for 5 days before bone marrow transplantation, then once daily until 100 days after transplantation, reduces the incidence of CMV interstitial pneumonia but not overall mortality at 6 months. CMV disease can be expected to occur in 10% to 15% of bone marrow transplant recipients within 60 days after discontinuation of prophylactic ganciclovir therapy. A strategy of pre-emptive ganciclovir use in those bone marrow transplant recipients with positive BAL cultures for CMV 35 days after transplantation who were not receiving ganciclovir prophylaxis reduced both the incidence of CMV interstitial pneumonia and the mortality rate at 180 days. The optimal approach to prevent CMV disease in bone marrow transplant recipients is not known at this time.

4.   Antiparasitics

a.   Pneumocystis carinii. TMP-SMX 1 double-strength tablet given twice daily on 2 or 3 consecutive days weekly is effective prophylaxis against this organism. Monthly aerosolized pentamidine may also be of value.

b.   Strongyloides stercoralis. Patients living in endemic areas should have stool cultures evaluated and treatment initiated (if necessary) before beginning immunosuppressive therapy.

D. Immunization
1. **Vaccines.** Live attenuated viral vaccines should not be used in immunocompromised patients. The efficacy of vaccines against *S. pneumoniae* and *H. influenzae* in immunocompromised patients is suspect. Nevertheless, many authorities recommend their use before immunosuppressive therapy.
2. **Biologic response modifiers**
   a. **Pooled immunoglobulin.** These preparations, given IV at doses of 0.1 to 0.2 g/kg at monthly intervals, have been used in patients with chronic lymphocytic leukemia, multiple myeloma, and other malignancies. Controlled trials appear to indicate some reduction in bacterial infections, but the preparations are expensive, and lifelong therapy is required.
   b. **Monoclonal antibodies.** Prophylactic administration of antibodies directed against virulence determinants of gram-negative bacteria (e.g., J-5 antisera) may be of value in reducing the incidence of infection. However, mortality has been unaltered in clinical trials.
3. **Varicella zoster virus immune globulin** (1 vial/10 kg body weight, to a maximum of five vials) is effective in reducing morbidity and mortality in seronegative immunocompromised patients exposed to VZV. The product should be given IM within 96 h of exposure.

E. Miscellaneous. IV catheters (nonsurgically placed) should be changed at least every 72 h. Rectal temperatures, rectal suppositories, and unnecessary rectal examinations should be avoided in neutropenic patients.

SELECTED READINGS

Berkman SA, Lee ML, Gale RP. Clinical uses of intravenous immunoglobulins. *Ann Intern Med* 1990;112:278–292.

Crawford J, Ozer H, Stoller R, et al. Reduction by granulocyte colony-stimulating factor of fever and neutropenia induced by chemotherapy in patients with small-cell lung cancer. *N Engl J Med* 1991;325:164–170.

EORTC International Antimicrobial Therapy Cooperative Group. Ceftazidime combined with a short or long course of amikacin for empirical therapy of gram-negative bacteremia in cancer patients with gram-negative bacteremia in cancer patients with granulocytopenia. *N Engl J Med* 1987;317:1692–1698.

Giamarellou H, Antoniadou A. Infectious complications of febrile leukopenia. *Infect Dis Clin North Am* 2001;15:457–482.

Goodrich JM, Bowden RA, Fisher L, et al. Prevention of cytomegalovirus disease after allogeneic marrow transplant by ganciclovir prophylaxis. *Ann Intern Med* 1993;118:173–178.

Goodrich JM, Mori M, Gleaves CA, et al. Early treatment with ganciclovir to prevent cytomegalovirus disease after allogeneic bone marrow transplantation. *N Engl J Med* 1991;325:1601–1607.

Hughes WT, Armstrong D, Bodey GP, et al. From the Infectious Diseases Society of America: guidelines for the use of antimicrobial agents in neutropenic patients with unexplained fever. *J Infect Dis* 1990;161:381–396.

Hughes WT, Armstrong D, Bodey GP, et al. 2002 guidelines for the use of antimicrobial agents in neutropenic patients with cancer. *Clin Infect Dis* 2002;34:730–751.

Klastersky J, Zinner SH, Calandra T, et al. Empiric antimicrobial therapy for febrile granulocytopenic cancer patients: lessons from four EORTC trials. *Eur J Cancer Clin Oncol* 1988;24(suppl 1):S35–S45.

MacArthur RD, Bone RC. Sepsis, SIRS, and septic shock. In: Bone RC, eds. *Pulmonary and critical care medicine, vol 3.* 4th ed. St. Louis: Mosby-Year Book, 1997:1–12.

Nichols CR, Fox EP, Roth BJ, et al. Incidence of neutropenic fever in patients treated with standard-dose combination chemotherapy for small-cell lung cancer and the cost impact of treatment with granulocyte colony-stimulating factor. *J Clin Oncol* 1994;12:1245–1250.

Pizzo P. Considerations for the prevention of infectious complications in patients with cancer. *Rev Infect Dis* 1989;11(suppl 7):S1551–S1563.

Pizzo P. Management of fever in patients with cancer and treatment-induced neutropenia. *N Engl J Med* 1993;328:1323–1332.

Steward WP. Granulocyte and granulocyte-macrophage colony-stimulating factors. *Lancet* 1993;342:153–157.

Disorders of Hemostasis and Transfusion Therapy

Mary R. Smith and NurJehan Stutz

Disorders of the hemostatic mechanisms are common in patients with malignancy. Abnormalities associated with thromboembolic events cause significantly more morbidity and mortality than disorders leading to hemorrhage.

I. Thromboembolism in cancer

A. Pathophysiology. The thromboembolic risk associated with neoplasia reflects an imbalance between platelet number, platelet function, levels of coagulation factors, and generation of thromboplastins compared with the levels of inhibitors of hemostasis and fibrinolytic activity. Thrombosis may be minor and localized or widespread and associated with multiple-organ damage. There may also be hemorrhage of varying degrees of severity in association with the thromboembolic events.

1. Factors that may affect the risk of thromboembolism vary widely from patient to patient and include the following:

- Specific type of tumor
- Nutritional status of the patient
- Type of chemotherapy
- Response to chemotherapy (e.g., tumor lysis syndrome)
- Liver and renal function
- Patient immobility and venous stasis

2. Factors that can initiate thrombus formation are common to many cancers:

- Circulating tumor cells adhere to the vascular endothelium and form a nidus for clot formation.
- Tumors may penetrate the vessel, destroying the endothelium and promoting clot formation.
- Neovascularization associated with many tumors may stimulate clotting.
- Arterial thrombosis associated with tumors may result from vasospasm.
- A systemic hypercoagulable state develops (e.g., decreased protein C).
- External compression of vessels by tumor masses impedes blood flow and leads to stasis and clot development.

3. Platelet abnormalities associated with an increased risk of thromboembolism include thrombocytosis and increased platelet adhesion and aggregation. Tumors may produce substances that cause increased platelet aggregation with subsequent release of platelet factor III and ensuing acceleration of coagulation.

B.   Clinical syndromes. A variety of noteworthy clinical syndromes are associated with the "hypercoagulable state" of malignancy and of its treatment.

   1.   Disseminated intravascular coagulation. Disseminated intravascular coagulation (DIC) is a syndrome with many signs, symptoms, and laboratory abnormalities (Table 28.1). As many as 90% of patients with metastatic neoplasms have some laboratory manifestation of DIC, but only a small fraction of these patients suffer morbidity from the coagulation process or subsequent depletion of coagulation factors and consequent bleeding due to DIC. The initiating factor for DIC is apparent in some situations but unknown in others.

   Among the common initiators of DIC are the following:

- Thromboplastic substances in granules from promyelocytes of acute promyelocytic leukemia (DIC may worsen with therapy). There is a significant concomitant fibrinolysis in many patients.
- Sialic acid from mucin produced by adenocarcinomas of the lung or gastrointestinal tract.
- Trypsin released from pancreatic cancer.
- Impaired fibrinolysis associated with hepatocellular carcinoma.

Table 28.1.   Laboratory diagnosis of disseminated intravascular coagulation (DIC)

Laboratory tests	Acute DIC	Chronic DIC
Screening		
PT, aPTT	Usually prolonged	Normal
Platelets	Usually decreased	Normal or slightly decreased
Fibrinogen	Usually decreased but may be normal[a]	Usually normal[a]
Confirmatory[b]		
Fibrin monomer	Positive	Positive
FDP	Strongly positive	Positive
D-Dimer	Positive	Positive
Thrombin time	Normal or abnormal	Usually normal
Factor assays	Decreased factors V and VIII	Normal factors V and VIII
Antithrombin III	May be reduced	Usually normal

PT, prothrombin time; aPTT, activated partial thromboplastin time; FDP, fibrinogen degradation products.

[a]Fibrinogen is usually elevated in advanced malignancy or acute leukemia that is not complicated by DIC. Thus, a normal fibrinogen level may actually be decreased for the physiologic state of the patient.

[b]Changes indicated are confirmatory if present; the absence of the indicated findings in some of the confirmatory tests does not exclude the diagnosis.

- DIC in any patient may be fostered by sepsis or other causes of the systemic inflammatory response syndrome (SIRS).

2.   Lupus anticoagulant in neoplastic disease. The lupus anticoagulant is an antiphospholipid antibody (immunoglobulin G or M). Antiphospholipid antibodies are reported to be associated with a number of malignant disorders including hairy-cell leukemia, lymphoma, Waldenström's macroglobulinemia, and epithelial neoplasms. The lupus anticoagulant leads to a prolonged activated partial thromboplastin time (aPTT) but is paradoxically associated with an increased risk of thrombosis.

3.   Trousseau's syndrome (tumor-associated thrombophlebitis). Suspect the possibility of neoplasia in the following circumstances:

- An unexplained thromboembolic event occurs after the age of 40.
- Thromboses occur in unusual sites.
- The thromboses affect superficial as well as deep veins.
- The thromboses are migratory.
- The thromboses tend not to respond to the "usual" anticoagulant therapies.
- An unexplained thrombosis occurs more than once.

4.   Thrombotic events that occur after surgery for tumors of the lung, ovary, pancreas, or stomach.

5.   Nonbacterial thrombotic endocarditis may be found in association with carcinoma of the lung. These thrombi are formed from accumulations of platelets and fibrin. The mitral valve is the most frequent site of origin of these thrombi, which frequently embolize.

6.   Thrombotic thrombocytopenic purpura. Thrombotic thrombocytopenic purpura (TTP) is a poorly understood syndrome characterized by thrombocytopenia, microangiopathic hemolytic anemia, fever, fluctuating neurologic signs and symptoms, and acute renal failure. TTP and the hemolytic–uremic syndrome (thrombocytopenia, hemolysis, and acute renal failure) have been associated with untreated malignancies as well as with a number of drugs used for treating malignant disease. The agent most often reported is mitomycin, but other drugs including bleomycin, cisplatin, cyclophosphamide, gemcitabine, and vinca alkaloids may also be associated with these syndromes. TTP may be difficult to diagnose in this setting because the chemotherapy suppresses platelet production, some agents may impair renal function, and many of the features of DIC are similar to those of TTP. Careful review of the peripheral blood smear is required to identify the changes in red blood cells (RBCs) that are associated with a microangiopathic hemolytic process.

There is growing evidence that damage to the endothelium is seen in association with TTP. For many patients with TTP, von Willebrand–cleaving protease levels are very low or absent, leading to the presence of unusual ultralarge multimers of von Willebrand factor (vWF). The von Willebrand–cleaving proteolytic activity is thought to be inhibited by an anti–vWF-cleaving protease immunoglobulin G.

The prognosis of patients with TTP is poor, and its therapy has been varied. Plasmapheresis and transfusion with fresh-frozen plasma appear to be the best modalities of therapy. Plasmapheresis and fresh-frozen plasma infusion replace the von Willebrand–cleaving protease missing in patients with TTP. In patients who are nonresponders to plasmapheresis or plasma transfusion, immunoadsorption of the patient's plasma by staphylococcal protein A columns has been used.

Complications from platelet transfusions are not as common in TTP associated with malignancy and bone marrow transplantation as in other cases of TTP; thus, platelet transfusion can be used especially if there is a threat of bleeding.

7.   Thromboembolism associated with chemotherapy

    a.   The use of **central arterial or venous catheters** has markedly facilitated the delivery of chemotherapy, but all such catheters are associated with a significant risk of vascular thrombosis. The empiric use of low doses of warfarin (1 mg/day) decreases the risk of thrombosis without inducing a hemorrhagic state. It is not necessary to follow the prothrombin time (PT) with low-dose warfarin.

    b.   Many **chemotherapy agents** cause significant chemical phlebitis. The most common offending agents are mechlorethamine (nitrogen mustard), anthracyclines, nitrosoureas, mitomycin, fluorouracil, dacarbazine, and epipodophyllotoxins.

    c.   L-Asparaginase inhibits the synthesis of proteins, including coagulation factors. This inhibition may cause either hemorrhage or thrombosis. Patients with pre-existing hemostatic disorders are at particular risk for complications when using L-asparaginase. L-Asparaginase also decreases antithrombin III (AT-III) activity.

    d.   **Tamoxifen** has been associated with thromboembolic events. This effect may be magnified when tamoxifen is combined with chemotherapeutic agents.

    e.   **Estrogens** may increase the risk of thromboembolism. This is likely due, at least in part, to a decrease in protein S and an increase in coagulation factors.

    f.   **Superior vena cava syndrome** is nearly always associated with thrombosis in the thoracic venous system cephalad to the site of obstruction and may lead to upper-extremity thrombosis.

C.   Principles of therapy for thrombosis associated with neoplasia

    1.   Discrete vascular thrombosis

        a.   General guidelines. Therapy should be directed at controlling the neoplasm. As an anticoagulant, heparin is superior to warfarin in these patients. Warfarin and antiplatelet drugs have been used with varying degrees of success in some patients with thromboembolism associated with tumors. The use of heparin, warfarin, and antiplatelet agents alone or in combination may be associated with normalization of hemostatic parameters. Despite this, patients with malignant disease are often resistant to anticoagulant therapy and may continue to have thrombotic events even while receiving what appears to be adequate anticoagulant therapy. Great care must be exercised in the use of both heparin and warfarin in patients with malignant disease because hemorrhage into areas of necrotic tumor can be hazardous. The use of anticoagulant therapy is generally contraindicated in patients with central nervous system metastases. Bulky disease is a relative contraindication, especially if central necrosis of the tumor is suspected and particularly if the lesion is in the mediastinum or pleural spaces.

The decision to treat thromboembolism occurring in a patient with malignancy may be difficult. One must carefully weigh the risks of therapy against expected benefits. The patient's life expectancy, concurrent therapy, and type of malignancy also influence the decision.

b.   Heparin. Low doses of heparin (5,000 U given SC every 12 h) can be used to protect patients with malignant disease from thromboembolism during perioperative periods. Heparin may be used as the initial or long-term therapy for thromboembolic events in patients with malignant disease. Heparin may be administered either IV or by the SC route. Generally, the IV route is preferred for initial therapy so that the anticoagulant effect begins at once and adjustment of doses can be easily achieved. An initial dose of 5,000 U (70 U/kg) of heparin is given as an IV bolus followed by 1,000 to 1,200 U (15 U/kg)/h as a continuous infusion. One should check the aPTT 1 h after the heparin bolus to ensure that the patient is heparinizable (i.e., not AT-III deficient), 6 h after beginning therapy, and 6 h after any change in the dose of heparin. Some patients with malignant disease may appear to be refractory to heparin; in all likelihood, this reflects low levels of AT-III, owing to poor production or increased consumption, both of which may occur in patients with malignant disease. (*Note:* Infusion therapy with L-asparaginase has been associated with reduced levels of AT-III.) As long as the AT-III activity is above 50% of normal, it is usually possible to achieve the desired anticoagulant effect if adequate doses of heparin are given. If AT-III activity is less than 50% of normal, AT-III may be replaced using AT-III concentrates or fresh-frozen plasma.

Heparin may be administered by the SC route for both the acute and the chronic management of thromboembolism associated with malignancy. Using the SC route may be less desirable when treating acute events because the onset of anticoagulant effect is somewhat slower (2 to 3 h), and adjusting the therapeutic effect may be more difficult. SC heparin can be considered for chronic therapy provided that the patient can manage the twice-daily injection and weekly monitoring of the aPTT. In a patient who has been receiving IV heparin, half the total dose of IV heparin received in the previous 24 h should be given SC twice a day (e.g., 1,000 U/h by IV infusion equals 12,000 U SC b.i.d.). For the patient being started on SC heparin, the initial dose is 7,500 to 10,000 U SC b.i.d. The aPTT should be checked 6 h after the third dose of heparin. Otherwise, the aPTT should be checked 6 h after an SC dose of heparin. The goal for the aPTT should be similar to that of IV heparin, namely, 1.5 to 2 times the patient's baseline aPTT.

Low molecular weight (LMW) heparin(s) can be used for thromboembolism and for primary prevention. The selection of drug and its dosing schedule should be made by the treating physician. If monitoring of the drug is indicated owing to liver or kidney dysfunction in the patient, one must use anti-Xa levels as the aPTT is not indicative of the anticoagulant effect of LMW heparins.

c.   Warfarin is often selected as the therapy of choice for the chronic management of thromboembolic events associated with malignant disease. The use of warfarin in this setting is of concern because patients with malignant disease are frequently taking multiple medications that can alter the patient's response to warfarin. An additional concern about the use of warfarin in patients with malignancy is the development of purpura fulminans. This complication may be due to lower-than-normal protein C levels in patients who had DIC before initiation of warfarin therapy. Warfarin should not be used if there is laboratory evidence of DIC.

Despite these caveats, warfarin is often used for the prevention and treatment of clotting problems in patients with cancer. For most patients, an international normalized ratio (INR) of 2 to 3 is required; for patients with mechanical prosthetic valves, recurrent systemic embolism, or lupus anticoagulant with thrombosis, an INR of 2.5 to 3.5 is necessary (Table 28.2). Table 28.3 also gives the recommended vitamin K dose necessary to reduce the INR to therapeutic levels in patients who are taking warfarin and have INR values higher than 5. Care must be taken to balance the risks of bleeding in patients with elevated INRs—with or without thrombocytopenia—against the risks of clotting and thrombosis if the reversal of the anticoagulation is too vigorous.

d.   The use of platelet-inhibiting drugs such as aspirin, other nonsteroidal anti-inflammatory agents, and dipyridamole has met with varying degrees of success in the prevention of repeated thromboembolic events in patients with malignant disease. Care must be taken with the use of such drugs, especially in thrombocytopenic patients, because the risk of bleeding associated with thrombocytopenia is increased.

e.   Fibrinolytic therapy. Systemic malignancy is a relative contraindication to fibrinolytic therapy.

f.   Vascular interruption devices such as Greenfield filters may be used in patients who cannot tolerate anticoagulant therapy or who develop emboli while on adequate anticoagulant therapy.

2.   Disseminated intravascular coagulation. Therapy for DIC includes the following:

• Urgently correct shock (if present).
• Treat the underlying disease process.

Table 28.2. Clinical indications and international normalized ratio (INR) goals: using the INR for anticoagulation monitoring

A. Clinical indications requiring an INR of 2.0–3.0

Prophylaxis

Postoperative deep vein thrombosis (general surgery)

Postoperative deep vein thrombosis during hip surgical procedures and fractures

Myocardial infarction to prevent venous thromboembolism

Transient ischemic attacks

Tissue heart valves

Atrial fibrillation

Valvular heart disease

Recurrent deep vein thrombosis and pulmonary embolism

Arterial disease including myocardial infarction

Treatment

Venous thrombosis

Pulmonary embolism

B. Clinical indications requiring an INR of 2.5–3.5

Prophylaxis

Mechanical prosthetic valves

Recurrent systemic embolism

Lupus anticoagulant with thrombosis

Table 28.3. Vitamin K_1 administration for patients on warfarin doses of vitamin K_1 to reduce INR in patients on warfarin

INR	Vitamin K_1 dosage (slow IVP)[a]	Time expected for response to vitamin K or to repeat INR
>3.5 but <5	None, hold warfarin	24 h
≥5 but <10.0	0.5–1.0 mg; may repeat dosage if INR still high at 24 h	Reduction of INR expected at 8 h; therapeutic INR expected at 24–48 h
≥10.0 but <20	3–5 mg; may repeat dosage if INR is still high at 6–12 h	Reductions of INR expected at 6 h; repeat INR every 6–12 h
≥20	10 mg; may repeat dosage if INR is still high at 6–12 h (consider fresh-frozen plasma)	Reduction of INR expected at 6 h; repeat INR every 6–12 h

[a] If patient is bleeding, a procedure is planned, or patient has just had a procedure, consider the use of fresh-frozen plasma or prothrombin concentrates.
Modified from Hirsh J, et al. Oral anticoagulants. Mechanism of action, clinical effectiveness, and optimal therapeutic range. *Chest* 1992; 102 (suppl):312.

- Replace depleted blood components (e.g., platelets, cryo-precipitated antihemophilic factor [AHF] for fibrinogen and factor VIII, fresh-frozen plasma for other factors) if clinically significant bleeding is present.
- Consider the use of heparin only in the following situations:
  - In patients with acute promyelocytic leukemia (see Chapter 18).
  - When there is evidence of ongoing end-organ damage due to microvascular thrombosis.
  - If venous thrombosis occurs.

These latter two complications of DIC are most likely to occur as a component of the SIRS, and the treatment of the underlying cause of the SIRS is necessary in addition to treatment with heparin. There is no evidence that chronic warfarin therapy is of value for treating the chronic DIC seen in some patients with neoplasia if thromboses are absent. Warfarin may predispose to the development of purpura fulminans in the presence of chronic DIC.

II. Bleeding in patients with cancer
A. Tumor invasion. It is well recognized that bleeding may be a warning sign of cancer. Bloody sputum may indicate carcinoma of the lung, blood in the urine may be a sign of carcinoma of the bladder or kidney, blood in the stool may be due to carcinoma of the alimentary tract, and postmenopausal vaginal bleeding may be caused by endometrial carcinoma. In each of these instances, bleeding can be directly related to the invasive properties of cancer and disruption of normal tissue integrity.

B. Hemostatic abnormalities. Often bleeding in patients with cancer is not due to the direct effects of the neoplasm but rather to indirect effects of the cancer or its therapy on one of the components of the hemostatic system. Because of the frequency and the special management problems caused by abnormalities in the hemostatic system in patients with cancer and the frequency with which these problems occur, it is important to consider the possible causes and corrective measures in detail.

  1. Increased vascular fragility may be due to chronic corticosteroid therapy, chronic malnutrition, or "senile purpura." Bleeding is usually not severe, but bruising, particularly around IV sites, is common. Hemostatic therapy is not necessary.

  2. Thrombocytopenia may occur for a variety of reasons. Some of the more common causes are as follows:

  a. Chemotherapy and radiotherapy regularly cause depression of platelet production. Serial blood cell counts must be monitored while patients are being treated.

  b. Bone marrow invasion or replacement causing thrombocytopenia is commonly seen only with leukemias or lymphomas but may occur in other cancers that invade the bone marrow.

  c. Splenomegaly with splenic sequestration is most common with leukemia or lymphoma.

  d. Folate deficiency with decreased platelet production is common in patients with cancer because of poor nutrition. Dietary history should provide the clues to the diagnosis.

e. Neoplasm-induced immune thrombocytopenic purpura. Patients with lymphoproliferative malignancies (e.g., chronic lymphocytic leukemia, Hodgkin's disease) often develop immune thrombocytopenic purpura (ITP). ITP may also be the presenting symptom of a nonhematologic malignancy. Usually, the ITP improves with prednisone 1 mg/kg/day followed by treatment of the malignancy.

f. Drug-induced immune thrombocytopenia. Many nonchemotherapy medications used to treat patients with malignancy can cause immune thrombocytopenia. Offending agents to consider are heparin, vancomycin, H_2-receptor antagonists, penicillins, cephalosporins, interferon, and sulfa-containing antibiotics, diuretics, and hypoglycemic agents.

g. Graft-versus-host disease developed after bone marrow transplantation may produce a chronic (often isolated) immune-mediated thrombocytopenia. The platelet count may respond to increased immunosuppression.

3. Abnormalities of platelet function must be suspected in patients who have a normal or near-normal platelet count but signs or symptoms of bleeding and a documented prolonged bleeding time. Most cases are secondary to drug effects including aspirin and other nonsteroidal anti-inflammatory agents, antibiotics (e.g., ticarcillin), antidepressants (e.g., tricyclic drugs), tranquilizers, and alcohol. Consider any drug that the patient is taking as a possible offender until proved otherwise. The presence of fibrin degradation products is a common cause of platelet dysfunction in patients with malignancy who also have DIC. Platelet dysfunction may occur in patients with malignant paraproteinemias as a result of the coating of the platelet surfaces by the immunoglobulin. When renal failure develops or is present in such patients, the platelet dysfunction is magnified.

4. Coagulation factor deficiencies may develop in patients with malignancy for several reasons:

- Acute (decompensated) DIC depletes most clotting factors but to variable degrees.
- Liver failure causes deficiency of all clotting factors except factor VIII.
- Malnutrition leads to deficiency of factors II, VII, IX, and X (the vitamin K–dependent factors).
- Fibrinolysis may be due to the release of urokinase in prostate cancer or secondary to DIC. This may produce hypofibrinogenemia as well as fibrin split products, which act as circulating anticoagulants.
- Functionally abnormal clotting factors are occasionally seen. The most commonly diagnosed abnormality is dysfibrinogenemia.

5. Acquired circulating anticoagulants may develop in patients with a number of different tumors. Many of these anticoagulants are heparinoid in nature. The most common associations are with carcinoma of the lung and myeloma. Other anticoagulants act as antithrombins; in this case, the most common association is with carcinoma of the breast.

6.   Chemotherapy and other drug-induced bleeding

Mithramycin, although rarely used now, may lead to platelet dysfunction and a reduction in multiple coagulation factors. Hemorrhage due to these effects may occur in up to half of patients treated with mithramycin.

Anthracyclines may be associated with primary fibrinolysis or fibrinogenolysis and hemorrhage.

Dactinomycin is a powerful vitamin K antagonist that causes defective synthesis of all vitamin K–dependent proteins (factors II, VII, IX, and X, protein C, and protein S).

Melphalan, cytarabine, doxorubicin, vincristine, and **vinblastine** are all associated with platelet dysfunction.

Mitomycin, daunorubicin, cytarabine, bleomycin, CDDP, methyl-CCNU, tamoxifen, deoxycoformycin, gemcitabine, atorvastatin, clopidogrel, ticlopidine, cyclosporine, sulfonamides, tacrolimus, sirolimus, "crack" cocaine, penicillin, rifampin, penicillamine, oral contraceptives, arsenic, quinine, and **iodine** are all associated with TTP.

III.   Laboratory evaluation of hemostasis in patients with malignancy. About half of all patients with cancer and about 90% of those with metastases manifest abnormalities of one or more routine coagulation parameters. These abnormalities may be minor early in the patient's disease, but as the disease progresses, the hemostatic abnormalities become more pronounced. Serial coagulation tests may offer the clinician a clue to response to therapy or recurrence of malignant disease. Serial evaluations of coagulation tests are of more value in patients with no symptoms of hemostatic disruption than is a single determination.

A.   Screening tests for bleeding. The following tests provide an adequate screening battery: **Platelet count, bleeding time, aPTT, PT, thrombin time,** and **fibrinogen level.**

B.   Interpretation of screening laboratory studies. Abnormal results of the screening tests reflect hematologic problems caused by blood vessels, platelets, or coagulation factors. The following list provides clues to the interpretation of the screening test results that help determine the most likely cause or causes of the patient's bleeding.

1.   Platelet count

Normal: 150,000 to 450,000/μL.

If **thrombocytopenia** is less than 100,000/μL, consider the following:

- Bone marrow failure
- Increased consumption of platelets
- Splenic pooling of platelets

Thrombocytosis with a platelet count of more than 500,000/μL has the following characteristics:

- It is common in patients with neoplasms.
- It may be seen in association with iron deficiency (e.g., secondary to gut neoplasm).
- It usually poses no risk of arterial thrombosis unless the patient has a myeloproliferative disorder.

2.   Bleeding time. This is a useful screening test if the platelet count is normal and platelet dysfunction is suspected.

*   A normal bleeding time requires normal platelet number, normal platelet function, and normal function of the blood vessels and connective tissues.
*   A prolonged bleeding time may be due to thrombocytopenia, abnormal platelet function, and, rarely, inadequate vessel function. The bleeding time may be spuriously prolonged in elderly people with "tissue-paper" skin.
*   The following formula is a rough rule of thumb to be used to estimate what the bleeding time should be in patients who have platelet counts between 10,000 and 100,000/μL. Although it was derived using the Mielke template, the principle should still hold for contemporary bleeding time devices: bleeding time (min) = 30 − ([platelet count/μl]/4,000).

3.   Prolonged prothrombin time. This is seen in the presence of the following:

*   Deficiency of one or more of the following clotting factors: VII, X, V, II (prothrombin), or I (fibrinogen); oral anticoagulant therapy leads to a deficiency of factors II, VII, IX, and X.
*   Circulating anticoagulants against factor VII, X, V, or II.
*   Dysfibrinogenemia.

4.   Prolonged activated partial thromboplastin time

*   Deficiency of any of the following clotting factors: XII, XI, IX, VIII, X, V, II, or I. Factor XII deficiency is not associated with bleeding. Fletcher and Fitzgerald factor deficiencies (both rare) may also prolong the aPTT.
*   Circulating anticoagulants directed against the factors mentioned above or the lupus inhibitor.
*   Anticoagulant therapy with heparin or oral anticoagulants.

5.   Prolonged thrombin time. Prolongation of the thrombin time may be due to the following:

*   Hypofibrinogenemia (fibrinogen less than 100 mg/dL)
*   Some forms of dysfibrinogenemia
*   Fibrin–fibrinogen split products
*   Heparin therapy
*   Paraproteins

If the thrombin time is prolonged, further studies to clarify the cause may be required.

6.   Low fibrinogen level. When evaluating the results of a fibrinogen assay, one must be familiar with the assay method used. Many laboratories use immunologic assays, which measure both functionally normal and abnormal fibrinogens. If such an assay is in use, the thrombin time can be used to evaluate the functional integrity of the fibrinogen. A low functional fibrinogen level means that production is decreased, consumption is increased, or a dysfibrinogen is present. Fibrinogen is an acute-phase reactant and is often elevated with advanced malignancy. A fibrinogen level in the normal range may actually be relatively low for the patient's physiologic state and thus may be a sign of DIC (see Table 28.1).

C.   Laboratory findings in patients with disseminated intravascular coagulation. Acute DIC is often associated with significant hemorrhage, whereas chronic DIC may be asymptomatic or associated with thromboses. Screening and confirmatory laboratory tests are shown in Table 28.4.

D.   Review of peripheral smear for schistocytes and decrease numbers of platelets if TTP suspected.

IV.   Treatment of hemorrhagic syndromes in patients with malignant disease

A.   Transfusion therapy

1.   General guidelines

a.   Regard elective transfusion with allogeneic blood as an outcome to be avoided. Consider the factors that will influence the use of blood products, including the following:

- Alternative forms of therapy that could control bleeding (e.g., topical measures or desmopressin).
- *How symptomatic is the patient?* Do not treat an abnormal laboratory test in a symptom-free patient. For example, patients with chronic DIC may demonstrate prolongation of both the PT and the aPTT and mild to moderate thrombocytopenia. If there is no demonstrable bleeding, transfusion therapy is not necessary.

b.   Use the specific blood component needed by the patient.

Table 28.4.   Coagulation tests that may show an abnormality in patients with cancer without clinical bleeding or thrombosis

Test	Common results in patients with malignancy
Antithrombin III	Decreased
β-Thromboglobulin	Increased
Cryofibrinogen	Present
D-Dimer	Increased
Factor VIII	Increased
Fibronectin	Decreased
Fibrin monomer (soluble)	Present
Fibrinogen	Increased
Fibrin(ogen) degradation products	Present
Fibrinopeptide A	Increased
Fibrinopeptide B	Increased
Plasmin	Increased
Plasminogen	Decreased
Platelet count	Increased or decreased
Platelet factor 4	Increased
Protein C	Decreased

c.   Minimize complications of transfusion by using the following:

- Only the amount and type of blood product indicated for the patient in the specific clinical setting
- Leukoreduced blood products, irradiated blood, or both, when indicated

2.   Blood component therapy
  a.   Platelet transfusions
   (1)   Available forms of platelets for transfusion. Platelets may be ordered and transfused in various ways. Because most patients with an underlying malignancy have the potential for needing long-term platelet support, platelet products should be leukocyte reduced from the initiation of transfusion (see Section IV.A.3 below). In general, patients who need platelet support can be started with random-donor platelets. Given the added expense and the limited pools of platelet apheresis donors in many centers, single-donor and human leukocyte antigen (HLA)–matched platelets should be reserved for patients who have become refractory to random-donor platelets (see Section IV.A.2.a.(4) below). There are no solid data to suggest that starting with platelet apheresis products decreases the incidence of alloimmunization. In fact, the Trial to Reduce Alloimmunization to Platelets Study Group study (1997) did not show any benefit in the use of platelet apheresis products over platelet concentrates. Conversely, patients who are candidates for bone marrow transplantation should receive single-donor platelets (if available) from the initiation of platelet therapy. Many blood centers have geared up production of platelet apheresis, and this product may be more readily available in some places than in others. Patients who are candidates for transplantation with bone marrow from an HLA-matched sibling should not receive apheresis products from the potential donor before the transplantation.
    (a)   Random-donor platelets or platelet concentrates. Four to 6 U (usually pooled in one bag) are considered an adequate dose for a 70-kg adult.
    (b)   Platelets obtained by apheresis (single-donor platelets) and human leukocyte antigen–matched platelets obtained by apheresis. These come as a single pack and represent the platelets obtained by apheresis from a single donor. One unit of platelets obtained by apheresis is equivalent to 4 to 6 U of platelet concentrate.
   (2)   Check platelet count 10 min to 1 h, and then 24 h, after platelet transfusion to estimate survival of platelets in the patient. Each unit of platelet concentrate should increase the platelet count by about 7,000/µL. The expected 1-h posttransfusion rise in platelets is 15,000 platelets/µL divided by the patient's body surface area in square meters for each unit of platelet concentrate (Thus, for a person of 2 m^2, 6 U should produce a rise of 45,000/µL [6 × 15,000/2]).

(3) Criteria for transfusing platelets
(a) For patients with **reduced platelet production,** criteria for transfusion are shown in Table 28.5.
(b) Increased platelet destruction. Platelet transfusions are of limited benefit in patients with thrombocytopenia due to increased destruction as a result of either antibodies or consumption. If potentially life-threatening bleeding complicates thrombocytopenia due to increased destruction, platelet transfusions may be given; however, small increments in the platelet count usually occur. IV γ-globulin 1 g/kg IV daily × 2 days given before the platelet transfusions might improve the response.
(c) Dysfunctional platelets. One must stop any drugs known to cause platelet dysfunction. Although

Table 28.5. Guidelines for platelet transfusion in patients with reduced platelet production

Platelet count	Recommendation
0–5,000/μL	Transfuse with platelets even if there is no evidence of bleeding
6,000–10,000/μL	Transfuse with platelets if there is: Fresh minor hemorrhage Temperature of 38°C or active infection Rapid decline in platelet count (>50%/d) Headache Significant gastrointestinal blood loss Recent chemotherapy that may be expected to cause severe stomatitis or gastrointestinal ulceration Presence of confluent petechiae (as opposed to scattered petechiae) Continuous bleeding from a wound or other sites Planned minor procedure such as a bone marrow biopsy
11,000–20,000/μL	Transfuse with platelets if there is more rapid bleeding or if more complicated procedures are anticipated
>20,000/μL	If major surgery is planned or when life-threatening bleeding occurs, the platelet count should be increased to at least 50,000/μL For intracranial surgery or opthalamic surgery, transfuse to a platelet count of at least 100,000/μL (bleeding time must be checked before surgery and must be normal) In fully anticoagulated patients, is advisable to keep the platelet count to at least 50,000/mL

the use of platelet transfusions should be considered, pharmacologic methods of enhancing platelet function, such as desmopressin, should be used if possible (see Section IV.B.1).

(4) Refractoriness to platelet transfusions (platelet rise less than 5,000/µL after 5 to 6 U of platelet concentrates or 1 U of platelets obtained by apheresis on two separate occasions) is a common problem in multiply transfused patients. Alloimmunization is the most difficult form to treat and therefore is best prevented (see Section IV.A.3). Apparent refractoriness to platelets may be due to shortened platelet lifespan from fever, septicemia, DIC, splenomegaly, drugs, infections, or bleeding.

　　(a) Evaluation. Patients who become refractory to platelet transfusions should have a laboratory evaluation for alloimmunization. They should also be evaluated for infection and DIC. Further, all potentially offending medications should be stopped.

　　(b) Therapy. The therapeutic modalities for ITP (corticosteroids, IV globulin, danazol) are generally ineffective for platelet refractoriness due to alloimmunization. Two therapeutic options exist:

　　　　(i) Human leukocyte antigen–matched platelets

　　　　(ii) Cross-matched platelets. Because platelets are available at most blood centers, if a blood center performs cross-matching, it is often easier to obtain cross-matched platelets because no specific donor requirement is required. This product is as effective as HLA-matched platelets in producing a platelet response in the alloimmunized patient. Either platelet concentrates or apheresed platelets can be cross-matched with the recipient. Nonreactive or, in extenuating circumstances, the least reactive platelets can then be selected for transfusion.

b. Coagulation factor support

　　(1) Fresh-frozen plasma contains all clotting factors (but not platelets) and should be used for multiple coagulation factor deficiencies. Fresh-frozen plasma requires 20 to 30 min to thaw and must be thawed at 37°C.

　　(2) Cryoprecipitated antihemophilic factor is a source of factor VIII–vWF complex, fibrinogen, and factor XIII. Each bag of cryoprecipitated AHF contains about 50% of the factor VIII–vWF complex (minimum of 80 U) and 20% to 40% of the fibrinogen (minimum of 150 mg) harvested from 1 U of blood. Cryoprecipitated AHF is stored in a frozen state and has the advantage of concentrating the clotting factors in a small volume (10 to 15 mL/bag). It is used primarily in deficiencies of fibrinogen. The goal is to keep the fibrinogen level higher than 100 mg/dL. The usual dosage of cryoprecipitated AHF to correct hypofibrinogenemia is 1 bag of cryoprecipitated AHF for every 5 kg of body weight. Because 50% is recovered after transfusion, this may raise the fibrinogen level only by about 50 mg/dL. Larger doses may be needed for severe hypofibrinogenemia or "flaming" DIC. The patient is evaluated to determine if the laboratory values have been corrected.

(3)   Factor IX concentrates are available as factor IX complex concentrates, which contain factors II, VII, IX, and X, or as coagulation factor IX concentrates. The latter are highly purified factor IX concentrates with few or no other coagulation factors. Several precautions are worth noting regarding the factor IX concentrates:

(a)   This concentrate is made from pooled plasma but is treated with viral attenuation processes such as dry or vapor heat in the case of factor IX complex concentrates (therefore, the risk of hepatitis is significant) and solvent–detergent or monoclonal antibody in the case of coagulation factor IX concentrates. The dose depends on the preparation to be used. The goal is to bring the factor concentration to no more than 50% of normal.

(b)   There is a small risk of DIC resulting from the use of factor IX complex concentrates. Patients with liver dysfunction and newborns are at increased risk. The coagulation factor concentrates are far less thrombogenic and should be used in cases at increased risk for venous thrombosis or DIC.

(c)   Factor IX concentrates are stored in the lyophilized state. Do not shake when reconstituting.

3.   Leukocyte reduction. Patients who have not previously received transfusions and who will need long-term blood product support should receive leukocyte-reduced (less than 5×10^6 leukocytes/bag) blood products. Leukocyte reduction may prevent febrile transfusion reactions, prevent cytomegalovirus (CMV) infections, and delay alloimmunization. Controversy still exists as to whether tumor recurrence and infections are a result of immunomodulatory effects of blood transfusion and if they can be reduced by leukoreduction. Two methods of leukocyte reduction by filtration are currently available: bedside and prestorage.

a.   Bedside filtration involves leukocyte reduction at the time of transfusion. Disadvantages include plugging of the filter, the presence of leukocyte breakdown products, bag breakage, and lack of consistency of products. Filters are available for RBCs and platelets.

b.   AS-1 or AS-3 prestorage filtered red blood cells are RBCs that have been leukocyte reduced generally within 8 to 24 h of collection. Advantages are fewer leukocyte breakdown products, ease of administration, and consistent quality (guaranteed less than 5×10^6 leukocytes/bag). Cost may be perceived as a disadvantage. However, this is offset by the expense of stocking filters, training of staff in the use of filters, and breakage. There is ongoing controversy as to whether leukocyte-reduced blood products should be provided to all patients, not just patients at risk.

4.   Cytomegalovirus-negative blood. Only patients known to be anti-CMV negative with impaired immunity should be considered for the use of CMV-negative blood. This group includes children, for the most part. The use of CMV-negative blood seriously restricts the potential donor pool for these patients. Leukocyte-reduced blood products (less than 5.0×10^6/bag) are equivalent to CMV-negative screened products.

White blood cell (WBC) depletion filters also remove CMV since CMV resides in the WBCs. Irradiation of blood products does not render them CMV-free. Frozen deglycerolized blood is considered free of CMV contamination.

5. Irradiated blood products. These prevent the development of graft-versus-host disease. Irradiated blood products, in the case of patients with cancer or hematologic malignancies, are indicated in the following situations:

- Congenital immunodeficiency
- Bone marrow, peripheral blood stem cell, or umbilical cord stem cell transplantation
- Directed blood donations to blood relatives
- Granulocyte transfusions
- High-dose chemotherapy with growth factor or stem cell rescue
- Hodgkin's disease
- Leukemia and non-Hodgkin's lymphoma (relative indication)

B. Other forms of therapy

1. Desmopressin. Desmopressin 0.3 µg/kg IV over 30 min every 12 to 24 h for 2 to 4 days may be used to elevate factor VIII and vWF levels as well as improve platelet function. Tachyphylaxis may occur if therapy is continued for longer periods. Intranasal desmopressin 0.25 mL b.i.d. using a solution containing 1.3 mg/mL has been given for minor bleeding episodes.

2. Fibrin glue. This is a topical biologic adhesive. Its effects imitate the final stages of coagulation. The glue consists of a solution of concentrated human fibrinogen, which is activated by the addition of bovine thrombin and calcium chloride. The resulting clot promotes hemostasis and tissue sealing. The clot is completely absorbed during the healing process. The best adhesive and hemostatic effect is obtained by applying the two solutions simultaneously to the open wound surface. Fibrin glue has been used primarily in surgical settings. It has been most effective when used for surface, low-pressure bleeding. There is a small risk of anaphylactic reaction because of the bovine origin of the thrombin.

3. Antifibrinolytic agents. ϵ-Aminocaproic acid (EACA) and tranexamic acid have been used to control bleeding associated with primary fibrinolysis as seen in patients with prostatic carcinoma and in a small number of patients with refractory thrombocytopenia. Great care must be taken in the use of these agents because of a possible increased risk of thrombosis. EACA may be used topically to control small-area, small-volume bleeding.

4. Oprelvekin (interleukin-11). Oprelvekin has recently been approved by the U.S. Food and Drug Administration for the treatment and prevention of chemotherapy-related thrombocytopenia. Oprelvekin is a thrombopoietic growth factor that directly stimulates the proliferation of hematopoietic stem cells and megakaryocyte progenitor cells as well as megakaryocyte maturation, resulting in increased platelet production. It may cause substantial fluid retention and should be used with caution in patients who have congestive heart failure (CHF), those with a history of CHF, and those being treated for CHF. One must also be cautious using this agent in patients who are receiving diuretic therapy or ifosfamide because sudden deaths have been reported as a result of severe hypokalemia. Oprelvekin should be used to prevent thrombocytopenia, which would be severe enough to require platelet transfusions. Therapy usually begins 6 to 24 h after the completion of chemotherapy, and patients should be monitored for any signs or symptoms of allergic reactions or cardiac dysfunction.

SELECTED READINGS

Anand SS, Wells PS, Hunt D, et al. Does this patient have deep vein thrombosis? *JAMA* 1998;279:1094–1099.

Baker WF Jr. Thrombosis and hemostasis in cardiology: review of pathophysiology and clinical practice. II. Recommendations for antithrombotic therapy. *Clin Appl Thromb Hemost* 1998;4:143–147.

Bauer KA, et al. Tumor necrosis factor infusions have a pro-coagulant effect on the hemostatic mechanism of humans. *Blood* 1989;74:165.

Bern MM, Lokich JJ, Wallach SR, et al. Very low doses of warfarin can prevent thrombosis in central venous catheters: a randomized prospective trial. *Ann Intern Med* 1990;112:423.

Beutler E. Platelet transfusions: the 20,000/μl trigger. *Blood* 1993; 81:1411–1413.

Brennan M. Fibrin glue. *Blood Rev* 1991;5:240.

Dzik S. Leukodepletion blood filters: filter design and mechanisms of leukocyte removal. *Transfusion Med Rev* 1993;7:65.

Dzik WH. Leukoreduced blood components, laboratory and clinical aspects. In: Rossi EC, et al., eds. *Principles of transfusion medicine.* 2nd ed. Baltimore, Williams & Wilkins, 1996:353–373.

Esparaz B, Kies M, Kwaan H. Thromboembolism in cancer. In: Kwaan HC, Samama MM, eds. *Clinical thrombosis.* Boca Raton: CRC Press, 1989:317–333.

Friedberg RC. Clinical and laboratory factors underlying refractoriness to platelet transfusions. *J Clin Apheresis* 1996;11:143–148.

Gelb AB, Leavitt AD. Crossmatch compatible platelets improve corrected count increments in patients who are refractory to randomly selected patients. *Transfusion* 1997;37:624–630.

Ginsberg JS. Management of venous thromboembolism. *N Engl J Med* 1996;335:1816–1828.

Griffin MR, Stanson AW, Brown ML, et al. Deep venous thrombosis and pulmonary embolism: risk of subsequent malignant neoplasms. *Arch Intern Med* 1987;147:1907–1911.

Hillyer CD, Emmens RK, Zago-Novaretti M, et al. Methods for the reduction of transfusion transmitted cytomegalovirus infection: filtration versus the use of seronegative donor units. *Transfusion* 1994;34:929–934.

Hirsh J, et al. Oral anticoagulants. Mechanism of action, clinical effectiveness, and optimal therapeutic range. *Chest* 1992;102(suppl):312.

Hull RD, Pineo GF. Prophylaxis of deep vein thrombosis and pulmonary embolism: current recommendations. *Clin Appl Thromb Hemost* 1998;4:96–104.

Humphries JE. Transfusion therapy in acquired coagulopathies. *Hematol Oncol Clin North Am* 1994;8:1181–1201.

Kunkel LA. Acquired circulating anticoagulants in malignancy. *Semin Thromb Hemost* 1992;18:416–423.

Lane TA. Leukocyte reduction of cellular blood component: effectiveness, benefits, quality control and costs. *Arch Pathol Lab Med* 1994;118:392–404.

Legler TJ, Fischer I, Dittman J, et al. Frequency and course of refractoriness in multiply transfused patients. *Ann Hematol* 1997;74:185–189.

Mannucci DM. Desmopressin: a non-traditional form of treatment for congenital and acquired bleeding disorders. *Blood* 1988;72:1449–1455.

McCarthy PM. Fibrin glue in cardiothoracic surgery. *Transfusion Med Rev* 1993;7:173–179.

Murgo A. Thrombotic microangiopathy in the cancer patient including those induced by chemotherapy agents. *Semin Hematol* 1987;24:161–177.

O'Connell, Lee EJ, Schiffer CA. The value of 10 min posttransfusion platelet counts. *Transfusion* 1988;28:66–67.

Pisciotto PT, Benson K, Hume H, et al. Prophylactic versus therapeutic platelet transfusion practices in hematology and/or oncology patients. *Transfusion* 1995;35:498–502.

Poon M. Cryoprecipitate: uses and alternatives. *Transfusion Med Rev* 1993;7:180–192.

Practice parameter for the use of fresh-frozen plasma, cryoprecipitate, and platelets. *JAMA* 1994;271:777–781.

Przepiorka D, LeParc GF, Stovall MA, et al. Use of irradiated blood components: practice parameter. *Am J Clin Pathol* 1996;106:6–11.

Przepiorka D, LeParc GF, Werch J, et al. Prevention of transfusion associated CMV infection: practice parameter. *Am J Clin Pathol* 1996;106:163–169.

Schafer A. The hypercoagulable state. *Ann Intern Med* 1985;102:814–828.

Slichter SJ. Algorithm for managing the platelet refractory patient. *J Clin Apheresis* 1997;2:4–9.

Sorenson HT, Mellemkjaer L, Steffensen FH, et al. The risk of the diagnosis of cancer after primary deep venous thrombosis or pulmonary embolism. *N Engl J Med* 1998;338:1169–1173.

Tefferi A, Silverstein MN, Hoagland HC. Primary thrombocythemia. *Semin Oncol* 1995;22:334–340.

Trial to Reduce Alloimmunization to Platelets Study Group. Leukocyte reduction and ultraviolet B irradiation of platelets to prevent alloimmunization and refractoriness to platelet transfusions. *N Engl J Med* 1997;337:1861–1869.

Platelet transfusion for patients with cancer: clinical practice guidelines of the American Society of Clinical Oncology. *J Clin Oncol* 2001;19:1519–1538.

29

Critical Care Issues in Oncology and Bone Metastasis

Roland T. Skeel

Spinal cord compression, cerebral edema, superior vena cava syndrome (SVCS), anaphylaxis, respiratory failure, tumor lysis syndrome, and bone metastasis can be major causes of morbidity and, in some cases, potential mortality in patients with cancer. Because of the critical nature of these complications of cancer and its treatment, oncologists, oncology nurses, and other oncology health professionals must be prepared to recognize the signs and symptoms of these disorders promptly, so that appropriate therapy can be instituted without delay.

I. Spinal cord compression

A. Tumors. The most common tumors resulting in spinal cord compression are breast cancer, lung cancer, prostate cancer, and renal cancer, although it may also occur with sarcoma, multiple myeloma, and lymphoma. Purely intradural or epidural lesions are uncommon because more than three-fourths of cases arise from either metastasis to a vertebral body or other bony parts of the vertebra or, less commonly, direct extension from a paravertebral soft tissue mass. Seventy percent of the bone lesions are osteolytic, 10% osteoblastic, and 20% mixed. More than 85% of patients with metastases to the vertebra have lesions that involve more than one vertebral body.

B. Symptoms and signs. The most common early symptoms seen in patients with spinal cord compression are localized vertebral or radicular pain. These are not from the cord compression per se but rather from involvement of the vertebral structures and nerve roots at the level of the compression. Localized tenderness to pressure or percussion over the involved vertebrae is often found on physical examination. Because pain is seen initially in up to 90% of patients, localized back pain, radicular pain, or spinal tenderness in a patient with cancer should evoke the clinical suspicion of the physician and prompt further evaluation to determine whether the patient has potential or early cord compression. Muscle weakness, evidenced by subjective symptoms or objective physical findings, is present in 75% of patients by the time of diagnosis. The clinician must be aware that progression of this symptom can vary from a gradual increase in weakness over several days to a precipitous loss of function over several hours that may worsen rapidly to the point of paraplegia. If muscle weakness is present, it is incumbent on the physician to act urgently to obtain consultation with the neurosurgeon and the radiotherapist. It is not appropriate to wait until the next morning! By the time there is muscle weakness, most patients also have sensory deficits below the level of the compression and often have changes in bladder and bowel sphincter function. When compression is diagnosed late or if treatment is not started emergently, only 25% of patients who are unable to walk when treatment is started regain full ambulation.

C.   Diagnosis. Magnetic resonance imaging (MRI) is the diagnostic modality of choice, although high-resolution computed tomography (CT) with myelography is an alternative. Plain radiographs and bone scans give evidence of metastases to vertebrae but in and of themselves are not diagnostic of spinal cord involvement.

When there is evidence of bony involvement of the spine on a plain radiograph, CT scan, or bone scan, our approach is to obtain an MRI for those patients who have subjective or objective evidence of weakness, radicular pain, paresthesia, or sphincter dysfunction because these patients are at highest risk of spinal cord compression. Routine MRIs in patients who have completely asymptomatic bony spine metastases (without pain, tenderness, or neurologic findings on a comprehensive clinical examination) are not cost effective. In patients with only localized pain or tenderness to correspond with the bone scan or radiographic findings, the yield of additional tests is also low. Thus, the clinical determination of whether to obtain additional invasive or costly diagnostic tests is more difficult and requires a careful assessment of all clinical features of the patient. All patients with metastasis to the spine require close follow-up, and they and their families must be urged to report relevant symptoms immediately.

D.   Treatment

1.   Corticosteroids. When a radiologic study identifies the level of cord compression or a neurologic deficit is detected on physical examination, dexamethasone may be started to reduce spinal cord edema. A recommended dose is 10 to 20 mg IV as a loading dose and then 4 to 6 mg PO or IV every 6 h to be continued through the initial weeks of radiation therapy. Thereafter, the dexamethasone therapy may be tapered.

2.   Radiotherapy

a.   Although the preferences of individual centers vary, we generally recommend the **immediate initiation of radiotherapy** once cord compression is diagnosed. This is based on both randomized and nonrandomized studies showing no significant improvement in outcome for patients treated with surgery plus radiation versus those treated with radiation alone. In addition, metastatic disease to the spine is often not totally resectable, so that follow-up radiation therapy is frequently required. Third, because patients with evidence of spinal metastases frequently have either overt or microscopic evidence of metastases elsewhere that would likely grow during the postoperative recuperation period after surgery, the use of radiotherapy instead allows the initiation of some form of systemic therapy concurrently.

b.   Radiation therapy is most frequently given to a total dose of 40 to 45 Gy with daily dose fractions of 200 to 250 cGy. Alternatively, 400 cGy daily may be given initially for the first 3 days of therapy and then subsequently decreased to standard-dose levels for the completion of the radiation course.

c.   The clinical response to radiation is dependent not only on the degree of cord involvement and the duration of symptoms but also on the underlying cell type. In general, patients with severe deficits such as complete paraplegia or a long duration of neurologic deficit are unlikely to have return to normal function. This underscores the need to diagnose and treat these patients rapidly. Lymphoma, myeloma, and other hematologic malignancies, along with breast and small cell lung carcinoma, tend to be more responsive than adenocarcinomas of the gastrointestinal tract, renal cancer, and others.

3.   Surgery. Surgery (whether decompressive laminectomy for posterior lesions or anterior approaches for other lesions) still plays a crucial role in selected patients. Indications for surgery include worsening of neurologic signs or symptoms or the appearance of new neurologic findings during the course of radiation treatment, vertebral collapse at presentation, a question of spinal stability, and disease recurrence within a prior radiation port. In selected patients, the use of surgery to remove disease in the vertebral bodies followed by stabilization can result in dramatic improvement in pain and function.

II.   Cerebral edema
A.   Clinical evaluation

1.   Neurologic signs and symptoms. Intracranial metastases are commonly manifested by a variety of neurologic symptoms and signs, including headache, change in mentation, visual disturbances, cranial nerve deficits, focal motor or sensory abnormalities, difficulty with coordination, and seizures. In the more critical condition of brainstem herniation, there may be gradual to rapid loss of consciousness, neck stiffness, unilateral or bilateral pupillary abnormalities, ipsilateral hemiparesis, or respiratory dysfunction; the specific findings depend on whether there is uncal, central, or tonsillar herniation. Any new neurologic complaint from a patient with cancer should be viewed by members of the oncology team with a high index of suspicion that it represents metastasis, especially if metastasis to the brain is commonly associated with the patient's tumor type.

The history and physical examination provide the first clue to the presence of a metastatic lesion or associated cerebral edema. In general, a history of gradual progression of neurologic symptoms before the development of a significant deficit is more consistent with a metastatic lesion, whereas the absence of symptoms followed by the abrupt onset of a severe deficit is suggestive of a cerebrovascular event.

2.   Radiologic studies. MRI is the imaging modality of choice because it has greater sensitivity than CT in detecting the presence of metastatic lesions and in determining the extent of cerebral edema. CT is substituted for MRI in many institutions because of availability, ease of administration, with shorter test time and less cost. However, although CT is sufficient to detect the presence of cerebral edema in most patients, it is necessary to realize that CT fails to diagnose some lesions and may underestimate cerebral edema. If CT of the brain reveals no definite abnormality in the presence of persistent neurologic findings, MRI is the recommended next step. Delay of appropriate imaging studies (either CT or MRI) to examine plain skull radiographs or to obtain radionuclide studies in patients experiencing neurologic difficulties is not warranted.

Warning: In a patient with cancer who has focal neurologic signs or symptoms, headache, or alteration in consciousness, a lumbar puncture to evaluate for possible neoplastic meningeal spread should not be done until a CT scan or MRI shows no evidence of mass, midline shift, or increased intracranial pressure. To do the lumbar puncture without this assurance could precipitate brainstem herniation, which is often rapidly fatal.

B. Treatment

1. Symptomatic therapy. Once the presence of cerebral edema is established, dexamethasone 10 to 20 mg IV to load followed by 6 mg IV or PO four times daily should be started. The rationale for the use of steroids centers around the etiology of cerebral edema. It appears that the invasion of malignant cells releases leukotrienes and other soluble mediators responsible for vasodilation, increased capillary permeability, and subsequent edema. Dexamethasone inhibits the conversion of arachidonic acid to leukotrienes, thereby decreasing vascular permeability. Additionally, steroids appear to have a direct stabilizing effect on brain capillaries. There is some evidence to suggest that patients who do not have lessening of cerebral edema with the dexamethasone dose just described may respond to higher doses (50 to 100 mg/day). Because of the risk of gastrointestinal bleeding and other side effects of doses higher than 32 mg/day, higher doses are usually not given for more than 48 to 72 h.

Patients with severe cerebral edema leading to a life-threatening rise in intracranial pressure or brainstem herniation should also receive mannitol 50 to 100 g (in a 20% to 25% solution) infused IV over about 30 min. This may be repeated every 6 h if needed, although serum electrolytes and urine output must be monitored closely. Patients with severe cerebral edema should be intubated to allow for mechanical hyperventilation to reduce the carbon dioxide pressure to 25 to 30 mm Hg in order to decrease intracranial pressure.

2. Therapy of the intracerebral tumor. Once the patient has been stabilized, appropriate therapy for the cause underlying the cerebral edema should be implemented. Radiation is the usual modality for most metastases, but surgery may be considered in addition for suitable candidates with easily accessible lesions; combined surgery and radiotherapy may result in a longer disease-free and total survival if there are only one or two metastatic lesions and the systemic disease is controlled.

3. Nonmalignant causes of cerebral edema, such as subdural hematoma in thrombocytopenic patients and brain abscess in immunocompromised patients, must always be considered.

III. Superior vena cava syndrome. The superior vena cava is a thin-walled vessel located to the right of the midline just anterior to the right main-stem bronchus. It is ultimately responsible for the venous drainage of the head, neck, and arms. Its location places it near lymph nodes that are commonly involved by malignant cells from primary lung tumors and from lymphomas. Lymph node distention or the presence of a mediastinal tumor mass may compress the adjacent superior vena cava, leading to superior vena cava syndrome (SVCS). Similarly, the presence of a thrombus due to a hypercoagulable state secondary to underlying malignancy or a thrombus developing around an indwelling central venous catheter may also lead to the development of this syndrome.

A.   Symptoms and signs. Patients who develop SVCS commonly complain of dyspnea, orthopnea, paroxysmal nocturnal dyspnea, and facial, neck, and upper-extremity swelling. Associated symptoms may include cough, hoarseness, and chest or neck pain. Headache and mental status changes also may be seen. A patient's symptoms may be gradual and progressive, with only mild facial swelling being present early in the course of this disorder. These early changes may be so subtle that the patient is unaware of them. Alternatively, if a clot develops in the superior vena cava in association with narrowing of the vessel, the signs and symptoms may appear suddenly. Physical examination may reveal a spectrum of findings from facial edema to marked respiratory distress. Neck vein distention, facial edema or cyanosis, and tachypnea are commonly seen. Other potential physical findings include the presence of prominent collateral vessels on the thorax, upper-extremity edema, paralysis of the vocal cords, and mental status changes.

B.   Radiologic evaluation. Patients may often be diagnosed by physical findings plus the presence of a mediastinal mass on chest radiographs. Although previously it was thought that the superior venocavogram was required to establish the diagnosis and delineate the extent of obstruction, current opinion now appears to favor the use of CT instead. CT permits a more detailed examination of surrounding anatomy, including adjacent lymphadenopathy; may differentiate between extrinsic compression and an intrinsic lesion (primary thrombus); poses less risk to the patient; aids in treatment planning for radiation therapy; and allows for possible percutaneous biopsy of a compressing mass.

SVCS may occur in patients with subclavian or internal jugular IV catheters. The injection of contrast material into these catheters is useful to determine the presence of a thrombus. However, a thrombus forms in the venous vasculature distal to the caval obstruction in most patients with SVCS secondary to external compression. Thus, a clot may be primary or secondary; determination of the cause and the appropriate treatment depends on both the clinical situation and the radiologic findings.

C.   Tissue diagnosis. Although some patients present with such severe respiratory compromise as to require emergent treatment, most patients are clinically stable and may undergo biopsy for a tissue diagnosis if they are not previously known to have cancer. Tissue may be acquired through multiple methods including bronchoscopy, CT-guided biopsy, mediastinoscopy, mediastinotomy, and thoracoscopy. Thoracotomy is the most invasive option and is rarely needed. Because of increased venous pressure and dilated veins distal to the obstruction, extreme care must be taken to ensure adequate hemostasis after any biopsy procedure.

D.   Treatment. Initially, patients with SVCS may be treated with oxygen for dyspnea, furosemide 20 to 40 mg IV to reduce edema, and dexamethasone 16 mg IV or PO daily in divided doses. The benefit of dexamethasone is not clear. In patients with lymphoma, there is probably a lympholytic effect with resultant decrease in tumor mass; in patients with most other tumors, the effect is probably limited to decreasing any local inflammatory reaction from the tumor and from subsequent initial radiotherapy.

    1. Neoplasms. Therapy for SVCS ultimately involves radiation therapy for most tumors but possibly chemotherapy as a single modality for particularly sensitive tumor types such as small cell lung cancer, lymphomas, and germ cell cancers. Radiation therapy may be given in relatively high-dose fractions (e.g., 4 Gy) for several days, followed by a reversion to "standard doses" thereafter. Dexamethasone is continued for about 1 week after the start of radiation treatment.

    2. Thrombi. SVCS secondary to vascular thrombi may require the use of thrombolytic therapy, though this is not necessary in most cases. Both streptokinase 250,000 U by IV bolus over 30 min and urokinase 4,400 U/kg by IV bolus over 10 min have been used. Recombinant tissue plasminogen activator (rt-PA) 0.5 mg/kg/day × 2 days has also been used for SVCS, but there are fewer reported studies or cases. Although 50% to 75% of patients have resolution of clots with thrombolytic therapy when treated within 7 days of occurrence, thrombi that have been present for longer than 7 days are unlikely to be treated successfully. Avoid thrombolytic therapy in patients with a tumor that might bleed. Anticoagulation with heparin after thrombolytic therapy is recommended; patients whose catheters become patent and functional should receive low-dose warfarin (1 mg/day PO) thereafter at a minimum. Depending on the situation, therapeutic doses of warfarin may be indicated.

    For patients with thrombi secondary to external superior vena cava pressure from neoplasms, thrombolytics are not usually used, but patients are commonly anticoagulated with heparin and then warfarin to prevent propagation of the clot (see Chapter 28).

IV. Anaphylaxis

A. Causes. Anaphylaxis, although infrequent, is one of the most catastrophic potential side effects of biologic and chemotherapy. Anaphylaxis is a hyperimmune reaction mediated by the release of immunoglobulin E. This emergency situation may arise in oncology patients who are exposed to serum products, bacterial products such as L-asparaginase, certain cytotoxic agents (such as paclitaxel [Taxol] or the Cremophor component of paclitaxel), antibiotics such as penicillin, iodine-based contrast material, latex, and monoclonal antibodies (which have murine components). However, virtually any drug can lead to a hyperimmune response resulting in anaphylaxis.

B. Clinical manifestations. Patients may display anxiety, dyspnea, and presyncopal symptoms. Urticaria, generalized itching, and evidence of bronchospasm and upper-airway angioedema may occur. Peripheral vasodilation may be manifest by facial flushing or pallor, can result in significant hypotension, and may lead to syncope.

C. Management. Prompt recognition and treatment can be invaluable in blunting an adverse response and may prevent a reaction from becoming life threatening. Patients must be assessed rapidly to ensure that an open airway is present and maintained. Supplemental oxygen should be given for respiratory symptoms. Endotracheal intubation may be necessary. If severe laryngeal edema rather than bronchospasm is the cause of respiratory distress, tracheostomy or cricothyrotomy is necessary.

1. Epinephrine 0.3 to 0.5 mg (0.3 to 0.5 mL of 1:1,000 epinephrine or 3 to 5 mL of a 1:10,000 solution) IV is given every 10 min for severe reactions with laryngeal stridor, major bronchospasm, or severe hypotension, for a maximum of three doses (1 mg) or until the episode resolves, whichever occurs first. For milder reactions, a dose of 0.2 to 0.3 mL of 1:1,000 epinephrine may be given SC and repeated every 15 min twice. In the event of life-threatening anaphylaxis, 0.5 mg (5 mL of a 1:10,000 solution) should be given IV; this dose may be repeated once in 10 min if needed. Because of the cardiovascular stress associated with epinephrine, its use in relatively minor allergic reactions, such as pruritus alone, should be avoided. Alternatively, epinephrine may be administered through the endotracheal tube if IV access is unavailable.

2. Intravenous fluids (either normal saline or lactated Ringer's solution) may be given for hypotension. Hypotension unresponsive to these measures requires the use of vasopressors such as dopamine.

3. Albuterol or metaproterenol aerosol treatments can be used to treat bronchospasm.

4. Diphenhydramine 25 mg IV may be followed by a second dose, if necessary. Blood pressure must be monitored because hypotension can result.

5. Corticosteroids have a slow onset of action measured in hours. Although their administration may be reasonable for their later effects, they do not have a primary role in the acute management of this emergent condition. Hydrocortisone 100 to 500 mg IV or methylprednisolone 125 mg IV may be given for their later effects.

6. Cimetidine 300 mg IV or other H_2-blocker may be given for urticaria; it has no significant role in acute, severe episodes, although it has a preventive role in averting reactions from paclitaxel along with dexamethasone (Decadron) and diphenhydramine.

V. Respiratory failure

A. Causes. Respiratory failure in patients with cancer may have many potential causes:

- Bacterial or other pneumonias, especially in patients who are neutropenic due to therapy
- Sepsis (and other causes of the systemic inflammatory response syndrome)
- Interstitial pulmonary spread of cancer
- Overwhelming parenchymal pulmonary metastases
- Radiation injury
- Lung damage from chemotherapy agents (such as bleomycin, high-dose cyclophosphamide, or methotrexate)

- Pulmonary edema secondary to cardiac damage from cytotoxic agents (like doxorubicin), or
- Biologic agents ("capillary leak syndrome" with interleukin-2 [IL-2])
- Retinoic acid syndrome from tretinoin (all-*trans*-retinoic acid) therapy of acute promyelocytic leukemia
- Pulmonary emboli, either multiple small or single large

B. Management. The management of severe respiratory failure requires intubation and mechanical ventilation, which is usually managed by pulmonologists or critical care specialists. However, because the prognosis of most patients with advanced solid tumors who develop respiratory failure is poor, careful consideration of a patient's entire medical situation must be made. Relevant factors include the patient's underlying medical illnesses, such as concurrent cardiopulmonary disease, and their particular tumor type and potential for response to antineoplastic therapy. It is prudent—some would say imperative—to ascertain well in advance of the emergency the goals of the patient and the wishes of patients and their families regarding intensive care unit support and full resuscitative measures.

C. Prevention. If possible, progressive steps to prevent or lessen the possibility of the development of respiratory failure should be undertaken. These include the following:

1. Careful monitoring of granulocyte counts to be aware of patients at risk for bacterial infection.

2. Routine lung auscultation of patients receiving agents with potential pulmonary toxicity followed by appropriate action in the event of pulmonary findings. This may include giving furosemide if indicated and discontinuing offending agents (like bleomycin) before the development of serious symptoms. Reasons for discontinuing bleomycin therapy include unexplained exertional dyspnea, fine bibasilar rales, fine bibasilar reticular shadows on chest radiograph, and significant fall in pulmonary function tests from pretreatment levels.

3. Ensuring that patients are ambulatory or that antithrombotic precautions are taken for hospitalized patients who are bedridden.

4. Consideration of underlying cardiopulmonary disease, prior chest irradiation, and so forth before patients are considered to be candidates for systemic therapy is most important. Concurrent illnesses may proscribe the selection of or modify the dosing of cytotoxic agents (such as cisplatin, which requires substantial IV hydration) and biologic agents (like IL-2, before which patients' cardiac and pulmonary function should be tested).

VI. Tumor lysis syndrome. This syndrome may be seen with any tumor that is undergoing rapid cell turnover as a result of high growth fraction or high cell death due to therapy. In general, acute leukemia, high-grade lymphoma, and, less commonly, solid tumors such as small cell lung cancer and germ cell cancers undergoing therapy are the most commonly associated tumor types. Tumor lysis syndrome is characterized by the metabolic abnormalities of hyperuricemia, hyperkalemia, and hyperphosphatemia leading to hypocalcemia. Severe clinical situations, including acute renal failure, and serious cardiac dysrhythmia, including ventricular tachycardia and ventricular fibrillation, may develop. It is therefore important for physicians to be aware of which patients might be at risk for this syndrome, attempt to prevent its onset, monitor patients' blood chemistry values carefully, and initiate treatment promptly.

A. Prevention. It is useful to start all patients who have tumor types that predispose to this complication on allopurinol 600 mg/day PO for 1 or 2 days at least 24 h before initiating chemotherapy. Thereafter, patients may receive allopurinol 300 mg/day PO.

For patients who must be treated immediately, allopurinol is started at the same dose just described, urine should be alkalinized (pH 7), and IV fluid hydration with a "brisk diuresis" of about 100 to 150 mL/h of urine maintained. This can be achieved through the use of IV crystalloid, with 1 ampule (44.6 mEq) of sodium bicarbonate in each liter of IV solution. If the desired urine output is not reached after adequate hydration, furosemide 20 mg IV may be given to facilitate diuresis. If routine monitoring of urine shows pH less than 7.0, an additional ampule of sodium bicarbonate may be added to each liter of infused fluid. Acetazolamide 250 mg PO q.i.d. may also be added to keep urine alkaline.

B. Monitoring. During the course of chemotherapy for patients at risk of tumor lysis syndrome, serum electrolytes, phosphate, calcium, uric acid, and creatinine levels should be checked before therapy and at least daily thereafter. Patients at high risk (e.g., high-grade lymphoma with large bulk) should have these parameters checked every 6 h for the first 24 to 48 h. In addition, patients who show any initial or subsequent abnormality in any of these parameters should have appropriate therapy initiated and have measurements of abnormal parameters repeated every 6 to 12 h until completion of chemotherapy and normalization of laboratory values.

C. Treatment. Patients who have evidence of tumor lysis syndrome must have adequate hydration with half-normal saline solution. Oral aluminum hydroxide can be used to treat hyperphosphatemia.

Hyperkalemia may be treated in multiple ways. However, the clinician must differentiate between methods that reduce serum potassium by driving this ion intracellularly (as is done with dextrose and insulin or sodium bicarbonate) and methods that lead to actual potassium loss out of the body (as with furosemide through the urine and with sodium polystyrene sulfonate resin [Kayexalate] through the gut). If hyperkalemia or hypocalcemia occurs, an electrocardiogram should be obtained, with continuous monitoring of the cardiac rhythm until these abnormalities are corrected. In addition, because of the potential cardiac arrhythmias secondary to hyperkalemia with hypocalcemia, cardioprotection could be achieved through the use of IV calcium.

We recommend the following:

1. For patients with mild elevation of potassium (serum potassium no higher than 5.5 mEq/L), increasing IV hydration using normal saline solution with a single dose (20 mg) of IV furosemide is often sufficient. An alternative to normal saline is the use of 2 ampules of sodium bicarbonate (89 mEq) in 1 L of 5% dextrose/water, although alkalinization per se is probably not beneficial.

2. For patients with serum potassium levels between 5.5 and 6.0 mEq/L, increased IV fluids, furosemide, and oral sodium polystyrene sulfonate resin 30 g with sorbitol may be used.

3. For patients with serum potassium levels of more than 6.0 mEq/L or evidence of cardiac arrhythmia, several options may be combined. IV calcium gluconate, 10 mL of a 10% solution or 1 ampule, is given first, followed by increased IV fluids, furosemide, plus 1 ampule of 50% dextrose and 10 U of regular insulin IV. Albuterol may be used to augment the effect of the insulin. Oral sodium polystyrene sulfonate resin with sorbitol also may be used except in patients with a history of congestive heart failure or reduced left ventricular function. Dialysis may be necessary for refractory hyperkalemia.

VII. Hypercalcemia

  A. Causes of tumor hypercalcemia

   1. Associated tumors. Hypercalcemia is relatively common in patients with malignancy. In one study, it was shown that the most common cause of hypercalcemia in hospitalized patients is malignancy. Hypercalcemia of malignancy can be associated with bone metastasis, or it may occur in the absence of any direct bone involvement by the tumor. Based on the findings of study on 433 patients with hypercalcemia of cancer, 86% of the patients had identifiable bone metastasis. More than one-half (n = 225) of the cases were accounted for by patients with breast carcinoma, and cancer of the lung and kidneys accounted for a smaller proportion. Patients with hematologic malignancies accounted for approximately 15% of the cases. These patients usually had hypercalcemia in the presence of diffuse tumor involvement of bone, although in a small percentage there was no evidence of bone involvement.

   2. Humoral mediators. In approximately 10% of the cases of malignancy, hypercalcemia develops in the absence of radiographic or scintigraphic evidence of bone involvement. In this group of patients, the pathogenesis of hypercalcemia appears to be secondary to humoral mediators, including parathyroid hormone (PTH)–related peptide, and a number of osteoclast-activating factors (OAFs). A number of cytokines with potent bone-resorbing activities have been identified. These cytokines may account for the previously designated OAF. There is evidence indicating that prostaglandins (PGs) play a role in the hypercalcemia of malignancy. PGs are potent stimulators of bone resorption. There may also be the coexistence of tumor with primary hyperparathyroidism or other cause of hypercalcemia (e.g., vitamin D intoxication, sarcoidosis).

 B. Symptoms, signs, and laboratory findings. Hypercalcemia often produces symptoms in patients with cancer and, in fact, may be the patients' major problem. Polyuria and nocturia, resulting from the impaired ability of the kidneys to concentrate the urine, occur early. Anorexia, nausea, constipation, muscle weakness, and fatigue are common. As the hypercalcemia progresses, severe dehydration, azotemia, mental obtundation, coma, and cardiovascular collapse may appear. In addition to hypercalcemia, the laboratory studies may reveal hypokalemia and increased blood urea nitrogen (BUN) and creatinine levels. Patients with hypercalcemia of malignancy frequently have hypochloremic metabolic alkalosis, whereas with primary hyperparathyroidism, metabolic acidosis is more common. The concentration of serum phosphorus is variable. PTH levels may be normal, low, or high, but marked elevations are rarely seen. Bone involvement is best evaluated by a bone scan, which is often positive in the absence of radiographic evidence of bone involvement.

C.   Treatment. The management of hypercalcemia of malignancy has two objectives: reducing elevated levels of serum calcium and treating the underlying cause. When hypercalcemia is mild to moderate (serum calcium less than 12 to 13 mg/dL) and the patient is not symptomatic, adequate hydration and measures directed against the tumor (e.g., surgery, chemotherapy, or radiation therapy) may suffice. Severe hypercalcemia, on the other hand, is a life-threatening condition requiring emergency treatment. Therefore, for more severe degrees of hypercalcemia, other measures must be taken, including enhancement of calcium excretion by the kidney in patients with adequate renal function and the use of agents that decrease bone resorption.

The agents used for treatment of hypercalcemia have differences in the time of onset and duration of action as well as in their potency. Therefore, effective treatment of severe hypercalcemia requires the use of more than one modality of therapy.

A suggested approach to the treatment of severe hypercalcemia is as follows:

- Rehydration with 0.9% sodium chloride
- Bisphosphonate therapy—either pamidronate or zoledronic acid
- Continuing saline diuresis (0.9% sodium chloride + furosemide)

1.   Rehydration. Rehydration and restoration of intravascular volume comprise the most important initial step in the therapy of hypercalcemia. Rehydration should be accomplished using 0.9% sodium chloride (normal saline) and often requires the administration of 4 to 6 L over the first 24 h. Rehydration alone causes only a mild decrease of the serum calcium levels (about 10%). However, rehydration improves renal function, facilitating urinary calcium excretion.

2.   Saline diuresis. After adequate restoration of intravascular volume, forced saline diuresis may be used. Sodium competitively inhibits the tubular resorption of calcium. Therefore, the IV infusion of saline causes a significant increase in calcium clearance. Because of the large amounts of saline that may be required to correct hypercalcemia, it is advisable to monitor the central venous pressure continuously. The infusion of normal saline (0.9% sodium chloride) at a rate of 250 to 500 mL/h, accompanied by the IV administration of 20 to 80 mg of furosemide every 2 to 4 h, results in significant calcium diuresis and mild lowering of the serum calcium in the majority of patients. This type of therapy requires strict monitoring of cardiopulmonary status to avoid fluid overload. Also, it requires ready access to the laboratory to prevent electrolyte imbalance, since the urinary losses of sodium, potassium, magnesium, and water must be replaced to maintain metabolic balance. In some cases, the infusion of saline at rates of 125 to 150 mL/h plus the addition of furosemide 40 to 80 mg IV once or twice a day may reduce the serum calcium until other measures aimed at inhibiting bone resorption take effect.

3. **Bisphosphonates**
   a. **Mechanism of action.** The bisphosphonates are potent inhibitors of normal and abnormal osteoclastic bone resorption. They bind to the surface of calcium phosphate crystals and inhibit crystal growth and dissolution. In addition, they may directly inhibit osteoclast resorptive activity.
   b. **Pamidronate (Aredia) and zoledronic acid (Zometa).** Pamidronate and zoledronic acid are very potent inhibitors of bone resorption and highly effective agents for the treatment of hypercalcemia of malignancy. Pamidronate has been the treatment of choice for hypercalcemia of malignancy for several years. Zoledronic acid, which has recently become available, is at least as effective in the treatment of hypercalcemia. Because it can be given over 15 min rather than over 2 h or more, it is likely to replace pamidronate in most formularies.
      (1) **Dosage and administration.** For symptomatic, moderate hypercalcemia (corrected serum calcium 12 to 13.5 mg/dL), the recommended dose of pamidronate is 60 to 90 mg given IV as a single dose over 4 to 24 h. The maximum recommended dose of zoledronic acid in hypercalcemia of malignancy is 4 mg, given as a single-dose IV infusion over **no less than 15 min.**
      (2) **Side effects.** Pamidronate and zoledronic acid are usually well tolerated, and no serious acute side effects have been reported. Mild fever with temperature elevations of 1°C have been noted occasionally in patients after drug administration. The transient fever is presumed to be due to release of cytokines from osteoclasts. Pain, redness, swelling, and induration at the site of infusion occur in approximately 20% of patients. Hypocalcemia, hypophosphatemia, or hypomagnesemia may be seen in 15% of the patients. Both should be used with caution in patients with decreased renal function.

4. **Glucocorticoids.** Large initial doses of hydrocortisone 250 to 500 mg IV q8 h (or its equivalent) can be effective in the treatment of hypercalcemia associated with lymphoproliferative diseases such as non-Hodgkin's lymphoma and multiple myeloma and in patients with breast cancer metastatic to bone. However, it may take several days for glucocorticoids to lower the serum calcium level. Maintenance therapy should be started with prednisone 10 to 30 mg/day PO. The mechanisms by which glucocorticoids lower the serum calcium are multiple and involved.

5. **Oral phosphate supplements** (Neutra-Phos or Fleet Phospho-Soda). Oral phosphate therapy is an adjunct for the chronic treatment of hypercalcemia of malignancy. Oral phosphate decreases the intestinal absorption of calcium and enhances the deposition of insoluble calcium salts in bone and

tissue. Oral phosphate supplements at dosages of 1.5 to 3.0 g/day of elemental phosphorus can result in mild lowering of the serum calcium levels as well as a reduction in urinary calcium excretion. Diarrhea usually limits the amount of phosphate that can be given. Phosphate supplements should never be given to patients with renal failure or when hyperphosphatemia is present, since soft tissue calcification may occur. Monitoring of the level of calcium and phosphorus as well as the calcium times phosphorus ion product is important to prevent metastatic calcifications.

6.   Prostaglandin inhibitors. Nonsteroidal anti-inflammatory agents inhibit cyclo-oxygenase and thereby block PG synthesis. Inhibitors of PG synthesis have been effective in rare cases of metastatic renal cell carcinoma and squamous cell carcinoma of the lung. Indomethacin 50 mg t.i.d. is the most potent inhibitor of PG synthesis. Aspirin 1 g t.i.d. has also been shown to be effective in selected cases.

VIII.   Bone metastasis. Metastases to bone occur frequently from many types of tumors and have great potential for morbidity. Bone involvement can be a source of constant pain, limiting a patient's activity and quality of life. The consequences of spinal involvement have been discussed already. The occurrence of a pathologic fracture in a weight-bearing bone has catastrophic implications: Patients who are consequently immobilized or bedridden are predisposed to a variety of complications including deep venous thrombi, pulmonary emboli, aspiration pneumonia, and decubitus ulcers as well as psychosocial consequences, including depression.

A.   Clinical findings. Bone involvement with metastatic disease can be manifested by a spectrum of clinical presentations. This can vary from constant aching pain through nocturnal exacerbations of pain to sharp pains brought on by pressure, weight bearing, other use, or range of motion of the affected site. Tenderness of an affected bone area may or may not be present. Tenderness or sharp pain with weight bearing often implies a greater degree of disruption of the bony architecture and thus a greater potential for fracture, particularly in a weight-bearing area.

B.   Radiologic findings. These often depend on the type of malignancy involved as well as the extent of the metastases. Multiple myeloma is a prime example of a malignancy that leads to pure osteolytic lesions. Consequently, radionuclide bone scans are rarely useful in the evaluation of patients with this disease. Rather, a metastatic skeletal survey (plain radiographs) is preferable. In contrast, prostate cancer most commonly has purely osteoblastic lesions. Therefore, a radionuclide bone scan would be the diagnostic test of choice. In general, most tumor types have the potential to yield either type of bone lesion or both. A radionuclide bone scan may be done to permit a "global view" in these patients.

The presence of "hot spots" in the spine, in weight-bearing bones such as the femur, or in other major long bones such as the humerus should lead the clinician to assess the patient further with plain radiographs of these bones. Patients who display significant cortical thinning of long bones or large lytic bone metastases are at high risk of developing pathologic fractures with great morbidity. These patients should be evaluated both by orthopedic surgery for consideration of prophylactic surgery to stabilize the affected bone and by radiation oncology for treatment of the tumor to permit regeneration of normal bone.

C. Treatment

1. **Surgery.** Because rapid return of the patient to as normal a life as possible is an overriding concern when treating patients with metastatic disease, surgical stabilization is most often the initial step in treating pathologic fractures of long bones. If the fracture is the initial manifestation of tumor relapse, biopsy confirmation can also be obtained. Whereas fractures at sites of significant residual bony architecture can be satisfactorily stabilized with an intramedullary rod or pin, marked lytic destruction may necessitate additional structural support such as methylmethacrylate cement to fill the intramedullary canal and cortical defects. Pathologic fractures of non-weight-bearing bones can be managed by splinting (ribs) or sling immobilization (humerus or clavicle) while delivering radiotherapy to promote healing. Fixation may also be used in the upper extremities to speed recovery of function, particularly of the humerus. Surgical stabilization of the spine may also be used in selected circumstances (provided the patient has an anticipated survival time of more than 3 months) and can result in significant pain relief and reduction in risk of cord and nerve root compression.

2. **External-beam therapy.** Radiation doses of 15 to 20 Gy in three to five fractions lead to complete relief of pain in about 50% of patients, with an additional 30% of patients having some decrease in pain, whereas 80% to 90% show significant improvement with 30 to 40 Gy. The alleviation of symptoms can be expected within 2 to 3 weeks. For patients who may be expected to have more prolonged survival, higher doses over a larger number of fractions may be used. Most patients receive optimal results from courses of 30 Gy in 10 fractions (2 weeks) or 40 Gy in 15 fractions (3 weeks).

Radiotherapy fields should include the area of evident bone involvement, as shown on radiograph and bone scan, with a sufficient extension to prevent relapse at the portal margin. It is seldom necessary to treat the entire bone unless the entire bone is involved because encroachment on marrow reserve may compromise any systemic chemotherapy that might also be indicated.

3. **Strontium-89 therapy.** A different approach to the therapy of symptomatic bone metastases is through the use of radioisotopes, such as strontium-89, which is given by IV injection. This isotope is highly selective for bone, is an emitter of beta radiation, and has low penetration into surrounding tissue. Strontium's affinity to metastatic bone disease is reported to be 2 to 25 times greater than its affinity to normal bone. This therapy is especially useful in patients with breast or prostate cancer who have many metastatic bone sites or who have received maximal external-beam irradiation to a specific site. Palliative effects may be seen in other types of tumors as well. Pain relief may occur as early as 1 to 2 weeks after the

first injection. Multiple studies indicate that 10% to 20% of patients experience complete pain relief, whereas another 50% to 60% have at least a moderate reduction in symptoms. Responses last 3 to 6 months. Patients who experience some relief of symptoms may receive multiple doses at 3-month intervals if there has been adequate hematologic recovery.

The toxicity of strontium-89 is primarily hematologic, involving both leukocytes and platelets. About 10% of patients may experience a transient "flare" of their bone pain, similar to what is seen with tamoxifen therapy in breast cancer. This flare reaction often foreshadows a response to treatment. Other radioisotopes for the palliation of painful bone metastases include samarium-153 and rhenium-186.

4.   Biphosphonates. Pamidronate and zoledronic acid are specific inhibitors of osteoclastic activity. They not only are effective for the treatment of hypercalcemia associated with malignancy but can reduce bone pain and reduce fractures, especially in multiple myeloma, breast cancer, and prostate cancer. Some improvement in survival may be seen in multiple myeloma.

SELECTED READINGS

Allen KL, Johnson TW, Hibbs GG. Effective bone radiation as related to various treatment regimens. *Cancer* 1986;37:984.

Allon M, Shanklin N. Effect of bicarbonate administration on plasma potassium in dialysis patients: interactions with insulin and albuterol. *Am J Kidney Dis* 1996;28:508–514.

Arrambide K, Toto RD. Tumor lysis syndrome. *Semin Nephrol* 1993; 13:273–280.

Bern MM, Lokich JJ, Wallach SR, et al. Very low dose of warfarin can prevent thrombosis in central venous catheters. *Ann Intern Med* 1990;112:423–428.

Ciesielski-Carlucci C, Leong P, Jacobs C. Case report of anaphylaxis from cisplatin/paclitaxel and a review of their hypersensitivity reaction profiles. *Am J Clin Oncol* 1997;20:373–375.

Coleman RE, Purohit OP. Osteoclast inhibition for the treatment of bone metastases. *Cancer Treat Rev* 1993;19:79–103.

Comis RL. Bleomycin pulmonary toxicity: current status and future directions. *Semin Oncol* 1992;19:64–70.

Cooper PR, Errico TJ, Martin R, et al. A systematic approach to spinal reconstruction after anterior decompression for neoplastic disease of the thoracic and lumbar spine. *Neurosurgery* 1993;32:1–8.

Escalante CP. Causes and management of superior vena cava syndrome. *Oncology* 1993;7:61. (In this same issue are three reviews of this article that lend further perspective to this disorder.)

Fleisch H. Bisphosphonates: a new class of drugs in diseases of bone and calcium metabolism. In: Brunner KW, Fleisch H, Senn H-J, eds. *Recent results in cancer research, vol 116: bisphosphonates and tumor osteolysis.* Berlin: Springer-Verlag, 1989:1–28.

Garmatis CJ, Chu FC. The effectiveness of radiation therapy in the treatment of bone metastases from breast cancer. *Radiology* 1978; 126:235.

Gray BH, Olin JW, Graor RA, et al. Safety and efficacy of thrombolytic therapy for superior vena cava syndrome. *Chest* 1991;99:54–59.

Greenberg A. Hyperkalemia: treatment options. *Semin Nephrol* 1998;18:46–57.

Hauser MJ, Tabak J, Baier H. Survival of patients with cancer in a medical critical care unit. *Arch Intern Med* 1982;142:527.

Johnston FG, Uttley D, Marsh HT. Synchronous vertebral decompression and posterior stabilization in the treatment of spinal malignancy. *Neurosurgery* 1989;25:872.

Kanis JA, McCloskey EV, Taube T, et al. Rationale for the use of bisphosphonates in bone metastases. *Bone* 1991;12(suppl 1):S13–S18.

Katin MJ, et al. Hematologic effects of 89-strontium treatment for metastases to bone. *Proc Am Soc Clin Oncol* 1993;3:12.

Man Z, Otero AB, Rendo P, et al. Use of pamidronate for multiple myeloma osteolytic lesions. *Lancet* 1990;335:663.

McAfee PC, Bohlman HH. One-stage anterior cervical decompression and posterior stabilization with circumferential arthrodesis. *Am J Bone Joint Surg* 1989;71:78.

Porter AT, Davis LP. Systemic radionuclide therapy of bone metastases with strontium-89. *Oncology* 1994;8:93.

Samarian-153 lexidronam for painful bone metastases. *Med Lett Drugs Ther* 1997;39:83–84.

Seifert V, Zimmerman M, Stolke D, et al. Spondylectomy, microsurgical decompression and osteosynthesis in the treatment of complex disorders of the cervical spine. *Acta Neurochir (Wien)* 1993;124:104–113.

Soffen EM, Greenberg A, Boumann J, et al. The role of strontium-89 systemic radiotherapy in the management of osseous metastases from prostate cancer. *Techn Urol* 1997;3:76–80.

Thiebaud D, Leyvraz S, von Fliedner V, et al. Treatment of bone metastases from breast cancer and myeloma with pamidronate. *Eur J Cancer* 1991;27:37–41.

Weissman DE. Steroid treatment of CNS metastases. *J Clin Oncol* 1988;6:543–551.

Woods JA, Lambert S, Platts-Mills TA, et al. Natural rubber latex allergy: spectrum, diagnostic approach, and therapy. *J Emerg Med* 1997;15:71–85.

30

Malignant Pleural, Peritoneal, and Pericardial Effusions and Meningeal Infiltrates

Walter D. Y. Quan, Jr.

Malignant pleural, peritoneal, and pericardial effusions and malignant meningeal infiltrates are uncommon early in the course of the malignancy. They occur more frequently with disseminated disease and often herald a poor prognosis. Although pleural and peritoneal effusions may initially have little adverse effect on quality of life, when progressive, they (as well as pericardial effusions and meningeal infiltrates) can result in incapacitating disability and death. It is therefore necessary for the clinician to have a high index of suspicion for these problems and to be prepared to take appropriate action and deliver palliative treatment promptly.

I. Pleural effusions

A. Causes. Malignant pleural effusions arise in association with malignant cells lining the pleura, exuded into the pleural space, or blocking veins or lymphatics. The most common malignancy associated with pleural effusions in women is carcinoma of the breast, whereas in men, it is carcinoma of the lung. Other causes of malignant pleural effusions include lymphoma, mesothelioma, and carcinomas of the ovary, gastrointestinal tract, urinary tract, and uterus. Malignancy is not the only cause of effusions, even in patients with known neoplastic disease; therefore, it is important to attempt to exclude other possible causes such as congestive heart failure, infection, and pulmonary infarction.

B. Diagnosis

1. Clinical diagnosis. Effusions may be asymptomatic or may be suspected because of respiratory symptoms such as shortness of breath with exertion or at rest, orthopnea, paroxysmal nocturnal dyspnea, or occasionally chest pressure or cough. The patient may feel more comfortable when lying on one side when the effusion is unilateral. On physical examination, dullness to percussion, decreased tactile fremitus, diminished breath sounds, and egophony are typical signs over the area of the effusion.

2. A chest radiograph should be obtained to confirm the clinical impression. If fluid appears to be present, a lateral decubitus film must be obtained to help estimate the volume of the effusion and how free it is within the pleural space.

3. Diagnostic thoracentesis should be performed. Ultrasonographic guidance is helpful if loculation is present. Fluid should be obtained for bacterial, acid-fast, and fungal cultures, for cytologic examination, and for determining protein concentration (greater than 3 g/dL in most exudates), lactate dehydrogenase (LDH) level, specific gravity, and cell count. The cytologic examination is important because if the results are positive, as in 50% to 70% of patients with malignant effusion, the diagnosis is established. Other parameters of the pleural fluid that may be helpful in establishing that the fluid is an exudate and not a transudate include a specific gravity of more than 1.015, protein concentration that is more than 0.5 times the serum protein concentration, LDH level more than 0.6 times the serum LDH level, and low glucose level. A cytologic examination of fluid from a newly discovered pleural effusion is wise, regardless of whether the patient is known to have malignancy, because for nearly half of all malignant effusions, this finding is the first sign of malignancy. Analyzing pleural fluid for carcinoembryonic antigen (CEA) may be helpful in some patients. Levels higher than 20 ng/mL are suggestive of adenocarcinoma, although they do not substitute for a tissue diagnosis in patients who have no history of malignancy. CEA elevations may be seen in adenocarcinomas from various primary sites including the breast, lung, and gastrointestinal tract. Elevated levels between 10 and 20 ng/mL may reflect malignancy or benign disorders such as pulmonary infection. The role of assessing other tumor markers on a routine basis has not been established. Likewise, the utility of monoclonal antibodies and gene rearrangement studies in patients with lymphomas to distinguish reactive mesothelial or lymphocytic cells from malignant cells has yet to be determined. The routine use of a "panel of tumor markers" is costly and time consuming.

4.   Pleural biopsy may be helpful in establishing the diagnosis in up to 20% of patients for whom the pleural fluid cytology results are negative.

5.   Thoracotomy or pleuroscopy with direct biopsy may be done in patients who have negative cytology and pleural biopsy results but in whom there is still high suspicion of malignancy.

C.   Treatment. As malignant pleural effusions are generally a sign of systemic rather than localized disease, the best therapy is treatment that effectively treats the malignancy systemically. Unfortunately, effective systemic treatment is often not possible, particularly when the malignancy is commonly refractory to systemic treatment (e.g., in non–small cell carcinoma of the lung) or in patients who have previously been heavily treated and in whom systemic therapy is no longer effective. In these circumstances, locoregional therapy is required for palliation of the patient's symptoms.

1.   Drainage. Many malignant pleural effusions recur within 1 to 3 days after simple thoracentesis; about 97% recur within 1 month. Chest tube drainage (closed tube thoracotomy) allows the pleural surfaces to oppose each other and, if maintained for several days, may result in obliteration of the space and improvement in the effusion for several weeks to months. It does not appear to be as effective when used alone as when a cytotoxic or sclerosing agent is added, and therefore, one of these agents is commonly instilled into the space while the chest tube is in place.

2.   Cytotoxic and sclerosing agents. The most widely used agents for intrapleural administration are bleomycin, doxycycline, and talc. Other agents including fluorouracil, interferon-α, and methylprednisolone acetate have been less commonly used. Recent randomized studies have suggested that bleomycin may be more effective than doxycycline (in part because doxycycline sometimes requires multiple dose administrations) and that talc is either equal to or slightly better than bleomycin in terms of recurrence. The agents vary in toxicity, ease of administration, and cost. Additionally, institutional experience often determines the agent utilized. Nevertheless, for optimal effectiveness, drainage of pleural fluid as completely as possible is required before instillation.

    a.   Method of administration. The drug to be used is diluted in 50 to 100 mL of saline and instilled through the thoracostomy tube into the chest cavity after the effusion has been drained for at least 24 h and the rate of collection is less than 100 mL/24 h. Throughout the procedure, care must be taken to avoid any air leak. The thoracostomy tube is clamped, and the patient is successively repositioned on his or her front, back, and sides for 15-min periods during the next 2 to 6 h. The tube is then reconnected to gravity drainage or suction for at least 18 h to ensure that the pleural surfaces remain opposed and to prevent the rapid accumulation of any fluid in reaction to the instillation. Some clinicians repeat the instillation daily for a total of 2 to 3 days. For most of the agents, this has no proven benefit. Exceptions include methylprednisolone acetate and doxycycline, which appear to be more effective with additional doses. If the drainage is less than 40 to 50 mL over the previous 12 h, the tube may be removed and a chest radiograph obtained to be certain that pneumothorax has not occurred during removal of the tube. If the thoracostomy tube continues to drain more than 100 mL/24 h after the last instillation, it may be necessary to leave it in place for an additional 48 to 72 h to ensure that a maximum amount of adhesion between the pleural surfaces has taken place. Because the use of sclerotic agents can be painful, it is prudent for the clinician to consider the use of scheduled narcotic analgesia, particularly during the initial 24 h.

    b.   Recommended agents. Efficacy, side effects, cost, and institutional (operator) experience must be considered when choosing a sclerosing agent. Bleomycin, in one prospective study, was shown to be more effective than tetracycline. It is also more expensive per dose than the other agents. Talc is the least expensive, but this must be balanced against the costs of related procedures, including thoracoscopy and anesthesia. A recent prospective study showed talc to be superior to bleomycin in terms of recurrence rate of effusions at 90 days and later.

    (1)   Bleomycin 1 mg/kg or 40 mg/m^2 has relatively little myelosuppressive effect and is highly effective.

    (2)   Talc 5 g is given typically as a powder (poudrage). It is highly effective but requires thoracoscopy and general anesthesia. Rarely, adult respiratory distress syndrome has been reported, primarily with doses greater than 10 g.

(3) **Doxycycline** 500 mg may cause pleuritic chest pain. An injection of 10 mL of 1% lidocaine (100 mg) through the chest tube may reduce this symptom.

c. **Alternative agents**

(1) **Fluorouracil** 2 to 3 g (total dose) may have a theoretical advantage in sensitive carcinomas, but whether that advantage is significant has not yet been established. Pain is generally minimal. Occasional patients may experience a depressed white blood cell count, especially at the higher dose.

(2) **Interferon-α** 50×10^6 U typically causes influenza-like symptoms. Lower doses appear to be ineffective. Patients treated with interferon should be premedicated with acetaminophen 650 mg before administration and then repeated in 6 h. Meperidine 25 mg IV by slow push may be given for rigors from interferon.

(3) **Methylprednisolone acetate** 80 to 160 mg appears to be well tolerated.

d. **Responses.** A combination of chest tube drainage and instillation of one of the agents discussed in Section I.C.2.b or c controls pleural effusions more than 75% of the time. The durations of response are often short, with a median between 3 and 6 months unless the patient's systemic disease comes under adequate control. In that circumstance, the effusion may not recur for years or at least until the systemic disease once more emerges.

e. **Side effects** common to most agents include chest pain, fever, and occasional hypotension. These effects are usually not severe and may be controlled by standard symptomatic management. Fever after pleurodesis is usually not due to infection.

3. **Thoracotomy and pleural stripping** may be tried subsequently for effusions refractory to medical treatment.

II. Peritoneal effusions

A. **Causes.** Malignant peritoneal effusions usually occur in association with diffuse seeding of the peritoneal surface with small malignant deposits. The impairment of subphrenic lymphatic or portal venous flow may result in peritoneal effusions. Alternatively, it has been postulated that a "capillary leak" phenomenon mediated by tumor cells or immune effector cells could be a contributing factor. Carcinoma of the ovary is the most commonly associated malignancy in women, whereas in men, gastrointestinal carcinomas are most common. Other neoplasms that may cause peritoneal effusions include carcinoma of unknown primary, lymphoma, mesothelioma, and carcinomas of the uterus and breast. Liver metastasis by itself, unless it is far advanced, is not usually associated with symptomatic peritoneal effusions.

B. **Diagnosis**

1. **Symptoms and signs.** Patients may be completely symptom-free or have so much fluid that they have severe abdominal distention, abdominal pain, and respiratory distress. In the presence of peritoneal metastases, there may be abnormal bowel motility that at times resembles a paralytic ileus and may result in loss of appetite, early satiety, nausea,

and vomiting. On examination, the lower abdomen and flanks bulge when the patient is supine. Confirmatory signs include shifting dullness, a fluid wave, diminished bowel sounds, or the "puddle sign" (periumbilical dullness when the patient rests on knees and elbows).

2. Radiographic studies. Ascites may be suggested on a recumbent film of the abdomen, although radiographs are less sensitive than computed tomography (CT) or ultrasound in detecting fluid. CT is also helpful in defining whether there are enlarged retroperitoneal nodes, tumor masses in the abdomen or pelvis, or liver metastases in association with the ascites.

3. Paracentesis is used to distinguish malignancy from other causes of peritoneal effusions, including congestive heart failure, hepatic cirrhosis, and peritonitis. Malignant cells are found in about half of patients in whom the effusion is due to malignancy. Other tests are less reliable, and treatment decisions must often be based on incomplete data. Elevated LDH and protein levels, along with a negative gram stain and cultures, are supportive but nonspecific for malignancy. The use of monoclonal antibodies to identify tumor cells is still experimental.

C. Therapy. As with malignant pleural effusions, malignant peritoneal effusions as a rule are optimally treated with effective systemic therapy. (The possible exception to this is peritoneal effusions from carcinoma of the ovary. In this circumstance, there may be advantage to IP therapy because most systemic disease is on the peritoneal surface.) If the patient is resistant to all further systemic treatment, regional treatment should be tried, but the likelihood of success is less and the complications greater with peritoneal effusions than with pleural effusions. Success probably is less because of the greater likelihood of loculations to areas inaccessible to therapy and the impossibility of obliterating the peritoneal space in the same way that the pleural space can be obliterated. Complications are greater because of the increase in adhesions caused by instillation therapy and the resultant increase in obstructive bowel problems.

1. Paracentesis may be helpful in acutely relieving intraabdominal pressure. If the ascites has caused impairment of respiration, paracentesis may give temporary relief. Rapid withdrawal of large volumes of fluid (more than 1 L) can result in hypotension and shock, however, and if frequent paracenteses are performed, severe hypoalbuminemia and electrolyte imbalance may result. Repeated procedures could also subject the patient to increased risk of peritonitis or bowel injury. This procedure thus results in only temporary benefit.

2. Bed rest and dietary salt restriction, although helpful in the treatment of various nonmalignant causes of ascites, are of less benefit in malignant ascites.

3. Diuretics may be helpful in reducing ascites, but care must be taken not to be too vigorous in attempts at diuresis because of the possibility of dehydration and hypotension. A reasonable choice of diuretic is a combination of either furosemide 40 mg or hydrochlorothiazide 50 to 100 mg/day and spironolactone 50 to 100 mg/day.

4. Intracavitary therapy. Radioisotopes, cytotoxic drugs, and sclerosing agents have been used with some benefit for treating malignant ascites, but overall probably fewer than half of patients have a satisfactory response. The utility of these agents has less to do with direct tumor cytotoxicity and more with the induction of a local inflammatory response with subsequent sclerosis. The radioactive isotopes gold-198 and phosphorus-32 should be used only by those with experience and appropriate certification. Cytotoxic agents such as fluorouracil are associated with less risk to the person administering the therapy.

　a. Method. The peritoneal fluid should be drained slowly through a Tenckhoff catheter over a 24- to 36-h period. The potential distribution of the therapeutic agent can be determined by instilling ^{99m}Tc-glucoheptonate macroaggregated albumin in 50 mL of saline and obtaining an abdominal scintigram. Two liters of warmed 1.5% peritoneal dialysate solution is instilled, allowed to remain for 2 h, and then drained. The chemotherapeutic agent is next mixed with 2 L of fresh 1.5% dialysate solution containing 1,000 U of heparin/L. After warming, this solution is instilled through the Tenckhoff catheter. For some agents, draining after 4 h is recommended.

　b. Agents

　　(1) Cisplatin 50 to 100 mg/m^2 (especially for carcinoma of the ovary). Drainage is optional. Saline diuresis is recommended. Dosages higher than 100 mg/m^2 should not be used without protection by IV sodium thiosulfate. Cisplatin is repeated every 3 weeks.

　　(2) Fluorouracil 1,000 mg (total dose) in normal saline with 25 mEq of sodium bicarbonate/L. Drainage is optional. Treatment is given on days 1 to 4 monthly.

　　(3) Mitoxantrone 10 mg/m^2. Drainage is optional. This dose has been administered on a weekly basis, although white blood cell counts must be monitored.

　　(4) Interferon-α 50 × 10^6 U (for ovarian cancer). Drainage is optional. This dose has been administered weekly for 4 weeks or longer. Patients should be premedicated with acetaminophen before and every 4 h on the day of therapy.

　　(5) Floxuridine (FUDR) 3 g in 1.5 to 2 L of normal saline given daily for 3 days every 3 to 4 weeks has been used in colon, gastric, and ovarian cancer.

　　(6) Other agents that have been used IP include carboplatin, methotrexate, cytosine arabinoside, etoposide, bleomycin, thiotepa, and doxorubicin. High-dose interleukin-2 (IL-2) with lymphokine-activated killer cells has shown activity in ovarian and colorectal cancer but at the cost of significant toxicity, including peritoneal fibrosis, which in general has prevented the administration of more than one or two cycles. Lower-dose IL-2, 6 × 10^6 IU, on days 1 and 7 has been used successfully.

5. Peritoneal–venous shunts (Denver shunt, LeVeen shunt) may offer palliative relief for refractory ascites because recurrent paracentesis leads to infection and leakage of peritoneal fluid through the paracentesis sites. Potential disadvantages are shunt occlusion, the systemic dissemination of cancer, and disseminated intravascular coagulation.

III.   Pericardial effusions. Although 5% to 10% of patients dying with disseminated malignancy have cardiac or pericardial metastases, far fewer have symptomatic pericardial effusion. However, although malignant pericardial effusions are not particularly common, they are of great importance because of their potential to cause acute cardiac tamponade and death.

A.   Causes. The most common neoplasms causing pericardial effusions are carcinomas of the lung and breast, lymphomas, and melanoma.

B.   Diagnosis

1.   Clinical diagnosis. Patients with developing cardiac tamponade may exhibit a variety of grave symptoms including extreme anxiety, dyspnea, orthopnea, precordial chest pain, cough, and hoarseness. On examination, they are likely to have engorged neck veins, generalized edema, tachycardia, distant heart tones, lateral displacement of the cardiac apex, a low systolic blood pressure and low pulse pressure, and a paradoxical pulse. They may also have tachypnea and a pericardial friction rub.

2.   Electrocardiogram (ECG) may show nonspecific low-voltage, T-wave abnormalities, elevation of ST segments, and ventricular alternans or the more specific total electrical alternans. Premature beats and atrial fibrillation also occur.

3.   Chest radiograph typically shows an enlarged cardiac silhouette, often with a bulging appearance suggestive of an effusion ("water-bottle heart"). There is frequently an associated pleural effusion.

4.   Echocardiography can confirm the diagnosis and provide important information on the location of the effusion within the pericardium.

5.   Pericardiocentesis reveals neoplastic cells on cytologic examination in more than 75% of patients.

C.   Treatment

1.   Volume expansion and vasopressor support are applied (if necessary) to maintain blood pressure. Adequate oxygenation must be maintained. Diuretics are contraindicated.

2.   Pericardiocentesis under ECG and blood pressure monitoring should be done in emergent circumstances. If the patient can be stabilized or in cases of pericardial effusion without tamponade, pericardiocentesis under two-dimensional ECG is preferable because it significantly reduces the incidence of cardiac laceration, arrhythmia, and tension pneumothorax as a complication of the procedure.

3.   Instillation of chemotherapeutic or sclerosing agents. Because pain may be associated with the intrapericardial therapy, lidocaine (Xylocaine) 100 mg may be administered intrapericardially as a local anesthetic. (Check with the cardiologist on the safety for each patient.) After the cytotoxic or sclerosing agent is instilled, the pericardial catheter is clamped for 1 to 2 h and then allowed to drain. One of the following agents may be used:

   a.   Fluorouracil 500 to 1,000 mg in aqueous solution as supplied commercially. This dose is generally not repeated.
   b.   Thiotepa 25 mg/m^2 in 10 mL of normal saline may be preferred in tumor deemed sensitive to alkylating agents. Myelosuppression may occur. The dose is usually not repeated.
      Complications of intrapericardial therapy include arrhythmias, pain, and fever.
4.   Radiotherapy with radioisotopes or 2,000 to 4,000 cGy of external-beam therapy may help control effusions.
5.   Systemic chemotherapy (with standard regimens) after pericardiocentesis is a possible alternative for newly diagnosed, potentially responsive malignancies such as lymphomas. Chemotherapy, intrapericardial or systemic, or radiotherapy controls the effusion for at least 30 days in 60% to 70% of patients. If they are ineffective,
6.   Surgery to create a pericardial window may be necessary and can be effective for several months. It is not recommended, however, unless simpler measures fail.
IV.   Malignant subarachnoid infiltrates
A.   Causes. Leptomeningeal involvement with non–central nervous system cancer is an uncommon complication of most neoplasms, although in children with acute lymphocytic leukemia who have not received prophylactic treatment, the incidence approaches 50%. Of the nonleukemic diseases, breast carcinoma and lymphomas (primarily Burkitt's and T-cell lymphoblastic) account for about 30% each in cases of malignant subarachnoid infiltrates. Carcinoma of the lung and melanoma account for 10% to 12% each.
B.   Diagnosis
   1.   Clinical diagnosis. Patients commonly present with headache, change in mental status, cranial nerve dysfunction, or spinal root–derived pain, paresthesia, or weakness. Any onset of change in neurologic status, particularly of cerebral, cranial nerve, or spinal root origin, should alert the clinician to the possibility of subarachnoid infiltrates.
   2.   Diagnostic studies
      a.   CT of the head should be done to look for any intracranial mass. If none is present, a lumbar puncture should be done.
      b.   A lumbar puncture is done, and the following are evaluated or performed:

   * Opening pressure
   * Cytology of centrifugal specimen for malignant cells
   * Total cell count and differential
   * Cerebrospinal fluid (CSF) chemistry, including glucose and protein
   * Microbiologic studies: India ink or cryptococcal antigen determination, gram stain, cultures (routine, acid-fast, fungi), and special studies as indicated by the clinical situation

      c.   Magnetic resonance imaging or myelography with computed tomography follow-up is performed if signs or symptoms of cord compression are present.

C.   Treatment. Malignant subarachnoid infiltrates may be treated with radiotherapy, intrathecal chemotherapy, or a combination of the two.

1.   Radiotherapy. The radiation field is usually limited to the most involved field (frequently the brain), and intrathecal chemotherapy is used to control the infiltrates elsewhere. This technique is used even though the entire neuraxis is usually involved because total craniospinal irradiation causes severe myelosuppression, which limits the patient's tolerance to concurrent or subsequent cytotoxic chemotherapy.

2.   Chemotherapy may be administered by lumbar puncture or preferably into a surgically implanted (Ommaya) reservoir that communicates with the lateral ventricle. The latter has the advantages of being easily accessible in patients who require repeated treatments and of giving a better distribution of drug than can be obtained through lumbar puncture. When the Ommaya reservoir is used, a volume of CSF equal to that to be injected (6 to 10 mL) should be removed through the reservoir with a small-caliber needle. The chemotherapy should then be given as a slow injection. When the chemotherapy is given through lumbar puncture, the volume of injection (usually 7 to 10 mL) should be greater than that of the CSF withdrawn, so as to have a higher closing than opening pressure. This method facilitates distribution of the drug and minimizes post–lumbar puncture headache. The most commonly used drugs for intrathecal therapy are the following:

a.   Methotrexate 12 mg/m^2 (maximum 15 mg) twice weekly until the CSF clears of malignant cells, then monthly.

b.   Cytarabine 30 mg/m^2 (maximum 50 mg) twice weekly until the CSF clears of malignant cells, then monthly.

c.   Liposomal cytarabine 50 mg (total dose) is given every 14 days for 2 doses. If the CSF clears, give 50 mg every 14 days for two additional doses. Then give 50 mg every 4 weeks for two additional doses (total of six doses).

d.   Thiotepa 2 to 10 mg/m^2 twice weekly until the CSF clears of malignant cells, then monthly.

Each of the agents is given in preservative-free saline or, if available, buffered preservative-free diluent similar to Elliot's B solution. Any subsequent flush solution should be of similar composition. **Other drugs used to treat effusions (e.g., fluorouracil, mechlorethamine, or radioisotopes) must not be used to treat meningeal disease.**

D.   Response to treatment. Most patients with meningeal leukemia or lymphoma respond to a combination of radiotherapy and intrathecal chemotherapy. Carcinomas are less likely to improve, but mild to moderate improvement may be seen in up to 50% of patients.

E.   Complications. Aseptic meningitis or arachnoiditis, seizures, acute encephalopathy, myelopathy, leukoencephalopathy, and radicular neuropathy may result from intrathecal chemotherapy with or without radiotherapy. Bone marrow suppression is not usually severe unless the patient undergoes spinal irradiation or systemic chemotherapy as well. Oral leucovorin can be given after the intrathecal methotrexate (10 mg leucovorin PO every 6 h for six to eight doses, starting either at the same time or 24 h after the methotrexate) to prevent marrow toxicity. Serious complications are infrequent, however, and in patients with advanced metastatic disease, they usually are not a major problem.

SELECTED READINGS

Pleural Effusions

Andrews CO, Gora W. Pleural effusions: pathophysiology and management. *Ann Pharmacother* 1994;28:894–903.

Chernow B, Sahn SA. Carcinomatous involvement of the pleura: an analysis of 96 patients. *Am J Med* 1977;63:695.

de Campos JR, Vargas FS, de Campos Werebe E, et al. Thoracoscopy talc poudrage: a 15-year experience. *Chest* 2001;119:801–806.

Diacon AH, Wyser C, Bollinger CT, et al. Prospective randomized comparison of thoracoscopic talc poudrage under local anesthesia versus bleomycin instillation for pleurodesis in malignant pleural effusions. *Am J Respir Crit Care Med* 2000;162:1445–1449.

Fuller DK. Bleomycin versus doxycyclines: a patient-oriented, approach to pleurodesis. *Ann Pharmacother* 1993;27:794.

Goldman CA, Skinnider LF, Maksymiuk AW. Interferon instillation for malignant pleural effusions. *Ann Oncol* 1993;4:141–145.

Hamed H, Fentiman IS, Chaudary MA, et al. Comparison of intracavitary bleomycin and talc for control of pleural effusions secondary to carcinoma of the breast. *Br J Surg* 1989;76:1266–1267.

Herrington JD. Chemical pleurodesis, with doxycycline 1 g. *Pharmacotherapy* 1996;16:290–295.

Johnson WW. The malignant pleural effusion: a review of cytopathologic diagnoses of 584 specimens from 472 consecutive patients. *Cancer* 1985;56:905.

Kessinger A, Wigton RS. Intracavitary bleomycin and tetracycline in the management of malignant pleural effusions: a randomized study. *J Surg Oncol* 1997;36:81–83.

Ostrowski MJ. Intracavitary therapy with bleomycin for the treatment of malignant pleural effusions. *J Surg Oncol (Suppl)* 1989;1:7–13.

Patz EF Jr, McAdams HP, Erasmus JJ, et al. Sclerotherapy for malignant pleural effusions: a prospective randomized trial of bleomycin vs. doxycyline with small-bore catheter drainage. *Chest* 1998;113:1305–1311.

Surland LG, Weisberger AS. Intracavitary 5-fluorouracil in malignant effusions. *Arch Intern Med* 1965;116:431.

Van Hoff DD, LiVolsi V. Diagnostic reliability of needle biopsy of the parietal pleura: a review of 272 biopsies. *Am J Clin Pathol* 1975;64:200.

Walker-Renard PB, Vaughan LM, Sahn SA. Chemical pleurodesis for malignant pleural effusions. *Ann Intern Med* 1994;120:56–64.

Weissberg D. Bleomycin and talc for control of pleural effusions. *Br J Surg* 1990;77:955.

Peritoneal Effusions

Baker AR. Treatment of malignant ascites. In: DeVita S, Hellman, Rosenberg SA, eds. *Cancer: principles and practice of oncology*. 3rd ed. Philadelphia: Lippincott, 1989:2317.

Berek JS, Hacker NF, Lichtenstein A, et al. Intraperitoneal recombinant alpha-interferon for "salvage" immunotherapy in stage III epithelial ovarian cancer. A Gynecologic Oncology Group study. *Semin Oncol* 1986;13(suppl 2):61.

Lacy JH, Wieman TJ, Shivley EH. Management of malignant ascites. *Surg Gynecol Obstet* 1984;159:397.

Leichman L, Silberman H, Leichman CG, et al. Preoperative systemic chemotherapy followed by adjuvant postoperative intraperitoneal therapy for gastric cancer: a University of Southern California pilot program. *J Clin Oncol* 1992;10:1933–1942.

Lissoni P, Mandala M, Curigliano G, et al. Progress report on the palliative therapy of 100 patients with neoplastic effusions by intracavitary low-dose interleukin-2. *Oncology* 2001;60:308–312.

Markman M, Hakes T, Reichman B, et al. Phase II trial of weekly or biweekly intraperitoneal mitoxantrone in epithelial ovarian cancer. *J Clin Oncol* 1991;9:978–982.

Muggia FM, Jeffers S, Muderspach L, et al. Phase I/II study of intraperitoneal floxuridine and platinums (cisplatin and/or carboplatin). *Gynecol Oncol* 1997;66:290–294.

Muggia FM, Liu PY, Alberts DS, et al. Intraperitoneal mitoxantrone or floxuridine: effects on time-to-failure and survival in patients with minimal residual ovarian cancer after second-look laparotomy: a randomized phase II study by the Southwest Oncology Group. *Gynecol Oncol* 1996;61:395–402.

Nicoletto MO, Fiorentino MW, Viante O, et al. Experience with intraperitoneal alpha2a interferon. *Oncology* 1992;49:467–473.

Speyer JL, Beller U, Colombo N, et al. Intraperitoneal carboplatin: favorable results in women with minimal residual ovarian cancer after cisplatin therapy. *J Clin Oncol* 1990;8:1335–1341.

Steis RG, Urba WJ, VanderMolen LA, et al. Intraperitoneal lymphokine-activated killer cell and interleukin-2 therapy for malignancies limited to the peritoneal cavity. *J Clin Oncol* 1990;8:1618–1629.

Sugarbaker PH, Gianola FJ, Speyer JC, et al. Prospective, randomized trial of intravenous versus intraperitoneal 5-fluorouracil in patients with advanced primary colon or rectal cancer. *Surgery* 1985;95:414.

Pericardial Effusions

Buzaid AC, Garewal HS, Greenberg BR. Managing malignant pericardial effusion. *West J Med* 1989;150:174–179.

Callahan JA, Seward JB, Nishimura RA, et al. Two-dimensional echocardiographically guided pericardiocentesis: experience in 117 consecutive patients. *Am J Cardiol* 1985;55:476–479.

Helms SR, Carlson MD. Cardiovascular emergencies. *Semin Oncol* 1989;16:463.

Liu G, Crump M, Gross PE, et al. Prospective comparison of the sclerosing agents doxycycline and bleomycin for the primary management of malignant pericardial effusion and cardiac tamponade. *J Clin Oncol* 1996;14:3141–3147.

Maher ER, Buckman R. Intrapericardial installation of bleomycin in malignant pericardial effusion. *Am Heart J* 1986;111:613–614.

Shepherd FA, Ginsberg JS, Evans WK, et al. Tetracycline sclerosis in the management of pericardial effusion. *J Clin Oncol* 1985;3:1678–1682.

Malignant Subarachnoid Infiltrates

Glantz MJ, Jaeckle KA, Chamberlain MC, et al. A randomized controlled trial comparing intrathecal sustained-release cytarabine (Depocyt) to intrathecal methotrexate in patients with neoplastic meningitis from solid tumors. *Clin Cancer Res* 1999;5:3394–3402.

Gutin PH, Levi JA, Wiernik PH, et al. Treatment of malignant meningeal disease with intrathecal thiotepa: a phase II study. *Cancer Treat Rep* 1977;61:885–887.

Jaeckle KA, Phuphanich S, van den Bent MJ, et al. Intrathecal treatment of neoplastic meningitis due to breast cancer with a slow-release formulation of cytarabine. *Br J Cancer* 2001;84:157–163.

Olson ME, Chernik NL, Posner JB. Infiltration of the leptomeninges by systemic cancer. *Arch Neurol* 1974;30:122–137.

Managing Cancer Pain

Michael J. Fisch and Charles S. Cleeland

Patients should not suffer needlessly from cancer pain. Most pain from cancer can be adequately controlled with analgesics given by mouth. When this is not possible, a variety of more sophisticated pain management techniques can provide good pain control. It is estimated that about 85% of patients could be free of significant pain with the techniques we have available today. Unfortunately, many patients do not benefit from adequate pain control. Estimates based on surveys in the United States indicate that less than half of all patients with cancer obtain optimal pain control. Poorly controlled pain has such catastrophic effects on the quality of life of patients and their families that proper management of pain must have the highest priority for those who take care of patients with cancer. For example, symptoms such as depressed mood, fatigue, anorexia, and sleep disturbance are associated with poor pain control. Indeed, overall performance status and adherence to anticancer treatment regimens may deteriorate in the presence of persistent severe pain. Desperate patients and families may seek relief through alternative or complementary medicine or even from physician-assisted suicide. Improving the practice of anticipating, evaluating, and treating pain will benefit most patients.

I. Prevalence, severity, and risk for pain. Most cancer patients with terminal disease need expert pain management; between 60% and 80% of such patients have significant pain. Pain is also a problem for many patients much earlier in the course of their disease. Patients with months or years to live may be compromised by poorly controlled pain. Sometimes chronic pain will be expressed by the patient in confusing terms ("stiffness," "nagging") or masquerade as some other symptoms (fatigue, apathy, anxiety, anorexia). For this reason, the estimates of the prevalence and impact of chronic pain in this population are probably conservative. Nevertheless, in the United States, 60% of all outpatients with metastatic disease have cancer-related pain, and one-third report pain so severe that it significantly impairs their quality of life. Multicenter studies indicate that about 40% of outpatients with cancer pain do not receive analgesics potent enough to manage their pain. Minority patients, female patients, and older patients are at greater risk for poorly controlled pain.

II. Etiology of cancer pain

A. Direct tumor involvement is the most common cause of pain, present in about two-thirds of those with pain from metastatic cancer. Tumor invasion of bone is the physical basis of pain in about 50% of these patients. The remaining 50% of these patients experience tumor-related pain that is due to nerve compression or infiltration or involvement of the gastrointestinal tract or soft tissue.

B. Persistent posttreatment pain, from long-term effects of surgery, radiotherapy, and chemotherapy, accounts for an additional 20% of all who report pain with metastatic cancer, with a small residual group experiencing pain from non–cancer-related conditions.

C. Complex, chronic pain. Most patients with advanced cancer have **pain at multiple sites** caused by multiple mechanisms. Pain **production** occurs either by stimulation of peripheral pain receptors or by damage to afferent nerve fibers. Peripheral pain receptors can be stimulated by pressure, compression, and traction as well as by disease-related chemical changes. Pain due to stimulation of pain receptors is called *nociceptive pain*. Damage to visceral, somatic, or autonomic nerve trunks produces *neurogenic* or *neuropathic pain*. Neuropathic pain is thought to be caused by spontaneous activity in nerves damaged by disease or treatment. Patients with cancer often have nociceptive and neuropathic pain simultaneously. In addition to evaluating the broad possible causes of pain production, the evaluating clinician should also consider the relevant mechanisms of pain **perception** and **expression** (see Fig. 31-1). Pain perception refers to the transmission of the nociception to the central nervous system (CNS). Peripheral nerve fibers include myelinated Aδ fibers that are responsible for the transmission of sharp pain and unmyelinated C fibers that carry dull and burning pain. These primary sensory afferents have their cell bodies in the dorsal horn, where the pathways decussate and ascend along the spinothalamic tracts to the thalamus and cortex. Repetitive or continuous stimulation of the peripheral nerves can increase the excitability of the secondary neurons and spread the neurologic region of pain perception and transmission. The N-methyl-D-aspartate (NMDA) receptor is involved in the neurobiology of this "wind-up" phenomenon as well as in the development of tolerance to opioid analgesics. Understanding this

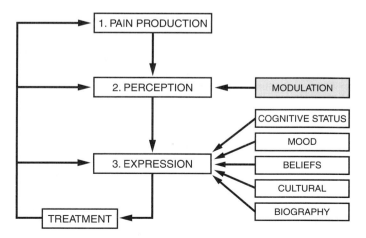

Fig. 31-1. Schema of the pain construct. (Courtesy of Dr. Eduardo Bruera).

biology of pain perception helps one account for the observation that some patients experience pain that endures even after the tumor or injury has resolved, and sometimes the pain is more severe than one might expect from the nerve or tissue insult itself. Of course, the clinician can directly observe only pain expression; the production and perception of the pain can only be inferred from indirect clues. Pain expression can be influenced by multiple factors (mood, cultural beliefs, etc.). For this reason, effective pain assessment and management require a comprehensive understanding of the patient as a person.

III. Assessment of pain. Proper pain management requires a clear understanding of the characteristics of pain production, perception, and expression as described above. The changing expression of cancer pain demands repeated assessment because new causes of pain can emerge rapidly and pain severity can increase quickly. In patients with advanced disease, pain from multiple causes is the rule and not the exception. A careful history includes questions concerning the location, severity, and quality of the pain as well as the aspects of the patient's daily routine that may be adversely affected by the pain experience.

A. Pain severity. Inadequate pain assessment and poor physician–patient communication about pain are major barriers to good pain care. Physicians and nurses tend to underestimate pain intensity, especially when it is severe. Patients whose physicians underestimate their pain are at high risk for poor pain management and compromised function. A small minority of patients with cancer may complain of pain in a dramatic fashion, but many more patients underreport the severity of their pain and the lack of adequate pain relief.

Several studies have confirmed that there are multiple reasons for this reluctance to report pain, including the following:

- Not wanting to acknowledge that the disease is progressing
- Not wanting to divert the physician's attention from treating the disease
- Not wanting to tell the physician that pain treatments are not working
- Patients may not want to be put on opioid analgesics because of the following reasons:
  - Not wanting to become addicted
  - Fearing the psychoactive components of opioids
  - Being concerned that using opioids "too early" will endanger pain relief when they have more pain
  - Fearing that being placed on opioids signals that death is near
  - Having accepted religious or societal norms or teachings that pain should be endured

Presenting information that addresses these concerns in a straightforward manner will allay most of these fears and should be considered as an essential step in providing pain control. It is important that patients understand that they will function better if their pain is controlled. Patient education materials available from state cancer pain initiatives and from the National Cancer Institute, American Cancer Society (ACS), the National Comprehensive Cancer Network (NCCN), and the Agency for

Health Care Policy and Research (AHCPR) can be very useful for both patients and families and should be given to patients when they develop pain.

Communication about pain is greatly aided by having patients use a scale to rate the severity of their pain. A simple rating scale ranges from 0 to 10, with 0 being "no pain" and 10 being pain "as bad as you can imagine." Used properly, pain severity scales can be invaluable in titrating analgesics and in monitoring for increases in pain with progressive disease. Mild pain is often well tolerated with minimal impact on a patient's activities. However, there is a threshold beyond which pain is especially disruptive. This threshold has been reached when patients rate the severity of their pain at 5 or greater on a 0 to 10 scale. When pain is too great (7 or greater on this scale), it becomes the primary focus of attention and prohibits most activity not directly related to pain. Although it may not be possible to eliminate pain totally, reducing its severity to 4 or less ought to be a minimum standard of pain therapy.

In some instances, patients may develop chronically high levels of pain expression that do not respond to appropriate analgesic dosing and/or invasive pain procedures. The proper care of this small set of patients often requires a multidisciplinary approach and includes regular administration of pain medication plus counseling and sometimes use of antidepressants or anxiolytic agents. In such cases, the focus of the clinician tends to be on the functional outcome of treatment, and the patient's expression of pain intensity is less useful.

B. Diagnostic steps. Those who treat patients with cancer should be familiar with the common pain syndromes associated with the disease:

1. Having the patient show the area of pain on a drawing of a human figure aids identification of the syndrome. This can be particularly helpful in indicating areas of referred pain, common with nerve compression.

2. Careful questioning concerning the characteristics of the pain is essential for physical diagnosis. For example, pain characterized as "burning" or "shooting" may indicate neuropathic pain.

3. In addition to severity, these characteristics include the temporal pattern of the pain (constant or episodic) and its quality. Episodic or "incident" pain (such as severe pain when standing) requires a different strategy for management compared with chronic pain.

4. Other important characteristics of pain are its relationship to physical activity and what seems to alleviate the pain.

5. The physical examination includes examination of the painful area as well as neurologic and orthopedic assessment. A brief assessment of mood and cognition is also appropriate. Impaired cognition can confound symptom assessment dramatically.

6. Because bone metastases are a common cause of pain and pain can occur with changes in bone density not detectable on radiographs, bone scans can be helpful. Magnetic resonance imaging (MRI) is useful in the evaluation of retroperi-

toneal, paravertebral, and pelvic areas as well as the base of the skull.
7. Diagnostic nerve blocks can provide information concerning the pain pathway. Diagnostic blocks can also determine the potential effectiveness of neuroablative procedures that destroy the pain pathway. Nerve blocks are difficult to study in a controlled fashion, and for that reason, there is significant variation in the practice patterns of pain specialists with regard to the use of nerve blocks and other interventional pain procedures.

C.   The impact of pain on the patient. When pain is of moderate or greater severity, we can assume that it has a negative impact on the patient's quality of life. That impact, including problems with sleep and depression, must be evaluated and treated when appropriate. A reduced number of hours of sleep compared with the last pain-free interval, difficulties with sleep onset, frequent interruptions of sleep, and early morning awakening suggest the need for appropriate pharmacologic intervention. Just as patients hesitate to report severe pain, they may hesitate to report depression. Family caregivers can often provide important clues regarding the presence or absence of a mood disturbance. Significant depression should be treated. Treatment approaches may include use of antidepressants, counseling, and/or referral to a behavioral health specialist. Sometimes a patient will accept only one of the suggested options, thus requiring some degree of flexibility on the part of the clinician in order to achieve the best results.

It is important to make an attempt to differentiate between physical pain and psychological stress. Accurate pain assessment in patients who are cognitively impaired, particularly those with agitation, may be extremely difficult. A small number of patients in severe psychosocial distress express their concerns as a report of physical pain. These patients present with symptoms that may be attributable to either agitated delirium or pain. Although it is important to recognize severe somatization and to provide psychiatric referral or counseling to these patients, it is equally important to recognize true physical pain. Often, the treatment approach for this difficult situation includes both pain medication and treatment of the underlying psychological distress.

D.   The addicted patient. Some patients with severe alcoholism or drug addiction may request analgesics for their psychological effects. This is unlikely to occur in patients without a clear history of severe addictive behavior. Patients who are recovered alcoholics or drug abusers may be difficult to treat because of their resistance to taking analgesics. In any case, if this diagnosis is suspected, the issue should be discussed openly with the patient and an agreement should be reached about the use of opioids for the management of pain as opposed to mood alterations. With this group of patients, long-acting opioids or continuous infusion is preferable to short-acting opioids or patient-controlled analgesia. Prescriptions by a single physician would make the negotiation process with a patient much simpler. Although their care is more complex, patients with drug or alcohol addiction should never be denied appropriate pain medications.

IV. Treatment

A. General aspects. All health care professionals who see patients with cancer should be familiar with standard guidelines for management of cancer pain such as those published by the NCCN or AHCPR. An example of a cancer pain practice guideline is shown in Table 31.1. This guideline incorporates basic principles of cancer pain assessment, initial treatment, and routine management of opioid side effects.

The prompt relief of pain from cancer frequently involves the use of simultaneously rather than serially administered combinations of drug and other adjunctive therapies. Identification of a treatable neoplasm as a factor in pain production calls for appropriate radiotherapy (e.g., to bone metastases), chemotherapy, or, in some instances, surgical debulking. Until such treatment can be effective (this may take days to weeks), the patient's pain must be managed with analgesics. In many instances, analgesics are the only pain treatment available because of the patient's condition, the physical basis of the pain, or limited treatment options. The principles of pharmacologic management of pain are evolving through studies of analgesic effectiveness and research on the use of combinations of palliative medications.

There is a growing consensus concerning the types of drugs to use, their routes of administration, and how best to schedule them. The first step is the choice of analgesic drug to be used (nonopioid, opioid, or a combination of both). The second step is the choice of adjuvant drugs, which can increase analgesic effectiveness and can produce other palliative effects to counter the disruptive consequences of pain.

B. Nonsteroidal anti-inflammatory drugs

1. Mechanism of action and selection of agents. Nonsteroidal anti-inflammatory drugs (NSAIDs) constitute the majority of nonopioid analgesics. Their effect on the inflammatory process is a key to their analgesic property. Tumor growth produces inflammatory and mechanical effects in adjacent tissues that can trigger the release of prostaglandins, bradykinin, and serotonin, which in turn may precipitate or exacerbate pain in the surrounding tissues. Prostaglandin-mediated actions on peripheral receptors probably include both direct activation and sensitization to other analgesic substances. Prostaglandins are frequently associated with painful bone metastasis because of their involvement in bone reabsorption. The NSAIDs appear to exert their analgesic, antipyretic, and anti-inflammatory actions by blocking the synthesis of prostaglandins. Table 31.2 gives the usual starting doses and dose ranges for several commonly used NSAIDs.

By virtue of their different mechanisms of action and toxicity profiles, the NSAIDs and opioids are often administered together. Enteric-coated aspirin is one of the first-choice drugs for mild to moderate cancer pain. Other NSAIDs such as ibuprofen, diflunisal, naproxen, and choline magnesium trisalicylate (Trilisate) have established value in the management of clinical pain. These drugs are better tolerated than aspirin but are usually significantly more expensive. Individual differences in

Table 31.1.   An example of a pain practice guideline

A. Comprehensive pain assessment
   1. Evaluation of pain. Determine level using 0–10 intensity scale, location, onset, duration, frequency, quality (somatic, visceral, neuropathic), history, etiology, associated symptoms, what modifies the pain, side effects associated with treatment of pain, and response to other pain medications.
      No pain (0)   Mild (1–3)   Moderate (4–6)   Severe (7–10)
   2. Evaluation of past medical history (oncologic or other significant medical illnesses) to include medication history
   3. Physical examination
   4. Evaluation of relevant laboratory and imaging studies
   5. Evaluation of risk factors for undertreatment of pain, including underreporting, extremes of age, gender, cultural barriers, communication barriers, and a history of substance abuse
   6. Evaluation of psychosocial issues (patient distress, family support, psychiatric history, special issues relating to pain [meaning of pain for patient/family, patient/family knowledge of and beliefs surrounding pain])
B. Overall management plans
   1. If pain = 0, reassess at each subsequent visit or interaction
   2. Manage pain related to oncologic emergencies, if any
      a. Such pain requires assessment and treatment (e.g., surgery, steroids, radiotherapy, antibiotics) along with an emergent consultation
      b. Oncologic emergencies include
         • Bowel obstruction/perforation
         • Brain metastasis
         • Leptomeningeal metastasis
         • Fracture or impending fracture of weight-bearing bone
         • Epidural metastasis/spinal cord compression
         • Pain related to infection
   3. Manage non-emergency-related pain
C. Management of non-emergency-related pain
   1. If pain = 1–3
      • Nonsteroidal anti-inflammatory drugs (including COX-2 agents) and acetaminophen. If ineffective: opioids (hydrocodone scheduled or as needed)
      • Overall reassessment at each subsequent visit or interaction
   2. If pain = 4–6
      • Oral opioids
      • Morphine 10 mg orally every 4 h as needed or scheduled
      • Oxycodone 5 mg orally every 4 h as needed or scheduled
      • Adjuvants: nonsteroidal anti-inflammatory drugs, antidepressants, antiepileptics, etc.
      • Overall reassessment in 24–48 h

Continued

Table 31.1. *Continued*

3. If pain = 7–10 (possible pain crisis)
- Oral opioids: morphine 20 mg orally every 4 h as needed (opioid naive)
- 30% increase in current opioid regimen (sustained and immediate release [rescue] opioids)
- Morphine, hydromorphone, or oxycodone for rescue dosing
- Consider intravenous opioid titration (PCA pump may be used to titrate)
- Reassess frequently, based on clinical situation

D. Additional steps for pain that was rated 4–10
   1. Re-evaluate opioid titration
   2. Re-evaluate pain diagnosis
   3. Consider consults from specialty services[a]
   4. All patients receiving opioids should begin
   - Bowel regimen (such as oral Senna 1 tablet twice daily)
   - Antiemetics as needed (such as metoclopramide 10 mg 30 min before meals and at bedtime)
   - Educational activities regarding pain management
   - Psychosocial support as needed

E. At the time of re-evaluation for patients whose pain was 4–10
   1. If pain now = 1–3
   - Consider conversion to a sustained-release agent with rescue medications
   - Continue adjuvants or add them as needed
   - Reassess and modify side effects of pain treatment
   - Provide psychosocial support
   - Provide educational activities
   - Reassess pain every week until comfortable, then every visit
   2. If pain now = 4–6
   - Continue opioid titration
   - Consider specific pain problems
   - Consider consults from specialty services[a]
   - Continue psychosocial support
   - Continue educational activities
   3. If pain now = 7–10[b] (possible pain crisis)
   - Continue opioid titration
   - Re-evaluate working diagnosis
   - Consider specific pain problems
   - Obtain consults from specialty services[a]
   - Continue psychosocial support

---

[a] Postoperative Pain Service, Cancer Pain Section, Department of Symptom Control and Palliative Care, or other specialties as needed (i.e., Radiotherapy).
[b] Some patients with chronic pain syndromes will report high pain scores on an ongoing basis. Generally, this situation is not a crisis.
This practice guideline was created by the National Comprehensive Cancer Network (NCCN) and modified by the University of Texas M.D. Anderson Cancer Center under the supervision of Allen Burton, M.D., and Charles Cleeland, Ph.D.

Table 31.2. **Starting doses and dose ranges of some nonsteroidal analgesic agents**

Drug	Starting dose (mg)	Frequency	Dose range
Aspirin	650	q4–6 h	Up to 1,300 mg q6 h
Choline magnesium trisalicylate	500	q6 h	Up to 1,000 mg q6 h
Diflunisal	500	q8–12 h	Up to 1,500 mg daily
Ibuprofen	400	q4–6 h	Up to 2,400 mg daily
Naproxyn	250	q8–12 h	Up to 1,250 mg daily
Piroxicam	10	q12–24 h	Up to 20 mg daily
Tolmetin	400	q8 h	Up to 1,800 mg daily
Rofecoxib[a]	25	q24 h	Up to 50 mg daily
Celecoxib[a]	100	q24 h	Up to 400 mg daily

[a] These agents are COX-2 selective.

analgesic response to the various NSAIDs clearly occur but are not yet well understood.

A new generation of cyclo-oxygenase-2 (COX-2) NSAIDs have become available (rofecoxib and celecoxib). These agents are inhibitors of COX-2, the enzyme expressed in inflamed tissues, and have minimal or no effects on COX-1 (the enzyme expressed normally in the stomach and kidney). These newer NSAID drugs have been widely used because of their once- or twice-daily dosing schedule and the roughly 50% relative reduction in significant gastrointestinal adverse events compared with other NSAIDs. These drugs are considerably more expensive than other NSAIDs, and this can interfere with proper adherence to the medication in some patients. The COX-2 inhibitors have some unique and important drug interactions. Rofecoxib is known to interact with warfarin and causes a roughly 10% increase in the prothrombin time international normalized ratio. Celecoxib does not interact with warfarin, but it is metabolized by the cytochrome P-450 enzyme system (particularly 3A4) in the liver and interacts with other agents that utilize this metabolic pathway. The clinical implication of the difference in the way these drugs are metabolized is that clinicians should consider the potential for drug interactions before choosing a specific COX-2 inhibitor.

Acetaminophen is a peripherally acting analgesic that does not inhibit peripheral prostaglandin synthesis. Therefore, it does not have anti-inflammatory effects or the side effects associated with the use of NSAIDs. Acetaminophen should be considered in patients who have contraindications to the use of NSAIDs.

Commercial preparations containing codeine or oxycodone and acetaminophen or aspirin are among the most widely prescribed scheduled analgesics and are frequently administered to patients with cancer. This is generally appropriate because of the synergistic effects of the combination. Such a combination is reported to be particularly effective for bone pain.

2. Side effects. NSAIDs have a number of potentially serious side effects, including gastritis and gastrointestinal hemorrhage, bleeding due to platelet inhibition, and renal failure. Most of these side effects are related to the prostaglandin-inhibitory effect of these drugs and are therefore common to all these drugs. Renal failure due to the inhibition of renal medullary prostaglandins can be of particular concern in patients who might also be receiving opioids. Decreased renal elimination of active opioid metabolites might result in somnolence, confusion, hallucinations, or generalized myoclonus. Therefore, kidney function should be monitored in patients receiving a combination of NSAIDs and opioids.

Gastrointestinal complications include gastric pain, nausea, vomiting, hemorrhage, and, in extreme cases, perforation. Gastrointestinal damage is mediated by prostaglandin inhibition. The most common form of nephrotoxicity associated with NSAIDs is renal failure, related to prostaglandin inhibition and consequent vasodilation. Hepatic injury has been reported with the use of aspirin, benoxaprofen, and phenylbutazone and, less commonly, with diclofenac, ibuprofen, indomethacin, naproxen, pirprofen, and sulindac. Sulindac, however, appears to be associated with a higher incidence of cholestasis.

NSAID use is also associated with a variety of hypersensitivity reactions involving the skin (rash, eruption, itching), blood vessels (angioneurotic edema, vasomotor disorders), and respiratory system (rhinitis, asthma). In particular, aspirin may cause anaphylactic crisis, a syndrome characterized by dyspnea, sudden weakness, sweating, and collapse. Undesirable hematologic effects of NSAIDs include platelet dysfunction, aplastic anemia, and agranulocytosis. Factors often considered in the empiric selection of an NSAID for a given patient include its relative toxicity, cost, and dosage schedule and the patient's prior experience. The use of certain aspirin analogs (choline magnesium trisalicylate) has been suggested to be associated with a low incidence of gastropathy and platelet dysfunction. The effects of NSAIDs used as single agents in the management of cancer pain are characterized by a ceiling effect, beyond which further increases in dose do not enhance analgesia.

C. Opioid analgesics

1. When to start therapy. The choice of an opioid analgesic as opposed to a nonopioid analgesic follows from an assessment of the severity of pain. The decision is relatively easy when pain is mild (choose nonopioid) or severe (choose opioid, usually in combination with a nonopioid). The choice is more difficult when the patient reports moderate pain, especially when there is reason to suspect that the patient may be underreporting pain severity. Several studies have documented that many patients with cancer are inadequately managed because of the physician's reluctance to use opioids in dosages and with schedules known to be sufficient to relieve moderate pain.

Opioid analgesics should be prescribed promptly as soon as there is evidence that pain is not well controlled with nonopioid analgesics. Usually, nonopioid analgesics can be continued as a way of maximizing analgesia because their site of action is different from that of the opioids.

2.   Schedule of treatment and selection of dose. Except in a minority of patients whose pain is clearly episodic, analgesics should be given on an around-the-clock basis, with the time interval based on the duration of effectiveness of the drug and the patient's report of the duration of effectiveness. There is evidence that total opioid requirement is lower when opioids are given on a scheduled basis, thereby preventing peaks of pain. Putting patients in the position of having to ask for medication or continually making a judgment about whether their pain is severe enough to take analgesics focuses their attention on pain, reminds them of their need for drugs, and allows pain to reach a severity not readily controlled by the same doses that would be effective with scheduled administration. Nevertheless, there may be large individual differences in the required dose of opioid, depending on such factors as the patient's opioid use history, activity level, and metabolism. The patient's report of pain severity and pain relief is the best guideline for opioid titration.

3.   The so-called weak opioids, including codeine and hydrocodone, usually formulated in combination with acetaminophen or aspirin, can provide active patients with good pain relief for long periods of time. As disease advances, oral administration of the more potent opioids provides most patients with pain relief. Recent data demonstrate that oxycodone as a single entity should be considered a potent opioid. There is considerable agreement that propoxyphene is not ideal for chronic use because of its low efficacy at commercially available doses and the presence of a toxic metabolite at higher doses that is a CNS stimulant, has a long serum half-life, and has no analgesic properties. Oral administration is preferred, but the physician must remain flexible to changes that are dictated by the patient's ability to use orally administered drugs. This may include the use of opioid and nonopioid suppositories and other alternative routes of administration (transdermal, sublingual, rectal, subcutaneous).

4.   Oral morphine, either in immediate- or sustained-release preparation, is the analgesic of choice for moderate to severe cancer pain. Long-acting formulations of morphine and other opioids are convenient for both the patient and the health care staff. Immediate-release morphine is much cheaper, however, and is as effective. A typical starting dose for immediate-release oral morphine is 10 to 30 mg every 4 h in patients not currently receiving opioids. When a patient is switching from another opioid (usually codeine or oxycodone) to morphine, it is important to calculate the equianalgesic morphine dose as a basis for determining what morphine-equivalent doses are the threshold for pain control (Table 31.3). The starting dose may not be sufficient, and relatively rapid upward titration may be needed, especially if pain is severe.

The upward titration of morphine and other oral opioid analgesics can be done by giving a supplemental "boost" using 50% of the scheduled dose 2 h after the scheduled dose if there

Table 31.3. Dose equivalence of selected opioids

Drug	Approximate equianalgesic dose	
	Oral	Parenteral
Morphine	30 mg q3–4 h[a]	10 mg q3–4 h
Hydromorphone	4–8 mg q3–4 h	1.5 mg q3–4 h
Levorphanol	4 mg q6–8 h	2 mg q6–8 h
Codeine[b]	130 mg q3–4 h	
Hydrocodone[b]	30 mg q3–4 h	
Oxycodone[b]	20 mg q3–4 h	
Transdermal fentanyl	25-μg/h patch = 8–22 mg/24 h IV or IM morphine sulfate = roughly 50 mg/d of oral morphine sulfate; 50-μg/h patch = roughly 60 mg MS-Contin q12 h	

[a] Slow-release formulations of oral morphine that are available have 8- to 12-h durations of analgesic action.
[b] Codeine, hydrocodone, and oxycodone are often given as combination products with aspirin, acetaminophen, or both.
Adapted from Weissman DE, et al. *Handbook of cancer pain management.* 4th ed. Madison: Wisconsin Cancer Pain Initiative, 1993.

is still significant pain and the patient is not overly sedated or lethargic. The scheduled dose is then set at 150% of the initial scheduled dose. Because of the time it takes to achieve a steady state, there may need to be some readjustment downward if the patient is unduly sleepy or is lethargic at the time of the scheduled dose. The supplemental dose may be given after any scheduled dose (even if there was an increase in the scheduled dose) as long as a sufficient time has passed for the drug to be absorbed from the stomach. An alternative way to titrate is simply to add 50% to the next scheduled dose, but staying with the previously determined schedule (usually every 4 h). When the doses of opioid are higher (e.g., morphine 100 mg every 4 h), some clinicians use less, for example, 20% to 30% (20 to 30 mg) as the boost, but incrementally add to the dose with each scheduled treatment until adequate pain relief has been achieved. Depending on the understanding of the patient and family, it is often best to have the patient check in with a physician or nurse after every other dose increase to be sure the treatment plan is understood, safe, and effective.

5. Long-acting preparations. When an effective dose of short-acting morphine has been established, the required 24-h dose for a long-acting preparation can be calculated. An additional supply of short-acting morphine, given when necessary, will help the patient manage "breakthrough" pain. Consistent need for this additional short-acting morphine (e.g., three or four doses daily) dictates an upward adjustment of the dose of sustained-release drug. Orders for immediate-release morphine should allow for some upward titration of dose by the patient or by the nurse. Each dose of short-acting morphine for breakthrough pain is usually 15% to 20% of the 24-h dose of long-acting morphine. If more than this is required, it is usually an indication for increasing the dose of the long-acting preparation.

6. Although the **opioid agonist–antagonist analgesics** have established effectiveness in the control of acute (especially procedurally related) pain, their use in chronic cancer pain is limited by the possibility of precipitous withdrawal in the patient who has been taking morphine-type drugs, by their analgesic ceiling effect (when the drug does not provide more pain relief), and by the lack of an oral form of administration.

7. **Methadone** is an agonist opioid analgesic that has the advantages of extremely low cost (often 10- to 30-fold less expensive than other strong opioids), efficacy in neuropathic pain, slow development of tolerance, and lack of known active metabolites. Because of its long and unpredictable half-life and relatively unknown equianalgesic dose as compared with other opioids, methadone was generally used by pain specialists with experience in its use. More recently, however, the utility of this agent in cancer pain has become more widely appreciated and it is being used in hospital and hospice settings. The methadone preparation widely used in the United States is a racemic mix of the D-isomer and L-isomer of methadone. The D-isomer has antagonist activity at the NMDA receptor, and this produces clinically relevant benefits in the control of neuropathic pain.

The relative potency of methadone increases with higher morphine-equivalent doses. Thus, when converting from another opioid to methadone, the calculated equianalgesic dose of methadone should be decreased by 75% to 90%. A guideline for choosing an appropriate initial dose of methadone based on the oral morphine-equivalent daily dose of the previous opioid is shown in Table 31.4. For example, a patient who has been using sustained-release morphine at 80 mg every 8 h (240 mg/day) would be appropriately switched to methadone at a dose of 10 mg every 8 h (30 mg/day, an 8:1 conversion ratio). In contrast, a patient who is taking sustained-release morphine at a total daily dose of 60 mg/day might be switched to an oral methadone dose of 5 mg every 8 h (15 mg/day, a 4:1 conversion ratio).

Methadone is available as a pill, an elixir, and for parenteral use. The oral bioavailability of the drug is excellent (50% to 80%). Methadone is roughly twice as potent IV or IM compared with orally. Thus, a patient with well-controlled pain on a stable oral methadone dose of 10 mg every 8 h would be switched to IV methadone at 5 mg every 8 h if necessary. SC use of methadone may cause skin irritation in some patients.

8. **Alternative potent opioids** include levorphanol, which has a longer half-life than morphine, and single-entity oxycodone and hydromorphone, which has a half-life similar to morphine. Equivalent starting doses can be selected from Table 31.3, but if the patient has been on high doses of morphine, care must be taken to reduce the dose to 50% to 75% of the calculated equianalgesic dose to account for incomplete

Table 31.4.   Suggested dosing of oral methadone based on morphine-equivalent daily dose (MEDD)

Oral MEDD (mg/d)	Initial dose ratio (oral morphine/oral methadone)
<30	2:1
30–99	4:1
100–299	8:1
300–499	12:1
500–999	15:1
≥1,000	≥20:1[a]

[a] Great caution must be used when converting to methadone when very high opioid doses have been used. Often, only a portion of the total opioid dose is converted initially, with further conversions taking place over several days to weeks.

cross-tolerance that may increase the relative potency of the newly prescribed agent.

9.   Alternative routes. About 70% of patients benefit from the use of an alternative route for opioid administration sometime before death. The duration for which patients need these routes varies between hours and months. Although intermittent injections can be effective for a brief period of time, this method is painful for the patient, time consuming for the nursing staff, and difficult to manage at home.

a.   Intravenous infusion. A number of studies have shown that IV infusions of opioids produce stable blood levels of drug and that they are safe and effective for treating both postoperative and cancer pain. IV infusion using a patient-controlled analgesia pump may be very effective in gaining rapid control over pain that has gotten out of hand. It may also be of value when the patient cannot take medications orally and does not wish to take suppositories. The main problem associated with continuous IV infusions is the prolonged maintenance of an IV line. Patients may need to be subjected to numerous venipunctures when peripheral IV lines are used. Totally implantable IV catheters represent a major improvement, permitting long-term IV access. However, these catheters are expensive and need to be surgically implanted, and their maintenance requires considerable nursing expertise and patient teaching. If such a catheter is already available in a patient with advanced cancer who has pain, it certainly could be used for the administration of opioids. Starting doses of morphine for severe pain are 2 to 3 mg hourly as a continuous infusion, with patient-controlled boosts of 1 mg every 6 to 15 min. At the end of 24 h, 50% of the patient boosts can be added to the total 24-h dose of the continuous infusion until the patient is requiring less than one boost hourly. At that time, a shift to oral analgesics can be started, if the patient is able to take oral medications. If the doses of IV morphine are high, the shifting to appropriate oral doses may take several days. It is usually safe and effective to give a 24-h dose of long-acting morphine orally that is equal in milligrams (not equianalgesic) to the 24-h requirement IV and simultaneously to reduce the IV dose (continuous infusion rate) by half. Boosts can be given by mouth, but the patient should have the IV boost option as reassurance. The next day, the 24-h IV dose required (continuous plus boosts) can be added orally to the previous day's oral dose (long acting plus short acting) and the infusion further reduced. The same process is repeated until the patient is getting adequate pain relief with the oral morphine. The infusion can usually be stopped and needed boosts given orally by the third or fourth day.

b.   Subcutaneous route. This route has been found to be safe and effective for the administration of morphine and hydromorphone. SC opioids can be administered as a continuous infusion using a pump (use as small a volume as possible, e.g., less than 5 mL/h) or as an intermittent injection. A butterfly needle can be left under the skin for about 7 days, making both intermittent injections and continuous infusion painless. The needles are frequently inserted in the subclavicular region, anterior chest, or abdominal wall. This allows patients to have free limbs.

c.   Rectal route. Most of the experience reported in the literature is with the short-term use of rectal opioids for the management of acute pain. Both solid and liquid solutions have been used. Although there is considerable interindividual variation in the bioavailability of rectally administered morphine, there is general consensus that this drug is well absorbed after rectal administration. A number of authors have treated terminally ill patients with cancer with rectal morphine, with good pain control until death. Advantages of the rectal route include the absence of the need for the insertion of needles and the use of portable pumps. However, rectal administration can be uncomfortable or psychologically distressing for some patients; absorption may be decreased by the presence of stool in the rectum, by diarrhea, or simply by normal bowel movements; and progressive titration may be difficult because of the limited availability of different commercial preparations.

d.   Transdermal route. The recent development of a transdermal preparation of fentanyl citrate has revitalized an interest in this route. Pharmacokinetic data suggest that transdermal fentanyl is well absorbed, although there is considerable delay in reaching steady-state blood levels and a slowly declining plasma concentration after removal of the patch. The 72-h dosing of the patch makes it convenient to use, and treatment appears to be well tolerated. The transdermal route is generally worth avoiding if the enteral route is readily available. Transdermal preparations are generally more expensive and more difficult to titrate compared with oral opioids. However, this route is quite useful for patients with chronic malignant bowel obstruction or similar chronic problems with the oral route.

e.   Transmucosal route. Fentanyl citrate can also be formulated in a candied matrix to allow it to be administered orally as a lozenge on a stick. Oral transmucosal fentanyl citrate (OTFC) appears to be rapidly effective for breakthrough pain or for procedures. Dose-equivalency studies have suggested that OTFC is about 10 times more potent than parenteral morphine. Starting doses are usually 200 μg, with dosing intervals of 4 to 6 h. Drug dose requires titrating up as with other agents with single doses of up to 1,600 μg. This transmucosal route has been used sparingly because the lozenges are expensive and patients often try to use them sparingly, thus limiting their effectiveness.

f. Spinal route. Some patients suffering from localized pain syndromes might benefit from intraspinal administration of opioids. The advantage of this route is the lack of systemic side effects of opioids and the fact that a relatively small dose of drugs is necessary. The disadvantage is the need for the insertion of catheters into the epidural or intrathecal space, the need for expensive infusion pumps, and, in many patients, the rapid development of tolerance to the analgesic effect of different opioids. To overcome this rapid development of tolerance, some clinicians have used a combined infusion of opioids and local anesthetic. Because of the complexity associated with this route, it should only be considered in selected patients and after an adequate trial of systemic opioids and adjuvant drugs. The insertion of the catheter and the maintenance of the spinal analgesic regimen should be under the control of a pain specialist.

10. Adverse effects of opioids. Fear of the inability to manage side effects is one of the main reasons cited by oncologists that they limit their use of opioids. Yet, most of the agents used in chemotherapy are associated with more potent side effects than the opioids. The analgesic and side effects of opioid agonists are not identical for all patients. Some patients may require a higher equivalent dose of a certain opioid agonist to achieve adequate analgesia. This higher equivalent dose may result in a higher incidence of side effects such as nausea or sedation. Therefore, when significant toxicity occurs in a patient treated with a certain opioid agonist such as morphine, it may be appropriate to change to another opioid. In addition, after prolonged treatment, high dosages, or renal failure, patients may experience the accumulation of active metabolites of opioid agonists. Active metabolites have been identified for morphine, hydromorphone, oxycodone, and fentanyl. This accumulation results in CNS side effects such as sedation, generalized myoclonus, confusion, and, in some patients, agitated delirium or grand mal seizures. In these patients, it is also useful to change from one opioid to another.

This so-called opioid rotation (or "opioid switching") can produce better analgesia and fewer adverse effects. Most often, such a switch occurs from morphine to a more potent opioid such as methadone, hydromorphone, fentanyl, or oxycodone. The dose guidelines for switching to methadone are shown in Table 31.4. When switching from morphine to hydromorphone or oxycodone, the initial dose should be 50% to 75% of the calculated equianalgesic dose. When switching from morphine to transdermal fentanyl, dose reduction is not needed because the dosing guidelines already incorporated the safety factor necessary for opioid rotation.

It is important to understand the side effect liability of these analgesics and be prepared to deal with side effects prophylactically or when they do occur. *Most patients develop tolerance for side effects much more rapidly than they develop tolerance for the analgesic effects of the opioids.*

a.   Sedation. This occurs in most patients during the beginning of opioid treatment or after a major increase in dose. Most patients develop rapid tolerance to this side effect, and while the sedation disappears within 3 to 5 days, the analgesic effect persists. When sedation occurs in patients with cancer receiving a stable dose of opioid, it is necessary to suspect the potential accumulation of active opioid metabolites such as morphine-6-glucuronide. This occurs more frequently in patients who are receiving high doses of opioids or present with renal failure. It is also important to suspect other non–opioid-related causes such as hypercalcemia, because these patients are frequently very ill. Opioid-induced sedation can be managed by opioid rotation (some opioids have a higher ratio of analgesic effects to sedation than others) or by the addition of amphetamine derivatives such as methylphenidate, starting with 5 mg PO b.i.d. daily (last dose no later than 3 P.M. to avoid insomnia).

b.   Nausea and vomiting. Most patients present with these symptoms after initial administration or a major increase in dose. Some authors propose the use of prophylactic antiemetics on a regular basis during the first days of treatment because in most patients, nausea disappears after that period. The mechanism for the nausea is central. These side effects can be well antagonized by a prokinetic agents such as metoclopramide 10 mg PO q.i.d. Dexamethasone 2 to 4 mg PO q.i.d. is also a useful antiemetic that potentiates metoclopramide in these patients but has significant side effects when used for more than 1 or 2 weeks. As with sedation, nausea is a syndrome with multiple possible etiologies in patients with cancer who are receiving opioids: Severe constipation, cancer-induced autonomic failure, gastritis, increased intracranial pressure, and opioid metabolite accumulation are all possible causes of nausea.

c.   Constipation. This is probably the most common adverse effect of opioids, and it is necessary to anticipate constipation when opioid therapy is started. Opioids act at multiple sites in the gastrointestinal tract and spinal cord. The result is decreased intestinal secretions and peristalsis. Although tolerance to both sedation and nausea develops quickly, it develops very slowly to the smooth muscle effects of opioids, so that constipation persists when these drugs are used for chronic pain. At the same time that the use of opioid analgesics is initiated, provision for a regular bowel regimen, including stimulants and stool softeners, should be instituted to diminish this adverse effect (see Chapter 26).

d.   Respiratory depression. This is the most serious adverse effect of opioid analgesics. Opioids can cause increasing respiratory depression to the point of apnea. In humans, death due to overdose of opioids is nearly always due to respiratory arrest. At equianalgesic doses, the morphine-like agonists produce an equivalent degree of respiratory depression. When respiratory depression occurs, it is usually in opioid-naive patients after acute administration of an opioid and is associated with other signs of CNS depression including sedation and mental clouding. Tolerance quickly develops to this effect with repeated drug administration, allowing the opioid analgesics to be used in the management of chronic cancer pain without significant risk of respiratory depression. If respiratory depression occurs, it can be reversed by the administration of the specific opioid antagonist naloxone. In patients chronically receiving opioids who develop respiratory depression, naloxone in a 1:10 dilution should be titrated carefully to prevent the precipitation of severe withdrawal syndromes while reversing the respiratory depression. Long-acting drugs such as methadone, fentanyl patches, or slow-release morphine are likely to cause a higher incidence of respiratory depression. The accumulation of active opioid metabolites and the simultaneous use of other depressants such as benzodiazepines or alcohol are risk factors for respiratory depression. Although this is the most feared side effect of opioid analgesics, it occurs seldom in patients receiving chronic opioid therapy for the treatment of cancer pain.

e.   Allergic reactions. These occur infrequently with opioids. However, it is common that patients are described as "allergic" to a number of opioid analgesics. This commonly results from a misinterpretation by the patient or clinician of some of the common side effects of opioids, such as nausea, sedation, vomiting, or sweating. In most instances, a simple discussion with the patient is enough to clarify this issue.

f.   Urinary retention. The increase in the tone of smooth muscle of the bladder induced by opioids results in an increase in the sphincter tone leading to urinary retention. This is most common in elderly patients. Attention should be directed to this potential transient side effect, and catheterization may be necessary for management.

g.   "Newer" side effects. During recent years, as a result of increased education in the assessment and management of cancer pain, patients have been receiving higher doses of opioids for longer periods of time than ever before. This more aggressive use of opioids is associated with additional side effects, usually seen only in patients with late-stage disease receiving high doses of opioids.

   (1)   Cognitive failure. Patients can experience a transient decrease in concentration and psychomotor coordination after starting opioids or after a sudden increase in the opioid dose. In some patients, the opioid-induced cognitive failure can be permanent. Some of the cognitive effects can be reversed by the administration of amphetamine derivatives such as methylphenidate. Cognitive screening tools (such as the Mini-Mental State Examination and other similar bedside assessments) are useful in patients receiving high doses of opioids.

(2)   Other central effects. Organic hallucinations, myoclonus, grand mal seizures, and even hyperalgesia have been observed in patients receiving high doses of opioids for long periods. These effects are likely due to the accumulation of active opioid metabolites. Sometimes, the development of these problems in a previously stable patient heralds the onset of renal insufficiency or renal failure. Improvement is frequently seen after the renal function improves and/or there is an opioid rotation. Hallucinations may be treated symptomatically with low doses of haloperidol 0.5 to 2 mg b.i.d. while the underlying problem is being addressed. Myoclonus can be treated with clonazepam 0.5 mg PO b.i.d. to start, with titration every 3 days up to a maximum daily dose of 20 mg.

(3)   Severe sedation and coma. When coma occurs in patients receiving a stable dose of opioids for a long period of time, it should be suspected that accumulation of active opioid metabolites has occurred. These patients usually improve quickly after discontinuation of opioids.

(4)   Pulmonary edema. Although noncardiogenic pulmonary edema is a well-recognized complication of opioid overdose in addicts, it had not been recognized until recently as a potential complication of cancer pain treatment. Pulmonary edema usually occurs when patients have undergone rapid increases in dose, usually as a result of severe neuropathic pain. Even though the mortality of the syndrome is very low among patients presenting with acute opioid overdoses, because of the conservative nature of the treatment of terminally ill patients with cancer, the mortality of pulmonary edema is much higher within this population.

V.   Adjuvant drugs. Opioid analgesics are the most important drugs for the treatment of cancer pain. Although these drugs can, in most patients, control severe pain even when they are used appropriately, they may produce new symptoms or exacerbate pre-existing symptoms, most notably nausea and somnolence. This aspect of treatment with opioid compounds is particularly problematic in patients with advanced cancer. The combination of severe pain, anorexia, chronic nausea, asthenia, and somnolence is a frequent finding in patients with advanced cancer. The term *adjuvant drug* has been used in a variety of ways, even in the context of cancer pain management. For the purposes of the following paragraphs, an adjuvant drug meets one or more of the following criteria:

- Increases the analgesic effect of opioids (adjuvant analgesia)
- Decreases the toxicity of opioids
- Improves other symptoms associated with terminal cancer

Most symptomatic patients with cancer receive more than one or two adjuvant drugs. Unfortunately, there is still limited consensus on the type and dose of the most appropriate adjuvant drugs.

Claims have been made for the adjuvant analgesic effect of many drugs, but unfortunately, most of the evidence for these effects is anecdotal. Controlled clinical trials are needed to define more clearly the indications and risk-to-benefit ratios. These agents, some of which have the potential to produce significant toxicity, can aggravate the toxicity of opioids.

A.   Tricyclic antidepressants. Despite the frequent use of these agents in British hospices and South American and European cancer centers, the use of tricyclics in North American cancer centers has been uncommon. Tricyclic antidepressants have been found to be useful for a variety of neuropathic pain syndromes, especially when pain has a prominent dysesthetic or burning character. Both amitriptyline and desipramine have been found to be effective in the management of postherpetic neuralgia, diabetic neuropathy, and other neurologic conditions. There is, however, only limited evidence for a significant analgesic effect in cancer pain. Clinical experience and expert consensus suggest that tricyclics should be tried for the management of pain of central, deafferentation, or neuropathic origin.

The optimal drug and dosing regimens are unknown. Amitriptyline or imipramine (25 mg at bedtime) may be started at low doses; if the drug is not overly sedating and the patient does not experience bothersome anticholinergic side effects, the dose may be increased every 3 days to a total daily dose of 150 mg or higher. The effects of newer antidepressants, such as the selective serotonin uptake inhibitors or specific monoamine oxidase inhibitors, on pain control have not been clearly established. Until further evidence is available, the more traditional tricyclics should be used as adjuvant analgesics. The toxic effects of these drugs are mainly autonomic (dry mouth, postural hypotension) and centrally mediated (somnolence, confusion). Cardiovascular side effects are also possible at therapeutic dosing levels, including increased heart rate, prolonged PR interval, intraventricular conduction delays, increased corrected QT interval (QTc), and flattened T waves. Because their use may contribute to symptoms already present in debilitated patients, they should be administered cautiously in those who are very ill.

B.   Anticonvulsants. Carbamazepine, phenytoin, valproic acid, and clonazepam, alone or in combination with the tricyclic antidepressants, have been used successfully to treat neuropathic pain. Based on the well-documented efficacy for the treatment of trigeminal neuralgia, considerable experience and expert consensus suggest the use of these agents for neuropathic cancer pain syndromes, including neural invasion by tumor, radiation fibrosis or surgical scarring, herpes zoster, and deafferentation. Based on clinical observations, improvement can be expected in a proportion of patients whose predominant complaint is pain of a shooting, lancinating, burning, or hyperesthetic nature.

Gabapentin has been proposed in recent years as an effective and well-tolerated agent in advanced cancer patients. The effective dose of gabapentin is generally 900 to 1,800 mg/day. It is given in divided doses, three times a day. Titration to an effective dose can take place rapidly, over about 2 weeks (see Table 31.5). To minimize potential side effects, especially somnolence, dizzi-

Table 31.5. Suggested dose titration for gabapentin when used for neuropathic pain

Day 1:	Take 1 capsule[a] at bedtime.
Days 2–4:	Take 1 capsule in the morning and 1 capsule at bedtime.
Days 5–7:	Take 1 capsule in the morning, 1 capsule at midday, and 1 capsule at bedtime.
Days 8–10:	Take 2 capsules in the morning, 2 capsules at midday, and 2 capsules at bedtime.
Days 11–14:	Take 3 capsules in the morning, 3 capsules at midday, and 3 capsules at bedtime.

[a] 100 mg.

ness, fatigue, and ataxia, the first dose on day 1 may be administered at bedtime. Effective doses in the treatment of neuropathic pain in patients with cancer are not well established.

Side effects of therapy with this group of agents are potentially serious, particularly in patients with advanced cancer, and can include bone marrow depression, hepatic dysfunction, somnolence, ataxia, diplopia, and lymphadenopathy. Periodic monitoring of complete blood cell count and liver function is recommended.

C. Corticosteroids. Controlled studies suggest that the administration of corticosteroids to selected patients with advanced cancer results in decreased pain and improved appetite and activity. Unfortunately, the duration of the effects is probably short lasting. The mechanism by which corticosteroids appear to produce beneficial symptom effects in patients with terminal cancer is unclear but may involve their euphoriant effects or the inhibition of prostaglandin metabolism. The optimal drug and dosing regimens have not been established. For the treatment of painful conditions, prednisone or dexamethasone is often administered in doses totaling 30 to 60 mg PO daily and 8 to 16 mg PO daily, respectively. As soon as symptomatic relief is obtained, attempts should be made to decrease the dose progressively to the minimally effective dose. Although long-term side effects are not an important consideration in many patients with advanced cancer, treatment may produce limiting side effects in these patients, particularly immunosuppression (candidiasis occurs in most patients), proximal myopathy, and psychiatric symptoms. The incidence of psychologic disturbances ranges from 3% to 50%, with severe symptoms occurring in about 5% of patients. The spectrum of disturbances ranges from mild to severe affective disorders, psychotic reactions, and global cognitive impairment.

D. Clonidine. Clonidine, an α_2-adrenergic agonist developed for treatment of hypertension, can be administered orally or as part of an epidural regimen for control of cancer-related pain, especially neuropathic pain.

E. Approaches to metastatic bone pain

1. Strontium-89. Strontium-89 and a number of other isotopes have been found to be useful in the treatment of pain in patients with bony metastases. This agent is more useful in patients with multiple pain locations who might not benefit from radiation therapy. The main limitations of this agent are its high cost and the potential for severe and prolonged hematologic toxicity, mainly thrombocytopenia.

2.   Bisphosphonates. These agents have been found to be significantly better than placebo in patients with bone pain due to a variety of primary tumors. Pamidronate, clodronate, and zoledronate are the agents that have been most frequently studied. Because of their poor oral bioavailability, these drugs are most useful when given IV. In addition to pain control, these drugs can significantly reduce a number of other complications of osteolysis, such as hypercalcemia, fractures, and need for radiation therapy. A new generation of bisphosphonates with increased oral bioavailability will be available in the near future.

3.   External-beam radiotherapy. Radiation therapy can effectively control bone pain in about 70% of patients within 2 to 4 weeks. This treatment is most useful in patients with a single or small number of painful areas. A single administration may be as effective as multiple smaller fractions, reducing the cost and discomfort of transportation back and forth associated with multiple doses.

VI.   Neuroablative procedures. Evaluation of the physical basis of the pain may indicate that a neuroablative procedure, in which the pain pathway is destroyed, would be of benefit for pain control. As aggressive opioid analgesia becomes more accepted, most patients with cancer do not require these neuroablative interventions. Destruction of the pain pathway can be accomplished surgically or through destructive nerve blocks using an agent such as phenol. The major barrier to the more widespread application of these techniques is the limited number of practitioners expert in their use. The most frequently used neurosurgical procedure is the anterolateral or spinothalamic cordotomy. This is often performed as closed percutaneous cordotomy by stereotactically placing a radiofrequency needle in the anterolateral quadrant of the cervical spinal cord. Unilateral pain control can unmask significant pain on the opposite side of the body. For pain of head and neck cancer, procedures such as percutaneous radiofrequency coagulation of the glossopharyngeal nerve may be used. Nevertheless, performance of such procedures does not eliminate the need to administer and monitor the effectiveness of analgesics. Because of afferent regeneration, destructive procedures have had their greatest application in patients whose expected life span is only a few months.

Destructive anesthetic block of the celiac plexus has been used for several decades in the management of pain in the abdominal region. This block, which can be preceded by reversible diagnostic block, is a boon to many patients suffering from the severe pain accompanying cancer of the pancreas and may also be helpful for pain from cancers of the liver, gallbladder, or stomach. The effectiveness of the destruction of the celiac plexus for pain relief is supported by at least one randomized clinical trial. If success is achieved with the diagnostic block, lasting disruption of the pain pathway can be achieved using alcohol or phenol. Pain from rib metastases or tumors of the chest wall can be relieved with intercostal nerve blocks.

Intrathecal and epidural nerve blocks have provided pain relief, but those procedures carry a risk of sensory and motor deficit.

VII.   Coping or behavioral skill techniques. Teaching specific skills to manage pain can be of help to many patients, especially those who face pain for months to years. Evaluation and prescription of the specific skills most beneficial to the individual can often be obtained through consultation with a behavioral psychologist, psychiatrist, or nurse pain specialist. Such techniques should never be used as a substitute for appropriate analgesia. The skills include relaxation, self-hypnosis, and other distraction and cognitive control techniques. These measures can affect the sensation of pain by reducing muscle tension on pain-generating lesions as well as by maximizing the patient's ability to cope with the pain and remain as active as the disease permits. All patients need education about the nature of their pain, the methods that can be used to relieve it, and how they can cooperate with their health care providers to achieve good pain control.

SELECTED READINGS

Bennett G, Serafini M, Burchiel K, et al. Evidence-based review of the literature on intrathecal delivery of pain medication. *J Pain Symptom Manage* 2000;20:S12–S36.

Bruera E, Belzile M, Pituskin E, et al. Randomized, double-blind, cross-over trial comparing the safety and efficacy of oral controlled-release oxycodone with controlled-release morphine in patients with cancer pain. *J Clin Oncol* 1998;16:3222–3229.

Bruera E, Pereira J, Watanabe S, et al. Opioid rotation in patients with cancer pain. A retrospective comparison of dose ratios between methadone, hydromorphone, and morphine. *Cancer* 1996; 78:852–857.

Cherny NI, Arbit E, Jain S. Invasive techniques in the management of cancer pain. *Hematol Oncol Clin North Am* 1996;10:121–137.

Cherney N, Ripamonti C, Pereira J, et al. Strategies to manage the adverse effects of oral morphine: an evidence-based report. *J Clin Oncol* 2001;19:2542–2554.

Cleeland CS, Gonin R, Hatfield AK, et al. Pain and its treatment in outpatients with metastatic cancer. *N Engl J Med* 1994;330:592–596.

Corbo M, Balmaceda C. Peripheral neuropathy in cancer patients. *Cancer Invest* 2001;19:369–382.

Foley KM, Gelband H, eds. *Improving palliative care for cancer: summary and recommendations.* Washington, D.C.: National Academy Press, 2001.

Grossman SA, Benedetti C, Payne R, et al. NCCN practice guidelines for cancer pain. *Oncology* 1999;13:33–44.

Indelicato RA, Portenoy RK. Opioid rotation in the management of refractory cancer pain. *J Clin Oncol* 2002;20:348–352.

Mercadante S, Casuccio A, Agnello A, et al. Morphine versus methadone in the pain treatment of advanced cancer patients followed up at home. *J Clin Oncol* 1998;16:3656–3661.

Pereira J, Lawlor P, Vigano A, et al. Equianalgesic dose ratios for opioids: a critical review and proposals for long-term dosing. *J Pain Symptom Manage* 2001;22:672–677.

Portenoy RK. Issues in the economic analysis of therapies for cancer pain. *Oncology* 1995;9(suppl 11):71–78.

Portenoy RK, Hagen NA. Breakthrough pain: definition and management. *Oncology* 1989;3(suppl 8):25–29.

Ripamonti C, Groff L, Brunelli C, et al. Switching from morphine to oral methadone in treating cancer pain: what is the equianalgesic dose ratio? *J Clin Oncol* 1998;16:3216–3221.

Rowlingson JC. Interventional cancer pain management. *Anesth Analg* 1998;suppl:106–113.

Weissman DE, et al. *Handbook of cancer pain management.* 4th ed. Madison: Wisconsin Cancer Pain Initiative, 1993.

Emotional and Psychiatric Problems in Patients with Cancer

Kathleen S. N. Franco-Bronson and
Kristi S. Williams

I. General principles. Clinical psychiatric disorders occur in up to half of patients with cancer at some point during their treatment. Delirium, depression, and anxiety are those most frequently seen and may coexist in the same patient. Vigilant monitoring for early symptoms of psychiatric distress is important to the care of these patients. The clinician should inquire regularly about symptoms in the affective and cognitive domains. Symptom clusters help differentiate anxiety, depression, and acute confusional states from other psychiatric disorders. Once an accurate diagnosis is made, appropriate treatment that may include medication can be directed toward target symptoms. More than one psychiatric diagnosis may be present, requiring a hierarchical approach. For example, if both delirium and depression are present, the cause of the delirium should be determined and treated before starting antidepressant therapy (which could worsen the delirium). Once the delirium has improved, treatment for the depression can be considered. When major depression and an anxiety disorder coexist, treatment for the depression is started first and may adequately manage both disorders.

II. Acute confusional states

A. Precepts. Psychiatrists are often asked to assist in the care of "agitated" patients. The initial request may be for medication advice, but prescribing psychotropic drugs without understanding the cause of the patient's distress can have serious consequences. Delirium is characterized by fluctuating levels of alertness and consciousness, shortened attention and concentration, rapidly changing moods, irregular sleep–wake cycles, garbled or slurred speech, hypervigilance, and behavior not consistent with good judgment. The delirious patient may also have delusional ideas or hallucinations or appear depressed. Visual, auditory, tactile, and occasionally olfactory hallucinations can be present. The more sensory modalities that are involved in the hallucinations, the greater is the likelihood that the patient is experiencing an acute confusional state.

B. Etiologies

1. Medications remain the most common reason for acute confusional states. The most frequently identified medications to cause delirium are sedatives, narcotic analgesics, anxiolytics, anticholinergic drugs, and corticosteroids.

2. Metabolic causes are often seen in patients with cancer and include hypernatremia and hyponatremia, hyperthyroidism and hypothyroidism, poorly controlled diabetes mellitus, vitamin deficiencies (B_{12}, folate, thiamine), and hypercalcemia.

3. Infections of the respiratory, urinary, central nervous, and other systems are common, especially in immuno-suppressed patients.

4. Chemical withdrawal from benzodiazepines, alcohol, and other drugs can induce delirium.

5. Medical illness such as tumors, cardiac arrhythmias, congestive heart failure, liver disease, trauma, strokes, renal failure, and a variety of other conditions can cause acute changes in mental status.

C. Therapeutic approach. Once an acute confusional state is identified, the primary therapeutic approach is to treat the cause. The key is to determine when symptoms of delirium first occurred and to look for preceding changes in medications, vital signs, laboratory studies, or imagery/radiology. This helps to determine how to best proceed with treatment, for example, withdrawing a medication or treating a urinary tract infection found on a urinalysis. Antipsychotic medications may be helpful for managing symptoms such as hallucinations, delusions, and extreme agitation, but they do not treat the cause of the delirium.

1. Orientation (frequent reconnection) of the patient aids in reduction of confusion.

a. It is helpful to orient the patient frequently to place, time, and why they are at the hospital and to give current explanations of procedures. This routine should be done once or more per shift when the delirious patient is awake. Because patients' attention, concentration, and recent memory are frequently impaired, they often do not recall instructions given to them earlier. Leaving a large, legibly written note card with the patient's name, date, hospital name, and other data is beneficial in some instances.

b. A large calendar, a clock, and family pictures or mementos can assist the patients in feeling less estranged from their environment.

c. Some patients are reassured by a small night light in their room, which cuts down on illusions or misinterpretations. Patients with compromised vision or hearing are particularly distraught when they are even less able to discern what is happening around them, and they should be provided with their hearing aids and glasses.

2. Medication helps to control hallucinations, delusions, and psychotic agitation. The lowest dose to control symptoms is usually preferable.

a. Haloperidol (Haldol; Table 32.1) is a butyrophenone, an antipsychotic agent with potent dopamine-blocking action. It is less likely to produce cardiovascular, respiratory, gastrointestinal, and general anticholinergic side effects than many of the other antipsychotic medications. However, moderate doses may cause extrapyramidal symptoms. The starting dose in a patient with an acute confusional state is 0.25 to 2 mg PO or IM, on an as-needed or regular dosing schedule every 4 to 6 h. A marked advantage of haloperidol is that sedation is minimized while controlling agitation. There are exceptions to the usually preferred low doses of antipsychotic medications. For example, if patients

Table 32.1. Antipsychotic medications: prominent characteristics and dosage for patients with cancer

Agent	Starting dose (mg)[a]	Characteristics
Phenothiazines		
Chlorpromazine (Thorazine)	10–25	Significant hypotension risk, lowers seizure threshold, highly sedating, anticholinergic
Thioridazine (Mellaril)	10–25	Similar to chlorpromazine but more likely to alter electrocardiogram, not available IM
Perphenazine (Trilafon)	4	Moderate sedation and hypotension
Trifluoperazine (Stelazine)	2	High frequency of extrapyramidal side effects
Others		
Haloperidol (Haldol)	0.5–2.0	Good for acute delirium, high frequency of extrapyramidal side effects, available IV, IM, or PO
Risperidone (Risperdal)	0.5–1.0	Some α-adrenergic effects, mild extrapyramidal side effects as dose increases, PO form only
Olanzapine (Zyprexa)	5	More sedation, weight gain, less extrapyramidal side effects, PO form only, available as tablet that dissolves on tongue
Quetiapine (Seroquel)	25–50	More sedation, less extrapyramidal effects
Ziprasidone (Geodon)	20	Less weight gain, contraindicated with QT prolongation, less extrapyramidal effects

[a] Dose generally can be repeated every 4–6 h (other than risperidone, olanzapine, quetiapine, ziprasidone), on either an as-needed or a regular schedule (e.g., b.i.d.).

tolerate higher doses with few side effects, they may benefit by having improved pain control. IV haloperidol has not been approved by the U.S. Food and Drug Administration, although it is commonly used in the seriously agitated patient. Half the oral dosing is prescribed when the medication is given IV. Some patients require larger IV doses to control symptoms. Avoid very high doses in patients with alcoholic cardiomyopathy, those prone to torsades de pointes or similar arrhythmias, and those with an excessively long QTc interval. Extrapyramidal side effects are minimal with IV administration.

b. Risperidone (Risperdal) is less likely to produce extrapyramidal side effects but is available only in oral form. **Olanzapine** (Zyprexa, Zydis) is sedating and can be given in a tablet that dissolves on the tongue.

c. **A delirious patient** with vision or hearing impairment is likely to hallucinate during periods of excessive sedation.
d. If the patient demonstrates a **predictable period of confusion,** such as during the early evening ("sundowning") when there is less environmental activity, a once-a-day dose at that time may be adequate.
e. **When increasing the dose of antipsychotic drugs,** muscle spasms, restlessness, or pseudo-parkinsonian symptoms may occur. Adding a small amount of trihexyphenidyl (Artane) 1 to 2 mg b.i.d., benztropine (Cogentin) 1 mg b.i.d., or diphenhydramine (Benadryl) 25 mg b.i.d. can often reduce the side effects. However, increasing the level of anticholinergic activity with these choices may cause an atropinic-like psychosis. Constipation, urinary retention, dry mouth, tachycardia, and increasing confusion are warnings of this potential problem, especially when multiple anticholinergic medications (e.g., antiemetics, analgesics) are being prescribed. Therefore, antiparkinsonian drugs are not prescribed prophylactically but only if clearly indicated. Ondansetron (Zofran), granisetron (Kytril), or dolasetron (Anzemet) may be substituted for other antiemetics, reducing extrapyramidal symptoms and avoiding the need for an antiparkinsonian medication. Some antiemetics (e.g., droperidol) are also antipsychotics, but these, like metoclopramide, can lead to extrapyramidal symptoms.
f. **Benzodiazepines** such as lorazepam (Ativan) can be given 0.5 to 2.0 mg every 8 h. They can be administered in small doses to a patient who needs some sedation without added anticholinergic activity or those whose cardiac status is at risk (i.e., heart block) if some antipsychotic medications were increased. Using both benzodiazepines and antipsychotics is sometimes helpful. One pattern might be 0.5 to 2 mg haloperidol IV or PO at 4 P.M., 1 to 2 mg of lorazepam IV or PO at 8 P.M., and so forth if the patient is agitated.
g. **Increasing delirium.** Too much medication may have been given if the patient's agitation increases with higher doses. High blood levels of longer-acting medications can accumulate, particularly if serum protein is low and hepatic and renal functioning are compromised.
h. **Hypotension.** Avoid adding other antipsychotics, for example, thorazine, as they predispose to hypotension and shock. If the blood pressure does drop significantly, norepinephrine bitartrate (Levophed) or a similar choice may be necessary because the antipsychotic medications like haloperidol block the action of dopamine. The half-life of the antipsychotic is generally 24 to 48 h.
III. **Depression.** Patients with cancer have various emotional responses to their diagnoses. The mourning period for some is brief, does not inhibit their ability to interact with family and friends, and does not hinder participation in their own treatment. Support from others, acceptance of their feelings, and time may be all that is necessary for them to continue the emotional work ahead. However, about one-fourth of patients with cancer develop longer, more severe depression. The greatest risk of depression is at the time of first relapse. There are many variables that influence this process, including emotional conflicts with loved ones,

disproportionate guilt, previous losses that were never resolved, long-standing debilitating illness, individual personality characteristics such as dependency, and inadequate support systems. Any of these factors, along with a family history of depression, are warnings for the physician to heed.

A.   Therapeutic approach

1.   Emotional support at frequent intervals from the physician is generally needed. Some patients explore old emotional conflicts, whereas others just need a safe person to whom they can express their feelings. It is important for patients to be able to hold on to hope. A degree of denial is acceptable, normal, and upheld. Only when this denial makes it impossible for a patient to make informed treatment decisions is it necessary to probe into the denial.

Psychotherapy of a supportive nature is often provided by the primary care physician, oncologist, psychiatrist, clergy, nurse, family, or friend individually or in any combination. For patients who wish to explore ambivalence, a professional psychotherapist trained in psychodynamic or interpersonal therapy is a good option. Cognitive therapy is helpful in letting go of detrimental interpretations while increasing one's ability to deal with emotional pain.

2.   Psychiatric care may be particularly instrumental when the patient's pre-existing personality style is interfering with treatment. Anniversary responses to previous losses, important family events, or past hospitalizations may have a great impact on the presentation of the depression and deserve exploration by a psychotherapist if a pattern is found. If there is a designated psychiatric consultant, this individual must work closely with the rest of the oncology team, communicating in a helpful way to the patient, family, and staff.

If a patient has felt depressed, distressed, or irritable for some time or describes a loss of pleasure from formerly enjoyable relationships or activities, inquiry about the following symptoms is necessary: insomnia or hypersomnia; alteration in appetite with expected weight change; reduced interest in family, sexuality, work, or hobbies; increased guilt; low energy level; poor concentration; thoughts of death or suicide; frequent crying episodes; and psychomotor hypoactivity or hyperactivity. When the diagnosis of depression in the medically ill patient is being made, the emphasis is placed on psychological features as opposed to physical ones. These include rumination or repetitive negative thoughts, increased tearfulness, hopeless–helpless feelings, withdrawal from family or friends, and anhedonia. These symptoms are characteristic of a major depressive disorder for which antidepressant medications in addition to psychotherapy are recommended. In some studies, group therapy for patients with breast cancer has improved quality of life and may prolong survival.

3.   Medications. In the past, patients with cancer were often undertreated for major depression that was mistaken as an "understandable" consequence of their illness or as simple grief. Now, evidence exists that psychosocial adjustment and improved life adaptation, in general, occur when patients with cancer and major depression are treated with antidepressant medications.

a. Selection of agents and their side effects. In addition to efficacy, an antidepressant medication should be selected on the basis of its safety and tolerability, including any tendency to sedate or activate, cause orthostatic changes, or produce anticholinergic effects. Medication selection should also be tailored to the patient's symptom cluster such as the need for sedation or weight gain versus the need for activation (Tables 32.2 and 32.3). Route of metabolism and elimination, as well as an increased risk for seizures, should affect the choice.

Highly anticholinergic medications frequently produce dry mouth, blurred vision, tachycardia, and constipation. They can also produce urinary retention, ileus, and acute confusion. Antihistaminergic drugs can increase sedation and appetite and worsen hypotension. Both H_1- and H_2-blocking agents can cause delirium, while a proton pump inhibitor will not. Medications that produce α-adrenergic receptor blockade are associated with increased orthostatic hypotension, dizziness, and reflex tachycardia.

b. Dosages (Table 32.4). Weak, debilitated, or elderly patients need protection from side effects of psychotropic agents. Starting out with small doses and gradually increasing the dose is prudent. Splitting doses may also be helpful for minimizing side effects and maximizing pain relief from antidepressant medications.

Table 32.2. Characteristics of commonly used heterocyclic antidepressants

Antidepressant	Sedation[a]	Anticholinergic actions[b]	Other characteristics
Amitriptyline (Elavil, Endep)	+4 to +5[c]	+4 to +5	Also available IM, orthostasis, quinidine-like, good for neuropathic pain
Doxepin (Sinequan, Adapin)	+4	+3 to +4	Highest appetite increase, orthostasis, good for neuropathic pain
Nortriptyline (Pamelor, Aventyl)	+3	+3	Less likely to cause orthostasis than other tricyclic antidepressants

Note: Do not use tricyclic if QTc >450. Tricyclics can also suppress respiratory drive and reduce seizure threshold.
[a] Associated with histaminergic blockade; appetite increase follows somewhat similar trends.
[b] Constipation, dry mouth, and urinary retention.
[c] Scale of 1–5, where 1 is least and 5 is most.

Table 32.3.   Characteristics of commonly used nonheterocyclic antidepressants

Antidepressant	Sedation[a]	Anticholinergic actions[b]	Other characteristics
Bupropion (Wellbutrin)	+1[c]	+1	Associated with increased seizure risk especially if organic brain pathology or eating disorder is present, more activating, less weight gain
Fluoxetine (Prozac)	+1	+1	May cause restlessness and gastrointestinal upset, more activating, less weight gain, safe in patients with renal disease but may accumulate in those with liver disease, self-tapers when discontinued
Sertraline (Zoloft)	+1	+1	Similar to fluoxetine, more diarrhea, few drug interactions, short half-life, should be tapered if discontinued
Paroxetine (Paxil)	+1	+2	Similar to fluoxetine, more anticholinergic than other SSRIs, should be tapered if discontinued
Citalopram (Celexa)	+1	+1	Similar to Sertraline, few drug interactions
Venlafaxine (Effexor)	+2	+1	Both serotonin and norepinephrine reuptake inhibitor, increases blood pressure at higher doses, augments pain relief
Mirtazapine (Remeron)	+4	+2	Weight gain, potential increase in cholesterol, sedation, available as tablet that dissolves on tongue
Nefazodone (Serzone)	+3	+2	Some sedation, fewer sexual side effects, mild orthostasis, possible liver toxicity in some

[a] Associated with histaminergic blockade; appetite increase follows somewhat similar trends.

[b] Constipation, dry mouth, and urinary retention.

[c] Scale of 1–5, where 1 is least and 5 is most.

Table 32.4.   Dosages for antidepressant therapy

Drug	Starting daily dose (mg)	Average daily dose for patient with cancer (mg)
Amitriptyline	10–25	75–150
Bupropion	75–150	300
Citalopram	10–20	20–40
Doxepin	25	75–150
Fluoxetine	10–20	20
Mirtazapine	7.5–15	30+
Nefazodone	50	300
Nortriptyline	10–25	50–100
Paroxetine	10–20	20
Sertraline	25–50	100
Venlafaxine	25 or 37.5 (XR form)	75 mg (37.5 mg b.i.d.)

If a patient has a personal history, family history, or previous response to medication (e.g., steroids) that reflects manic or hypomanic symptoms, proceed carefully, perhaps utilizing a mood stabilizer such as lithium or an anticonvulsant, and/or consult psychiatry (Table 32.5).

c.   Monoamine oxidase inhibitors (MAOIs) may be used to treat major depression or panic disorder but are somewhat inconvenient owing to tyramine dietary restrictions and medication interactions requiring much attention. They are sometimes tried when other choices have failed.

IV.   Anxiety

A.   Approach to the problem. As grieving is described as normal, so is anxiety in patients with cancer. However, anxiety varies in its cause, severity, and treatment. A detailed history of the onset, characteristics, and length of distress is important. Knowledge of the patient's previous symptoms, current and past physical illness, substance abuse, and medication usage is essential to the evaluation process. Antianxiety agents may be helpful for alleviating patients' distress and helping them cope with other problems associated with their cancer (Table 32.6).

B.   Problems that present as anxiety. The duration of the symptoms is one of the first factors to assess in the anxious patient.

1.   Suspect an adjustment disorder when maladaptive anxious symptoms have persisted less than 6 months and apparently represent an adjustment to learning the diagnosis or reactions to the treatment. This kind of anxiety may benefit from supportive therapy, relaxation therapy, or benzodiazepines.

2.   Generalized anxiety. If the anxiety has been present for more than 6 months, continuing no matter what environmental alterations occur, and is accompanied by signs of physical tension or poor attention to conversation or other daily activities, the patient is likely to have generalized anxiety. Supportive therapy, relaxation tapes, biofeedback, buspirone, gabapentin, and benzodiazepines are useful.

(text continues on page 686)

Table 32.5. Other medications used to treat affective disorders

Stimulants[a] to increase level of alertness

Drug	Starting dose	Average dose for cancer patients	Disorders	Pretreatment work-up	Follow-up studies	Comment
Methylphenidate (Ritalin)	2.5–5.0 mg qa.m.	5–20 mg qa.m. + noon	Medically ill patient with depression and lethargy	CBC, check vital signs	CBC	Watch for increases in blood pressure, heart rate, and respiratory rate with all stimulants
Long-acting methylphenidate (Concerta)	8 mg qa.m.	36–54 mg	Medically ill patient with depression and lethargy	CBC, vital signs		
Pemoline (Cylert)	18.75 mg qa.m.	37.5–56.25 mg qa.m.	Medically ill patient with depression and lethargy	Liver function tests, check vital signs	Liver function tests	Can bite tab and absorb sublingually under tongue
Modafinil (Provigil)	100–200 mg qa.m.	200–400 mg qa.m.	Medically ill patient with depression and lethargy	ECG, liver function tests		Reduce dose with hepatic impairment; do not use with cardiac disease

Mood stabilizers

Lithium carbonate (Eskalith, Eskalith CR, Lithobid)	300 mg qh.s.	300 mg t.i.d.	Mania[b] (may need to add clonazepam or antipsychotic[b]); depression (may need to add antidepressant)	ECG, electrolytes, UA, BUN/Cr, thyroid (T₄ TSH), CBC (esp. WBC and platelets)	Lithium level initially 2 ×/wk; gradually lengthen to q3 mo; thyroid studies q6 mo or earlier if indicated; UA/BUN/Cr, CBC if infection	Monitor blood level 12 h after evening dose and before morning dose; 0.8–1.0 mEq/L is most effective; watch for hypothyroidism, diabetes insipidus, nephropathy, dehydration
Carbamazepine[c] (Tegretol)	100 mg b.i.d.	200 mg t.i.d.	Mania or depression	CBC, reticulocytes, serum iron, liver function tests, UA, BUN, ECG	CBC, thyroid studies, blood level	Watch for leukopenia, thrombocytopenia, hepatoxicity, decreased effect of warfarin (Coumadin)

Continued

Table 32.5. *Continued*

Drug	Starting dose	Average dose for cancer patients	Disorders	Pretreatment work-up	Follow-up studies	Comment
Gabapentin (Neurontin)	100–300 mg t.i.d. or q.i.d.	300–800 mg t.i.d.	Insomnia, pain, panic disorder or other anxiety disorder, augmentation for other mood stabilizers	Cr clearance	Cr clearance	Can give larger dose (300–1,200 mg) at bedtime; can induce oversedation, occasional tremor or ataxia; useful for neuropathic pain
Lamotrigine (Lamictal)	25–50 mg q.d. (decrease starting dose if on valproate)	150–250 mg b.i.d.	Mania, depression	Liver function tests, Cr clearance		Increase dose every other week; high risk of Stevens–Johnson rash; would use *only* if physician familiar with this medication
Valproic acid (Depakene, Depakote)	15 mg/kg/d	500–750 mg/d (divided into t.i.d. doses)	Mania, depression	Liver function tests, CBC	Liver function tests, CBC, blood level	Watch for hepatotoxicity, especially in young children

Benzodiazepines

Clonazepam (Klonopin)	0.5 mg qh.s.	≥2 mg	Mania, anxiety	CBC, liver function tests	CBC, liver function tests	Impaired hepatic function and respiratory distress; require extremely cautious use; do not withdraw rapidly
Alprazolam (Xanax)	0.5 mg qh.s.	≥1 mg t.i.d.	Anxiety, minor depression	Liver function tests		Do not withdraw rapidly (reduce daily dose by 0.25 mg weekly); use cautiously if respiratory impairment

CBC, complete blood cell count; ECG, electrocardiogram; UA, urinalysis; BUN, blood urea nitrogen; Cr, creatinine; TSH, thyroid-stimulating hormone.

[a] Check on weight, pulse, and blood pressure. Tolerance may develop, and doses may require adjustment.

[b] Natural or corticosteroid induced.

[c] Caution required because of multiple drug interactions.

Table 32.6.   Antianxiety agents and nighttime sedatives

Agent	Half-life (h)	Onset	Starting dose (mg)[a]
Benzodiazepines			
Triazolam (Halcion)	1.5–3.5	Rapid	0.125 (qh.s.)
Oxazepam (Serax)[b]	8–20	Moderate	10 (t.i.d.)
Lorazepam (Ativan)[b]	10–20	Rapid	0.5 (t.i.d.)
Temazepam (Restoril)[b]	12–24	Rapid	15 (qh.s.)
Alprazolam (Xanax)	12–24	Moderate	0.25 (t.i.d.)
Chlordiazepoxide (Librium)	12–48	Moderate	10 (b.i.d.)
Clonazepam (Klonopin)	20–30	Rapid	0.5 (b.i.d.)
Diazepam (Valium)	20–90	Rapid	2–5 (b.i.d.)
Clorazepate (Tranxene)	20–100	Rapid	7.5 (b.i.d.)
Flurazepam (Dalmane)	20–100	Rapid	15 (qh.s.)
Nonbenzodiazepine hypnotics			
Zolpidem (Ambien)[b]	1.5–4.5	Rapid	5 (qh.s.)
Zaleplon (Sonata)[b]	1.0	Rapid	5 (qh.s.)

Antidepressants (for panic disorder)
   Start at lower doses than for depression, i.e., an imipramine starting dose of 10 mg t.i.d.

β-Blockers (for autonomic symptom control)
   Propranolol (Inderal)   10–20 mg t.i.d.
   Atenolol (Tenormin)   25–50 mg daily

Antipsychotics (for anxiety associated with delirium)

Antihistamines
May be safer in some cases when respiratory impairment is a complication; also used for insomnia.
Diphenhydramine (Benadryl) 25 mg; starting doses b.i.d. or t.i.d.
Hydroxyzine (Vistaril) 50 mg; starting doses t.i.d. or q.i.d.

Note: Elderly or extremely debilitated patients should be given lower doses. Caution should be taken when prescribing long-acting sedating medications because they have been associated with a high incidence of falls and hip fracture.
[a] If chronic alcohol or benzodiazepine use exists, it is probable that the dose needed is at least double the starting doses listed.
[b] Preferred in the elderly.

   3.   Brief, isolated episodes of anxiety that come and go lead the examiner to consider other diagnoses.
   a.   Panic attacks. If the patient has repeated "attacks" that have a rapid onset and last 20 min to a few hours and if they are accompanied by tachycardia, palpitations, shortness of breath, hyperventilation, choking, sweating, dizziness, and the wish to flee, without a physical or chemical explanation, they are most likely panic attacks. They may be treated with benzodiazepines such as clonazepam and alprazolam; however, antidepressants such as tricyclics, selective serotonin reuptake inhibitors (SSRIs), MAOIs, or mirtazapine are also effective. Antidepressants must be started at a very low dose (e.g., sertraline 12.5 mg, paroxetine 5.0 mg, or imipramine 10 mg) and increased slowly

every 1 to 2 days to avoid increased anxiety. While the dose is brought up to that typically used in depression, benzodiazepines may be added if needed. Benzodiazepines with a short half-life, like alprazolam, can induce breakthrough panic if tolerance develops, so those with longer half-lives, like clonazepam, may be preferred if tolerated. β-Blockers to block autonomic symptoms may be tried if performance anxiety around specific activities is identified, but they are less effective for panic disorder, as is buspirone.

b. Organic causes are often responsible for the anxiety.

(1) **Hypoxia.** Repeating episodes of anxiety accompanied by alterations in intellectual functioning, poor orientation, reduced judgment, shortened attention, a rapidly fluctuating mood, and difficulty with memory suggest hypoxia. When anxiety is induced by hypoxia, it is wise to reduce central nervous system (CNS) depressant medications and give small doses of an antipsychotic drug if the anxiety is accompanied by delirium. However, older antipsychotic and antiemetic medications as well as metoclopramide often produce akathisia, an extrapyramidal restlessness that mimics anxiety. Alternating the antipsychotic drug with small doses of a short–half-life benzodiazepine is one option for organically induced anxiety— if respiratory status or arterial blood gas measurements do not worsen. Newer antipsychotic agents are less likely to produce extrapyramidal akathisia but still should be monitored with pulse oximetry measurements.

(2) **Liver disease and other physical disorders.** If anxiety is associated with liver disease, start by reducing CNS depressant medications. When needed, small, infrequent doses of a short-acting benzodiazepine that requires conjugation but not oxidation in the liver are prescribed. These include lorazepam, oxazepam, and temazepam. Many other physical disorders can also produce anxious symptoms, including various brain tumors, pheochromocytoma, carcinoid, hyperthyroidism, cardiac arrhythmias, drug or alcohol withdrawal, and hyperparathyroidism. Gabapentin, which is renally cleared, may help with anxiety, sleep, and pain. It can also help augment other medications for mood stabilization and panic disorder.

(3) **Medications** such as theophylline, corticosteroids, antidepressants, and antipsychotic drugs can produce anxiety. Anxiety is frequently one of multiple symptoms associated with benzodiazepine or narcotic analgesic withdrawal.

c. Precipitating events can be identified in patients with cancer that initiate the previously discussed adjustment disorder lasting generally no longer than 6 months. Posttraumatic stress disorder, less often seen in patients with cancer, follows a distressing event outside the range of usual human experience. More frequently observed, however, are patients who describe intense fears of needles, radiotherapy rooms, or confined-space scanning devices. Often, the history unfolds to describe previously existing phobias. These

patients, like those with anticipatory anxiety about procedures or chemotherapy, may be assisted with relaxation
or desensitization techniques, imagery, antianxiety medications, and assurance. If patients begin to experience procedures, treatments, or interpersonal situations as being
particularly stressful, anticipatory anxiety intensifies the
requirement for larger doses of as-needed medication to attain some relief. Therefore, regular scheduling of antianxiety medication similar to that of pain medication is in order.

V.   Insomnia

A.   Principles. Difficulty falling asleep may be associated
with anxiety, whereas awakening in the middle of the night is
generally more closely related to depression. In addition, there
are a variety of physical disorders that cause sleeping irregularities. The sleep–wake cycle is almost always disturbed in a
delirious patient, no matter what the cause. Pain often awak-
ens a patient with cancer. Medications can awaken some patients directly (e.g., fluoxetine) or indirectly (e.g., diuretics).
Aside from sorting out these influences, the physician must
take into account the environment. Is the patient too hot or
cold? Is the ward too brightly lit or too noisy? Do the patients
awaken each time they are checked by the night staff? When
any or several of these concerns are corrected, sleeping medication may not be necessary, although the need for sedatives
remains in some patients.

B.   Benzodiazepines (see Table 32.6). This class of drugs is
most often prescribed if a patient needs nighttime sedation. The
shorter–half-life benzodiazepines (i.e., lorazepam or temazepam)
with a rapid onset produce less daytime grogginess than those
with a longer half-life. Short-acting agents tend to accumulate
less and are safer for patients with liver disease. On the other
hand, longer–half-life drugs (i.e., diazepam or flurazepam) with
a rapid onset produce less unwanted awakening during the
very early morning.

C.   Nonbenzodiazepine hypnotics (see Table 32.6). The
two medications in this class help patients fall asleep quickly
and do not leave the patient groggy in the morning. Clinical
experience shows tolerance can also develop to these medications.

D.   Antihistamines (see Table 32.6). These medications may be
chosen if physicians are hesitant to prescribe benzodiazepines,
such as for patients with severe respiratory disease. A disadvantage may be the higher anticholinergic potential of these
drugs, compared with the benzodiazepine family, which can
increase the risk of delirium.

E.   Others. Chloral hydrate 500 to 1,000 mg, an old standby
hypnotic, is occasionally used as long as patients are free of
gastrointestinal or liver disease. Barbiturates such as amobar-
bital sodium are occasionally used to treat some refractory sleeping disturbances for a short time but are not routinely used
because they induce respiratory depression and have addictive
potential. Gabapentin, which is renally cleared and has few
drug interactions, has become increasingly popular. Doses may
vary from 300 to 1,200 mg at bedtime. It is always better to start
with a lower dose.

SELECTED READINGS

Bezchlibnyk-Butler KZ, Jeffries JJ, eds. *Clinical handbook of psychotropic drugs.* 11th ed. Seattle: Hogrefe and Huber, 2001.

Breitbart W. Identifying patients at risk for and treatment of major psychiatric complications of cancer. *Support Care Cancer* 1995;3:45.

Davidson JR, Waisberg JL, Brundage MD, et al. Nonpharmacologic group treatment of insomnia: a preliminary study with cancer survivors. *Psychooncology* 2001;10:389–397.

Fromer MT. *Surviving childhood cancer.* Washington, D.C.: American Psychiatric Press, 1995.

Holland JC. *Psycho-oncology.* New York: Oxford University Press, 1998.

Homsi J, Walsh D, Nelson KA. Psychostimulants in supportive care. *Support Care Cancer* 2000;8:385–397.

Jacobson SA, Pies RW, Greenblatt DJ. *Handbook of geriatric psychopharmacology.* Washington, D.C.: American Psychiatric Press, 2002.

Kane FJ, Remmel R, Moody S. Recognizing and treating delirium in patients admitted to general hospitals. *South Med J* 1993;86:985.

Koenig HG, McCullough ME, Larson DB. *Handbook of religion and health.* New York: Oxford University Press, 2001:292–317.

Lipowski ZJ. *Delirium: acute confusional states.* New York: Oxford University Press, 1990.

Luebbert K, Dahme B, Hasenbring M. The effectiveness of relaxation training in reducing treatment-related symptoms and improving emotional adjustment in acute non-surgical cancer treatment: a meta-analytical review. *Psychooncology* 2001;10:490–502.

Marmelstein H, Lesko L, Holland JC. Depression in the cancer patient. *J Psychooncol* 1992;1:199.

Massie MJ, Gagnon P, Holland JC. Depression and suicide in patients with cancer. *J Pain Symptom Manage* 1994;9:325.

Massie MJ, Holland JC. Depression and cancer. *J Clin Psychiatry* 1990;51(suppl):S12.

McDaniel JS, Musselman DL, Nemeroff CB. Cancer and depression: theory and treatment. *Psychiatr Ann* 1997;27:360.

McDaniel JS, Musselman DL, Porter MR, et al. Depression in patients with cancer: diagnosis, biology and treatment. *Arch Gen Psychiatry* 1995;52:89.

Olin J, Massand P. Psychostimulants for depression in hospitalized cancer patients. *Psychosomatics* 1996;37:57.

Patenaude AF, Last B. Cancer and children: Where are we coming from? Where are we going? *Psychooncology* 2001;10:281–283.

Roth AJ, Holland JH. Psychiatric complications in cancer patients. In: Brain MC, Carbone PP, eds. *Current therapy in hematology–oncology.* 5th ed. St. Louis: Mosby, 1995:609.

Roth AJ, McClear KZ, Massie MJ. Oncology. In: Stoudemire A, Fogel BS, Greenberg DB, eds. *Psychiatric care of the medically ill patient.* Oxford: Oxford University Press, 2000:733–756.

Spiegel D, Bloom JR, Kraemer HC, et al. Gottheil E. Effect of psychosocial treatment of patients with metastatic breast cancer. *Lancet* 1989;2:888–891.

Zonderman DB, Costa PT, McCrae PR. Depression as a risk for cancer morbidity and mortality in a nationally representative sample. *JAMA* 1989;262:1191–1195.

Appendix A

Nomogram for Determining Body Surface Area of Adults from Height and Mass[a]

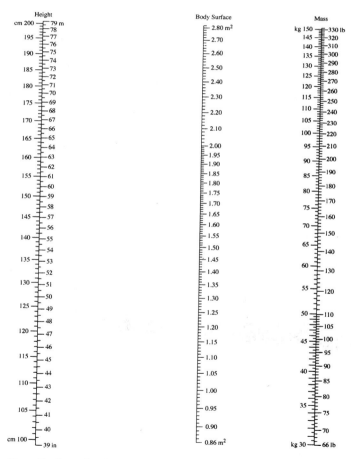

Height • Body Surface • Mass

[a] From the formula of Du Bois and Du Bois (*Arch Intern Med* 1916; 17:863): $S = M^{0.425} \times H^{0.725} \times 71.84$, or $S = \log M \times 0.425 + \log H \times 0.725 + 1.8564$, where S is body surface (cm^2), M is mass (kg), and H is height (cm). (From Lenter C, ed. *Geigy scientific tables, vol 1.* 8th ed. Basel: Ciba-Geigy, 1981:227).

Nomogram for Determining Body Surface Area of Children from Height and Mass[a]

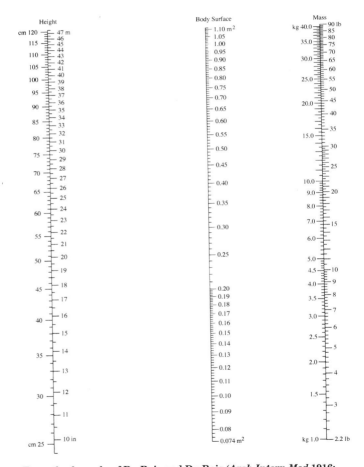

Height	Body Surface	Mass

[a] From the formula of Du Bois and Du Bois (*Arch Intern Med* 1916; 17:863): $S = M^{0.425} \times H^{0.725} \times 71.84$, or $S = \log M \times 0.425 + \log H + 0.725 + 1.8564$, where S is body surface (cm^2), M is mass (kg), and H is height (cm). (From Lenter C, ed. *Geigy scientific tables, vol 1.* 8th ed. Basel: Ciba-Geigy, 1981:226).

692

Appendix C

Cancer Screening Recommendations for Average Risk, Asymptomatic People by the American Cancer Society

Cancer screening recommendations for average-risk, asymptomatic people by the American Cancer Society

Test or procedure	Sex	Age	Frequency
Fecal occult blood testing (FOBT) and flexible sigmoidoscopy[a]	Men and women	50 and above	Annual FOBT, every 5 y flexible sigmoidoscopy
or			
Flexible sigmoidoscopy			Every 5 y
or			
FOBT			Annually
or			
Colonoscopy			Every 10 y
or			
Double-contrast barium enema (DCBE)			Every 5 y
Digital rectal exam (DRE) and prostate-specific antigen test (PSA)	Men	50 and over if life expectancy of at least 10 y	Annually[b]

Population

Pap test and pelvic examination	Women	18 and older	Annually until 3 or more consecutive satisfactory normal exams, then less frequently at discretion of physician
Breast self-examination	Women	20 and older	Monthly
Clinical breast examination	Women	20–39	Every 3 y
		40 and older	Annually
Mammography	Women	40 and older	Annually
Cancer-related check-up[c]	Men and women	20–39	Every 3 y
		40 and older	Yearly

[a]Preferred over either alone.

[b]Information should be provided to men about the benefits and limitations of testing.

[c]Includes exam for thyroid, testicles, ovaries, lymph nodes, oral cavity, and skin; health counseling about tobacco, sun exposure, diet and nutrition, risk factors, sexual practices, and environmental and occupational exposures.

From Smith RA, Cokkinides V, von Eschenbach AC, et al. American Cancer Society guidelines for the early detection of cancer. CA. *Cancer J Clin* 2002;528b–22.

Selected Oncology Web Sites—Cancer and Other

1. American Society of Hematology
   http://www.hematology.org/index.cfm
2. American Cancer Society (ACS statistics, other information, links to states)
   http://www.cancer.org/
3. American Society of Clinical Oncology (ASCO; physician site)
   http://www.asco.org
4. ASCO—People living with cancer (patient site)
   http://www.plwc.org
5. Agency for Health Care Research and Quality
   http://www.ahrq.gov
6. PubMed, National Library of Medicine (search medline and get abstracts)
   http://www.ncbi.nlm.nih.gov/entrez/query
7. Harvard Center for Cancer Prevention
   http://www.hsph.harvard.edu/cancer/
8. Health Services/Technology Assessment Text (a helpful collection of HSTAT guidelines, surgeon general reports, technology assessments, and reviews)
   http://hstat.nlm.nih.gov/
9. American Pain Society
   http://www.ampainsoc.org/
10. American Academy of Hospice and Palliative Medicine
    http://www.aahpm.org/
11. National Cancer Institute's Cancer Information home page (NCI information, including PDQ, clinical trials information, statistics)
    http://www.cancer.gov/
12. Cancer Therapy Evaluation Program (CTEP) home page (includes common toxicity criteria)
    http://ctep.cancer.gov/
13. Cancer Trials
    http://www.cancer.gov/clinicaltrials
    http://www.cancertrialshelp.org
14. Centers for Disease Control and Prevention (CDC)
    http://www.cdc.gov/
15. National Guideline Clearinghouse (guidelines for over 800 diseases and conditions, including many for cancer)
    http://www.guideline.gov/index.asp
16. National Comprehensive Cancer Network (NCCN) Complete Library of Clinical Practice Guidelines in Oncology, for health professionals (free registration required) and patients.
    http://www.nccn.org
17. Association of Community Cancer Centers (includes the Compendia-Based Drug Bulletin)
    http://www.accc-cancer.org/

18. Rxlist—Internet Drug Index (primarily for patients; includes alternative medicines)
    http://www.rxlist.com
19. FDA Oncology Tools web site (contains information about approved cancer therapies, product labels, approval summaries, what drugs are approved for what diseases, and considerations for making decisions about therapies, including advice on when to contemplate using unapproved drugs and how to obtain access to unapproved drugs)
    http://www.fda.gov/cder/cancer/
20. Newspapers, TV, and the weather (to keep some attachment to the real world)
    a. Weather Channel (if in case, like the editor, you have no windows in your office)
       http://www.weather.com
    b. CNN Interactive
       http://www.cnn.com
    c. *New York Times*
       http://www.nytimes.com
    d. Newspapers around the world
       http://www.newspapers.com

Subject Index

Subject Index

A

Absolute neutrophil count, 63–64, 464

ABVD regimen, Hodgkin's disease, 496t, 496–499

AC regimen, breast cancer, 282–289

Acetaminophen, 658–659

Acquired immunodeficiency disease. *See* HIV-associated malignancies

Acquired resistance, 14

Acral lentiginous melanoma, 361

Actinomycin D. *See* Dactinomycin

Activated protein C, 598

Activated prothrombin time, and heparin therapy, 607–608

Acute confusional states, 674–677

Acute drug toxicity, 61–62

Acute lymphoblastic leukemia, 438–454
  allogeneic transplantation, 439–442
  and central nervous system leukemia, 452–455
  chemotherapy principles, 417–418
  diagnosis and classification, 413–414
  experimental strategies, 453–454
  growth factors adjunctive treatment, 456
  hematopoietic stem cell transplantation, 439–442, 451–452
  and hyperleukocytosis, 455–456
  and impaired cardiac function, 446–447
  initial chemotherapy support, 414–417
  and minimal residual disease, 447
  in older adults, 446
  prognostic features, 438
  relapse, 450–452

therapeutic options, 439, 440t, 442–447

Acute megakaryocytic leukemia, 423

Acute mixed-lineage leukemia, 414

Acute myeloblastic leukemia, 483

Acute myeloid leukemia, 411–438
  and central nervous system leukemia, 452–455
  chemotherapy principles, 417–418, 418t
  cytogenetics, 412, 413t, 421–423, 428
  diagnosis and classification, 411–413
  growth factor adjunctive treatment, 456
  hematopoietic stem cell transplantation, 181–182, 435–437
  induction therapy, 419–421, 428–429
  postremission therapy, 421–423, 429–430
  in pregnancy, 435
  reinduction therapy options, 424
  relapse, 423–427, 430
  secondary form of, 43–44, 434
  therapeutic options, 418t

Acute promyelocytic leukemia, 430–434

Acyclovir, 596, 600

Adenocarcinoma of unknown origin, 539–544

ADIC regimen, soft tissue sarcomas, 395–396

Adjuvant therapy, 30. *See also under specific cancers*

Adrenocortical carcinoma, 350–355
  arterial embolization, 355
  chemotherapy, 353–355
  clinical picture, 350–351
  incidence and etiology, 350
  radiotherapy, 352–353
  in small intestine, 242